AF326827

E–Health and Telemedicine:

Concepts, Methodologies, Tools, and Applications

Information Resources Management Association
USA

Volume I

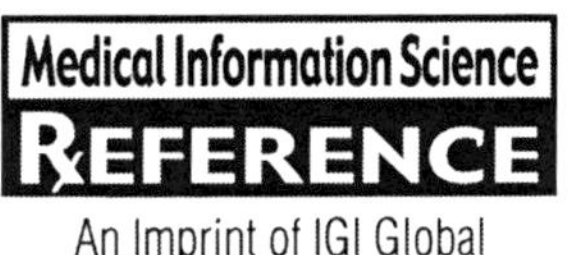

Managing Director:	Lindsay Johnston
Managing Editor:	Keith Greenberg
Director of Intellectual Propery & Contracts:	Jan Travers
Acquisitions Editor:	Kayla Wolfe
Production Editor:	Christina Henning
Multi-Volume Book Production Specialist:	Deanna Jo Zombro
Cover Design:	Samantha Barnhart

Published in the United States of America by
Medical Information Science Reference (an imprint of IGI Global)
701 E. Chocolate Avenue
Hershey PA, USA 17033
Tel: 717-533-8845
Fax: 717-533-8661
E-mail: cust@igi-global.com
Web site: http://www.igi-global.com

Library of Congress Cataloging-in-Publication Data

E-Health and telemedicine : concepts, methodologies, tools, and applications / Information Resources Management Association, editor.
    pages cm
 Includes bibliographical references and index.
 Summary: "This reference explores recent advances in mobile medicine and how this technology impacts modern medical care"-- Provided by publisher.
 ISBN 978-1-4666-8756-1 (hardcover) -- ISBN 978-1-4666-8757-8 (ebook) 1. Medical care--Technological innovation. 2. Medical informatics. 3. Telecommunication in medicine. I. Information Resources Management Association.
 R858.E223 2016
 610.285--dc23
                              2015019904

British Cataloguing in Publication Data
A Cataloguing in Publication record for this book is available from the British Library.

All work contributed to this book is new, previously-unpublished material. The views expressed in this book are those of the authors, but not necessarily of the publisher.

For electronic access to this publication, please contact: eresources@igi-global.com.

List of Contributors

Table of Contents

Volume I

Section 1
Fundamental Concepts and Theories

This section serves as a foundation for this exhaustive reference tool by addressing underlying principles essential to the understanding of E-Health and Telemedicine. Chapters found within these pages provide an excellent framework in which to position E-Health and Telemedicine within the field of information science and technology. Insight regarding the critical incorporation of global measures into E-Health and Telemedicine is addressed, while crucial stumbling blocks of this field are explored. With 15 chapters comprising this foundational section, the reader can learn and chose from a compendium of expert research on the elemental theories underscoring the E-Health and Telemedicine discipline.

Section 2
Frameworks and Methodologies

This section provides in-depth coverage of conceptual architecture frameworks to provide the reader with a comprehensive understanding of the emerging developments within the field of E-Health and Telemedicine. Research fundamentals imperative to the understanding of developmental processes within E-Health and Telemedicine are offered. From broad examinations to specific discussions on methodology, the research found within this section spans the discipline while offering detailed, specific discussions. From basic designs to abstract development, these chapters serve to expand the reaches of development and design technologies within the E-Health and Telemedicine community. This section includes 11 contributions from researchers throughout the world on the topic of E-Health and Telemedicine.

Section 3
Tools and Technologies

This section presents an extensive coverage of various tools and technologies available in the field of E-Health and Telemedicine that practitioners and academicians alike can utilize to develop different techniques. These chapters enlighten readers about fundamental research on the many tools facilitating the burgeoning field of E-Health and Telemedicine. It is through these rigorously researched chapters that the reader is provided with countless examples of the up-and-coming tools and technologies emerging from the field of E-Health and Telemedicine. With 21 chapters, this section offers a broad treatment of some of the many tools and technologies within the E-Health and Telemedicine field.

Section 4
Cases and Applications

This section discusses a variety of applications and opportunities available that can be considered by practitioners in developing viable and effective E-Health and Telemedicine programs and processes. This section includes 13 chapters that review topics from case studies to best practices and ongoing research. Further chapters discuss E-Health and Telemedicine in a variety of settings. Contributions included in this section provide excellent coverage of today's IT community and how research into E-Health and Telemedicine is impacting the social fabric of our present-day global village.

Volume III

Section 5
Issues and Challenges

This section contains 17 chapters, giving a wide variety of perspectives on E-Health and Telemedicine and its implications. Within the chapters, the reader is presented with an in-depth analysis of the most current and relevant issues within this growing field of study. Crucial questions are addressed and alternatives offered along with theoretical approaches discussed.

Section 6
Emerging Trends

*This section highlights research potential within the field of E-Health and Telemedicine while exploring
uncharted areas of study for the advancement of the discipline. Introducing this section are chapters that
set the stage for future research directions and topical suggestions for continued debate, centering on
the new venues and forums for discussion. A pair of chapters on space-time makes up the middle of the*

Preface

The constantly changing landscape of E-Health and Telemedicine makes it challenging for experts and practitioners to stay informed of the field's most up-to-date research. That is why Medical Information Science Reference is pleased to offer this three-volume reference collection that will empower students, researchers, and academicians with a strong understanding of critical issues within E-Health and Telemedicine by providing both broad and detailed perspectives on cutting-edge theories and developments. This reference is designed to act as a single reference source on conceptual, methodological, technical, and managerial issues, as well as provide insight into emerging trends and future opportunities within the discipline.

E-Health and Telemedicine: Concepts, Methodologies, Tools and Applications is organized into six distinct sections that provide comprehensive coverage of important topics. The sections are:

1. Fundamental Concepts and Theories;
2. Frameworks and Methodologies;
3. Tools and Technologies;
4. Cases and Applications;
5. Issues and Challenges; and
6. Emerging Trends.

The following paragraphs provide a summary of what to expect from this invaluable reference tool.

Section 1, "Fundamental Concepts and Theories," serves as a foundation for this extensive reference tool by addressing crucial theories essential to the understanding of E-Health and Telemedicine. Introducing the book is *Project Initiation for Telemedicine Services* by Cynthia M. LeRouge, Bengisu Tulu, and Suzanne Wood; a great foundation laying the groundwork for the basic concepts and theories that will be discussed throughout the rest of the book. Another chapter of note in Section 1 is titled *Principles of Information Accountability: An eHealth Perspective* by Randike Gajanayake, Tony Sahama, and Renato Iannella. Section 1 concludes, and leads into the following portion of the book with a nice segue chapter, *Telemedicine Program for Management and Treatment of Stress Urinary Incontinence in Women: Design and Pilot Test* by Anna Abelló Pla, Anna Andreu Povar, Jordi Esquirol Caussa, Vanessa Bayo Tallón, Dolores Rexachs, and Emilio Luque.

Section 2, "Frameworks and Methodologies," presents in-depth coverage of the conceptual design and architecture of E-Health and Telemedicine. Opening the section is *Information Architecture for Pervasive Healthcare Information Provision with Technological Implementation* by Chekfoung Tan and Shixiong Liu. Through case studies, this section lays excellent groundwork for later sections that will get into present and future applications for E-Health and Telemedicine. The section concludes with an excellent work by Sabah Al-Fedaghi, titled *Design Principles in Health Information Technology: An Alternative to UML Use Case Methodology.*

Section 3, "Tools and Technologies," presents extensive coverage of the various tools and technologies used in the implementation of E-Health and Telemedicine. Section 3 begins where Section 2 left off, though this section describes more concrete tools at place in the modeling, planning, and applications of E-Health and Telemedicine. The first chapter, *Healthinfo Engineering: Technology Perspectives from Evidence-Based mHealth Study in WE-CARE Project* by Anpeng Huang and Linzhen Xie, lays a framework for the types of works that can be found in this section. Section 3 is full of excellent chapters like this one, including such titles as *A System for the Semi-Automatic Evaluation of Clinical Practice Guideline Indicators* by Alexandra Pomares Quimbaya, María Patricia Amórtegui, Rafael A. González, Oscar Muñoz, Wilson Ricardo Bohórquez, Olga Milena García, and Melany Montagut Ascanio; and *Ambulance Dispatching System with Integrated Information and Communication Technologies on Cloud Environment* by Jian-Wei Li, Chia-Chi Chang, Yi-Chun Chang, and Yung-Fa Huang. The section concludes with *Using a Smartphone as a Track and Fall Detector: An Intelligent Support System for People with Dementia* by Chia-Yin Ko, Fang-Yie Leu, and I-Tsen Lin. Where Section 3 described specific tools and technologies at the disposal of practitioners, Section 4 describes the use and applications of the tools and frameworks discussed in previous sections.

Section 4, "Cases and Applications," describes how the broad range of E-Health and Telemedicine efforts has been utilized and offers insight on and important lessons for their applications and impact. The first chapter in the section is titled *The Role and Use of Telemedicine by Physicians in Developing Countries: A Case Report from Saudi Arabia* written by Dana Alajmi, Mohamed Khalifa, Amr Jamal, Nasria Zakaria, Suleiman Alomran, Ashraf El-Metwally, Majed Al-Salamah, and Mowafa Househ. This section includes the widest range of topics because it describes case studies, research, methodologies, frameworks, architectures, theory, analysis, and guides for implementation. The breadth of topics covered in the chapter is also reflected in the diversity of its authors, from countries all over the globe, such as: *A Case for Enterprise Interoperability in Healthcare IT: Personal Health Record Systems* by Mustafa Yuksel, Asuman Dogac, Cebrail Taskin, and Anil Yalcinkaya. The section concludes with *Political Attitudes on the Dutch Electronic Patient Record* by Evert Mouw, a great transition chapter into the next section.

Section 5, "Issues and Challenges," presents coverage of academic and research perspectives on E-Health and Telemedicine tools and applications. The section begins with *Detection of Pre-Analytical Laboratory Testing Errors: Leads and Lessons for Patient Safety* by Wafa Al-Zahrani and Mohamud Sheikh. Chapters in this section will look into theoretical approaches and offer alternatives to crucial questions on the subject of E-Health and Telemedicine. For example, *Operative Role Management in Information Systems* written by Taina Kurki and Hanna-Miina Sihvonen. The section concludes with *Approaches to Evidence-Based Management and Decision-Making in Healthcare Organizations: Lessons for Developing Nations* by Nouf Al Saleem and Mohamud Sheikh.

Section 6, "Emerging Trends," highlights areas for future research within the field of E-Health and Telemedicine, opening with *Mobile Health Services: A New Paradigm for Health Care Systems* by Nabila Nisha, Mehree Iqbal, Afrin Rifat, and Sherina Idrish. This section contains chapters that look at what might happen in the coming years that can extend the already staggering amount of applications for E-Health and Telemedicine. The final chapter of the book looks at an emerging field within E-Health and Telemedicine, in the excellent contribution, *Coalitions: The Future of Healthcare in Public Private Partnerships* by Erinn N. Harris.

Although the primary organization of the contents in this multi-volume work is based on its six sections, offering a progression of coverage of the important concepts, methodologies, technologies, applications, social issues, and emerging trends, the reader can also identify specific contents by utilizing the extensive indexing system listed at the end of each volume. As a comprehensive collection of research on the latest findings related to using technology to providing various services, *E-Health and Telemedicine: Concepts, Methodologies, Tools and Applications*, provides researchers, administrators and all audiences with a complete understanding of the development of applications and concepts in E-Health and Telemedicine. Given the vast number of issues concerning usage, failure, success, policies, strategies, and applications of E-Health and Telemedicine in countries around the world, *E-Health and Telemedicine: Concepts, Methodologies, Tools and Applications* addresses the demand for a resource that encompasses the most pertinent research in technologies being employed to globally bolster the knowledge and applications of E-Health and Telemedicine.

Section 1
Fundamental Concepts and Theories

This section serves as a foundation for this exhaustive reference tool by addressing underlying principles essential to the understanding of E-Health and Telemedicine. Chapters found within these pages provide an excellent framework in which to position E-Health and Telemedicine within the field of information science and technology. Insight regarding the critical incorporation of global measures into E-Health and Telemedicine is addressed, while crucial stumbling blocks of this field are explored. With 15 chapters comprising this foundational section, the reader can learn and chose from a compendium of expert research on the elemental theories underscoring the E-Health and Telemedicine discipline.

Chapter 1
Project Initiation for Telemedicine Services

Cynthia M. LeRouge
Saint Louis University, USA

Bengisu Tulu
Worchester Polytechnic Institute, USA

Suzanne Wood
Saint Louis University, USA

ABSTRACT

This study investigates project initiation for telemedicine, a technology innovation in healthcare organizations that manifests both intra- and inter-organizational collaboration. Moving from a telemedicine project to a sustainable telemedicine service line can be a challenge for many organizations (LeRouge, Tulu, & Forducey, 2010). Project definition (a.k.a., initiation) sets the strategic vision for a project and has been categorized as the most important stage in a project (C. Gray & Larson, 2008) and a key element for project success (Stah-Le Cardinal & Marle, 2006). Although project management best practices have been applied in many domains, there are few studies that link published best practices to the telemedicine domain. This study first presents a model, resulting from a review of project management literature that specifies the recommended components project definition. Using this model as a foundation, the authors explore how project definition is deployed in the telemedicine domain, using the instantiation of telestroke projects for this study. The authors base their findings on a multi-case qualitative data set, with each case representing a distinct telemedicine business model. Findings from this study explicate how the telestroke project initiation process is collaboratively managed and how this process impacts the overall success of the telemedicine programs through the lens of the five distinct telemedicine business models. Specifically, this study contributes insights on key elements of project initiation in the telemedicine context as well as the effects of the varying business models (focusing on commonalities and differences).

DOI: 10.4018/978-1-4666-8756-1.ch001

INTRODUCTION

Health Information Technology (HIT) is one area where governments and healthcare organizations continue to spend money with the hopes of improved outcomes and reduced costs. Taken alone, a project characterized as information technology (IT), healthcare, or inter-organizational, would likely be classified as a complex project. When these characteristics are aggregated under one project, we have a formidable challenge, particularly when the project goal is to produce a sustainable service or work flow. It was reported in the literature that 91% of HIT projects fail (Maxfield 2007). These HIT projects affect not only those employed in the healthcare industry, but also the majority of citizens that seek healthcare for themselves or loved ones.

Various business best practices, such as LEAN and project management tenants promoted by the Project Management Book of Knowledge (PMBOK) are increasingly being applied to the healthcare context to support the success of change efforts. Research in applying and adapting these best practices grounding in other domains is still in the early stages in the healthcare sector (Chiocchio et al., 2012; LeRouge et al., 2010), though the value of project management best practices for the healthcare sector is increasing in recognition (Deutsch, Georg Duftschmid, & Dorda, 2010; Gertner et al., 2010). Telemedicine service lines are among these complex HIT projects. The start or expansion of a telemedicine service line is intrinsically collaborative as it requires both intra- (IT, administration, clinical) and inter- (hospital A, hospital B) collaboration efforts coming together to provide distance-based medical care using telecommunications technology. In addition, these initiatives operate within a complex legal, policy, and standards environment that can impose constraints as well as ambiguities. Different components, some inside the organization and others in the external environment, need to be orchestrated

from the beginning of the telemedicine project to avoid issues in implementation and to provide a foundation for a service line that is sustainable beyond the project end date (where project activities are moved into standard operational process). The recommended first stage in any project is the initiation, also called project definition or conceptualization. This stage (or process group as referenced by the Project Management Institute) has been categorized as the most crucial step in the project (J. Knutson, 1999) and a key element for project success (Merla., 2009). Project definition moves organizations from strategy to execution.

The project management discipline provides best practices and guidelines for project initiation. Although project management tenants are applicable for different fields, the telemedicine field includes few studies that link project management concepts to the application of programs. Further investigation is necessary to determine the need for contextualization and adaptation of these tenants to best suit and benefit the healthcare sector. Telemedicine initiatives may be short-lived, if they are not built on a strong strategic foundation (LeRouge et al., 2010), which starts with project initiation activities and decisions. Unfortunately, little is known about the underlying nature of project initiation in telemedicine projects.

Moreover, it is not enough to understand key project initiation components; organizations also need to align these components to their business models to enhance contextualizing and application. A business model tells the story about how an organization will leverage a generic value chain and structure its operations so as to generate sustainable margins (Magretta, 2002). The business model (or story) associated with telemedicine projects consists of variations on the same underlying theme of delivering more efficient and effective healthcare (Strauss & Corbin, 1990). Understanding the type of business model employed (e.g., formal health network, alliance of health organizations, outsource service) is important because it enables us to see how context, structure, and profit incentive interplay with stakeholder interests are mediated by a specific initiative or way of operating (Baden-Fuller, 2010).

The purpose of this study is to investigate the relationship between traditional project initiation best practices and telemedicine (i.e. telestroke) project initiation practices associated with various business models. Some variance exists among the nature of various types of telemedicine service specialties. To minimize variance, this study uses one instantiation of a telemedicine service line, telestroke programs.

Telestroke programs facilitate time-sensitive, critical diagnosis and decision making through rapid linkages between patients where specialized care may not be available (remote, rural, or awkward locations) to expert stroke care (often in major urban centers) via telecommunications equipment in a very time sensitive situation. Given the time sensitivity of stroke care and published statistics indicating that stroke is one of the leading causes of death and disability in countries, such as the United States where stroke is the fourth leading cause of death (Towfighi & Saver, 2011) and third leading organ and disease specific cause of death (Towfighi, Ovbiagele, & Saver, 2010), successful telestroke programs can literally represent the difference between life and death and merit research attention. A telestroke encounter is a collaborative encounter among patients, on-site clinicians, and remote providers who use telecommunications tools to share data, analysis, diagnosis, and treatment directives with the goal of reducing stroke-related permanent disability and death. Emergency room videoconference access and patient data are passed to a remote stroke specialist who assists with diagnosis and providing directives for appropriate treatment (frequently, whether the patient condition is suited to administering receive tissue plasminogen activator, tPA, which may greatly reduce the effects of stroke, under suitable conditions). This promising form of telemedicine is growing in popularity (Silva,

Farrell, Shandra, Viswanathan, & Schwamm, 2012) due to societal need and reports of the clinical success of telestroke encounters (Joshi et al., 2013).

The impact of telemedicine on the efficiency and effectiveness of stroke care will ultimately be determined by the technology architecture, the systems developed around it, and strategy for implementing it. "The efficacy of the architecture will determine the efficacy of the system, and the efficacy of the system will determine the efficacy of the strategy" (Paul, Ramaprasad, & Wickramasinghe, 2012). Telemedicine efficacy seems to be more of a question of system (socio-technical system) and strategy than of architecture in the current climate (Pruitt, 2013). The efficacy of a telemedicine service's system and strategy is first rooted in the project initiation process. When we look at telestroke project initiation through the lens of competing business models, we have an opportunity to understand how project initiation can be structured to achieve best results. Therefore, this study seeks to address the following research questions:

- How is project initiation enacted in the telemedicine domain, within the confines of telestroke project initiatives?
- What commonalities and differences exist in this telemedicine context under the condition of various telemedicine business models?

We address these research questions through a qualitative multi-case study by 1) specifying a model of the recommended components of the project initiation phase resulting from a review of project management literature 2) describing the key characteristics for each business model case context, 3) providing findings that analyze the process that the initiation phase follows in the telestroke context and 4) comparing the various telemedicine business model implications for key components of the project initiation phase as part of the analysis of results. Our analysis highlights both commonalities and differences in project initiation across the various business models.

BACKGROUND AND PROJECT INITIATION FRAMEWORK

Telemedicine is one type of service that healthcare organizations provide with the help of collaboration technologies (such as videoconferencing) and intra- and inter-organizational systems. As organizations explore harnessing technology to establish new forms of collaborative work in healthcare, such as telemedicine, work models and project management practices need to be validated, further refined, or constructed in light of cross-system realities for several reasons (LeRouge et al., 2010). First, participating units might differ significantly in their healthcare, management, and technical practices and maturity. Second, regulatory, social, and cultural environments may vary substantially over time and organization context. Third, various stakeholders in collaborative work may have different or even conflicting goals and ascribe to their own definitions of work or project success. In addition, managing cross-organizational projects and work teams involved in these forms of collaborative work requires a high level of coordination that exceeds the need for teams working within one, familiar organizational unit. Launching or expanding technology to establish or expand new forms of collaborative work in healthcare requires project success that transfers into sustainable services.

The recipe for project success has been identified to include the following key ingredients, executive support, user involvement, experienced project manager, clear business objectives, and minimized scope (Kaplan & Tripsas, 2008). The key questions raised in the initiation phase (the first phase or process group of the project life cycle) address idealization, strategy alignment, project goals and the way that the project responds to multiple stakeholders' interests (Preston & Karahanna, 2009) (Karlos Artto, Kujala, Dietrich, & Martinsuo, 2008) (Päivi Lehtonen & Miia Martinsuo, 2008). Project initiation includes the tasks and deliverables associated with defining a project's objectives and scope as well as gaining organizational leadership's approval of and dedication to the initiative. Each project requires careful analysis to link a project upwards to the organizational strategy and downwards to the work involved, before the journey begins. Project definition involves process, communication, politics, strategy alignment and multiple actors with a common interest in developing an idea (Preston & Karahanna, 2009) (Karlos Artto et al., 2008); in other words, project definition involves complex decisions and the adroit application of many soft skills (Merla., 2009; Preston & Karahanna, 2009).

Organizations that use project initiation best practices report easier application of lessons learned from past projects, stakeholder alignment, more realistic targets, and a structured path to gain project approval all leading to a great chance for project success (Morris, 2005; Rojas-Meluk, 2008). The current study proposes that analyzing this stage can provide a good opportunity to identify key foundational components that increase the probability of sustainable telemedicine programs and HIT, in general.

The Project Management Institute is a recognized professional project management association that provides practitioners and organizations with standards that describe good practices (manifested as the Project Management Book of Knowledge – PMBOK), globally recognized credentials that certify project management expertise, and resources for professional development, networking and community ("Project Management Institute,"). Neither the PMBOK (which has been approved by the American National Standards Institute) nor the International Standards Organization (ISO) on project management (ISO 21500:2012, released in September 2012) provides a ready list of project initiation components. The collective set of project initiation processes in both the PMBOK and the ISO guidelines consist of: 1) Develop Project Charter, 2) Identify Stakeholders, 3) Establish Project Team.

PRINCE2 is a process-based approach for project management that serves as the de-facto project management standards for project management in Europe; PRINCE2 complements the PMBOK. The project charter, the main deliverable of the project initiation phase, helps to join strategy with project execution and solidify the relationship between the project and the project's owner within the organization. PRINCE2 does not provide a project initiation model that depicts components, but does provide a list of initiation objectives that include: 1) assessing project justification, 2) establishing a stable management basis on which to proceed, 3) ensuring a firm and accepted foundation to the project, 4) committing resources, 5) encouraging project leadership to take project ownership, 6) providing a baseline for decision-making processes throughout the project's life, and 7) ensuring the project's investment of time and resources is wise, taking project risks into account ("PRINCE2/ US,").

Though a detailed model of project initiation guiding points are not specified by PMI, ISO or PRINCE2, the detailed components of project initiation that accompany these standards can be found in the project management literature. To provide a research framework for this study, we used the aforementioned standards as a general guide and performed a review of project management literature (using variations of project management and project initiation as key words to search databases such as ABI Inform Complete) to develop our project initiation model presented in Figure 1.

Our model illustrates the project initiation activities carried out by the idea owner(s) that influence the evolution of the project charter (e.g., assess environment, secure project sponsor). The model also illustrates how the project charter can be strategically utilized once it is created by the project team lead by the project manager.. The model sets forth the collaboration and delegation of authority among key leadership roles involved in launching the project (namely, the idea owner, sponsor, and project manager) and the project initiation areas that generally begin to crystalize

Figure 1. Project initiation model

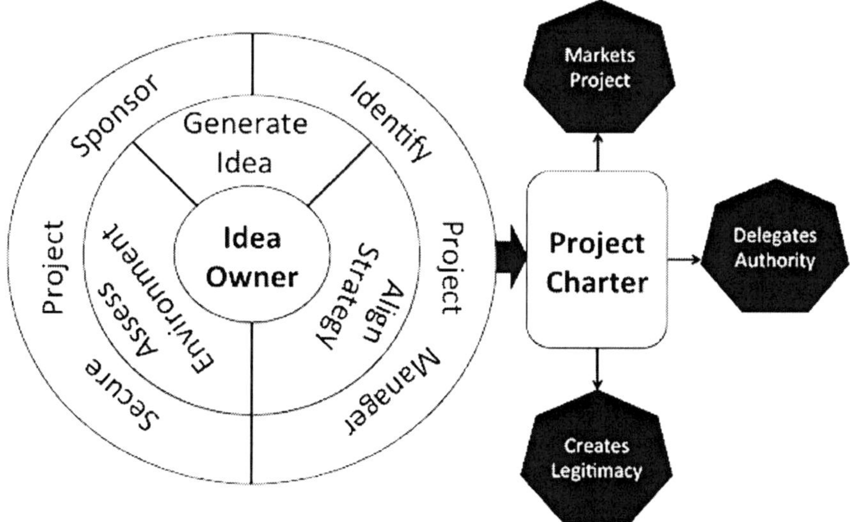

with their entry over time. Generating the project idea, aligning the project strategy, and assessing the project environment forms a recursive process to be revisited as more information becomes available and more stakeholders are engaged. For example, the identification of the project sponsor or manager may introduce additional insights or questions regarding the project idea or environment. Regarding recursiveness, it is also important to note that PMI prescribes the use of the term process groups, rather than phases to reflect that activities associated with each project group are not tied to a timeline, but are done as information becomes available, thus one can move to detailed planning though not all elements of project initiation are complete and elements of project initiation

may be revisited during detailed project planning or execution. In fact, the recursive process may be revisited and updated at intervals along the entire project life cycle to assess the viability of continuing the project as conceived and perhaps, to obtain a formal authorization for continuance.

Figure 2 provides key components for each aspect of the project initiation model based on our literature review. For example, the details provided in Figure 2 entail the key characteristics (decision factors) recommended in considering a project sponsor and project manager as components of related initiation activities. Figure 2 also illustrates the core components of the project charter (e.g., project approval and funding, constraints and assumptions) as reported in the literature. "The

Figure 2. Research framework: Project initiation model

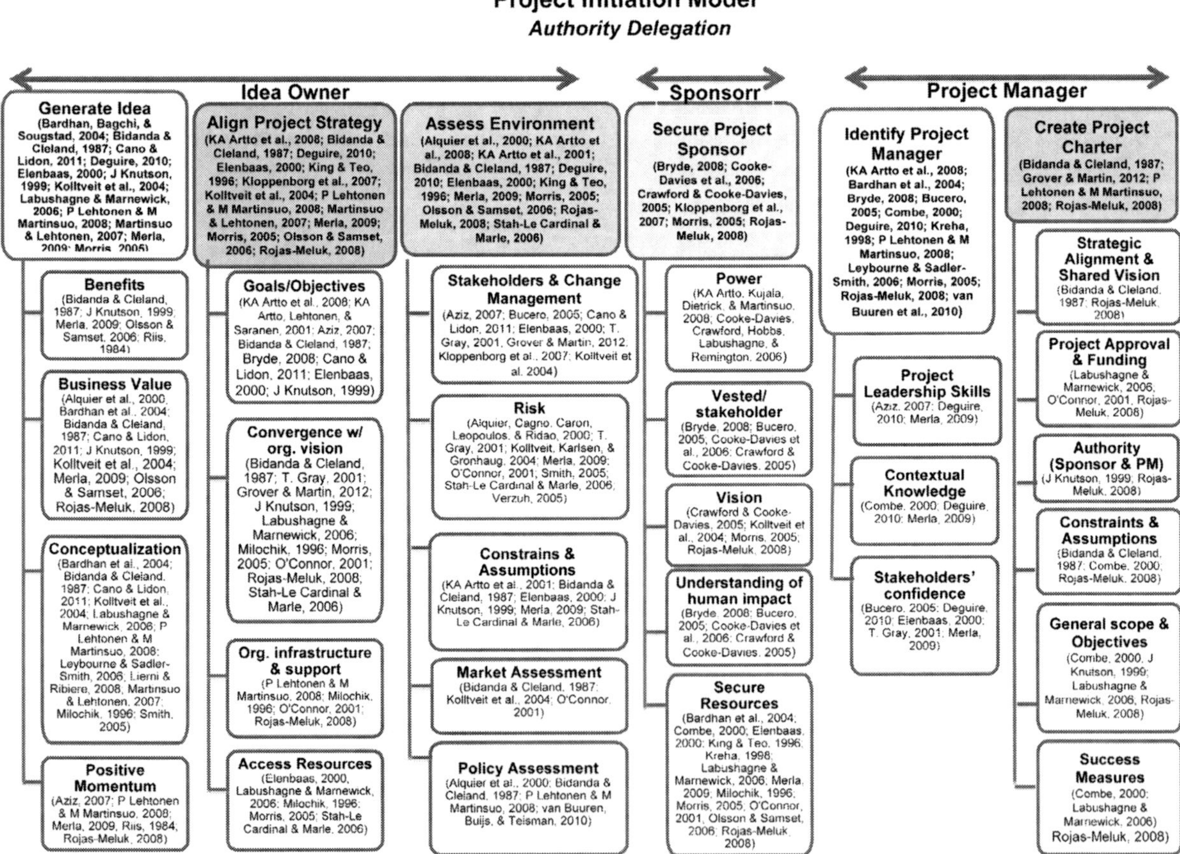

project management discipline is around different fields and industries. Although the same general framework is applicable in the different industries and projects, in the detailed execution each industry and each project tailors the framework according to their necessities" (Stah-Le Cardinal & Marle, 2006). Thus, this study will use this model as a research framework to study project initiation for telestroke projects and tailor insights to various business models within this context.

METHODOLOGY

Reviews of telemedicine in the healthcare domain call for qualitative approaches to better describe and explore telemedicine systems (Aoki, Dunn, Johnson-Throop, & Turley, 2003). To investigate the proposed research questions, we followed a comparative case study approach of five cases (Yin, 1994).

Case Study Business Models

We began our study in 2011 by identifying five distinct telestroke programs with different organizational configurations. We performed a content analysis of these programs using publically available documents and by attending telestroke conference presentations that referenced various other programs to provide background, determine key informants, and identify any statements regarding project initiation. To differentiate the five models one from another, each was labeled according to key characteristics using the following nomenclature: (1) outsourced; (2) alliance; (3) not-for-profit private hospital network; (4) not-for-profit university sponsored network; and (5) for-profit private hospital network. Table 1 provides a summary of key characteristics of five business models. Next, we provide a description of each model.

Table 1. Description of participant business models

Case	Model Name (Abbreviation)	Description	Participants	Telestroke Status (as of Paper Submission)
1	Outsourced (OUTSOURCE, or O)	A for-profit neurological consulting service comprised of 40 physicians who provided teleneurology specialty care to healthcare institutions	Private company contracting with domestic and international healthcare service organizations	On-going telestroke services and multiple new projects
2	Alliance (ALLIANCE, or A)	University-based statewide telehealth implementation initiative	Partnership led by a major university with a medical school that included private healthcare institutions and the state legislature	No operational telestroke services to date
3	Not-for-Profit Private Hospital Network (NFP NETWORK, or NFPN)	A not-for-profit private hospital coalition providing targeted neurological services to mostly underserved rural areas of a single state	Coalition of 14 hospitals: • 2 hub sites, • 10 in-network spoke sites, • 4 out-of-network spoke sites	On-going telestroke service line seeking to expand services and to increase community awareness
4	Not-for-Profit University Sponsored Network (NFP UNIVERSITY, or NFPU)	A not-for-profit university sponsored hospital coalition providing telestroke services to mostly underserved rural areas of a single state	Coalition of 24 hospitals: • 2 hub sites, • 22 spoke sites	On-going telestroke service line with continuing efforts to expand the number of spoke sites
5	For Profit Private Hospital Network (FOR PROFIT, or FP)	A benchmarked for-profit private health system with representation in multiple states	A single large healthcare system with hubs and spoke sites in multiple states	On-going telestroke service line exploring inter-state service possibilities

Outsourced

The outsourced (labeled OUTSOURCE, or O) business model was defined as a for-profit health-care company dedicated to providing state of the art neurological consulting services. The company provided virtual neurological services to both domestic and international clients in the following healthcare service domains: hospitals, rehabilitation centers, physician practices, mental health agencies, independent centers, and home health agencies. Nationally distributed teleneurologists, 40 in all, used advanced telemedicine technology to provide services to as many requesting institutions as appropriate. This business model was not focused on funding or capacity concerns; rather, the main goal was to deliver services to a particular healthcare institution, thus addressing issues associated with a defined population. Understanding the business involved identifying and measuring gaps in service delivery, then determining and recruiting necessary resources to fill such gaps.

Alliance

The alliance (labeled ALLIANCE, or A) was a university-based statewide telehealth implementation initiative that represented an attempt to design a regional system facilitating the receipt of health services, including neurological services, for underserved populations located in rural areas. This business model featured a partnership among university affiliates (to include a medical school), private health organizations, and state governmental representatives who sought to design and implement a statewide telemedicine program. At the time this manuscript was submitted, no operational telestroke services had been delivered.

Not-For-Profit Private Hospital Network

The not-for-profit private hospital network (labeled NFP NETWORK, or NFPN) was a coalition of hospitals designed to provide neurological consulting services to institutions located within a single state. Hence, this business model consisted of two (2) major hub sites capable of delivering teleneurology services to 14 receiving spoke sites. Of the receiving sites, ten (10) were positioned within the hubs' health network and another four (4) were institutions situated outside the health network. The coalition's purpose was to provide high quality healthcare to each area of the state, particularly its rural sites where specialty services were either limited or nonexistent. As such, a key program goal was to promote National Institute of Health Stroke Scale standards throughout the network; employing a Values Center of Excellence designation for stroke care at the spoke sites supported such standards. This not-for-profit private hospital network was supported through internal funding and a fee-based participation system. At the time of manuscript submission, the coalition had maintained an on-going telestroke service line and was seeking to expand services beyond the emergency department, to involve other forms of provider services (post stroke), and to expand community awareness through grant funding.

Not-For-Profit University Sponsored Network

The not-for-profit university sponsored network (labeled NFP UNIVERSITY, or NFPU) was a coalition of hospitals designed to provide telestroke services to institutions located within a single state. This business model consisted of two (2) major hub sites capable of delivering telemedicine services to 22 receiving spoke sites. Part of a statewide effort to combat stroke, this network's purpose was to provide targeted telemedicine services underserved areas within the state, particularly those in rural settings. The NFP UNIVERSITY model, facilitated through grant funding, represented an on-going telestroke service line with continuing efforts to expand the number of spoke sites within the state.

For-Profit Private Hospital Network

The for-profit private hospital network (labeled FOR PROFIT, or FP) represented a single large hospital system network serving multiple communities in several states. The FOR PROFIT model consisted of multiple within-state telestroke hubs and receiving spoke sites serving defined populations of the states in which they were located. The American Heart and American Stroke Associations (AHA and ASA respectively) had recognized selected sites within this network for delivering benchmark quality stroke care. The FOR PROFIT model, funded through the organizational network to generate additional revenue, constituted an ongoing telestroke service line that was exploring interstate expansion opportunities.

Data Collection

The authors conducted both unstructured interviews/meetings and structured interviews. Structured interviews were conducted via telephone with nine different key informants (who represent the five organizations). The interview protocol included 15 open-ended questions about the vision, mission of the organization, how telehealth is aligned with this vision, how the telestroke projects were initiated, the challenges and the best practices founded and the business model that was built as a result of the project. The interviews lasted between 1 to 1.5 hours with one researcher acting as the lead interviewer and a second researcher acting as a scribe and also posing insight and follow-up questions, as warranted. Informants included chief medical officers, project managers, telehealth directors. Two members of the research team performed a site visit at one site. All interviews and discussions during site visits were audio taped, transcribed and then reviewed for transcription errors before data analysis began using a qualitative data analysis application (Dedoose (c)).

In addition to the structured interviews, two researchers visited organizational booths and attended informants' presentations at national conferences. Unstructured interviews and meetings occurred both prior to the structured interviews to learn foundational information and identify key informants as well as after the structured interviews for supplemental material and updates.

Data Analysis

In general, we used guiding principles from Lee and Baskerville (2003) to move data to the description and thereby develop understanding and insights. Two researchers performed selective coding using the key components of the Project Initiation General Approach (see Figure 1) as a coding schema and discussed their coding for reconciling purposes on regular intervals. During the coding process, coding was not restricted to this group of codes. The research team was open to identifying project initiation concepts that are unique to telemedicine projects. As the research team discovered new concepts being addressed by the interviewee that did not map to the existing codes, we created a new code, typically a child code, to explain a finding or highlight a detailed characteristic of a case for each new concept. We also used these child codes to better understand the similarities and differences between the implementation modalities.

We used business model as one of the descriptors associated with each transcript. After selective coding was complete, we used mixed-method tables to provide a cross section of each code by the business model descriptor to discern differences and similarities across the five business models.

FINDINGS

We used previously discussed project initiation activities that were supported by literature to provide a structured discussion of project initiation in the telemedicine context and compare project initiation approaches among the five organizations, which represent five diverse business models. Table 2 provides a highlight of our findings discussed in this section.

Generate Idea

Generation of a project idea is the first initiation activity for which the idea owner is responsible. Although we use a singular form for idea owner, we should acknowledge that in large and complex projects like telemedicine, multiple idea owners exist. They carry out the initiation tasks collaboratively to initiate the project. As the project

Table 2. Project initiation phase and select telemedicine attributes by business model type

Project Initiation Phase	Select Telemedicine Attributes by Business Model Type
Generate Idea - Create Positive Momentum	• Enhanced quality & access (all); • Reaching underserved populations – (NFPP, NFPU) • Enhanced operational efficiency - prescriptive (O, FPP) • Co-branding partnership with health org & others (O)
Align Project Strategy	• Look beyond project - grant issue (A, NFPP) • Ownership issue (A) • Organizational readiness to adopt changes (all) • Quality of care – status; center of excellence (NFPU) • ROI (O, FPP)
Assess Environment - Stakeholders & Change Management	• Manage community relationships, rivalries (NFPP, NFPU) • Assess provider buy-in/complex approval process (A, NFPP, NFPU) • Clarify hub (A & NFPU) • Marketing to providers and patients (NFPU) • Education (NFPU, but O considering formalizing)
Assess Environment - Risk	• Technology "proof of concept" (all) • Recognize Clinical Complexities and Standards of Care (all) • Standard Protocols (NFPU, O) • Multiple Locations/ local politics and readiness levels (all)
Assess Environment - Policy Assessment	• Reimbursement Model – fees for transfers (A, NFPU external) • Credentialing – Certifications (O challenge) • State and Federal (all - & International for O) • Opportunity – Center of Excellence (NFPU)
Secure Project Sponsor - Power	• Often comes from clinical neurological champion (NFPU, O) & political connections (all) • Committee / board (NFPU)
Secure Project Sponsor - Secure Resources	• Conservative cost/benefit – no downstream (NFPU) • Grant (delay for NFPU, O not directly eligible) • Focus on quality of care/ excellence (A & NFPU)
Identify Project Manager	• Trained PMP (NFPU) • Telehealth coordinator may have more "power" (NFPU) • Business manager (O), but may move to PMP • Informal (A – expert vs. political power)
Create Project Charter - Project Approval & Funding	Formal project charter (NFPU); blueprint (A); contract (O) • Initial Funding → Promoting the service →ROI (all)
Create Project Charter - Success Measures	Qualitative and Quantitative Measures • Operational – number of sites up, transfer numbers (O, NFPU), provider productivity (FPP) • Learning – NIH stroke scale (O, NFPU)Satisfaction – Patient and provider (all), customer (O) Lag Indicators (NFPU): • Technical - % use, successful connections, downtime • Clinical - tPA utilization, pt. outcome, efficiency (door to needle)

initiation progresses, the roles and responsibilities of idea owners could transform into more formal roles in the project team.

Identify Benefits and Business Value of Telestroke

Developing a powerful vision and identifying why a project is necessary is a very important factor in selling a project proposal and getting the project off to a powerful start (Merla, 2009). All five organizations identified the same primary benefits inherent in establishing telestroke services: enhanced quality and access. These benefits included the improvement of neurological services available (quality), "The hospitals that call us… the ones that do not have neurologists on site basically call us for everything…for the most part it's emergency care, but it's definitely not limited to stroke." Additional benefits included expanding the availability of these services to a larger geographic region (access). For example, NFP NETWORK stated: "The mission… is to expand healthcare to our community, and [our state] is an extremely rural community… this technology allows access to some of these specialists to our rural counties where they don't have that luxury." Furthermore, respondents indicated that expansion through telemedicine also enhanced access to care through increased efficiency. According to the FOR PROFIT site, "… the chiefs of service [had to] come up with a way of making [their] department more efficient…so, in a six-minute interval, [visits were completed that] might take a dermatologist 20 minutes [for] in-person appointment(s)." Essentially, telemedicine was a means by which to improve patient satisfaction around access to quality care.

Though there were similarities, each case had a unique interest in the launch of a telestroke service, as its leadership designed it. The FOR PROFIT AND OUTSOURCE cases considered more traditional business concerns and opportunities. The not-for-profit organizations, (both the NFP NETWORK and NFP UNIVERSITY), discussed how to establish and sustain the initiative to meet community needs.

Identifying individual organization benefits (particularly for hub sites) created a unique challenge for the alliance. The leadership committee recommended to hospital systems that they invest in the appropriate equipment to participate in the telemedicine network, even though the investment and participation was not mandated. The governance structure had, in some ways, been a barrier to the model's implementation. There was not always an incentive for individual hospitals and systems to participate. Investing in the appropriate equipment was beneficial to these institutions, from a financial standpoint, if patients then used their services at increasing rates. Because of the need to share equipment and distribute patients throughout the state, participants did not always realize a high return on investment. According to an ALLIANCE informant:

So [the hospital's] whole model is that the patients get transferred to their hospital for more care, which increases their own revenue. The concern was that in an open telestroke network, if the hospital could choose any stroke provider in the state, the fear was that…if a patient called, or a physician called at a hospital that was usually sending their patients to [Location X], and for whatever reason that hospital's doctor ended up talking to a provider in [Location Y], that they would redirect the patient to be transferred to [Location Y] as opposed to [Location X]. So [Location X] was like, why would we invest in a system that we would potentially lose patients?

Conceptualize the Project

The project should be conceptualized in a way to help the decision makers do what they do best: make decisions on what ideas should become projects to bring the most value into the organization (Rojas-Meluk, 2008). Organizations within this study decided on the option to incorporate telestroke initiatives into their expansion strategies based on quality and access drivers, as previously outlined. Yet, it appeared that only the for-profit and Outsourced telemedicine providers approached their decision to move forward with the project with a prescriptive formula in mind. In these instances, the decision to provide telestroke services was based on each organization's defined business model for providing a variety of services in the virtual environment. The project was framed and conceptualized according to this prescriptive formula. For NFP NETWORK AND NFP UNIVERSITY, however, environmental factors such as persistently poor health outcomes and other pressures (state and federal policy) much more heavily influenced the chosen course of action, and projects were accordingly framed.

It is of note that most of the organizations studied desired a gold standard or best practice from which to model and conceptualize their initiatives in an effort to save valuable time and avoid substantial capital investments associated with initial project development.

Create Positive Project Momentum

Project momentum is defined as an energy pattern that needs to be recognized to move the project to a successful implementation path (Nelson & Jansen, 2009). Sometimes this is positive energy, and in other cases it is negative energy resulting from delays or problems related to the project (Nelson & Jansen, 2009). For the NFP NETWORK, the key challenge to creating momentum was to convince various stakeholders (administrators and clinicians) of the need for and value of telestroke service lines. The strongest marketing tool identified in this project was "word of mouth", particularly word of mouth from a physician champion. Secondarily, but no less important to creating positive momentum, were continuing education and training programs. Telestroke protocol and

process training coupled with ongoing National Institutes of Health (NIH) stroke scale training initiatives, led to enhanced interest and participation, thus increasing project momentum. At times, additional marketing materials were created and dispersed internally and within the external community detailing the services that were to be available at telestroke spoke facilities.

Although the OUTSOURCE company acknowledged that their healthcare client assumed greater responsibility for creating organizational momentum, they recognized the importance of stakeholder's communication, making contact as early as possible and continually updating stakeholders as necessary. The effort was focused on creating a "co-branded partnership" with the healthcare organization. To develop this "co-branded partnership", the focus of the communications was on process understanding, "Everyone in the project needs to understand the process before the service goes live."

In an effort to maintain dynamic collaboration, both the ALLIANCE and the OUTSOURCE organizations engaged in a number of continuing education initiatives internally and externally. All organizations sponsored, organized and/or participated in telemedicine conferences geared toward the sharing of tools, processes, and lessons learned. This also led to some dynamic collaboration. As a result of co-attendance, organizations' paths sometimes crossed and fueled momentum, as in the case of the NFP NETWORK exploring a business opportunity with the OUTSOURCE. Momentum was also enhanced through conference networking that led to an informal mentorship opportunity as happened between the NFP UNIVERSITY and the NFP NETWORK.

Creating momentum was not only seen as an internal effort among identified and potential project team members. Respondents indicated they wanted to get the message out to providers and the communities in which they wished to provide service.

Align Project Strategy

To support the decisions made, an organization must develop and collect measures based on goals that are aligned with the organization's key initiatives(Rojas-Meluk, 2008). This requires the idea owner to determine the goals and objectives of the project early in the project initiation process. It also requires the idea owner to have a good understanding of the organization's mission, vision and short-term goals.

Affirm That the Project Converges With the Organizational Vision

Ideally, a project's content and objectives aligned with the organization's mission and strategic goals. All respondents mentioned quality of care; as the representative from the NFP NETWORK said, "[the] hope is that no matter where you live in [the state] that you will be able to access the [appropriate] standard of care … and that there is no disparity for those rural residents." Even in the case of the OUTSOURCE organization, whose vision was to provide telemedicine services in as many facilities as possible; the underlying mission was to enhance the efficiency and efficacy of the care provided.

In the NFP NETWORK model, multiple missions and visions existed. Its mission was to assemble disparate hospitals into a cohesive healthcare network. Telestroke was a means to this end. As such, they desired to achieve "Center of Excellence" status (spoke sites could be classified as primary stroke centers) for multiple network facilities in congruence with the organization's vision. Additionally, informants indicated that the telestroke effort indirectly supported the vision to move towards closer collaborative associations among network components, which was an administrative goal: "…even though we're all one parent company, there are divisions… [yet] we talk a lot about 'systemness': How can we be more of a system? How can we leverage [the

organization as a whole]?" Finally, telestroke also supported educational goals regarding the NIH's stroke scale and related best practices and inter-professional education.

Assess Organizational Infrastructure, Support, and Policies to Access Resources

Organizational infrastructure refers to how companies organize the people side of their business (roles, responsibilities, authority, focus, and control within the organization) ("Organizational Infrastructure: Define, Analyze & Change," 2010). For the NFP NETWORK, defining the project's governing organization presented a challenge. The interactions between the system's central facilities and rural hospitals were complicated, and it was initially not clear which hospital should lead the project. There was also complexity surrounding who should own this initiative; it could be either an information technology initiative or a corporate initiative. IT group initially owned the project, but ownership shifted to a more centralized corporate team. It took time to determine the right owner for the initiative and to establish the role of IT in the project. The governance structure was further complicated by the organization's change in top leadership. The case demonstrated that a change in power could result in a shift in a project's vision.

For the outsource organization, a board of directors oversaw each project. The board had the ability to either enable or constrain the project's initiation according to its business model. The organization's goal was to be profitable in delivering a specific product to the market, and this goal guided decision-making.

Governance for the ALLIANCE project was achieved by a steering committee with representatives from the telemedicine group, affiliated university, and government. Government involvement and support was present because the project was designed to improve healthcare at the state level. The committee's main actions in the initial stage of the case were aligning the viewpoints and interests of the interested parties and committee members to establish a vision and general scope for the project.

Assess Environment

The telemedicine environment includes the environment of the hub sites and the spoke sites as well as the external telemedicine environment. Knowing the environment can help idea owner and the project team better address issues of constraints or culture (Merla, 2009).

Identify Stakeholders And Consider Change Management Issues

Regarding stakeholder analysis, each case study acknowledged neurologists were key to success and utilized key clinical stakeholders as champions in the change management process. Each hospital in the NFP NETWORK was a stakeholder in the project, and each advocated for its unique interests. Hospital directors or representatives were key players in decision-making and local implementation. Each of these facilities had its own governance structure, and collaboration among leadership teams was essential. Having access to decision-makers was viewed as a key determinant of successful hospital implementation. In large hospitals and hospital systems, the negotiation and decision making process took time, and many stakeholders were involved. Thus, hospital directors played a significant role within their institutions, garnering awareness and support for the project and collaborating with key administrators and physicians.

The ALLIANCE case featured stakeholders with differing roles from around the region, and each person on the panel offered a unique perspective and had a different agenda. The ALLIANCE found support in larger healthcare organizations in order to increase access to resources and be-

come part of higher-level political initiatives. Each player's differing views made universal buy-in more difficult to achieve and slowed the initiative's progress. With the growing interest in telemedicine due to recent governmental support, vendors were offering equipment and solutions at the state level. For this reason, dealing with local governments was important when trying to make the right investment decisions and avoid potential pitfalls.

Each organization acknowledged that successful change management was key during the initiation process. Workflow changes related to the new protocols and services were inevitable once telestroke services were fully implemented. Each of the five business models engaged in these processes, though the extent of effort varied. For the OUTSOURCE model, plans were in place to incorporate full-time personnel for training and change management purposes. Associated challenges were particularly exemplified through the NFP NETWORK: "... [within our system]... [Each] hospital has its departments and its specialties... historically, [we have] been very competitive with one another, even though we're still [one system]. And now we're trying to venture into our rural hospitals [which have] taken care of themselves... so you've got all these communities of practice and all of these different silos ... that are having to work together and share information, share resources, and ... open up. It's not been easy, to be honest. It's not been easy at all."

Change management endeavors in all cases introduced some new or enhanced face-to-face meetings and email among stakeholders that may not have worked together before. Furthermore, in the course of enabling the telemedicine service line, new and collaborative relationships were formed or reinforced among administrators, nurses, doctors, researchers, IT personnel and others either within or across participating healthcare facilities.

Determine Constraints and Assumptions

A common constraint for many organizations was that of limited resources, particularly with regard to neurologists available to provide consulting services in anticipation of future growth. As a result, the NFP NETWORK looked to the OUT-SOURCE company, who had anticipated greater demand, for support: "[Our state] was prime, a perfect storm in fact…for telestroke, and [the outsourcing company's CEO] went ahead and got all of their neurologists licensed…in anticipation that there's going to be… [a greater] need for it."

For the ALLIANCE, the project made some assumptions about different hospitals in the state, namely their current technological capacity and their utilization rates. For hospitals that did not have a strong technological foundation, additional considerations were made, and more steps were necessary during telemedicine program implementation.

Identify and Assess Risks

Identifiable risks for the ALLIANCE included both operational viability and technical feasibility. According to the ALLIANCE, "Issues such as community benefit, service availability, and payment structure must be addressed to establish support for and the sustainability of the program." In this case, finding a sustainable telemedicine model was the critical issue. Issues relating to reimbursement had been vague and complex. Furthermore, stakeholders needed proof that the concept was feasible, especially with regard to the alignment of clinical protocols for the purpose of meeting standards of care. The ability to form partnerships with healthcare organizations was found to be a critical piece of this program's success. Additionally, the technology involved was carefully considered as implementation was costly and a variety of technical standards had to be bridged across many hospitals within the network.

Associated risks varied by organization type and levels of readiness for implementation, yet each shared similarities, especially with regard to cost and quality. A cost risk identified by the NFP NETWORK was overdependence on grant funding. In this case, the organization recognized the need to look beyond grants, and was pursuing telemedicine in the absence of initial funding with the intent to pursue grant opportunities only when the effort showed signs of sustainability. For the NFP UNIVERSITY's program, each healthcare facility had to understand the model's capabilities and to align expectations accordingly. Facilities often wanted to rush the process, and organizational leadership had to temper the pace of implementation to meet quality assurance standards and incorporate risk mitigation techniques, which were integral to program success.

Conduct External Market Assessment

Within the external market, several respondents (NFP NETWORK, FOR PROFIT, NFP UNIVERSITY, and ALLIANCE) indicated that awareness of and interest in telemedicine had increased within recent years, particularly because increasing means of reimbursement. According to the ALLIANCE,:

… more entities [were] paying for the service. There [was] recognition of the quality, and… the concept [was] getting more acceptable to… [talk] about along multiple lines. So, clinical people [were] talking about it. The marketing people [were] talking about it. The CFO people [were] talking about it. So, across several lines of administration, telemedicine [was] becoming more of a hot-button conversation than it was three years ago.

Even with increased awareness, however, negotiating the external market was largely driven by how an organization defined its market and the environment in which it implemented the telemedicine project. For the statewide initiatives (NFP NETWORK, NFP UNIVERSITY, and ALLIANCE), markets were defined in terms of geography, owing to the structure of the systems combined with the projects' intent. Specifically, the NFP NETWORK and NFP UNIVERSITY functioned within the confines of predetermined boundaries; in both cases such limitations were defined by the state in which they operated and, for the NFP NETWORK, further by the health system to which they belonged. As a result, each project team found themselves serving as a negotiator or mediator between competing organizations within their respective states (and/or systems) in an effort to create project alignment and enhance participation.

Conduct Policy Assessment

Policy changes within the external market, both state and federal, had a significant impact on the success of telestroke projects for many respondents. Until only recently (within the past few years), telemedicine had been supported largely through grants. In a few key states, however, congressional earmarks had supported telemedicine, as with Arizona and Alaska. According to an ALLIANCE representative, "Very few other programs could create sustainable telemedicine service lines, because the reimbursement issues were so vague and unreliable." The political landscape appeared to have adapted, at least in part, to changes in the technological landscape. In particular, Medicaid and Medicare had begun reimbursing telemedicine services, and stakeholders were anticipating leveraging telemedicine in response to healthcare reform.

In spite of a few major advances in federal legislation, several pitfalls remained including some financial and others administrative. For example, the ALLIANCE, NFP NETWORK, AND NFP UNIVERSITY faced continuing in-state patient transfer fees, and some lamented having to charge

hub sites clinical fees in the absence of authorized reimbursements for certain services.

In addition, many informants commented on issues related to state-level credentialing and national certification, including the OUTSOURCE organization"…you need to have one telemedicine license which can be…approved by every state so that you can facilitate the work. And I think you need to be paid for what you do. You need to be able to bill, and that's it."

Secure Project Sponsorship

The project sponsor, who is essentially in charge of approving the project and channeling support and resources, was found to be a vital component of a project's success. As indicated in the Project Initiation Model (see Figure 1), literature prescribes that an individual's level of power in the organization, stake in project success, vision s/he developed for the project, level of understanding of the project's human impact, and ability of the individual to secure resources should be consider in identifying a project sponsor. Within the five telestroke projects studied, none mentioned a single formal project sponsor within their organization. As a result, manifestations of sponsorship demonstrated some interesting aspects of partnerships and negotiation.

The NFP UNIVERSITY and NFP NETWORK established project sponsorship through multi-disciplinary leadership committees who authorized projects and did much of the initial planning. Consensus amongst committee members, though, had to be formalized before a project was planned in detail. In the ALLIANCE, some committee members "…wanted to move forward with video supported telestroke, and the other half of the committee [thought] that this was probably not necessary, and everything was fine in their organizations…they didn't see any advantage for spending the time or effort in this kind of process." Using a separate approach that aligned with their business model, the FOR PROFIT organization opted to leverage collaboration between leading decision makers and new customers to reach formal agreements.

Within the FOR PROFIT, NFP UNIVERSITY, and NFP NETWORK models, access to resources and support were often derived through actions from the clinical practice champion(s) affiliated with the service line. Frequently, neurologists tended to take a leading role and/or were specifically targeted for support by others within the system that recognized the value in the provision of telestroke services for patients and service providers alike. Furthermore, within the NFP NETWORK, committee or board members, to include non-governmental associations, often took proactive roles, using political clout to gain support and enhance project momentum.

One possible implication of our results is that the aforementioned deciding criteria for choosing a project sponsor may be distributed among various individuals in the context of a telemedicine project. The concept of a sponsor takes on a new meaning for the OUTSOURCE organization, as they are looking for target client sponsors who can influence a business decision to enter into a contractual agreement; in their case identifying a sponsor represents a business opportunity.

Identify Project Manager

Project managers lead the project towards fulfilling time, budget/resource and scope goals. They are the day-to-day operational managers of the project. The model guiding this study indicates that an individual's project management skills, contextual knowledge of the project and organization, and ability to evoke stakeholder confidence are key criteria in selecting a project manager.

While project sponsors tended to be neurology clinical practice specialists, continued management support for telestroke programs was often delegated to other clinical staff or telemedicine coordinators (who may also be clinically trained)

who were trained expressly for the purpose of administering programs, as indicated by the NFP UNIVERSITY program respondent: "…we have a few physicians that are very big champions and they help drive it at their facilities but I will tell you, I would say 90% of the time, it is nurse driven. Those are people we trained." Alternatively, the OUTSOURCE organization hired a business manager who was supported by physician leadership, which was appropriate for that particular business model.

Although clinical specialists largely shouldered accountability for implementation in all cases, findings indicated responsibility for various aspects of program management was often divided. The FOR PROFIT respondent indicated, "…what really helped in implementing [the program] everywhere [was an] agreement that each medical center had to assign a project manager, and a medical lead, and a training and technology lead… those people were responsible for… really taking ownership of local implementation." Similarly, the NFP NETWORK stated, "We've had a project management team in place since day one. [We hired a] director of project management... [We sat] down with him at the outset and said what we wanted to do and what are the deliverables, both technologically as well as clinically."

Interestingly, informal power appeared to drive the project managers' success, regardless of organization type or structure. Underscoring this point, a NFP NETWORK informant commented: "… the most important skill set for telemedicine beyond clinical/technical is the ability to establish a relationship…you can have all the technology and be the most confident 'strokologist' in the world, but if you cannot connect and have a rapport with your end user, it doesn't matter." Thus, connecting with various stakeholders through skillful relationship management (informal power) was key to the successful negotiation of project initiation and implementation. Such management, therefore, was viewed as a means by which stakeholders could align seemingly divergent agendas in order to facilitate a win-win environment conducive to project sustainability. This highlights the criteria in the research model to identify a project manager that can evoke stakeholder confidence (and thereby influence stakeholders) while also highlighting that one of the most important project management skills is communication skills. An argument can be made that these two criteria may be critically important deciding factors when selecting a project manager in the case of telemedicine projects.

Create Project Charter

In essence, a charter is a manifestation of project strategy for the architecture and system. In the general project management literature, it was speculated that the presence of a charter in the project initiation stage was predictive of the project's success. We should note that we did not ask respondents directly if they had a project charter (after discerning that this may not be a term familiar to our informants); rather, we inquired as to how the project was managed and other governance-related questions and what was used to guide the project.

Of these five telestroke projects, only the NFP NETWORK mentioned having a project charter, by name. The OUTSOURCE organization created a blueprint for the project, which was largely a result of an advanced planning process. The blueprint developed was a general telemedicine business model for the company, and did not specify a plan for the telestroke initiative. And the OUTSOURCE organization also had a contract with their client health organization, which can instantiate a charter. These two projects seemed to progress much faster and produced measurable results more quickly than the FOR PROFIT or the NFP UNIVERSITY program, which did not have formal project charters.

Identify Sources of Funding

Funding sources also varied by organization type. Within the NFP NETWORK, project funding was generated by contracts between the hub and each of the spoke sites. Contracts covered the cost of services, to include the price per consult, and were renegotiated on twelve-month intervals. Similar legal contracts existed for the outsourcing organization as part of its business model. Within the FOR PROFIT system, funding for the project was sourced from the service line directly. In this case, funding levels were considered in terms of patient volume and provider productivity per full-time equivalent (FTE). According to the FOR PROFIT system respondent, "So, you know, they got extra chunks of money based on the fact that they saw a certain number of same-day visits, and the only way to really truly do 50 same-day visits was to do [telemedicine]…They started to implement that across other specialties as well." Grants also played a role within the NFP UNIVERSITY and the ALLIANCE. In such instances, the focus was on enhanced quality of care and excellence in service delivery, perhaps because the grants stipulated the fulfilling of specific objectives.

Develop Success Measures

Given the healthcare context, project success measurement ranged from clinical measures, to measure of satisfaction with the system or training, to utilization measures, to measures of efficiency to technical system metrics. Defining success through quantitative and/or qualitative tools also differed by organization type, particularly due to the divergence of purposes that drove program initiation. Some measured success using quantitative metrics, such as the number of sites with whom the organization contracted (OUTSOURCE) or the number of appropriate transfers that occurred within the system (NFP

NETWORK). As stated previously with regard to the FOR PROFIT system, it was patient volume and provider productivity that drove the program. Many organizations also used the NIH, American Heart Association, National American Heart and Stroke Association, as well as the Brain Coalition standards, to derive baseline metrics for tPA utilization and administration rates, "door-to-needle" time, and to document patient outcomes overall, particularly in terms of morbidity and mortality (particularly with the NFP NETWORK and the NFP UNIVERSITY programs). Additionally, some used technical data, as with percent use of telemedicine services, to include connectivity and network downtime.

Many respondents combined such quantitative metrics with qualitative input, predominantly with regard to organizational learning and customer satisfaction as it related to a number of stakeholders: patients, providers, and contracted customers. The NFP NETWORK representative reflected, "…We [had] a certain set of competencies and skills to teach clinically and technically, but my hope [was] that we [would] continue to learn from our spoke sites. The ultimate goal for stroke care [was] that the patient or the person out in the community [would] learn more how to recognize stroke symptoms and signs and, if they've had one stroke, how to be real involved in the management of their stroke and not to have a recurrent stroke. So the goal then [was] to…not be one of the leading states for stroke mortality… The ultimate goal [was] that we [would] learn from our stroke patients and they [would] learn from us and our metro physicians and staff [would] learn from spokes."

The OUTSOURCE organization revealed that each individual implementation, and the business model in the aggregate, were measures of success. Organizational leadership had not, however, identified any particular key performance indicator, aside from profitability, to gauge success.

CONCLUSION

Telemedicine is a technology innovation in healthcare organizations that manifests both intra- and inter-organizational collaboration. Moving from a telemedicine project to a sustainable telemedicine service line can be a challenge for many organizations(LeRouge et al., 2010). In this paper, we investigate project initiation process in various telemedicine programs through a multi-site case study, review existing project management literature on project initiation process, and present a Project Initiation Model (see Figure 1) that combines project initiation activities and components found in the literature and project initiation practices we identified in our multi-site case study. This is one of the first studies that link published best practices to the telemedicine domain, particularly for the critical process of project initiation. Our findings explicate the nuances of project initiation for the telemedicine context, specifically the instance of telestroke, using our model constructed from project management literature as a framework. Our findings also reveal commonalities and differences that exist in project initiation for telestroke projects under the condition of five distinct business models.

In general, this study supports that the elements of project initiation found in the literature are represented in the telestroke context, though manifested in unique ways. For example, although aspects of project sponsorship exist, the roles and guiding characteristics of a project sponsor seem to be distributed among multiple individuals in the context of telemedicine. In addition, factors associated with each business model influence the way that certain model components were exemplified as was the case for organizational infrastructure and much less for other components (e.g., elements of business value, risk, and assessing the environment). The underlying implication is that the Project Initiation Model presented can be used as a decision guide and aid as telemedicine projects move through project initiation and that its utility may be further enhanced by extending the model to include details specific to the telemedicine business model at play. These findings can help practitioners better manage the telemedicine project initiation process towards a sustainable service line. The findings can also help the research community describe and frame future studies of telemedicine projects.

The implied importance of the ultimate deliverable of project initiation, the project charter (or some related manifestation), also seems to be reflected in our findings. The authors encourage future work that can directly link the project initiation decisions and the existence of some representation of a project charter to program success in telemedicine environments. In addition, we call on researchers to further other stages of the project management process within the telemedicine context.

The limitations of our study, as with any qualitative case analysis, relate to generalizability and the potential of coding bias (though research methods were employed using structure and rigor to minimize bias). We derived our findings based on a single instance of telemedicine, telestroke, at five different sites distributed across the country. We picked this emerging service line because it allowed us to observe project initiation as it happened in these five sites. We invite future research of various telemedicine service lines and case sites to assess the boundaries of our findings.

In essence, the study contributes to the construction of a bridge between telemedicine practice and project management best practices found in the literature. As we begin to understand the relationships and nuances, we can expedite the development of best practices and gold standards that help to pave the way to success in these complex intra- and inter-organizational projects.

ACKNOWLEDGMENT

We would like to thank our former graduate students Dora Luz Mejia Arango and Allison Tuma for their support in this research project.

REFERENCES

Alquier, A., Cagno, E., Caron, F., Leopoulos, V., & Ridao, M. (2000). Analysis of external and internal risks in project early phase. In *Proceeding of PMI Research Conference*.

Aoki, N., Dunn, K., Johnson-Throop, K., & Turley, J. (2003). Outcomes and methods in telemedicine evaluation. *Telemedicine Journal and e-Health*, 9(4), 393–401. doi:10.1089/1530562203772744734 PMID:14980098

Artto, K., Kujala, J., Dietrich, P., & Martinsuo, M. (2008). What is project strategy? *International Journal of Project Management*, 26(1), 4–12. doi:10.1016/j.ijproman.2007.07.006

Artto, K., Kujala, J., Dietrick, P., & Martinsuo, M. (2008). What is project strategy? *International Journal of Project Management*, 26(1), 4–12. doi:10.1016/j.ijproman.2007.07.006

Artto, K., Lehtonen, J.-M., & Saranen, J. (2001). Managing project front-end: Incorporating a strategic early view to project management with simulation. *International Journal of Project Management*, 19(5), 255–264. doi:10.1016/S0263-7863(99)00082-4

Aziz, L. (2007). *Managing change in healthcare information technology projects: The role of the project manager.* Paper presented at the PMI Global Congress Proceedings, Atlanta, GA.

Baden-Fuller, C. M., & Morgan, M. S. (2010). M.S. business models as models. *Long Range Planning*, 43(2-3), 156–171. doi:10.1016/j.lrp.2010.02.005

Bardhan, I., Bagchi, S., & Sougstad, R. (2004). Prioritizing a portfolio of information technology investment projects. *Journal of Management Information Systems, 21*(2), 33–60.

Bidanda, B., & Cleland, D. (1987). Techniques to assess project feasibility. *Project Management Journal*, 68–71.

Bryde, D. (2008). Perceptions of the impact of project sponsorship practices on project success. *International Journal of Project Management, 26*(8), 800–809. doi:10.1016/j.ijproman.2007.12.001

Bucero, A. (2005). *Getting senior executive to buy into project methods, a case study.* Paper presented at the 2005 PMI Global Conference Proceedings, Edinburgh, Scotland.

Cano, J., & Lidon, I. (2011). Guided reflection on project definition. *International Journal of Project Management, 29*(5), 525–536. doi:10.1016/j.ijproman.2010.04.008

Chiocchio, F., Lebel, P., Therriault, P.-Y., Boucher, A., Hass, C., Rabbat, F.-X., & Bouchard, J.-F. (2012). *Stress and performance in health care project teams.* Project Management Institute.

Combe, M. (2000). *Making the link from strategy to projects - What's the payoff?* Paper presented at the Proceedings of the Project Management Institute Annual Seminars & Symposium, Houston, TX.

Cooke-Davies, T., Crawford, L., Hobbs, J., Labushagne, L., & Remington, K. (2006). *Exploring the role of the executive sponsor.* Project Management Institute.

Crawford, L., & Cooke-Davies, T. (2005). *Project governance: The pivotal role of the executive sponsor.* Paper presented at the 2005 PMI Global Congress Proceedings, Toronto, Canada.

Deguire, M. (2010). *Project versus program business case decisions.* Paper presented at the 2010 PMI Global Congress Proceedings, Melbourne, Australia.

Deutsch, E., Duftschmid, G., & Dorda, W. (2010). Critical areas of national electronic health record programs–Is our focus correct? *International Journal of Medical Informatics, 79*(3), 211–222. doi:10.1016/j.ijmedinf.2009.12.002 PMID:20079685

Elenbaas. (2000). *Staging a project: Are you setting your project up for success?* Paper presented at the Proceedings of the Project Management Institute Annual Seminars & Symposiums, Houston, TX.

Gertner, E. I., Sabino, J. N., Mahad, E., Deitric, L. M., Patton, J. R., & Grim, M. K. et al. (2010). Developing a culturally competent health network: A planning framework and guide. *Journal of Healthcare Management, 55*(3), 190–204. PMID:20565035

Gray, C., & Larson, E. (2008). *Project management: The managerial process.* New York, NY: McGraw-Hill Irwin.

Gray, T. (2001). Customers come first. *PM Network, December 2001.*

Grover, V., & Martin, G. D. (2012). The initiation, adoption, and implementation of telecommunications technologies in U.S. organizations. *Journal of Management Information Systems, 10*(1).

Joshi, P., Marino, M., Bhoi, A., Gaines, K., Allen, E., & Mora, J. (2013). Implementing telestroke to reduce the burden of stroke in Louisiana. *Journal of Cardiovascular Disease and Research, 4*(1), 71–73. doi:10.1016/j.jcdr.2013.02.015 PMID:24023480

Kaplan, S., & Tripsas, M. (2008). Thinking about technology: Applying a cognitive lens to technical change. *Research Policy, 37*(5), 790–805. doi:10.1016/j.respol.2008.02.002

King, W. R., & Teo, T. S. H. (1996). Key dimensions of facilitators and inhibitors for the strategic use of information technology. *Journal of Management Information Systems, 12*(4), 35.

Kloppenborg, T. J., Stubblebine, P. C., & Tesch, D. (2007). Project manager vs. executive perceptions of sponsor behaviors. *Management Research News, 30*(11), 803–815. doi:10.1108/01409170710832241

Knutson, J. (1999). *The first step can be the most important.* PMI Journal.

Knutson, J. (1999). That first step can be the most important. *PM Network,* 19-20.

Kolltveit, B., Karlsen, J. T., & Gronhaug, K. (2004). Exploiting opportunities in uncertainty during the early project phase. *Journal of Management Engineering, 20*(4), 134–139. doi:10.1061/(ASCE)0742-597X(2004)20:4(134)

Kreha, B. (1998). Marketing your project's successes: Spread the good news too! In *Proceedings of the 19th Annual Project Management Institute 1998 Seminars & Symposium*, Long Beach, CA.

Labushagne, L., & Marnewick, C. (2006). *A structured approach to derive projects from the organisational vision.* Paper presented at the 2006 PMI Research Conference.

Lee, A. S., & Baskerville, R. L. (2003). Generalizing generalizability in information systems research. *Information Systems Research, 14*(3), 221–243. doi:10.1287/isre.14.3.221.16560

Lehtonen, P., & Martinsuo, M. (2008). Change program initiation: Defining and managing the program–organization boundary. *International Journal of Project Management, 26*(1), 21–29. doi:10.1016/j.ijproman.2007.07.003

Lehtonen, P., & Martinsuo, M. (2008). Change program intiation: Defining and managing the program - organization boundary. *International Journal of Project Management, 26*(1), 21–29. doi:10.1016/j.ijproman.2007.07.003

LeRouge, C., Tulu, B., & Forducey, P. (2010). The business of telemedicine: A strategy primer. *Telemedicine Journal and e-Health, 16*(8), 898–909. doi:10.1089/tmj.2009.0178 PMID:20925561

Leybourne, S., & Sadler-Smith, E. (2006). The role of intuition and improvisation in project management. *International Journal of Project Management, 24*(6), 483–492. doi:10.1016/j.ijproman.2006.03.007

Lierni, P. C., & Ribiere, V. M. (2008). The relationship between improving the management of projects and the use of KM. *VINE: The Journal of Information and Knowledge Management Systems, 38*(1), 133-146.

Magretta, J. (2002). Why business models matter. *Harvard Business Review, 80*(5), 86–86. PMID:12024761

Martinsuo, M., & Lehtonen, P. (2007). Program and its initiation in practice: Development program initiation in a public consortium. *International Journal of Project Management, 25*(4), 337–345. doi:10.1016/j.ijproman.2007.01.011

Merla, E. (2009). Art of the project start. In *Proceedings of the PMI Global Congress*, Amsterdam, Netherlands.

Merla, E. (2009). Art of the project start. *PMI Congress.*

Milochik, J. A. (1996). *Setting priorities for new business projects in pharmaceuticals and healthcare.* Paper presented at the Project Management Institute 27th Annual Seminar/Symposium, Boston, MA.

Morris, P. W. G. (2005). *Managing the front-end: How project managers shape business strategy and manage project definition.* Paper presented at the 2005 PMI Global Congress Proceedings, Edinburgh, Scotland.

Nelson, R. R., & Jansen, K. J. (2009). Mapping and managing momentum in IT projects. *MIS Quarterly Executive*, *8*(3), 141–148.

O'Connor, E. A. (2001). Preparing an effective business plan for your project. In *Proceedings of the Project Management Institute Annual Seminars and Symposium*, Nashville, TN.

Olsson, N. O. E., & Samset, K. (2006). *Front-end management, flexibility, and project success.* Paper presented at the PMI Research Conference.

DS Performance Group. (2010). *Organizational infrastructure. Define, analyze & change.* Retrieved August 2, 2013, 2013, from http://www.ds-performancegroup.com/?submit=Infrastructure

Paul, S., Ramaprasad, A., & Wickramasinghe, N. (2012). *Introduction to technology mediated collaborations in healthcare minitrack.* Paper presented at the 45th Hawaii International Conference on System Sciences, Maui, HI. doi:10.1109/HICSS.2012.367

Preston, D., & Karahanna, E. (2009). How to develop a shared vision: The key to IS strategic alignment. *MIS QUARTERLY EXECUTIVE*, *8*(1), 1–8.

PRINCE2/ US. (2013). Retrieved August 1, 2013, from http://www.prince2.com/us/prince2-process-model.asp#prince2-starting-up-a-project

Project Management Institute. (2013). Retrieved August 1, 2013, from http://www.pmi.org/

Pruitt, S. (2013). The office for the advancement of telehealth. *Telemedicine Journal and e-Health*, *19*(5), 346–348. doi:10.1089/tmj.2012.0283 PMID:23343256

Riis, J. O. (1984). *Initiating industrial projects.* Paper presented at the Internet-MES Symposium, Cairo, Egypt.

Rojas-Meluk. (2008). *Project initiation and measurement: Laying the foundation for better projects.* Paper presented at the 2006 PMI Global Congress Proceedings, Santiago, Chile.

Silva, G. S., Farrell, S., Shandra, E., Viswanathan, A., & Schwamm, L. H. (2012). The status of telestroke in the United States a survey of currently active stroke telemedicine programs. *Stroke*, *43*(8), 2078–2085. doi:10.1161/STROKEAHA.111.645861 PMID:22700532

Smith, C. (2005). *Project initiation request (PIR) process and the project management board (PMB).* Paper presented at the 2005 PMI Global Conference Proceedings.

Stah-Le Cardinal, J., & Marle, F. (2006). Project: The just necessary structure to reach your goals. *International Journal of Project Management*, *24*(3), 226–233. doi:10.1016/j.ijproman.2005.10.002

Strauss, A. L., & Corbin, J. M. (1990). *Basics of qualitative research: Grounded theory procedures and techniques.* Newbury Park, CA: Sage Publications.

Towfighi, A., Ovbiagele, B., & Saver, J. L. (2010). Therapeutic milestone stroke declines from the second to the third leading organ-and disease-specific cause of death in the United States. *Stroke*, *41*(3), 499–503. doi:10.1161/STROKEAHA.109.571828 PMID:20075347

Towfighi, A., & Saver, J. L. (2011). Stroke declines from third to fourth leading cause of death in the United States historical perspective and challenges ahead. *Stroke*, *42*(8), 2351–2355. doi:10.1161/STROKEAHA.111.621904 PMID:21778445 van Buuren, A., Buijs, J.-M., & Teisman, G. (2010). Program management and the creative art of cooperation: Dealing with potential tensions and synergies between spatial development projects. *International Journal of Project Management, 28*(7), 672–682. doi:10.1016/j.ijproman.2009.12.002

Verzuh, E. (2005). *Stakeholder management strategies applying risk management to people.* Paper presented at the 2005 PMI Global Congress Proceedings Toronto, Canada.

Yin, R. K. (1994). *Case study research: Design and methods* (Vol. 5). Thousand Oaks, CA: Sage Publications.

Chapter 2
Computerisation of Clinical Pathways:
Based on a Semiotically Inspired Methodology

Jasmine Tehrani
University of Reading, UK

ABSTRACT

Patient safety incidents are becoming more common in medical situations. The challenge of achieving significant improvements in patient safety is one of the key tasks facing healthcare at the start of the 21st century. Clinical pathways and clinical guidelines provide a measure of standardisation to help reduce medical error, but are often manually created and also prone to human error. This chapter explores the error issues regarding clinical pathways. It presents a method for generating clinical pathways from a semiotic perspective that can addresses social and informal/safety factors which conspire to influence the outcome of patient interaction and safety.

1. INTRODUCTION

Large numbers of people continue to be successfully cared for and treated in the National Health Service, but a significant number of errors and other forms of harm occur. It is calculated that around 10% of patients admitted to NHS hospitals are subject to a patient safety incident and that up to half of these incidents could have been prevented (Chang, Schyve et al. 2005). Increasing costs of health care, fuelled by demand for high quality, cost-efficient health care has propelled hospitals to restructure their patient care delivery systems. One such systematic approach is the adaptation of an engineering project management methodology, the critical path method (CPM), as a tool to organise, standardise and improve the quality of healthcare delivery and hence patient outcomes (Yang, Liu et al. 2010). Clinical Guidelines (CG) are developed as a standard way to manage medical activities since the 1980's and are structured multi-disciplinary care plans or medical processes in which diagnostic and therapeutic interventions performed for a particular diagnosis are described.

DOI: 10.4018/978-1-4666-8756-1.ch002

However, the application and adaptation of CGs in local hospital setting, inevitably has some limitations of process management in practice. Despite the benefits, there are many instances which show that CGs fail to offer a clear description of activities, conditions, sequence and authorities of action of a care process. Therefore current application of CGs cannot very well handle situation where decisions are made solely on human judgement and do not specify a facility for specifying how decision making (exceptions) can be handled. This issue is mostly related to healthcare settings where processes are complex, less structured and are made up of social agents such as physicians, departments with goals that they actively pursue in constant interaction with a network of other social agents (Mould, Bowers et al. 2010). Healthcare settings are dynamic networks of interrelated activities. As a result, current adaptation of CGs becomes a source of patient safety incident (Carthey 2010). Viewing errors as the result of poorly designed systems more so than incompetent or misguided individuals introduces variables that operationalize dynamics seen process management levels. Workflow management has been cited as potentially important in addressing medical errors and patient safety in many publications like the "To Err Is Human" and "Crossing the Quality Chasm" (Corrigan 2005). For example, "To Err Is Human" places at the core of a successful systems-based approach to reducing error the need for a strong patient-safety culture, simplified process design, development of clear work flow of activities and use of patient-centric modelling approaches in adaptation of CGs to local settings (Carthey 2010).

The proposed modelling approach to generation of Clinical Pathways (CP), adopts organisational semiotics to capture and represent the CG knowledge by determining the underlying semantics and the relationship between agents and their patterns of behaviour. We use Norm Analysis Method (NAM), one of semiotics methods (Stamper, Liu et al. 2000) to extract and analyse patterns of care activities and informal safety norms that affect patient safety outcomes. NAM identifies responsibilities and rules that govern human behaviour in an explicit and articulate manner. It recognizes conditions and constraints of the actions driven by their responsibilities. The extended method aims to enable the generation of CP from a semiotic perspective by capturing all necessary knowledge from syntactic level to social level and guiding the modelling of clinical pathways using Business Process Modelling Notation (BPMN) best practice (Aguilar-Saven 2004). The extended method adopts a socio-technical approach to map informal safety norms in to CP. This will result in a rigorous control over the process of care ensuring completeness, consistency and comprehensiveness of clinical pathway knowledge representation.

2. PATIENT SAFETY

The challenge of achieving significant improvements in patient safety is one of the key tasks facing healthcare at the start of the 21st century. There is broad international agreement on the nature of the task faced and the importance of achieving improvements to quality in this area.

Large numbers of people continue to be successfully cared for and treated in the National Health Service, but a significant number of errors and other forms of harm occur. It is calculated that around 10% of patients admitted to NHS hospitals are subject to a patient safety incident and that up to half of these incidents could have been prevented (Vincent et al., 2001; NPSA, 2004). The Department of Health Expert Group in June 2000 estimated that over 850,000 incidents harm National Health Service hospital patients in the United Kingdom each year. On average forty incidents a year contribute to patient deaths in each NHS institution (Osborn and Williams 2004). It was estimated by the Bristol Royal Infirmary Inquiry (2001) that around 25,000 preventable deaths occur in the NHS each year due to patient safety incidents. These incidents also generate a significant financial burden that includes avoidably prolonged care, additional treatment and litigation costs.

Medical errors are also a serious and challenging issue in the United States. According to the Institute of Medicine's (IOM's) recent report, *To Err Is Human: Building a Safer Health System* (1999), between 44,000 and 98,000 people die in hospitals each year as the result of medical errors. Safety incident is defined by the National Patient Safety Agency (NPSA, 2004, p. 1) as: *Any unintended or unexpected incident which could have or did lead to harm for one or more patients receiving NHS funded care.*

These types of incidents are also referred to in the literature as adverse events/incidents, medical error, clinical error, and include the concept of near miss. The latter is a situation in which an error or some other form of patient safety incident is averted, such as noticing and therefore avoiding giving the wrong drug to a patient. Near miss events (this term can be used in a different sense in midwifery, have not commonly been reported in healthcare practice, largely because the staff involved fear they may be blamed or criticised, but are an integral aspect of safety improvement in other safety critical industries.

Interventions identified to decrease medical errors and enhance patient safety within the health care delivery setting focus less on ——active‖ errors that occur (i.e., the specific mistake that immediately precedes the adverse event) and more on the ——latent‖ errors that derive from failures or flaws existing at various points in an overall system of care (IOM 1999). Viewing errors as the result of poorly designed systems more so than incompetent or misguided individuals introduces variables that operationalize dynamics seen at three levels of analysis within the organization: individual, group or team and structural level factors (Ferlie and Shortell, 2001).

- **Individual-level factors**: Such factors within the organization that may affect medical errors and patient safety include leadership (e.g., physician champions), the level of education or training provided to workers, and individual responses to performance feedback or quality information.
- **Group-level factors**: Include team-related dynamics (e.g., team integration, team effectiveness, team membership, team communication), as well as a focus on culture.
- **Structural-level factors:** Pertinent structural variables include the levels of standardization, coordination, and formalization characterizing a health care process, as well as the use of decision making and key inputs such as technology in that process.

In publications like the *To Err Is Human (IOM 1999)* all three levels have been cited as potentially important in addressing medical errors and patient safety. For example, *To Err Is Human* places at the core of a successful systems-based approach to reducing error the need for a strong patient-safety culture, appropriate physician leadership and opinion leaders in attending to medical errors, the need for simplification and standardization of work flows such as medication administration, and the use of interdisciplinary team approaches in complex care delivery situations.

In other publications such as The *Crossing the Quality Chasm* report organizational factors such as the use of information technologies, development of effective team-based approaches to care, greater coordination of care, and use of standard operating procedures in the areas of evidenced-based clinical practice and performance accountability to promote enhanced patient safety and ——error-proof‖ systems of care delivery has been addressed (Corrigan 2005).

2.1 Organisational and Human Factors Affecting Patient Safety Outcome

Human factors encompass all those factors that can influence people and their behaviour. In a work context, human factors are the environmental, organisational and job factors, and individual characteristics which influence behaviour at work.

Every day in the NHS, tens of thousands of patients are treated safely by dedicated healthcare professionals who are motivated to provide high quality and safe clinical care. For the vast majority of patients, the treatment they receive alleviates or improves their symptoms and is a positive experience. However, an unacceptable number of patients are harmed as a result of their treatment or as a consequence of their admission to hospital. It is inevitable that errors will occur in healthcare, as they do in other safety critical industries, because they are an intrinsic human trait – to err is human (Kohn et al., 2000). An acceptance of this stance, for example in aviation, has led to the achievement of significant improvements in safety (Leape, 1999; Wiegmann and Shappell, 2003). The focus within adverse event analysis, situations in which error and other forms of harm occur, in safety critical industries has moved from a propensity for individual blame to a systems approach. If it is accepted that people are liable to make errors, system and equipment design, training and other aspects of the work environment are given priority in terms of initiating change to minimise the risk.

The systems approach cited as pivotal to solving the errors problem by publications like *To Err Is Human* and *Crossing the Quality Chasm* demands that health services researchers consider greater application of systems-focused theory to questions of how organizational factors shape patient safety. A systems approach views outcomes like safety as the result of interconnected processes and parts that combine to fulfil some common purpose (Altman, Clancy et al. 2004).

Moreover, health care systems, as they manifest in the everyday workplace of hospitals and physician offices, are felt to represent ——complex adaptive‖ rather than ——mechanical‖ systems. An adaptive system is one in which the ——parts, which include human beings, have potential to respond differently and unpredictably at a given point in time. These system parts can also move each other to act in specific ways.

3. CLINICAL PATHWAYS

Clinical pathways (CP), also known as care pathways, critical pathways, integrated care pathways, or care maps, are one of the main tools used to manage the quality in healthcare concerning the standardization of care processes. It has been proven that their implementation reduces the variability in clinical practice and improves outcomes. Clinical pathways promote organized and efficient patient care based on the evidence based practice. Clinical pathways optimize outcomes in the acute care and homecare settings. Below you can see an example of clinical pathway used in hospitals.

Generally clinical pathways refer to medical guidelines. However a single pathway may refer to guidelines on several topics in a well specified context. CP is a multidisciplinary management tool based on evidence-based practice for a specific group of patients with a predictable clinical course, in which the different tasks (interventions) by the professionals involved in the patient care are defined, optimized and sequenced either by hour (ED), day (acute care) or visit (homecare). Outcomes are tied to specific interventions.

CP Usually contains three main components: Events may be divided up into categories such as Nursing, specimens/tests, teaching etc. etc. Time may be just a sequence of events (e.g. as in a day case procedure) or an actual time period such as minutes (e.g. A&E) or days (e.g. ward based care) (Panella, Marchisio et al. 2003).

The comments are usually to report deviations from the path ('exception reporting'). These are usually provided with codes to facilitate analysis and computer data entry. Once again the codes may be divided up into categories such as Patient/family, Clinician, Hospital, Community (e.g. bed/transport availability). A separate variance sheet may be kept documenting where in the path each variance occurred, Problem code, Action(s) and signature (Audimoolam, Nair et al. 2005).

3.1 Initial Development of Process Management Tools in Other Industries

Critical pathway techniques were first developed for use in industry as a tool to identify and manage the rate-limiting steps in production processes (Buffa 1969, Wagner 1975). In industry, any variation in production process is suboptimal. Thus, by defining the processes and timing of these processes, managers could target areas that were critical, measure variation, and try to make improvements. Once steps were taken to improve the process, there would be a re measurement. In time, variation would decrease, the time it took to complete the pathway costs would decrease, and quality of production would improve (O'hare 2000).

3.2 Characteristics

Clinical pathways (integrated care pathways) can be seen as an application of process management thinking to the improvement of patient healthcare. An aim is to re-centre the focus on the patient's overall journey, rather than the contribution of each specialty or caring function independently. Instead, all are emphasised to be working together, in the same way as a cross-functional team. More than just a guideline or a protocol, a care pathway is typically crystallised in the development and use of a single all-encompassing bedside docu-

ment, that will stand as an indicator of the care a patient is likely to be provided in the course of the pathway going forward; and ultimately as a single unified legal record of the care the patient has received, and the progress of their condition, as the pathway has been undertaken (Gattnar, Ekinci et al. 2011).

The pathway design tries to capture the foreseeable actions which will most commonly represent best practice for most patients most of the time, and include prompts for them at the appropriate time in the pathway document to ascertain whether they have been carried out, and whether results have been as expected (Panella, Marchisio et al. 2003). In this way results are recorded, and important questions and actions are not overlooked. However, pathways are typically not prescriptive; the patient's journey is an individual one, and an important part of the purpose of the pathway documents is to capture information on "variances", where due to circumstances or clinical judgment different actions have been taken, or different results unfolded (Sonnenberg and Hagerty 2006). The combined variances for a sufficiently large population of patients are then analysed to identify important or systematic features, which can be used to improve the next iteration of the pathway (Staccini, Joubert et al. 2001).

3.3 Scope of a Care Pathway

The care pathway may only be developed for an individual specialty or be Multidisciplinary (Integrated Care Pathway ICP). It may encompass only part of the total treatment plan such as an assessment in psychiatry or, as in the case of an elective Hip replacement, may commence at the pre-hospital outpatient visit and end with the community nurse removing the stitches. The time span they cover can vary considerably, within the ITU/ICU situation care pathways can be developed on a individual basis for the following 24 period or even shorter time spans.

3.4 Clinical Pathways Affecting Patient Safety Outcomes

Limitations to a clinical pathway approach most importantly include the fact that many patients cannot be squeezed into a uniform pathway because of their unique problems and needs. All patients must be treated as individuals, and we emphasize that the pathway is a general guideline and not a rigid protocol. Pathways are not particularly applicable to small groups of patients that are cared for infrequently. Pathways are probably only a temporary solution to the problem of maintaining high quality care while reducing costs (Camreon D, et al 2001).

Clinical Pathways can be viewed as algorithms in as much as they offer a flow chart format of the decisions to be made and the care to be provided for a given patient or patient group for a given condition in a step-wise sequence (Basse, Jakobsen et al. 2000). Nevertheless, as a new way of clinical process management, most of existing clinical pathways is paper-based which are static, stand-alone, disease-specific, non-personalized, isolated from clinical applications and designed for the ideal patient (Kohn, Corrigan et al. 2000).

Consequently, the application of CPs inevitably has limitations in process management in practice. They are designed by evidence are standard based methods and most of them are static and non-personalized. CPs are applied rigidly in specific care conditions without taking into consideration the dynamic collaboration of their participants and the unpredictable situations. As a result, they do not respond well to unexpected changes in a patient's condition and suit standard conditions better than unusual or unpredictable ones. Therefore current CP management cannot very well adapt to less structured and more complex clinical processes in dynamic hospital setting, where the clinical process, unlike the static and rigidly executed CP, are made up of social agents such as physicians, departments with goals that they actively pursue in constant interaction with a network of other social agents (Kohn, Corrigan et al. 2000). Nevertheless, the architecture of clinical pathways can hardly cover the social, organisational and human actor factors, which are crucial in successful execution of clinical pathways.

As you can see form the above example taken from the annual the report by the Clinical Pathway Group, Northwest NHS, there is very limited information provided by the clinical pathway.

Some of the limitation are:

- It does not specify the authorities of actions (agents) and lack details of care process.
- Due to the static and rigid structure, it cannot adapt well to unexpected circumstances.
- The architecture of clinical pathways does not address the social, organisational and human actor factors, which are crucial in successful execution of clinical pathways.
- The standards and national guideline for care has been applied too broadly, reducing adaptability to complex situations or changing care processes in unforeseen ways (Wein, 2011).
- Each care process requires additional information, however, none of this has been presented on the clinical pathway and instead practitioners have to refer to other guides to get a broad understanding of the care involved (Wein, 2011).
- The application of clinical pathways are not standardised within the NHS, this is partly because of the less well-defined and un-optimised structure of care pathways.
- Clinical pathways do not address social agents involved in care process, never the less; give information about formal, Informal and behavioural norms (rules) that exist within the care setting.

Clinical pathways are high-level models with high granularity, which do not specify the authorities of actions and lack details of care process. Care pathways can target patient safety outcomes, but can also produce new hazards, through applying standards too broadly, reducing adaptability to complex situations or changing care processes in unforeseen ways. Further research should explore how best to standardise care processes, while evaluating how best to prevent and monitor hazards, allow for innovation and adaptability to customize care when appropriate, and continue to develop new methods for taking into consideration the social agents and their behavioural norms involved in a care process.

Therefore, there is a need to address patient safety hazards introduced by clinical pathways. To do this we will be looking into optimisation and enrichment of clinical pathways by transforming them into process models which can address social and human factors affecting patient safety.

4. HUMAN FACTORS

Human factors has been defined in many ways. One simple definition is design for human use (Chapanis 1996). Chapanis defines human factors as a body of information about human abilities, limitations and characteristics that are relevant to design process. Human factors encompass all factors that can influence people and their behaviour. In a work context, human factors are the environmental, organisational and job factors, and individual characteristics which influence behaviour at work.

Human rather than technical failures now represent the greatest threat to complex and potentially hazardous systems. This includes healthcare systems. Managing the human risks will never be 100% effective. Human fallibility can be moderated, but it cannot be eliminated. It is inevitable that errors will occur in healthcare, as they do in other safety critical industries, because they are an intrinsic human trait – to err is human (Kohn et al., 2000). An acceptance of this stance, for example in aviation, has led to the achievement of significant improvements in safety (Carthey 2010). The focus

within adverse event analysis, situations in which error and other forms of harm occur, in safety critical industries has moved from a propensity for individual blame to a systems approach. If it is accepted that people are liable to make errors, system and equipment design, training and other aspects of the work environment are given priority in terms of initiating change to minimise the risk. Furthermore, achieving improvement in patient safety is not possible unless human factors are placed at the heart of improving clinical, managerial and organisational practice leading to improvements in patient safety (Chapanis 1996; Carthey 2010).

Based on literature review, there are few attempts to propose a categorisation of human factors in adverse event. Preliminary work on human factors was undertaken by James Reason (1995) where he analysed conditions under which human factors can contribute safety failures followed by the proposal of a generic model of accident causation (Reason 1995). Chang et al (2005) conducted a series of similar studies and presented an evaluation of existing patient safety terminologies and classifications and grouped the findings into five complementary root nodes: impact, type, domain, cause and prevention.

4.1 Human Factors in Healthcare

Human rather than technical failures now represent the greatest threat to complex and potentially hazardous systems. This includes healthcare systems. Managing the human risks will never be 100% effective. Human fallibility can be moderated, but it cannot be eliminated. It is inevitable that errors will occur in healthcare, as they do in other safety critical industries, because they are an intrinsic human trait – to err is human an acceptance of this stance, for example in aviation, has led to the achievement of significant improvements in safety (Carthey 2010). The focus within adverse event analysis, situations in which error and other forms of harm occur, in safety critical industries has moved from a propensity for individual blame to a systems approach. If it is accepted that people are liable to make errors, system and equipment design, training and other aspects of the work environment are given priority in terms of initiating change to minimise the risk.

The systems approach cited as pivotal to solving the errors problem by publications like *To Err Is Human* and *Crossing the Quality Chasm* demands that health services researchers consider greater application of systems-focused theory to questions of how organizational factors shape patient safety. A systems approach views outcomes like safety as the result of interconnected processes and parts that combine to fulfil some common purpose (Forster 2003). Furthermore, achieving improvement in patient safety is not possible unless human factors are placed at the heart of improving clinical, managerial and organisational practice leading to improvements in patient safety (O'hare 2000).

5. CURRENT LIMITATION IN IMPLEMENTATION OF CLINICAL PATHWAYS

Clinical pathways (CP), also known as care pathways, critical pathways, integrated care pathways, or care maps, are one of the main tools used to manage the quality in healthcare concerning the standardization of care processes. It is proven that their implementation reduces the variability in clinical practice and improves outcomes. Clinical pathways promote organized and efficient patient care based on the evidence based practice. Clinical pathways optimize outcomes in the acute care and homecare settings. Below you can see an example of clinical pathway used in hospitals. Generally clinical pathways refer to medical guidelines. However a single pathway may refer to guidelines on several topics in a well specified context. CP is a multidisciplinary management tool based on evidence-based practice for a specific group of

patients with a predictable clinical course, in which the different tasks (interventions) by the professionals involved in the patient care are defined, optimized and sequenced either by hour (ED), day (acute care) or visit (homecare). Outcomes are tied to specific interventions. Clinical pathways (integrated care pathways) can be seen as an application of process management thinking to the improvement of patient healthcare. An aim is to re-centre the focus on the patient's overall journey, rather than the contribution of each specialty or caring function independently. Instead, all are emphasised to be working together, in the same way as a cross-functional team. A care pathway is typically crystallised in the development and use of a single all-encompassing bedside document, that will stand as an indicator of the care a patient is likely to be provided in the course of the pathway going forward; and ultimately as a single unified legal record of the care the patient has received, and the progress of their condition, as the pathway has been undertaken (Tehrani, Liu et al.).

Despite the substantial improvements in modelling and generation of CPs, there is very little account for human factors. Abidi and Chen (Abidi and Chen 2006) present a semantic web framework and rendered the technical basis for a services-oriented architecture to generate and orchestrate patient-specific healthcare plans. A number of methods have been proposed to support the development in computerized medical guidelines and CPs. More recently, various methods are proposed to represent the clinical guidelines which were originally paper based as Computer Interpretable Guidelines, most of which can be visualised in flowcharts (Sonnenberg and Hagerty 2006). Plege et al.(Mor Plege 2012) reviewed a number of CIG modelling methodologies and established a consensus on the common structure. Other authors (Hurley and Abidi 2007) represented clinical pathway knowledge as a clinical pathway ontology which offers a detailed ontological model describing the structure and function of clinical pathways.

The above methods describe clinical pathway from structure aspect comprising concepts, relationships between concepts, and properties that describe the concept. However, these methods lacks of the mechanism to address human factors that affect patient safety outcomes. This paper builds on previous work on clinical pathway modelling by presenting a normative approach to the analysis and integration of human factors in to clinical pathways in order to accommodate exceptions which have not been dealt with by other conventional methods (Tehrani J 2012). The proposed methodology provides a robust mechanism to analyse human factor failure points and to identify and model the controls in to formal process models e.g. CPs. Norm Analysis Method (NAM) is adopted to analyse patterns of behaviour and decision making models of clinicians and the condition under which the behaviour will occur. This mechanism is crucial for conceptualizing and developing personalized clinical pathways which describes the conditions and temporality of human factor failure modes.

5.1 Paper-Based Pathway Specification

Currently, CPs are implemented as paper-based pathway specifications in UK hospitals. Limitations to implementation and application of pathway specifications include the problems of a one-size fits all approach where many patients have unique needs. Pathways are not particularly applicable to small groups of patients that are cared for infrequently (Michell, Tehrani et al. 2012). Furthermore, research shows that pathways are applied rigidly in specific care conditions without taking into consideration the dynamic collaboration of their participants and the unpredictable situations and do not support events and unexpected changes in a patient's condition. These clashes with the culture of less structured and more complex clinical processes in dynamic hospital setting, where the clinical processes, are made up of social agents

such as physicians, departments with goals that they actively pursue in constant interaction with a network of other social agents (Carthey 2010). Within NHS hospitals, most clinical pathways are paper-based, designed for the ideal patient, and include both planning information as well as mechanisms to record variations in actual clinical interventions. A pathway specification is probably the nearest clinical document to a process map for a specific clinical intervention. Below we will address in more detail the limitation of current application of CPs.

Despite the widespread introduction of information technology into primary health care within the United Kingdom, medical practitioners continue to use the more traditional paper medical record often alongside the computerised system. The resilience of the paper document is not simply a consequence of an impoverished design, but rather a product of the socially organised practices and reasoning which surround the use of the record within day to day consultative work. The practices that underpin the use of the medical records may have a range of important implications, not only for the general design of systems to support collaborative work, but also for our conceptions of 'writers', 'readers', 'objects' and 'records' utilised in those designs (Heath and Luff 1996).

The result of our study in one of the largest UK health trusts, shows that clinical pathways are implemented as paper-based pathway specifications which act as guidelines by providing advisory knowledge about actions and reference information before the event. They are also a means of ensuring the right work was done via control norms and capturing precepts and evaluations of clinical conditions in terms of tables and forms to be completed by the nurse. Clinical notes of what work was done both in terms of the action taken and the patient status provided new knowledge and beliefs/facts for later clinical decision making and actions. A CP can be considered as the nearest clinical document to a process map for a specific clinical intervention (Tehrani, Liu et al.).

As a result, the current implementation and application of clinical pathways in NHS can target patient safety outcomes and subsequently produce new hazards, through applying standards too broadly, reducing adaptability to complex situations or changing care processes in unforeseen ways. Despite the benefits, there are many instances which show that clinical pathways fail to offer a clear description of activities, conditions, sequence and authorities of action of a care process (Tehrani, Liu et al. 2012). The conditions and consequences expressed in CGs are always bound and there is no capability to handle human discretion.

Subsequently, the paper-based implementation of CPs as pathway specifications cannot handle situations where decisions are made solely on human judgment. Hence, one cannot model dynamics of care activity and alternative procedures in which decision are made solely based on human judgment (Liu, Sun et al. 2003). This issue is mostly related to healthcare settings where processes are complex, less structured and are made up of social agents such as physicians, departments with goals that they actively pursue in constant interaction with a network of other social agents (Mould, Bowers et al. 2010). In this dynamic network of interrelated activities, the current adaptation of CGs becomes a source of patient safety incident (Carthey 2010).

5.2 Lack of Human Factors in CP

Based on literature review, there are few attempts to propose a categorisation of human factors in adverse event. Preliminary work on human factors was undertaken by James Reason (1995) where he analysed conditions under which human factors can contribute safety failures followed by the proposal of a generic model of accident causation (Reason 1995). Chang et al (2005), conducted a series of similar studies and presented an evaluation of existing patient safety terminologies and classifications and grouped the findings into five complementary root nodes: impact, type, domain, cause and prevention. In this paper, cause and type root nodes are further analysed for the purpose of better understanding of human factors and towards a generic taxonomy and classification schema of human factors influencing near misses and adverse events. Our classification of human factors is largely based upon literature review and critical analysis of current studies on human factors. The main goal of introducing human factor controls in to clinical pathways is not so much to minimise that particular error but to enhance human performance at different levels of system (Michell, Tehrani et al. 2012).

6. THE NECESSITY OF QUALITY HEALTHCARE INFORMATION SYSTEM TO SUPPORT IMPLEMENTATION OF CPS

The primary role of a clinical information system is to allow the care professionals to manage, record and trace the patients pathway by recording details of care activities. It requires the identification and specification of all the activities, the agent responsible for each activity and sequence of the elements of process. The need for subsequent improvements in healthcare delivery process stresses the need for continuous traceability of all care activities, the reduction of variation in practice (standardization) and the detection, measurement, management and prevention of adverse event occurring during healthcare process. To achieve this, hospitals have to combine resources, define techniques and methodologies and build tools along with information systems to support real-time risk and vigilance management systems closely relate to clinical data. A quality healthcare information system requires not only the measurement of outcomes of process of care such as clinical outcome and patient satisfaction, but also the description and assessment of each process (operational efficiency).

The primary objective of a clinical pathway is to help healthcare professionals including users, doctors and physicians to manage, document and trace the care provided for the patients. It requires identification of the sequence of care activities provided along with linkage with live clinical data reflecting ever changing patient status. Thus the demand for patient-centred and integrated clinical data have shifted towards process-oriented system design. Our proposed methodology consist of two core steps. The initial stage is a process-oriented analysis of care activities which leads to the identification of information requirements. The first step is to extract and structure the description of activities in order to be familiarized with the sequence and details of care process. It includes identification of who does what at what time, how and why is it done. The second step is the representation of the CG knowledge by determining the underlying semantics and the relationship between agents and their patterns of behaviour. We then use Norm Analysis Method (NAM), from organizational semiotics (Stamper, Liu et al. 2000) to extract and analyse patterns of care activities and informal safety norms that affect patient safety outcomes. NAM identifies responsibilities and rules that govern human behaviour in an explicit and articulate manner. It recognizes conditions and constraints of the actions driven by their responsibilities (Filipe and Liu 2000). The proposed method aims to enable the generation of CP from a semiotic perspective by capturing all necessary knowledge from syntactic level to social level and guiding the modeling of clinical pathways using Business Process Modeling Notation (BPMN) best practice and adopts a socio-technical approach to map informal safety norms in to clinical pathways.

7. COMPUTERISATION OF CLINICAL PATHWAYS: BASED ON A SEMIOTICALLY INSPIRED METHODOLOGY

Semantics-Oriented Method for Generation of Clinical Pathways (SOG-CP) is a method for generating clinical pathways. SOG-CP adopts organisat ional semiotics methods including Semantic Analysis Method (SAM) and Norm Analysis Method (NAM) to explicitly represent the semantics of the concepts and their relationships, patterns of behavior and norms governing the action taken. Human factors are believed to contribute to at least 40% of safety errors, therefore in order to improve patient safety it is necessary to capture and represent informal/ safety factors in CPs. SAM gives us a basis for analysing human/Informal factors in healthcare setting by providing the method for identifying and representing authorities of action and their pattern of behaviour. In following sections, we will discuss the main methods used in SOG-CP including SAM and NAM. This is followed by a detailed review of SOG-CP methodology. Since, processes in CPs are a lot less optimised, well-studied and poorly documented compared to their business counterparts; Business Process Modeling (BPM) and BPMN are adopted to model patient care delivery (Muthu, Whitman et al. 2006). For this purpose, CPs are transformed into normative business process models which can address social and human factors affecting patient safety and enables identification and modeling of temporal aspects of care delivery by integrating the results of SAM and NAM into process models. As it can be seen in Figure 1, the proposed method comprises three main phases.

Figure 1. Clinical pathway for appendicitis

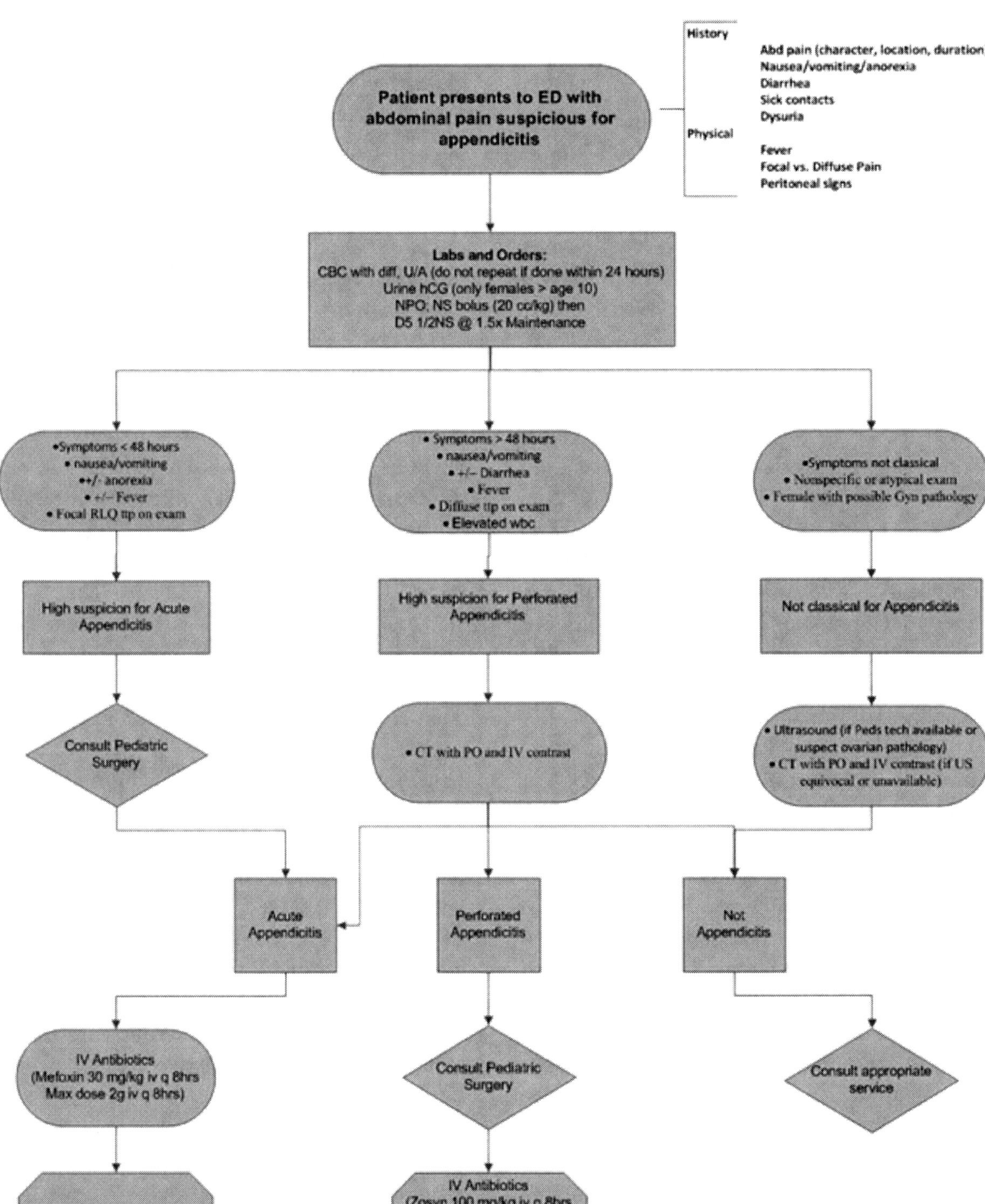

Figure 2. Instantiation of the 'ICOM box' to the final steps of the blood transfusion, representing attributes of a well-performed clinical activity

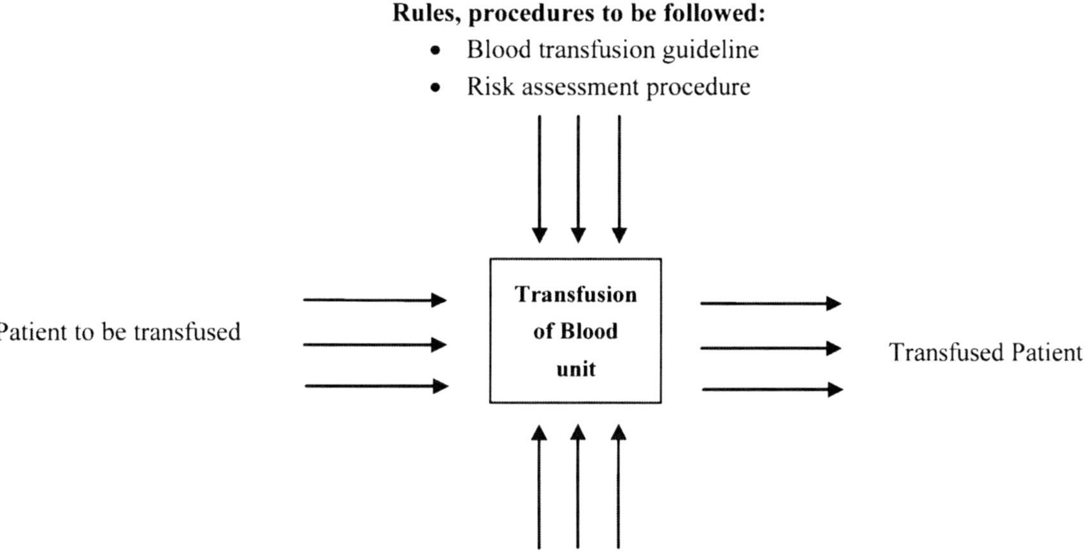

- **Knowledge engineering phase:** A knowledge management approach is taken to represent CP knowledge by ontologically modeling clinical guidelines in terms of possible patterns of behaviors, authorities of action, semantic units and their relationships
- **System's dynamics modelling phase:** Norm analysis is conducted to identify rules that govern the actions identified on the ontology chart. Norms, in addition to the knowledge already identified in sematic analysis and represented using ontology chart, specify the details of these possible behaviors. The final activity of this stage is transformation of CGs along with the knowledge captured during SAM and NAM to process models using BPMN standards.

- **Execution Phase:** Information collected during semantic analysis and norm analyses of clinical guideline are integrated to guide the generation of clinical pathways. The initial phase of this stage is to generate process models using BPMN to generate clinical pathway.

8. ORGANIZATIONAL SEMIOTICS

Organizational Semiotics (OS) is a discipline that has roots in Semiotics as applied to organizational processes. It studies the nature, characteristics, function and effect of information and communication within organizational contexts. An organization is a social system in which people behave in an organized manner conforming to a certain system of norms. These norms are regularities of perception, behavior, belief and value that are expressed as customs, habits, patterns of behavior and other cultural artifacts (Stamper *et al.*, 1988; Liu, 2000).

According to the OS perspective, an organization can be seen as an information system where agents employ signs to perform purposeful actions. Some of the organizational functions are of high regularity and have rules that can be clearly formalized.

Within the formalized part of the actions, a fraction of these may be very repetitive and can be automated by computer-based systems. In this sense, the software (technical system) is part of a whole information system and presupposes a formal system in which rules and formal procedures specify how the relations should be carried out and how the actions should be performed. Moreover, the formal system presupposes an informal system in which organizational culture, customs and values are reflected in the beliefs, habits and patterns of behavior of each individual member; at this level, meanings are agreed upon, intentions are understood and beliefs are formed. Therefore, OS provides a background that embodies knowledge and supports collaboration and reflection among people from the different disciplines involved in interaction design (Baranauskas and Bonacin, 2008).

Stamper proposed a set of methods to support the use of OS concepts for modelling information systems, named MEASUR - Methods for Eliciting, Analyzing and Specifying Users' Requirements (Stamper *et al.*, 1988). PLuRaL builds on three MEASUR methods: the Problem Articulation Method (PAM), the Semantic Analysis Method (SAM) and the Norm Analysis Method (NAM).

8.1 Problem Articulation Method (PAM)

PAM supports the identification of the main topics related to the context, e.g., stakeholders, action courses and bureaucracy, especially when the context is complex and still vague, allowing a more clear understanding of the problem (Kolkman, 1993). It aggregates several techniques as Unit System Definition, Collateral Analysis and Stakeholder Analysis.

Stakeholder Analysis proposes a model for identifying those who influence the (system) domain. Four main categories, presented in nested layers, represent the different information fields: actors and responsible parties (those who are directly involved with the problem), clients and suppliers (those who will effectively use the system or those who feed the system with information or services), partners and competitors (members of the market related to the system domain) and spectators and legislators (comprising not only those responsible for establishing the formal or informal rules but also the whole community that will receive the benefits or costs as a consequence of the implementation of the system). A chart can be used to support the stakeholders' identification.

8.2 Semantic Analysis Method (SAM)

SAM supports the analysis, specification and representation of an information system and is divided into four phases: problem definition, candidate-affordance generation, candidate grouping and ontology charting (Liu, 2000).

Affordance, a concept originally introduced to express the behaviour of an organism made available by some combined structure of the organism and its environment, was extended by Stamper (1993) to include patterns of behaviour related to social interactions. SAM also considers the concepts of agents and ontological dependencies. An agent is a special type of affordance, referring to those who are capable of assuming responsibilities. Ontological dependencies are links between affordances or agents, implying that the existence of an element drawn on the right depends on the existence of a corresponding element on the left in a ontology chart. Considering a statement that defines the (design) problem, the main affordances in the domain are elicited. After identifying the affordances and agents and grouping them, an ontology chart is drawn. In the chart, affordances are represented as rectangles, agents as ellipses and the lines establish the ontological dependencies.

8.3 Semantic Terminologies

Determiners are referred to attributes of an affordance like name of the person. Since some attribute like name may change, a separate table will be defined for them. That is, the start and finish time of the determiner is different from the related affordance.

Affordance is everything which stands for a real entity. According to Gibson 1986, affordance is a set of patterns of behaviour. In fact, it defines an object or a possible action which is available to agents in a society. These patterns of behaviour are meaningful only in the context of society. (Stamper 1985) ——The patterns of behaviour are defined within the context of the society and shared by members of that society‖. The main groups of affordances are agents, entities, determiners, relationships, and communication acts. As explained earlier, some affordances are agents. Agents take responsibilities. People and organizations are agents. Agents express patterns of behaviour. For instance, a person is born, communicates with others, takes responsibilities, gives responsibilities and dies. An entity or universal action type is something which is not belongs to other affordance types. In other words, it cannot take responsibility, such as a course or program of study. Moreover, it cannot be determiner, or relationship (Stamper 1994).

9. SEMANTIC ANALYSIS FOR BUSINESS DOMAIN MODELLING

The semantic analysis method (SAM) is a method for conceptualizing knowledge of a problem domain and to analyse the patterns of behaviours of various agents (i.e., physician or doctors) in an organization (Liu and Ong 1999). Semantic analysis consists of a negotiated understanding, between relevant process intervenient, of the meanings of domain specific signs, including agents, concepts, relationships, and other related aspects. The result of semantic analysis are provided in a graphical format, using what is called 'ontology chart'. The ontology chart models concepts and the responsible authorities of actions in the problem domain and captures domain knowledge supported by semantic units and ontological dependencies (Liu 2002). These concepts together with the ontological dependencies determine the semantics contextually (Li, Liu et al. 2008).

In this way, we can define the possible patterns of medical behaviour involved in CP such as operation and discharge and the people who perform these behaviours such as physicians or recovery nurses and the relationship between them as behaviours. Figure 3 is the result of SAM conducted for a major gynecology surgery guideline. An ontology chart introduces concepts as semantic units representing an agent, affordance or role label. An affordance is a possible pattern of behaviour available to a member of society, represented as rectangles. The affordance on the right is ontologically dependent on the one on left. This is called ontological dependency. For example, the antecedent *Recovery nurse* affords the *'evaluate rehabilitation status'* behaviour. A role label is associated with an agent that undertakes some specific responsibilities. A role is always defined with respect to the role carrier on its left and the concept determining the responsibility on its right (Liu 2000). An agent may have several roles. For example, when a person works in hospital, his role is staff; when a person is hospitalized in hospital, his role is patient. In addition, a concept may have properties prefixed by the hash sign (#) that capture descriptive information about the concept. For example, the concept of Ward has the properties of *#ward name* and *#ward number* in the following charts which are called determiners. Agents are represented as ellipses and represent those who can take responsibility for their actions. It could be an individual, a group of people e.g., *society*, *hospital* and *person*. A dependent concept, its immediate antecedent concepts and the ontological dependencies between them form a semantic context within which the behavioural patterns of the dependent concepts are defined. In addition, the ontology model can describe the generic-specific relationships. In Figure 2 for example, under the generic heading of staff, more specific items can be found: *AHP*, *Doctor* and *nurse*. Through SAM, possible patterns of behaviours in CP and their relationships are represented in an ontology chart which delineates the boundary of concern in the analysis and defines the meaning of terminology used in the clinical pathway model. Thus, misunderstanding caused by interdisciplinary communications is avoided. For a complete description of the syntax of ontology charts, reader may consult the article by Ronald Stamper (Stamper 1996) Furthermore semantic analysis places an emphasis on the ontological relationship which ensures a rigorous process of analysis and specification (Li, Liu et al. 2010). In doing so, a rigorous analytical principle of ontology constraint must be observed that a pattern of behaviour can be described only

Figure 3. Main stages of SOG-CP

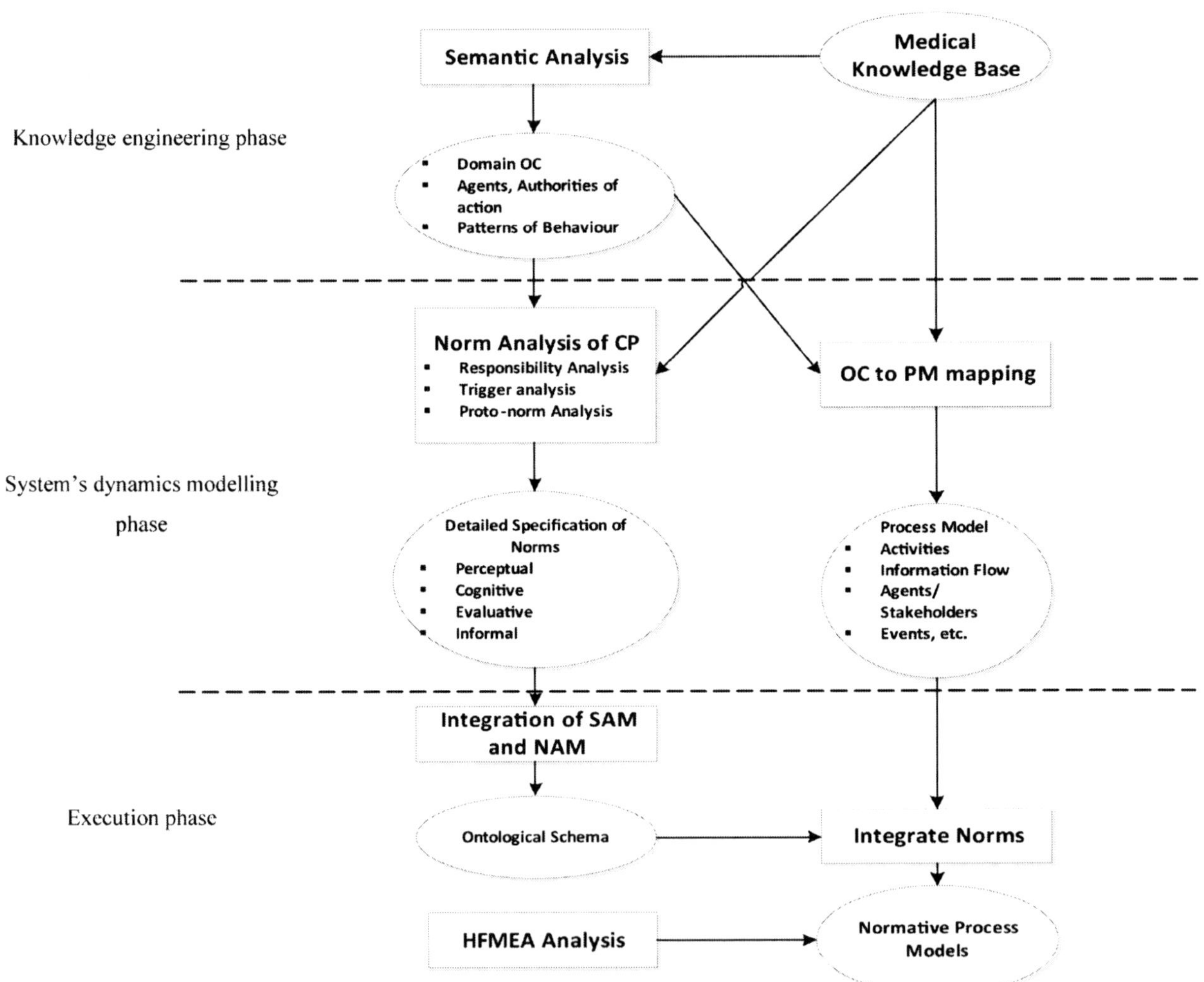

if the agent who acts is described in the model. This principle enables the correctness of clinical pathway generation.

From the above discussion, SAM can represent possible patterns of behaviors and their relationships (Figure 4). However, this is not enough to support generation of a CP because the mechanism to describe sequence and conditions determining when and how the medical behaviours will occur is not clarified, which will be discussed in next section.

9.1 Norm Analysis Method (NAM)

NAM is usually carried out on the basis of the results of SAM to specify the conditions and constraints on behaviors based on the norms concept. Norms are the rules that determine how social organisms interact and control affordances (Stamper 1993; Stamper *et al.*, 2000). They are related to how people behave, think, make judgments and perceive the world. Every norm can be written as IF <condition> THEN <consequence>. Behavioral norms, in particular, can be expressed in an extended format: WHENEVER <state> IF <condition> THEN <agent> IS <deontic operator: must, may, must not> TO <action>.

With this last structure, it is possible to complement the ontology chart to specify how agents deal with affordances. NAM consists of four steps for eliciting and formalizing norms: responsibility analysis, proto-norm analysis, trigger analysis and detailed norm specification (Liu, 2000). Each step assists the identification of parts of the norm. Specifically, responsibility analysis aims at assigning the agents in charge of each action. Trigger analysis focuses on the conditions that should happen and thus the action that will be performed and proto-norm analysis helps the analyst to identify relevant type of information

Figure 4. Semantic analysis for modelling of agents, patterns of behaviour and their relationships

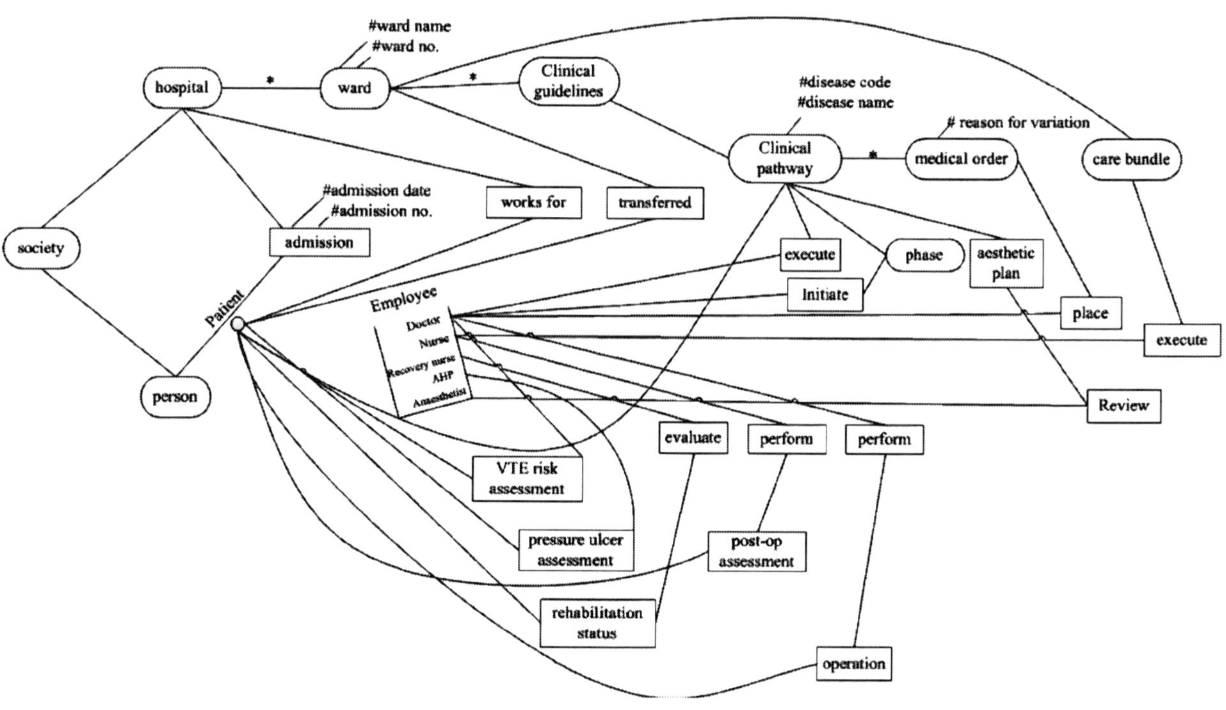

for making decisions concerning a certain type of behaviour. For example, a certain kind of information is needed to start or stop using a certain type of clinical pathway for a given patient (Liu, Al-rajhi et al.).

9.1.1 Taxonomy of Norms

In this section, we are attempting to present a summary of classifications of norms. Norms can be classified based on the following:

- Formality of norms
- Taxonomy of norms based on social psychology
- Taxonomy of substantive, communication and control norms

9.1.2 Norms Classified by Their Formality

One of the simplest norms relates directly to the automation of business procedures. To use a computer for anything more than a simple relay device for storing and forwarding signals, one must be able to instruct it in precise, mechanical detail what to do. Norms that are handled in this way or are so exactly specified as to be capable of automation fall into one class, Technical norms (Stamper et al, 2000). The second type of norms is the one that can be performed by people following explicit written norms or *rules* which they can be trained to implement in a rather mechanical way. But these are excluded from the first class because they do not exist in an explicit form that can be interpreted by a machine. These are the formal norms (Ades, 1998).

The third type comprises all other norms that are known by people who can live according to them without their being able to express them in writing. These taxa are the technical, formal and informal norms (Stamper et al, 2000). Informal norms may be classified according to the degree to which the norm subjects are aware of them. Broadly those which may be consciously held and capable of being discussed are separated from those that are tacit, and learned, used and passed on at an unconscious level of thought; suitable examples of these are the norms of fashion and the norms that govern a ballet performance (Liu et al, 2000). These three types of norms are related because *informal* norms are fundamental, *formal* norms can only operate by virtue of the informal norms needed to interpret them, while *technical* norms can play no role in an organisation unless embedded within a system of formal norms(Liu et al, 2000) (see Figure 5).

10. GENERATION OF CLINICAL PATHWAYS

The information collected during semantic analysis and norm analysis of clinical guideline is integrated to guide the generation of clinical pathways. Business process modelling notation best practice is adopted to generate clinical pathways. This will result in a rigorous control over the process of care ensuring completeness, consistency, comprehensiveness and adaptability of clinical pathway knowledge representation. We adopt process modelling techniques because it gives a rational means of organising information that is processed to perform care activities. In addition, it enables modelling of the complete end to end activities which results to a clear work-flow model. This improves interdisciplinary communication. On the other hand, process modelling facilitates the integration of information systems with the dynamics of CP in terms of action, roles and data exchange. In Figure 6, you can see part of the *Major Gynaecology pathways* modelled using BPMN techniques.

Figure 5. Taxonomy of norms

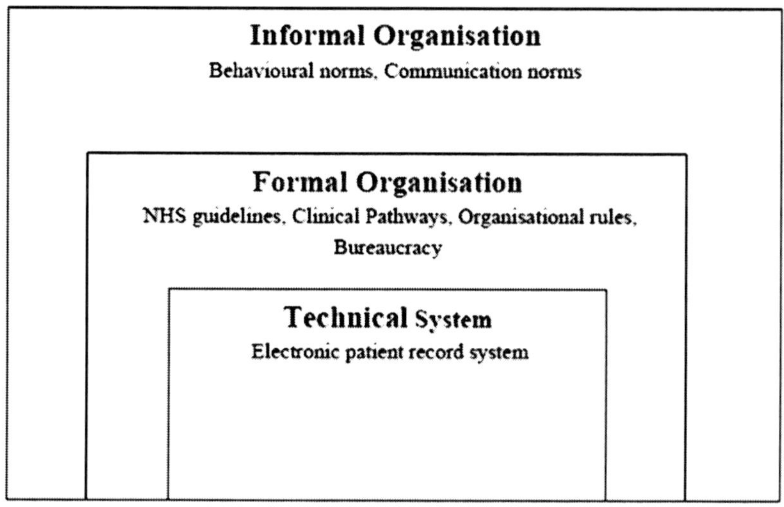

Figure 6. CP for major gynaecology surgery

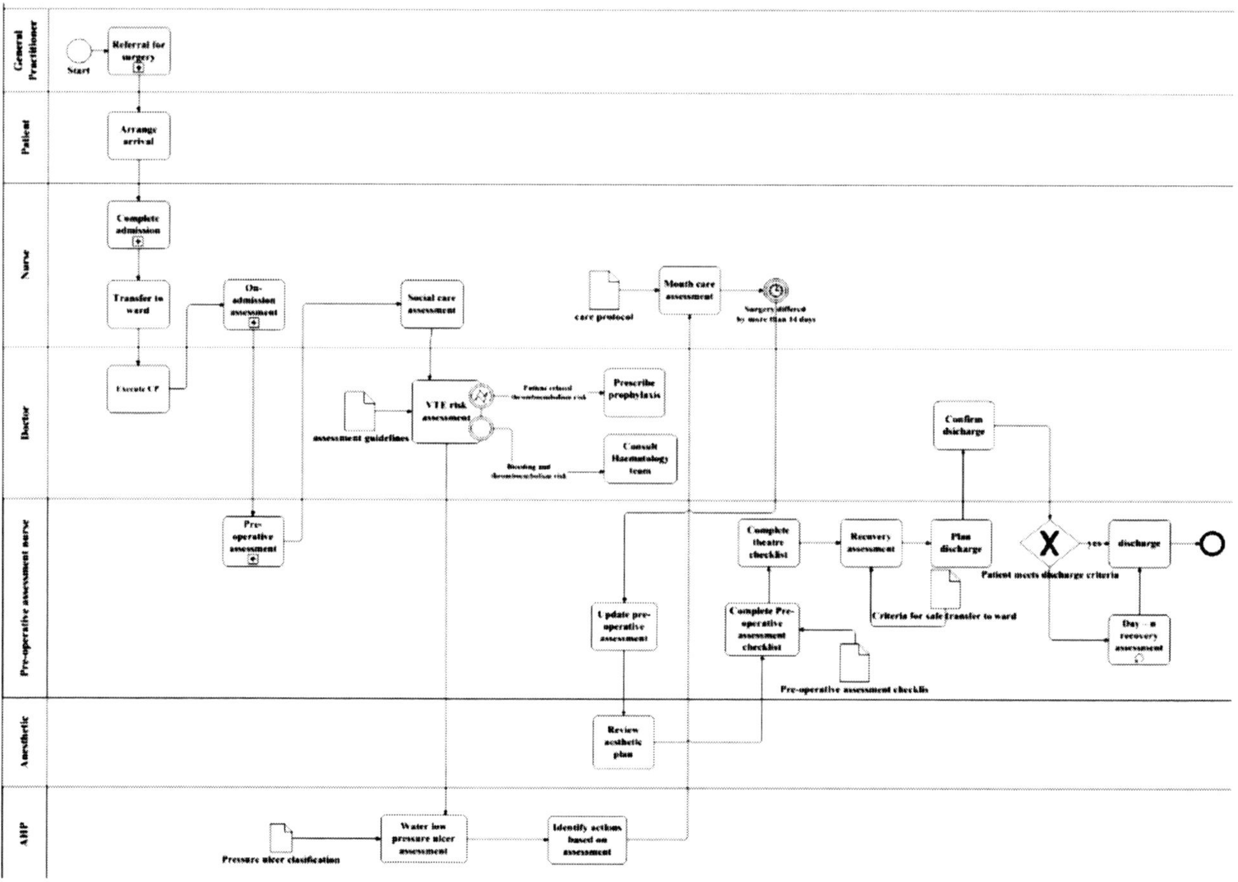

11. EXTENDING CLINICAL PATHWAYS BY CAPTURING BUSINESS DYNAMICS USING NORMS

Semantic analysis method provides all possible behaviours in CP which need further description by norms governing these behaviours. Norms, in addition to the knowledge represented in the semantic model, specify the details of these possibilities of behaviours; e.g., the conditions where certain clinical actions must happen or where they are actually impossible. Norm analysis (NA) is a method to identify and represent the norms in the ontology chart which govern the agent's behaviours in the social context by determining whether certain patterns of behaviours are acceptable or legal in the problem domain. The patterns of behaviour entailed in ontology chart as affordances can be formally specified by norms which describe constraints and rules an affordance must act upon during its existence as depicted in the ontological chart. The main steps of NAM are described in Table 1.

Norm specification uses the information collected in the previous stages to develop a formal specification of the norms. The norms are described as the following format (Liu 2000):

Whenever <condition> If <state> Then <agent> Is <deontic operator> To <action>

"Condition" and "state" are defined from the determined pre-conditions. The precondition for one of the norms in this case of affordance *Execution* being that "the patient is hospitalized for treatment", this makes up the whenever part of the norm. A second pre-condition determines the state part i.e. *"if there is a risk of bleeding"*, *"if surgery is delayed for more than 14 days"* which are usually indicated in trigger analysis. "Agent", as an authority, is responsible for executing defined action(s) or allocating them to other agents

Table 1. Main stapes of Norm Analysis Method

Step	Task	Outcome
1	Responsibility analysis	Identify responsible agents, i.e. norm subject
2	Proto-norm analysis	Select types of information required by the execution of the norm
3	Trigger analysis	Pre-condition: The conditions before invoking the norm
		Post-condition: The resultant after the successful execution of the norm
4	Detailed norm specification	Norms specified in the standard format

which is indicated in responsibility analysis. The entitlement is defined by the Deontic operators. "Deontic operator" is derived from Deontic Logic and can be one of the following: "obliged", "permitted" and "prohibited" which prescribe what people must, may, and must not do. It is essential to recognize that norms are not as rigid as logical conditions therefore they allow to model situations were decisions are made solely based on human judgement and there is a degree of flexibility in patterns of behaviour. For those actions that are "permitted", whether the agent will take an action or not is seldom deterministic. This elasticity characterizes the clinical processes and allows the subjective activity, therefore is of particularly value to support personalized clinical pathway.

The extension is carried out by incorporating norms into the business process diagram. In the diagram, each control condition is labelled as [N#] where # is the number for identification. The labels are then elaborated in the norm specifications to indicate the condition, the actor and action to be undertaken. Figure 4 depicts the extended business process for applying insurance policy, and Table 2 shows a list of norms for the control conditions of the care process. Phases in curly brackets are comments to help a reader to refer to the business process diagram in the corresponding figures.

Table 2. Norm analysis for major gynaecology care surgery

Norm N1 Whenever <the patient is assessed for venous thromboembolism> If <there is bleeding risk > Then <doctors> is <obliged> to <give prophylaxis>
Norm N2 Whenever <preforming post-op assessment> If <patient doesn't meet discharge criteria> Then <nurse> is <obliged> to <repeat post-op assessment in 2 days>
Norm N3 Whenever <performing pressure ulcer risk assessment> If <patient develops a pressure ulcer during this hospital stay > Then <nurse> is <permitted> to <arrange clinical photography>

On the list, the norms define business rules that are imposed on the particular process. For example, from the list in Table 1, Norm N1 reflects the straightforward rules that have to be followed after the post-operative assessment is completed. In addition, the norms allow exceptions to be specified in it. For example, Norm N2 includes both the business rules and an exception that will be triggered (caused) when the VTE assessment action has been invoked. Besides handling the business rules and exceptions, the norm provides a degree of flexibility that allows the analysts to introduce additional exceptions that may have been discovered in the later stage of analysis. For example, if patient for admission on day of surgery at pre-operative assessment the pre-operative nurse is obliged to perform MRSA screen or if the test screening is not carried out, the nurse is obliged to state reason for variance and actions taken. Using NAM it is possible to reflect the degree of flexibility actions in analysis (Figure 7).

12. DISCUSSION AND CONCLUSION

The challenge of achieving significant improvements in patient safety is one of the key tasks facing healthcare at the start of the 21st century. In this paper we propose a semiotics-oriented method to generate clinical pathways. Our approach adopts organisational semiotics and the methods such as SAM and NAM. We capture the knowledge of CG as ontology charts and specified norms. We use the information captured during semantic and norms analysis to guide the generation of clinical pathways using BPMN best practice. This will result in a rigorous control over the process of care ensuring completeness, consistency of clinical pathway knowledge representation.

This research has presented a method for generating clinical pathways from a semiotic perspective that can addresses social and informal/ safety factors which conspire together to influence the outcome of patient interaction and safety as compared to existing methods which fails to address these issues. This is achieved through modelling clinical pathways using SA and NA. In addition, it has been demonstrated that NAM allows the modelling of business dynamics, since

Figure 7. Extension of clinical pathway for major gynaecology surgery with norm

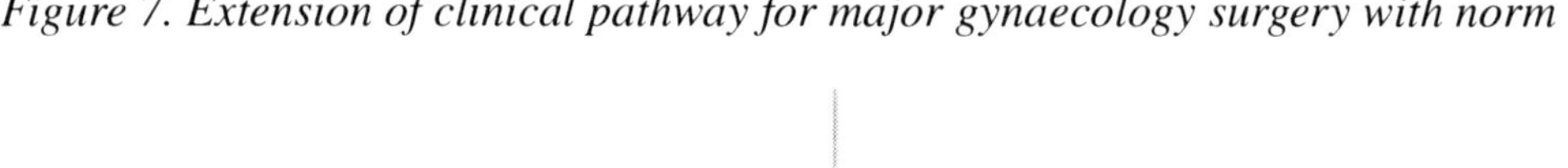
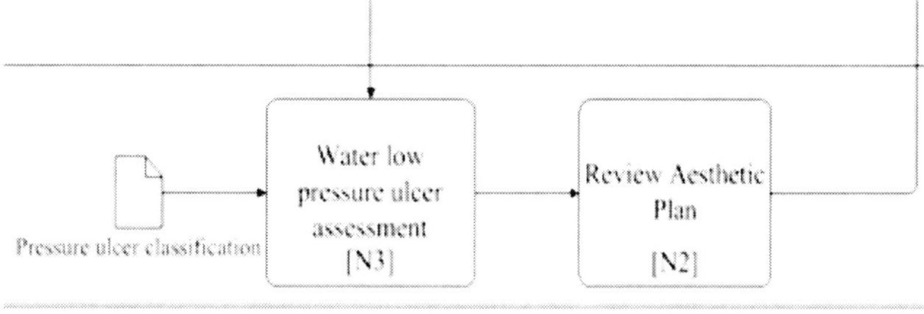

deontic operators facilitates modelling situations were decisions are made solely based on human judgement and there is a degree of flexibility in patterns of behaviour. Furthermore, the presented method enables a rigorous control over the process of knowledge articulation by embedding the results of ontology with norms which can ensure completeness, consistency and precise description of clinical pathways.

REFERENCES

Abidi, S. S. R., & Chen, H. (2006). Adaptable personalized care planning via a semantic web framework. In *Proceedings of 20th Intl Cong European Fed for Medical Informatics*. Maastricht: Academic Press.

Aguilar-Saven, R. S. (2004). Business process modelling: Review and framework. *International Journal of Production Economics, 90*(2), 129–149. doi:10.1016/S0925-5273(03)00102-6

Altman, D. E., Clancy, et al. (2004). Improving patient safety–Five years after the IOM report. *The New England Journal of Medicine, 351*(20), 2041–2043. doi:10.1056/NEJMp048243 PMID:15537902

Audimoolam, S. Nair, et al. (2005). The role of clinical pathways in improving patient outcomes. Academic Press.

Basse, L., Jakobsen, et al. (2000). A clinical pathway to accelerate recovery after colonic resection. *Annals of Surgery, 232*(1), 51. doi:10.1097/00000658-200007000-00008 PMID:10862195

Carthey, J., & Clarke, J. F. (2010). *Leadership for safety: Implementing human factors in healthcare*. London: NHS Institute for Innovation and Improvement.

Chang, A., Schyve, et al. (2005). The JCAHO patient safety event taxonomy: A standardized terminology and classification schema for near misses and adverse events. *International Journal for Quality in Health Care, 17*(2), 95–105. doi:10.1093/intqhc/mzi021 PMID:15723817

Chapanis, A. (Ed.). (1996). *Human factors in systems engineering*. Hoboken, NJ: John Wily & Sons.

Corrigan, J. (2005). Crossing the quality chasm. *Building a Better Delivery System.*

Filipe, J., & Liu, K. (2000). *The EDA model: An organizational semiotics perspective to norm-based agent design*. Citeseer.

Forster, P. (2003). To err is human. *Annals of Human Genetics, 67*(1), 2–4. doi:10.1046/j.1469-1809.2003.00002.x PMID:12556229

Gattnar, E. Ekinci, et al. (2011). Clinical process modeling and performance measurement in hospitals. Washington, DC: IEEE.

Heath, C., & Luff, P. (1996). Documents and professional practice: Bad organisational reasons for good. In *Clinical records*. New York: ACM. doi:10.1145/240080.240342

Helmreich, R. L. (2000). On error management: Lessons from aviation. *British Medical Journal, 320*(7237), 781. doi:10.1136/bmj.320.7237.781 PMID:10720367

Hurley, K. F., & Abidi, S. S. R. (2007). *Ontology engineering to model clinical pathways: Towards the computerization and execution of clinical pathways*. Washington, DC: IEEE. doi:10.1109/CBMS.2007.79

Kohn, L. T., & Corrigan, J. M. et al. (2000). *To err is human: Building a safer health system*. Washington, DC: National Academies Press.

Li, W. Liu, et al. (2008). Normative modeling for personalized clinical pathway using organizational semiotics methods. Washington, DC: IEEE.

Li, W., Liu, et al. (2010). A semiotic multi-agent modeling approach for clinical pathway management. *Journal of Computers*, 5(2), 266–273. doi:10.4304/jcp.5.2.266-273

Liu, K. (2000). *Semiotics in information systems engineering*. Cambridge, UK: Cambridge University Press. doi:10.1017/CBO9780511543364

Liu, K. (2002). Organizational semiotics: Evolving a science of information systems: IFIP TC8/WG8.1. In *Proceedings of Working Conference on Organizational Semiotics, Evolving a Science of Information Systems*. Boston: Kluwer Academic Publishers.

Liu, K., Sun, et al. (2003). Modelling dynamic behaviour of business organisations–Extension of DEMO from a semiotic perspective. *Knowledge-Based Systems*, 16(2), 101–111. doi:10.1016/S0950-7051(02)00077-1

Liu, K., Al-Rajhi, et al. (n.d.). *Modeling dynamic behavior of business organisations*. Academic Press.

Liu, K., & Ong, T. (1999). A modelling approach for handling business rules and exceptions. *The Computer Journal*, 42(3), 221–231. doi:10.1093/comjnl/42.3.221

Michell, V., Tehrani, et al. (2012). Are clinical documents optimised for patient safety? A critical analysis of patient safety outcomes using the EDA error model. *Health Policy and Technology Journal*.

Mor Plege, P. C., & Kumar. (2012). *Comparing computer-interpretable guideline models: A case study approach*. Academic Press.

Mould, G., Bowers, et al. (2010). The evolution of the pathway and its role in improving patient care. *Quality & Safety in Health Care*, 19(5), 1. PMID:20430932

Muthu, S., Whitman, et al. (2006). *Business process reengineering: A consolidated methodology*. Citeseer.

O'hare, D. (2000). The 'wheel of misfortune': A taxonomic approach to human factors in accident investigation and analysis in aviation and other complex systems. *Ergonomics*, 43(12), 2001–2019. doi:10.1080/00140130050201445 PMID:11191782

Osborn, S., & Williams, S. (2004). *Seven steps to patient safety: An overview guide for NHS staff*. London: The National Patient Safety Agency. Retrieved from http://www.npsa.nhs.uk/nrls/improvingpatientsafety/patient-safety-tools-and-guidance/7steps/

Panella, M., Marchisio, et al. (2003). Reducing clinical variations with clinical pathways: Do pathways work? *International Journal for Quality in Health Care*, 15(6), 509–521. doi:10.1093/intqhc/mzg057 PMID:14660534

Reason, J. (1995). Understanding adverse events: Human factors. *Quality in Health Care*, 4(2), 80–89. doi:10.1136/qshc.4.2.80 PMID:10151618

Sonnenberg, F., & Hagerty, C. (2006). Where are we and where are we going. *Computer-Interpretable Clinical Practice Guidelines,* 145-158.

Staccini, P., Joubert, et al. (2001). Modelling health care processes for eliciting user requirements: A way to link a quality paradigm and clinical information system design. *International Journal of Medical Informatics*, 64(2), 129–142. doi:10.1016/S1386-5056(01)00203-9 PMID:11734381

Stamper, R. (1994). *Social norms in requirements analysis: An outline of MEASUR*. Academic Press Professional, Inc.

Stamper, R., Liu, et al. (2000). Understanding the roles of signs and norms in organizations - A semiotic approach to information systems design. *Behaviour & Information Technology*, 19(1), 15–27. doi:10.1080/014492900118768

Stamper, R. K. (1996). *Signs, information, norms and systems*. Academic Press.

Tehrani, J. Liu, et al. (2012). Semiotics-oriented method for generation of clinical pathways. In *Proceedings of LISS 2012*. Springer.

Tehrani, J., Liu, et al. (2012). Ontology modeling for generation of clinical pathways. *Journal of Industrial Engineering and Management*, 5(2), 442–456. doi:10.3926/jiem.586

Tehrani, J. L. K., & Michel, V. (2012). Semiotics-oriented method for generation of clinical pathways. In *Proceedings of International Conference on Logistics, Informatics and Service Sciences (LISS)*. Beijing, China: Springer.

Yang, H., Liu, et al. (2010). Adaptive requirement-driven architecture for integrated healthcare systems. *Journal of Computers*, 5(2), 186–193. doi:10.4304/jcp.5.2.186-193

Chapter 3
The Role of Perceived Usefulness and Attitude on Electronic Health Record Acceptance

Randike Gajanayake
Queensland University of Technology, Australia

Tony Sahama
Queensland University of Technology, Australia

Renato Iannella
Queensland University of Technology, Australia

ABSTRACT

Information and communications technologies are a significant component of the healthcare domain, and electronic health records play a major role in it. Therefore, it is important that they are accepted en masse by healthcare professionals. How healthcare professionals perceive the usefulness of electronic health records and their attitudes towards them have been shown to have significant effects on the overall acceptance in many healthcare systems around the world. This paper investigates the role of perceived usefulness and attitude on the intention to use electronic health records by future healthcare professionals using polynomial regression with response surface analysis. Results show that the relationships between these variables are more complex than predicted in prior research. The paper concludes that the properties of the above determinants must be further investigated to clearly understand: (i) their role in predicting the intention to use electronic health records; and (ii) in designing systems that are better adopted by healthcare professionals of the future.

DOI: 10.4018/978-1-4666-8756-1.ch003

INTRODUCTION

The use of information and communications technology (ICT) in healthcare has become a significant aspect of the global healthcare agenda (Hackl, Hoerbst, & Ammenwerth, 2011; Protti & Johansen, 2010; Protti, Johansen, & Perez-Torres, 2009). Around the world, there are various approaches of implementing Health Information Technology (HIT), and electronic health records (EHR) are a significant component of this exercise, especially in patient information management (Hackl et al., 2011). Although most technological challenges have already been tackled, EHRs are yet to be fully integrated with the healthcare delivery process, and countries like Australia, New Zealand, Singapore, Denmark, Canada, USA and UK are investing significantly in this integration process. As a result of these efforts, the interaction with EHRs is bound to become a considerable part of a healthcare professional's (HCP) daily activities, and access to EHRs will be a critical requirement as more of the administrative and clinical processes are handled through EHR systems (Bramble et al., 2010). If adopted en masse by both HCPs and patients, EHRs and related technologies promise enviable benefits to healthcare delivery (Buntin, Burke, Hoaglin, & Blumenthal, 2011; Jha et al., 2009). However, HIT in general, and EHRs in particular, have suffered significant drawbacks due to dissatisfaction amongst HCPs (Hackl et al., 2011), which remains a significant barrier for the proliferation of EHRs in the care delivery process. Tackling this problem is both a timely and complex undertaking, and there is a need for studies that thoroughly identify the factors contributing to technology acceptance in the healthcare domain (Buntin et al., 2011).

Past studies on technology adoption have shown that adoption of EHRs is not as high as expected (Bramble et al., 2010; Ford, Menachemi, & Phillips, 2006; Gans, Kralewski, Hammons, & Dowd, 2005; Jha et al., 2009; Rao et al., 2011). Several reasons are said to be contributing factors for the low adoption and these have been clustered into eight categories by Boonstra and Broekhuis (Boonstra & Broekhuis, 2010): financial, technical, time, psychological, social, legal, organisational, and change process. According to Boonstra and Broekhuis, physicians have concerns regarding the use of EHRs that are based on their personal issues, knowledge, and perceptions. The perception of what an EHR system can deliver and the HCPs' attitudes towards it can significantly contribute to the acceptance of the system (Chau & Hu, 2002a). In past studies, this relationship has been considered to be linear and conclusions have been drawn accordingly about their significance in system adoption. With the development and availability of new technologies, however, they may be more complex than what was previously known. In regards to the intention to use EHR systems by future HCPs', this paper investigates the role played by perceived usefulness and attitudes towards EHRs as determinants. As a measure of each predictor and the dependent, the results of a quantitative survey conducted involving medical, nursing and health students from three education institutions in Queensland, Australia are utilised.

In what follows, first, a background on technology acceptance research and its role in the healthcare domain is discussed. Next, details pertaining to the theoretical foundations that underpin the hypotheses of the study are presented. Then, the details of the method employed in the study are given followed by the results and data analysis. The paper concludes with a discussion and conclusion, which summarizes the findings, identifies the limitations and makes recommendations for future work.

BACKGROUND

The use of ICT in the healthcare domain is gaining increasing importance around the world with the advancement of information systems and eHealth technologies (Meier, Fitzgerald, & Smith, 2013). In Australia, for example, the launch of the Personally Controlled Electronic Health Record

(PCEHR) (National E-Health Transition Authority, 2011) system laid the foundation for HCPs to interact with EHRs as a means of accessing healthcare information and communicating with patients. Similar initiatives elsewhere in the world have seen a clear move towards HIT becoming a significant aspect of day-to-day healthcare delivery. HCPs around the world are therefore destined to use EHRs as a key source of information for medical decision making. As a consequence, understanding how HCPs perceive EHRs and how those perceptions contribute to the overall intention to adopt EHRs have become an important aspect amongst today's HIT research community.

Technology Acceptance Research

Technology acceptance studies have been conducted in a vast range of domains. Early theories such as the technology acceptance model (TAM) have been widely used and several variations have been introduced. TAM was developed by Davis et al. (F.D. Davis, 1989; Fred D Davis, Bagozzi, & Warshaw, 1989) who argued that the key to increasing use of ICT was to, first, increase their acceptance. They showed that this can be assessed by asking them about their future intentions to use ICT. The foundations for TAM laid within the theory of reasoned action (TRA), a theory based in socio-psychological and behavioral theory. Following preliminary studies, several variables were established as measurements of ICT use behavior. Behavioral intention (BI) or acceptance and Attitude (ATT) were chosen as the principal determinants of ICT use. BI is influenced by one's attitude towards using ICT. Attitude, in turn, has two more determinants: perceived ease of use (PEOU) and perceived usefulness (PU). Furthermore, PU has an independent effect on BI and PEOU has an effect of PU and BI (Fred D Davis et al., 1989). These relationships have been further confirmed in studies which followed (Legris, Ingham, & Collerette, 2003; Venkatesh, Morris, Gordon, & Davis, 2003).

Technology Acceptance in Healthcare

Although TAM and related models have been applied in the study of ICT use in the healthcare domain since as far back as the 1990's (Holden & Karsh, 2010), its application is not as prominent as other fields (Schaper & Pervan, 2007). The study samples of the application of TAM in the healthcare domain include physicians, nurses, pharmacists, physiotherapists and medical technicians. Interestingly, support was not found for some of the key relationships in TAM-based models within the healthcare domain (Chau & Hu, 2002b; Holden & Karsh, 2010). As a result, Holden and Karsh (Holden & Karsh, 2010) recommended that the theories be augmented with additions and modifications to suit the healthcare domain.

THEORETICAL FOUNDATIONS AND HYPOTHESES

Considering the principal relationships in TAM and related models, research in the healthcare domain has shown strong statistical evidence for two of the relationships (Holden & Karsh, 2010): PU - BI and ATT - BI. In healthcare, PEOU showed mixed results for the relationship PEOU - BI (Holden & Karsh, 2010), indicating that the relationship may be moderated by factors in the study domains. Although previous studies have represented the relationships PU-BI and ATT-BI as linear relationships, in actuality it may be more complex. A reason for this complexity could be that, compared to a few years ago, ICT is closely related to the everyday activities of today's generation, especially young adults. As a result, the attitudes towards ICT and the usefulness people perceive may have evolved in recent times. In the healthcare context, these perceptions would transfer to the intention of EHRs use. Therefore, in this paper, these two relationships are investigated in detail.

Perceived Usefulness and Attitude

Perceived usefulness is defined as "the prospective user's subjective probability that using a specific application system will increase his or her job performance within an organizational context (Fred D Davis et al., 1989)." As reported in a recent review of the application of TAM in healthcare, perceived usefulness has been shown to be a significant factor in the intention to use ICT in all of the studies that were reviewed (Holden & Karsh, 2010). The report also reported that Attitude, which is defined as "an individual's overall affective reaction to using ICT (Venkatesh et al., 2003)", showed a significant relationship with the intention to use ICT in 5 out of 6 studies considered in this review. Attitude is said to tap into an individual's interest in and feelings of enjoyment and pleasure with ICT use (Venkatesh et al., 2003).

Considering what has been reported in prior research studies and the importance of the aforementioned relationships, the following hypotheses are made in this study:

H1a: Perceived usefulness is positively related to behavioral intention, such that future HCPs with positive (negative) perceptions of usefulness on EHRs will have high (low) intention to use EHRs in the future;

H1b: EHR Attitude is positively related to behavioral intention, such that future HCPs with positive (negative) attitudes on EHRs will have high (low) intention to use EHRs in the future.

Attitude is also said to mediate the effects of PU on BI (Venkatesh et al., 2003). This relationship has been well established in the technology acceptance literature and also in the healthcare domain (Schaper & Pervan, 2007). Therefore, the following is also hypothesized and tested in this study:

H2: EHR Attitude mediates the impact of perceived usefulness on behavioral intention.

METHOD

The method of data collection was an online questionnaire survey. The survey was administered via email and was left open for approximately four weeks with a reminder sent after two weeks. An online survey instrument and administration via email were seen as appropriate methods given that all participants had access to an Internet facility, owned email accounts and were considered to use email on a regular basis.

Survey Instrument

The survey instrument consisted of basic demographic details followed by a description of an EHR system that the respondents may use in their future professional activities. Table 1 shows the questionnaire items used to measure each of the constructs that are of focus in the paper. A 5-point Likert scale was used to measure the perceptions with 1 being "Strongly Disagree" and 5 being "Strongly Agree". All measurement items were reflective of the respective construct.

Participants

The participants of the survey were medical, nursing and health students from three academic institutions across Queensland, Australia. This cohort was chosen to represent the future HCP population because current HCPs' perceptions towards EHRs may be influenced by constraints such as institutional facilitating conditions, influence from governing bodies and other environmental conditions. Their perceptions on usefulness and attitudes may not entirely reflect what may be present when EHRs are implemented and become a part of everyday care delivery activities. The attitudes of a student cohort, on the other hand,

Table 1. Measurement items of constructs

Construct	Items[a,b]
Perceived Usefulness (PU)	PU1: I believe that this EHR system would be useful in my professional activities. PU2: I believe that this EHR system would help improve my patient care delivery. PU3: I think that this EHR system would improve my job performance. PU4: I feel that this EHR system can make health information sharing easier and more effective.
EHR Attitude (ATT)	ATT1: I believe that paper records can be better utilised to keep health information more secure than in EHRs. ATT2: Using this EHR system is a good idea. ATT3: I think EHRs are easy to work with than paper records. ATT4: I think I would enjoy working with this EHR system. ATT5: I think that EHR systems are expensive to implement and maintain. The expense could be better utilised to improve other healthcare facilities.
Behavioral Intention (BI)	BI1: I would use this EHR system in my professional activities for a few months. BI2: I would use this EHR system throughout my professional career.

[a] Measured in a 5 – point Likert scale. 1 = Strongly Disagree to 5 = Strongly Agree

[b] Primarily drawn from (Venkatesh et al., 2003) and have been altered to fit the context and cohort

are not motivated by such factors. However, it is recommended that the validity of this argument be established using data collected from current healthcare professionals in the presence of the moderating factors mentioned above.

RESULTS AND ANALYSIS

Results

A total of 334 valid responses were received from both undergraduate and postgraduate students and are used in the analysis. The demographics of the respondents are shown in Table 2. The age of the respondents ranged from 17 years to 60 with a mean age of 27.8 (SD = 10.1) years.

Analysis

First the measurement model was analyzed to test its validity and reliability using partial least square (PLS) analysis of structural equation modeling (SEM). The hypothesis testing was twofold: polynomial regression analysis was used to test hypotheses H1a and H1b whilst PLS was used to test H2.

Assessment of the Measurement Model

The construct reliability and construct validity were measured as an assessment of the measurement model. The statistical tools used were IBM SPSS 21 (SPSS Inc, 2012) and smartPLS 2.0 (Ringle, Wende, & Will, 2005).

In PLS, construct reliability is determined by the individual item reliability, internal composite reliability and the average variance extracted (AVE) (Barclay, Higgins, & Thompson, 1995). Individual item reliabilities were tested by producing individual item loadings for each construct. All measurement items showed acceptable item loadings (greater than 0.3 (Igbaria, Zinatelli, Cragg, & Cavaye, 1997)) as shown in Table 3. The internal composite reliability and AVE of each construct were of acceptable levels being higher than the thresholds of 0.707 and 0.5 respectively. The measurements for construct validity used

Table 2. Demographics of the respondents

Study Level	Medicine		Nursing		Other	
	M	*F*	*M*	*F*	*M*	*F*
Undergraduate	10	17	7	56	25	123
Postgraduate	3	7	4	23	15	44

Table 3. Item loadings, internal composite reliabilities and average variance extracted

Construct	Item	Item Loadings	AVE	Composite Reliability
Perceived Usefulness	PU1	0.8506	0.642	0.8768
	PU2	0.8550		
	PU3	0.8045		
	PU4	0.6828		
Attitude	ATT1	0.7067	0.5653	0.8659
	ATT2	0.6531		
	ATT3	0.8452		
	ATT4	0.8414		
	ATT5	0.6951		
Behavioral Intension	BI1	0.6671	0.6504	0.7838
	BI2	0.9251		

were discriminant validity and convergent validity. In PLS, correlations of the constructs and cross loading of constructs are used to determine the discriminant validity and convergent validity.

As seen in Table 4, the square roots of AVE (shown in bold) for each construct were greater than the correlation of constructs for each construct, indicating acceptable discriminant and convergent validity.

Cross loadings of the constructs were also calculated to determine how well individual indicators load on the latent variable compared to other variables. As seen in Table 5, the cross loading of each of the measurement items (shown in bold) are greater than the loading with other items indicating that the measures used in the study are more reflective of the constructs they were supposed to measure than the other constructs.

Table 4. Correlation of constructs and square root of AVE

	PU	ATT	BI
PU	**0.8012**		
ATT	0.7055	**0.7518**	
BI	0.6661	0.6091	**0.8065**

PU and ATT as Predictors of BI

Hypotheses H1a and H1b are tested here using response surface analysis. To test the hypotheses, polynomial regression with response surface analysis (Edwards, 2002) was employed. The polynomial equation used is as follows.

$$BI = \beta_0 + \beta_1 PU + \beta_2 ATT + \beta_3 PU^2 \\ + \beta_4 (PU * ATT) + \beta_5 ATT^2 + \varepsilon \tag{1}$$

Table 5. Cross loading of constructs

Indicators	PU	ATT	BI
PU1	**0.8506**	0.6451	0.5561
PU2	**0.8550**	0.6089	0.5350
PU3	**0.8045**	0.6707	0.5665
PU4	**0.6828**	0.5884	0.4697
ATT1	0.4965	**0.7067**	0.4121
ATT2	0.3723	**0.6531**	0.3560
ATT3	0.7824	**0.8452**	0.5760
ATT4	0.7010	**0.8414**	0.4940
ATT5	0.5129	**0.6951**	0.4147
BI1	0.3458	0.3012	**0.6671**
BI2	0.6665	0.6171	**0.9251**

The response surface methodology provides the means to examine (Shanock, Baran, Gentry, Pattison, & Heggestad, 2010): 1) how the degree of agreement/discrepancy between two predictor variables relate to an outcome variable; and 2) how the direction of discrepancy between two predictor variables relate to an outcome variable.

Table 6 summarizes the results of our polynomial regression analysis. Since the R^2 value (variance of BI explained by (1)) is significantly different from zero, the results of the regression analysis are evaluated using four surface test values (Edwards, 2002; Shanock et al., 2010): α_1, α_2, α_3 and α_4, where the slope of the line of perfect agreement (PU = ATT, shown as a straight line on the base of Figure 1) as related to BI is given by $\alpha_1 = \alpha_1 + \alpha_2$, the curvature along the same line as related to BI is given by $\alpha_2 = \alpha_2 + \alpha_3 + \alpha_5$, the slope of the line of incongruence (PU = -ATT, shown as a dotted line on the base of Figure 1) as related to BI, indicating the direction of the discrepancy, is given by $\alpha_3 = \alpha_1 - \alpha_2$, and the curvature of the line of incongruence indicating the discrepancy between PU, ATT and BI is given by $\alpha_4 = \alpha_3 - \alpha_4 + \alpha_5$.

Figure 1 shows the response surface pattern obtained from the polynomial regression analysis using (1). The results show in Table 6 shows a significant positive α_1 and α_2 (see (Shanock et al., 2010) for the equations used to calculate t-values for α terms). This indicates that when PU and ATT are in agreement, BI increases when PU and ATT

Table 6. Results from polynomial regression analysis: PU and ATT predictors of BI

Variables	Beta Coefficient (Std Err)[c]
Intercept/Constant (α_0)	3.09 (0.06)***
PU (α_1)	0.28 (0.10)**
ATT (α_2)	0.14 (0.09)
PU^2 (α_3)	0.201 (0.09)
PU*ATT (α_4)	-0.13 (0.14)*
ATT^2 (α_5)	0.09 (0.08)
R²	**0.41***
α_1	0.42 (0.08)***
α_2	0.17 (0.05)***
α_3	0.14 (0.18)
α_4	0.42 (0.18)*

* p < 0.05, ** p < 0.001, *** p < 0.0001

Figure 1. Behavioral intention as predicted by perceived usefulness and attitude

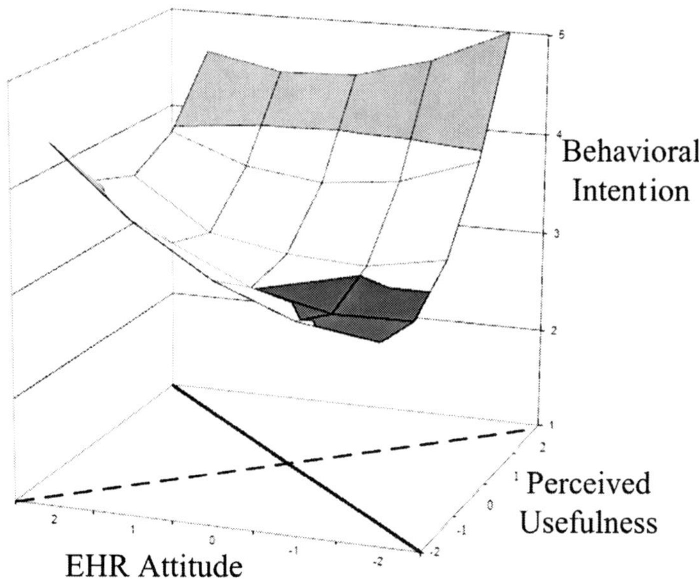

increase (indicated by the significant positive α_1) and that the relationship is curvilinear (indicated by the significant positive α_2). The curvature along the line of incongruence is significant and positive (indicated by a significant positive α_4) indicating that when PU and ATT are in disagreement, BI increases. An insignificant α_3 indicated that the direction of the discrepancy between PU and ATT does not significantly affect BI. The response surface analysis showed that PU and ATT are predictors of BI and the relationship is curvilinear. It also showed the perceived usefulness has the most significant effect on BI (indicated by the highest point of the graph).

Mediation by ATT

H2 was tested using PLS-SEM. To test the mediating effects of Attitude, the effect of PU on BI was tested with and without ATT. Table 7 shows the resulting path coefficients and t-values with their standard errors.

Sobel's mediation analysis (Sobel, 1982) was employed to eliminate the limitation of not testing the significance of the indirect paths. Sobel's test revealed that the relationship between PU and BI is mediated by ATT (Sobel test statistic = 3.753 (> 1.96), p < 0.0005). The direct effect of PU on BI decreased from 0.665 to 0.491 (p < 0.005) without and with ATT respectively, indicating a partial mediation.

DISCUSSION

This paper investigated the role of perceived usefulness and attitudes towards EHRs as predictors of the intention to adopt EHR systems by future healthcare professionals. The thesis of this paper is conceived as a critical success factor in HIT. The study hypothesized that perceived usefulness and attitudes of HCPs towards EHRs in general were positively related to the intention to adopt those types of systems. It also hypothesized that

attitude mediated the effect of perceived usefulness on intention to adopt EHR systems. Using the survey method, an online questionnaire survey was conducted with future healthcare professionals to measure the three constructs (PU, ATT and BI) and test the hypotheses. After establishing that the measurement model used was reliable and valid using partial least squares analysis, all hypothesized relationships were tested using response surface analysis and Sobel's mediation analysis.

Findings

In line with the general TAM, the study found that attitude and perceived usefulness were positive predictors of intention to adopt an EHR system. Unique to this study, the relationships between attitude and perceived usefulness with intention to adopt was shown to be curvilinear. It was also shown that attitude partially mediated the relationship between perceived usefulness and intention to adopt, which has been shown in later TAM studies conducted in the healthcare domain.

In previous TAM-based studies conducted in the healthcare domain, the relationships between constructs were assumed and treated as linear relationships. Although the results of those studies gave valuable insights for HIT researchers as well as health services, they were limited given the above assumption. Testing the relationships in more detail, as we have done here, require several considerations. Firstly, it is important to identify which aspects are the most prominent predictors of

Table 7. Test of mediation of attitude

Path	Path Coefficient	Std. Error	t-Value
PU – BI (With ATT)	0.4911	0.0588	8.353
PU – BI (Without ATT)	0.6654	0.0329	20.200
PU – ATT	0.7924	0.0236	33.551
ATT - BI	0.2213	0.0586	3.776

the intention to use EHR systems. In that regard, and as a first study, we considered perceived usefulness and attitude–the most significant predictors of intention to use in TAM. Secondly, it is important to identify an appropriate study cohort. Here, we used a student cohort. The results of this study make a significant contribution to the HIT literature by taking a student cohort who can be considered more technology aware or *digital natives*. It was shown that some relationships are in fact more complex than previously known. Thirdly, it is important to understand how the targeted population interact with technology in general because of the critical role technology plays in today's society. Although we see this as a limitation of the current study, its impact on our study is mitigated by the fact that we used a student cohort who, as stated above, we can assume to be aware and involved with modern Internet-based technologies.

Limitations

As with many empirical studies, the first limitation of this study relates to the sample size. The sample size, although sufficient enough for significant statistical analysis, was not very large and the sample was not representative of the Australian population of healthcare professionals. Secondly, we assumed that the students' knowledge and awareness of EHRs were uniform across the sample. To address this in future studies, it is advised that preliminary questions assess the respondents' EHR awareness or select a sample that has a known degree of experience working with EHRs.

Future Research Directions

Given that this is the first study that investigated the curvilinear relationship between predictors of intention to use EHR systems, there is grounds to suggest that similar studies are conducted to further validate the findings. Furthermore, to mitigate limitations associated with using a stu-

dent cohort, studies using students at prior and post exposure to EHR systems are recommended, which can be compared to results obtained from studies involving current healthcare professionals. The possibility of qualitative verification of the results using actual case studies is also noteworthy.

CONCLUSION

In the development of EHR systems, it is imperative to understand the complex relationships between how user perceptions on system capabilities, system usefulness and how user attitudes influence system acceptance. For example, an EHR system's usefulness and usability are seen as key aspects of "meaningful use" (Blumenthal & Tavenner, 2010) of EHR systems. User studies may be conducted to investigate how user perceptions evolve with continued use of systems such that appropriate pre-emptive measures can be taken to alter these changes, thus system acceptance and use are kept at optimal levels.

ACKNOWLEDGMENT

NICTA is funded by the Australian Government as represented by the Department of Broadband, Communications and the Digital Economy and the Australian Research Council through the ICT Centre of Excellence program. We thank Queensland University of Technology (QUT) for the funding support provided to conduct this research and the ethics review committee at QUT for their input during ethical clearance for conducting the survey.

REFERENCES

Barclay, D., Higgins, C., & Thompson, R. (1995). The partial least squares (PLS) approach to causal modeling: Personal computer adoption and use as an illustration. *Technology Studies*, 2(2), 285–309.

Blumenthal, D., & Tavenner, M. (2010). The "Meaningful Use" Regulation for Electronic Health Records. *The New England Journal of Medicine, 363*(6), 501–504. doi:10.1056/NEJMp1006114 PMID:20647183

Boonstra, A., & Broekhuis, M. (2010). Barriers to the acceptance of electronic medical records by physicians from systematic review to taxonomy and interventions. *BMC Health Services Research, 10*(1), 231. doi:10.1186/1472-6963-10-231 PMID:20691097

Bramble, J. D., Galt, K. A., Siracuse, M. V., Abbott, A. A., Drincic, A., Paschal, K. A., & Fuji, K. T. (2010). The relationship between physician practice characteristics and physician adoption of electronic health records. *Health Care Management Review, 35*(1), 55–64. doi:10.1097/HMR.0b013e3181c3f9ad PMID:20010013

Buntin, M. B., Burke, M. F., Hoaglin, M. C., & Blumenthal, D. (2011). The benefits of health information technology: A review of the recent literature shows predominantly positive results. *Health Affairs, 30*(3), 464–471. doi:10.1377/hlthaff.2011.0178 PMID:21383365

Chau, P. Y. K., & Hu, P. J. H. (2002a). Examining a model of information technology acceptance by individual professionals: An exploratory study. *Journal of Management Information Systems, 18*(4), 191–230.

Chau, P. Y. K., & Hu, P. J. H. (2002b). Investigating healthcare professionals' decisions to accept telemedicine technology: An empirical test of competing theories. *Information & Management, 39*(4), 297–311. doi:10.1016/S0378-7206(01)00098-2

Davis, F. D. (1989). Perceived usefulness, perceived ease of use, and user acceptance of information technology. *Management Information Systems Quarterly, 13*(3), 319–340. doi:10.2307/249008

Davis, F. D., Bagozzi, R. P., & Warshaw, P. R. (1989). User acceptance of computer technology: A comparison of two theoretical models. *Management Science, 35*(8), 982–1003. doi:10.1287/mnsc.35.8.982

Edwards, J. R. (2002). Alternatives to difference scores: Polynomial regression analysis and response surface methodology.

Ford, E. W., Menachemi, N., & Phillips, M. T. (2006). Predicting the Adoption of Electronic Health Records by Physicians: When Will Health Care be Paperless? *Journal of the American Medical Informatics Association, 13*(1), 106–112. doi:10.1197/jamia.M1913 PMID:16221936

Gans, D., Kralewski, J., Hammons, T., & Dowd, B. (2005). Medical groups' adoption of electronic health records and information systems. *Health Affairs, 24*(5), 1323–1333. doi:10.1377/hlthaff.24.5.1323 PMID:16162580

Hackl, W., Hoerbst, A., & Ammenwerth, E. (2011). Why the hell do we need electronic health records? *EHR acceptance among physicians in private practice in Austria: A qualitative study. Methods of Information in Medicine, 50*(1), 53–61. doi:10.3414/ME10-02-0020 PMID:21057716

Holden, R. J., & Karsh, B.-T. (2010). Methodological Review: The Technology Acceptance Model: Its past and its future in health care. *Journal of Biomedical Informatics, 43*(1), 159–172. doi:10.1016/j.jbi.2009.07.002 PMID:19615467

Igbaria, M., Zinatelli, N., Cragg, P., & Cavaye, A. L. M. (1997). Personal computing acceptance factors in small firms: A structural equation model. *Management Information Systems Quarterly, 21*(3), 279–305. doi:10.2307/249498

Jha, A. K., DesRoches, C. M., Campbell, E. G., Donelan, K., Rao, S. R., & Ferris, T. G. et al. (2009). Use of Electronic Health Records in U.S. Hospitals. *The New England Journal of Medicine*, *360*(16), 1628–1638. doi:10.1056/NEJMsa0900592 PMID:19321858

Legris, P., Ingham, J., & Collerette, P. (2003). Why do people use information technology? A critical review of the technology acceptance model. *Information & Management*, *40*(3), 191–204. doi:10.1016/S0378-7206(01)00143-4

Meier, C. A., Fitzgerald, M. C., & Smith, J. M. (2013). eHealth: Extending, enhancing, and evolving healthcare. *Annual Review of Biomedical Engineering*.

National E-Health Transition Authority. (2011). Concept of Operations: Relating to the introduction of a personally controlled electronic health record (PCEHR) system. Retrieved 20 August, 2013, from http://www.yourhealth.gov.au/internet/yourhealth/publishing.nsf/Content/PCEHRS-Intro-toc#.T9BeK8VIuSo

Protti, D., & Johansen, I. (2010). *Widespread Adoption of Information Technology in Primary Care Physician Offices in Denmark: A Case Study*. The Commonwealth Fund.

Protti, D., Johansen, I., & Perez-Torres, F. (2009). Comparing the application of Health Information Technology in primary care in Denmark and Andalucía, Spain. *International Journal of Medical Informatics*, *78*(4), 270–283. doi:10.1016/j.ijmedinf.2008.08.002 PMID:18819836

Rao, S. R., DesRoches, C. M., Donelan, K., Campbell, E. G., Miralles, P. D., & Jha, A. K. (2011). Electronic health records in small physician practices: Availability, use, and perceived benefits. *Journal of the American Medical Informatics Association*, *18*(3), 271–275. doi:10.1136/amiajnl-2010-000010 PMID:21486885

Ringle, C. M., Wende, S., & Will, S. (2005). SmartPLS 2.0 (M3) Beta (Version 2.0). Hamburg. Retrieved from http://www.smartpls.de

Schaper, L., & Pervan, G. (2007). ICT and OTs: A model of information and communication technology acceptance and utilisation by occupational therapists. *International Journal of Medical Informatics*, *76*, S212–S221. doi:10.1016/j.ijmedinf.2006.05.028 PMID:16828335

Shanock, L. R., Baran, B. E., Gentry, W. A., Pattison, S. C., & Heggestad, E. D. (2010). Polynomial regression with response surface analysis: A powerful approach for examining moderation and overcoming limitations of difference scores. *Journal of Business and Psychology*, *25*(4), 543–554. doi:10.1007/s10869-010-9183-4

Sobel, M. E. (1982). Asymptotic confidence intervals for indirect effects in structural equation models. *Sociological Methodology*, *13*, 290–312. doi:10.2307/270723

SPSS Inc. (2012). Statistical Package for Social Sciences (SPSS) (Version Version 21.0). Chicago, IL.

Venkatesh, V., Morris, M. G., Gordon, B. D., & Davis, F. D. (2003). User Acceptance of Information Technology: Toward a Unified View. *Management Information Systems Quarterly*, *27*(3), 425–478.

This work was previously published in the International Journal of E-Health and Medical Communications (IJEHMC), 5(4); edited by Joel J.P.C. Rodrigues, pages 108-119 copyright year 2014 by IGI Publishing (an imprint of IGI Global).

Chapter 4

The Impact of the Electronic Medical Records (EMRs) on Hospital Pathology Services:
An Organisational Communication Perspective

Andrew Georgiou
University of New South Wales, Australia

ABSTRACT

This chapter reviews what is currently known about the effect of the Electronic Medical Records (EMRs) on aspects of laboratory test ordering, their impact on laboratory efficiency, and the contribution this makes to the quality of patient care. The EMR can be defined as a functioning electronic database within a given organisation that contains patient information. Although laboratory services are expected to gain from the introduction of the EMRs, the evidence to date has highlighted many challenges associated with the implementation of EMRs, including their potential to cause major shifts in responsibilities, work processes, and practices. The chapter outlines an organisational communication framework that has been derived from empirical evidence. This framework considers the interplay between communication, temporal, and organisational factors, as a way to help health information technology designers, clinicians, and hospital and laboratory professionals meet the important challenges associated with EMR design, implementation, and sustainability.

INTRODUCTION

The chapter reviews what is currently known about the effect of the electronic medical record (EMR) on aspects of laboratory test ordering, its impact on laboratory efficiency and the contribution this makes to the quality of patient care. The chapter identifies the key challenges associated with the introduction of the EMR and the organisational context in which it is used in pathology laboratories. It examines how communication is undertaken within the laboratory and its effect on the way that work is carried out. Particular consideration is given to key concepts such as:

DOI: 10.4018/978-1-4666-8756-1.ch004

a) the synchronicity of communication required within sections of the laboratory (e.g., real time communication between the laboratory and clinicians versus asynchronous messages and notes); b) the role of feed-back mechanisms which provide confirmation of the receipt of information; and c) considerations of what (and how much) information is needed by different recipients. The chapter also incorporates an examination of temporal and spatial factors, particularly as they relate to where work is carried out, how it is allocated, prioritised and coordinated. The objective of the chapter is thus to outline an empirically-derived organisational communication framework, which can be used to help enhance the design, implementation and sustainability of EMR systems and hospital pathology services.

BACKGROUND

Hospital laboratory services are involved in the examination of clinical and pathologic data which are incorporated into a broader context and used to provide meaningful information to physicians and patients(Deeble & Lewis-Hughes, 1991). In the last few decades, this important task has become increasingly reliant on sophisticated information technology systems to assist in the management, storage and communication of data(Pantanowitz, Henricks, & Beckwith, 2007).

The EMR can be defined as a functioning electronic database that contains patient information within a given organisation (Aller, Georgiou, & Pantanowitz, 2012). EMRs can encompass a wide range of systems including computerised provider order entry (CPOE) systems that allow clinicians to place orders directly into computers (Birkmeyer, Lee, Bates, & Birkmeyer, 2002). They may also incorporate clinical information databases, which can be used to provide decision support to assist diagnosis, or to help understand and interpret laboratory results (Georgiou, Williamson, Westbrook, & Ray, 2007). The EMR

is therefore more than just a replacement for the previous paper-based medical record system, it has the potential to expand modes of communication and improve access to information and knowledge across the hospital and the wider community (Aller et al., 2012).

There is an expanding body of literature which has identified many benefits associated with the EMR, including the ability to provide timely access to patient information and electronic decision support to enhance clinical decision-making and the delivery of quality care(Buntin, Burke, Hoaglin, & Blumenthal, 2011). Nevertheless, there remain major international reservations about the slow pace of EMR diffusion amid concerns about the failure of the existing evidence base to clearly demonstrate benefits (Black et al., 2011). Literature reviews continue to point to the need to improve our knowledge of why some EMR implementations succeed and others do not (Jones, Rudin, Perry, & Shekelle, 2014). This has led to a growing international imperative to examine and improve our understanding of the context of EMR system implementations, particularly as regards the circumstances that may (or may not) contribute to their success and sustainability (Aarts, Ash, & Berg, 2007).

THE IMPACT OF THE EMR ON HOSPITAL LABORATORY SERVICES

Hospital pathology services are widely seen as an area where information and communication technologies (ICT) like the EMR can have a major impact on the efficiency and effectiveness of service delivery. Pathology laboratories are information-intense bodies that provide services across primary, secondary and tertiary care. It is estimated that pathology laboratory services are responsible for leveraging 60-70% of all critical decision-making involving admittance, discharge and medication (Forsman, 1996). Within this context the EMR has been identified as an important means to:

- Improve the efficiency and effectiveness of laboratory services.
- Increase the utilisation of evidence-based test ordering.
- Enhance the quality and safety of patient care.

Improve the Efficiency and Effectiveness of Laboratory Services

One of the most regularly used indicators of laboratory performance is the measure of turn-around times (TATs). TATs can be measured either from the time a test is ordered, a sample is taken, or the time the sample is presented at the laboratory reception area for processing, right up to the time a verified result has been issued and seen(A Georgiou, M Williamson, et al., 2007). TATs can influence how the quality of the pathology service is judged by clinicians (Hawkins, 2007). Research evidence has shown that EMR ordering (utilising a Computerised Provider Order Entry component) has contributed to significant reductions in TATs (Georgiou, Prgomet, et al., 2013; A Georgiou, M Williamson, et al., 2007). For instance, a 2002 study showed a 25% shorter laboratory TAT (measured from the time of receipt of a specimen in the laboratory to the electronic posting of the result) in a medical Intensive Care Unit (ICU)(Mekhjian et al., 2002). In 2006, a controlled before and after study in an Australian teaching hospital reported a significant average decrease of 15.5 minutes/test assay in laboratory TAT across intervention wards which used a CPOE system. This improvement in TAT was not found in the non-intervention wards (J.I. Westbrook, Georgiou, Dimos, & Germanos, 2006). Other studies have shown that these improvements have been consistent over time(J.I. Westbrook, Georgiou, & Rob, 2009) and across hospitals(J.I. Westbrook, Georgiou, & Lam, 2009).

Increase the Utilisation of Evidence-Based Test Ordering

Evidence-based medicine has meant a shift in the culture of health provision away from decisions based on opinion, past practices and precedent, towards a system that utilises science, research and evidence to guide decision making (Sackett, Rosenberg, Gray, Haynes, & Richardson, 1996). For pathology this has inspired greater emphasis on its role in the whole patient journey beginning with asking the right clinical questions, selecting the most appropriate test or investigation needed to diagnose the problem, across to providing appropriate clinical advice and treatment to encompass the whole spectrum of specialties involved in the patient pathway. The EMR can be seen as an important clinical aid, helping to provide the "end-to-end connectivity" to deliver effective order communication(Georgiou, Lang, Rosenfeld, & Westbrook, 2011; J.I. Westbrook et al., 2006) and decision support based on the linking of laboratory test results with evidence-based guidelines. Prior research in this area has provided potent examples of how guideline-based reminders can improve guideline compliance,(Overhage, Tierney, Zhou, & McDonald, 1997) or contribute to sustained and significant decreases in the proportion of troponin I test ordered in an Emergency Department in Melbourne, Australia(Georgiou, Lam, Allardice, Hart, & Westbrook, 2012). Even electronic prompts for basic information (e.g., specifying whether a gentamicin or vancomycin sample is random, peak or trough (J.I. Westbrook et al., 2006) or whether a patient is on heparin or warfarin when coagulation testing is undertaken(A Georgiou et al., 2011) can improve the efficiency and effectiveness of pathology services and their contribution to quality patient care.

Evidence-based test ordering is particularly relevant to issues concerning the volume of pathology test orders. The past few decades have seen a massive growth in pathology services with many more people receiving laboratory tests than previously, leading to a considerable increase in the volume of laboratory tests performed(Legg & Cheong, 2004). This has raised major concerns about excessive and redundant test ordering and the financial burden this may impose on health care resources. It also carries serious implications for patient safety, threatening to increase the number of false-positive test results associated with unnecessary and time-consuming diagnostic examinations(Axt-Adam, 1993).

Enhance the Quality and Safety of Patient Care

The World Health Organization's World Alliance for Patient Safety has highlighted the importance of pathology services to the global patient safety agenda, emphasising the role of the laboratory in ensuring that reliable and accurate results are delivered in a timely fashion to inform clinical management decisions (The World Alliance For Patient Safety Drafting Group et al., 2009). The main sources of laboratory errors have been shown to arise within the pre-analytic (doctor's test order) and post-analytic (laboratory report to the doctor) phases of the laboratory test order process (Bonini, Plebani, Ceriotti, & Rubboli, 2002). These are areas where the EMR can have a major positive impact. The addition of decision support functions can assist physicians to alleviate problems with test requisitions, for example, ordering incorrect tests, inaccurately specifying aspects of the test order, or neglecting a test altogether. The EMR may also help to promote appropriate test requests where there is a clear clinical question for which the result will provide an answer leading to the initiation of appropriate treatment (Price, 2003). For instance, a 1999 study carried out in the Brigham and Women's Hospital in USA, provided a powerful example where the introduction of electronic reminders about apparent redundant

tests led to significantly improved performance (27% in the intervention v 51% in the control) in the rate of redundant tests (Bates et al., 1999).

EMR: THE CHALLENGES ASSOCIATED WITH DESIGN, IMPLEMENTATION AND SUSTAINABILITY

Although laboratory services are expected to gain significantly from the introduction of the EMR, the evidence to date has also highlighted problems and inconsistencies (J. Callen, Paoloni, Georgiou, Prgomet, & Westbrook, 2010; J. L. Callen, Braithwaite, & Westbrook, 2008; Georgiou, Greenfield, Callen, & Westbrook, 2009; Andrew Georgiou et al., 2007; Georgiou, Morse, Timmins, Ray, & Westbrook, 2008; Georgiou & Westbrook, 2007; A Georgiou, J.I. Westbrook, et al., 2007; Georgiou, Westbrook, Callen, & Braithwaite, 2008; Johanna I. Westbrook, Georgiou, & Rob, 2008). One of the major limitations of the existing evidence base relates to the generalisability of existing research findings, along with concerns about the applicability of the findings to hospitals internationally (Black et al., 2011; Chaudhry et al., 2006). In part this has been linked to the preponderance of US-centred studies in the evidence base, (often from the same three or four hospitals), and the inclusion of a large number of early studies based on home grown applications prior to the worldwide proliferation of commercial "off-the-shelf" systems (Ash, Stavri, Dykstra, & Fournier, 2003; A Georgiou, M Williamson, et al., 2007).

Another major concern about the existing evidence base relates to the overwhelming focus on measures of process rather than patient care outcomes (Georgiou, Prgomet, et al., 2013). Measures of patient outcome usually involve the consideration of multiple and complex factors that can be difficult to identify and measure (A Georgiou, M Williamson, et al., 2007). Most studies that have considered the impact of electronic pathology ordering on indicators such as patient length of hospital stay, mortality or even readmission rates to ICU, report no significant changes (A Georgiou, M Williamson, et al., 2007). The generation of research evidence regarding clinical outcomes will likely need to employ more sophisticated statistical techniques to account for the many factors involved in considerations of patient outcome(J.I. Westbrook, Georgiou, & Lam, 2009; Johanna I. Westbrook et al., 2008).

The evidence also highlights major problems with implementing and sustaining electronic decision support features. There are often difficulties achieving agreement about standards (e.g., commonly agreed laboratory order sets or diagnostic algorithms relevant for specified patient conditions) (Bobb, Payne, & Gross, 2007). There is also the possibility of clinical resistance to particularly features of the EMR that may be related to problems with the usability of the system, its compatibility with existing applications or even a failure to complement the way that clinical and laboratory work is performed (A Georgiou, J.I. Westbrook, et al., 2007; L. Peute, Aarts, Bakker, & Jaspers, 2009; L. W. P. Peute & Jaspers, 2007).

FUTURE RESEARCH DIRECTIONS

Many health informatics researchers have noted that while information technology systems like the EMR can be designed and implemented, socio-material infrastructures (involving work processes, spatial locations and existing social settings) are hardly ever designed; instead they are generated dynamically and organically (Bygstad, 2010). In this way innovation associated with information technology should not be seen as a product of a single intervention, but part of a collective organisational and communication change process incorporating numerous stakeholders (e.g., care providers, patients, institutions, vendors, regulatory agencies) within tightly coupled clinical and social settings(Greenhalgh & Russell, 2010). The success or otherwise of the EMR should, therefore, be considered through a *multi-dimensional and system-oriented perspective* that takes into account the perspectives of the numerous stakeholders involved in the process (e.g., pathologists, laboratory scientists, doctors, nurses, patients, hospital managers etc.)(Georgiou, Westbrook, Braithwaite, & Iedema, 2005; A Georgiou, J.I. Westbrook, et al., 2007).

Generally, our understanding of the mechanisms by which information technology drives work practice change and improvements in service performance has been underdeveloped(Menou & Taylor, 2006). This is because many of the changes introduced by information technologies are undefined, complex or dynamic(Organisation for Economic Co-operation Development, 2011). While the EMR may be designed to facilitate improvements, evidence has shown that people may also decide not to use them, or may find their lack of integration with current work patterns difficult to handle, leading to situations where the full potential of the system is not realised(Clegg et al., 1997). Traditionally, information system research approaches have focused on the technological application, and struggled to appreciate the informational, organisational and communications infrastructure that underpins how work is performed (Chen, 1990).

As a consequence of widespread concerns about the applicability, sustainability and safety of the EMR and health information technology more generally, the US Committee on Patient Safety and Health Information Technology, Institute of Medicine has drawn attention to the critical importance of socio-technical factors involved in the adoption of information technology(Committee on Patient Safety and Health Information Technology; Institute of Medicine, 2011). Socio-technical approaches view social aspects (culture, values and politics) and technical elements (equipment, procedures and technology) as interdependent and interrelated (Coiera, 2004; J.I. Westbrook et al., 2007; Whetton & Georgiou, 2010).

Organisational Communication Framework

This chapter concludes by considering some of the key socio-technical factors identified by the Committee on Patient Safety and Health Information Technology(Committee on Patient Safety and Health Information Technology; Institute of Medicine, 2011) particularly in regards to the communication infrastructure that underpins each organisation. The chapter describes an organisational communication framework (see Figure 1) which considers the interplay between communication, temporal factors and organisational functions drawing heavily on empirical findings of the impact of the EMR on hospital laboratory services.

Organisational communication approaches emphasise the essential (constitutive) role that communication processes play in the make-up and functioning of an organisation (Putnam, Nicotera, & McPhee, 2009). The management of every organisation usually involves some combination

Figure 1. Diagrammatic conceptualisation of an organisational communication framework

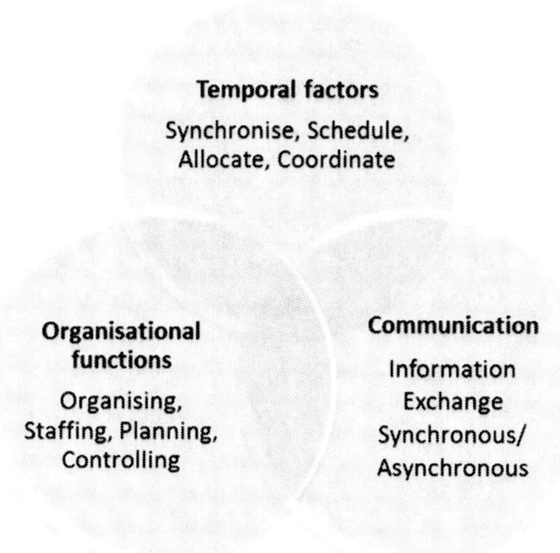

of the classic tasks related to the planning, organising, staffing and controlling of how work is performed(Fayol, 1967). Each of these functions is connected to a communication and temporal dimension (Georgiou, Westbrook, & Braithwaite, 2012). In order to *plan*, it is important to obtain information with which to organise future activities. The *organisation* of work requires people and resources to be set out according to specified communication networks. *Staffing* includes communication required for the management of human resources and *controlling* involves the coordination of resources using the exchange of information. The viability and eventual success of an EMR are therefore contingent on its suitability and fit within the particular organisational and communication setting in which it is installed (A. Georgiou et al., 2012).

Temporal Factors

One of the most challenging features of ICT systems is their effect on the *temporal landscape* that is how time is conceived, structured and organised, and the impact this has on how work is carried out (Adam, 2004). EMR systems are widely believed to facilitate major increases in the pace and volumes of data transfer, allowing for linkage and storage of information across multiple sites. They also have the ability to deliver efficiency gains that are often related to the speed and timeliness of information exchange and its effect on organisational output.

There is a general presumption that new technologies lead to an increase in the pace of activities, increasing reliance on some practices (e.g., computer entry) to the hindrance of others (e.g., manual tasks)(Georgiou, Tariq, & Westbrook, 2013). However, this supposition is overly simplistic because technologies, in and of themselves, are not necessarily the cause of this speed up (Wajcman, 2008). Often, what has changed is the way that work is *allocated, prioritised, sequenced* or *coordinated*(Georgiou, Westbrook, & Braithwaite, 2011). Take for instance the following example of the changes to pathology service blood collectors' (phlebotomists) work patterns that came about with the introduction of the EMR. In the past, the blood collectors' collection round involved their visiting each ward and immediately setting out on the task of sorting, verifying and validating each ward's blood collection requests. This task also involved identifying any duplicate blood collection requests that may have been made for the same patient. Once the EMR was implemented, practices changed dramatically to the point that the blood collector's job now started in the Central Specimen Reception area where a print-out was obtained that had all collection tasks already listed and included the identification of all duplicate requests. Aside from the obvious time savings involved, the new work practice procedure significantly altered the way that the blood collector's work was allocated, sequenced and coordinated (A. Georgiou et al., 2008; A Georgiou, JI Westbrook, & J Braithwaite, 2010).

The influence that temporal factors have on the EMR and organisations is complex and can be difficult to identify(Poole, 2004). For instance, in the past, "space" and "place" usually meant you were in the same place as the person with whom you needed to work with. However, information technology has fostered relations between people without face-to-face interaction(Giddens, 1990). This means that preparation for the introduction of the EMR needs to include an awareness of how the system may change the way that work is organised between professionals, departments and even within the community (A. Georgiou et al., 2011). For instance, will information exchange continue to happen in the same place or across distance? Will the exchange involve major shifts in responsibility among professionals?(Fernando, Georgiou, Holdgate, & Westbrook, 2009). Will the sequence of activity and allocation of tasks change between key professionals? Often it is these changes and shifts in responsibility which underpin

much of healthcare professionals concern about the implementation of new technologies like the EMR (Georgiou, Ampt, Creswick, Westbrook, & Braithwaite, 2009; J.I. Westbrook et al., 2007)

Communication

The introduction of the EMR is associated with the endeavour to ensure that the right data and information are provided to the right person when needed. Achieving these tasks can be much harder than expected. Communication across the "laboratory–hospital ward" interface can take on different forms, either as synchronous or asynchronous exchange. It is also linked to a complex array of actions involving many different groups and processes (Gorman, Lavelle, & Ash, 2003). Sometimes it is not easy to identify the right data or information needed, let alone when it is needed and by whom. Problems with communication across the hospital are often identified as a major cause of substandard quality of care. This is because the reasons for an adverse event (from a simple mishap to a more serious patient-related safety incident), are generally related to the role that communication plays in how things are planned and organised(Kuziemsky et al., 2009; Sutcliffe, Lewton, & Rosenthal, 2004).

The constitutive role that communication plays in how things are organised is illustrated by a case study of the Blood Bank. The Blood Bank provides compatible blood components for patients along with a range of tests (e.g., blood grouping, antibody screening and identification and pre-transfusion testing). Unlike other pathology laboratory departments, the Blood Bank does more than issue results; it also dispenses blood products(A. Georgiou et al., 2009). These tasks involve a large number of work processes and interrelationships across numerous professions (e.g., haematologists, laboratory scientists, physicians, nurses and technical officers). All these relationships are coordinated through the *synchronous* and coordinated exchange of vital information involving urgent patient-care situations (A. Georgiou et al., 2011).

The Blood Bank provides a valuable example of the importance of *synchronous* information to the safety and quality of care. In contrast, the Microbiology Department offers empirical evidence about *asynchronous* communication and the role that relevant patient information plays in the laboratory's processing and interpretation of test requests. A study that examined the impact of the EMR on the provision of information to the laboratory showed a significant improvement in the provision of relevant patient information that came about from: a) the laboratory's use of the EMR to access clinically relevant information about a patient's reason for admission; and b) improvements in the volume and nature of clinical information entered by physicians into the EMR (Georgiou, Prgomet, Toouli, Callen, & Westbrook, 2011).

CONCLUSION

There are many challenges for hospital laboratory services associated with the implementation and utilisation of the EMR. As a health technology, the EMR has the potential to bring about major shifts in responsibilities, procedures and even work practices (A Georgiou, J Westbrook, & J Braithwaite, 2010). The success or otherwise of EMR implementations are contingent on the conditions and circumstances in which they are placed. The EMR has to be negotiated and refined within each social and technical setting. Frameworks, like the organisational communications framework, derived from existing empirical evidence, provide an important theoretical lens which can help health information technology designers, clinicians and hospital and laboratory professionals deal with the important challenges associated with the implementation of the EMR.

REFERENCES

Aarts, J., Ash, J., & Berg, M. (2007). Extending the understanding of computerized physician order entry: Implications for professional collaboration, workflow and quality of care. *International Journal of Medical Informatics*, *76*(Supplement 1), S4–S13. doi:10.1016/j.ijmedinf.2006.05.009 PMID:16798068

Adam, B. (2004). *Time*. Cambridge, MA: Polity.

Aller, R., Georgiou, A., & Pantanowitz, L. (2012). Electronic Health Records. In L. Pantanowitz, J. M. Tuthill, & U. G. Balis (Eds.), *Pathology Informatics Theory and Practice* (pp. 217–230). Canada: American Society for Clinical Pathology.

Ash, J. S., Stavri, P. Z., Dykstra, R., & Fournier, L. (2003). Implementing Computerized Physician Order Entry: the importance of special people. *International Journal of Medical Informatics*, *69*(2-3), 235–250. doi:10.1016/S1386-5056(02)00107-7 PMID:12810127

Axt-Adam, P., van der Woulden, J. C., & van der Does, E. (1993). Influencing behaviour of physicians ordering laboratory tests: a literature study. *Medical Care*, *31*(9), 784–794. doi:10.1097/00005650-199309000-00003 PMID:8366680

Bates, D., Kuperman, G., Rittenberg, M., Teich, J., Fiskio, J., & Ma'luf, N. et al. (1999). A randomized trial of a computer-based intervention to reduce utilization of redundant laboratory tests. *The American Journal of Medicine*, *106*(2), 144–150. doi:10.1016/S0002-9343(98)00410-0 PMID:10230742

Birkmeyer, C. M., Lee, J., Bates, D. W., & Birkmeyer, J. D. (2002). Will electronic order entry reduce health care costs? *Effective Clinical Practice*, *5*(2), 67–74. PMID:11990214

Black, A., Car, J., Pagliari, C., Anandan, C., Cresswell, K., & Bokun, T. et al. (2011). The Impact of eHealth on the Quality and Safety of Health Care: A Systematic Overview. *PLoS Medicine*, *8*(1). doi:10.1371/journal.pmed.1000387 PMID:21267058

Bobb, A. M., Payne, T. H., & Gross, P. A. (2007). Viewpoint: controversies surrounding use of order sets for clinical decision support in Computerized Provider Order Entry. *Journal of the American Medical Informatics Association*, *14*(1), 41–47. doi:10.1197/jamia.M2184 PMID:17068352

Bonini, P., Plebani, M., Ceriotti, F., & Rubboli, F. (2002). Errors in laboratory medicine. *Clinical Chemistry*, *48*(5), 691–698. PMID:11978595

Buntin, M., Burke, M., Hoaglin, M., & Blumenthal, D. (2011). The benefits of Health Information Technology: A review of the recent literature shows predominantly positive results. *Health Affairs*, *30*(3), 464–471. doi:10.1377/hlthaff.2011.0178 PMID:21383365

Bygstad, B. (2010). Generative mechanisms for innovation in information infrastructures. *Information and Organization*, *20*(3-4), 156–168. doi:10.1016/j.infoandorg.2010.07.001

Callen, J., Paoloni, R., Georgiou, A., Prgomet, M., & Westbrook, J. (2010). The rate of missed test results in an Emergency Department. *Methods of Information in Medicine*, *49*(1), 37–43. PMID:19893851

Callen, J. L., Braithwaite, J., & Westbrook, J. I. (2008). Contextual Implementation Model: A Framework for Assisting Clinical Information System Implementations. *Journal of the American Medical Informatics Association*, *15*(2), 255–262. doi:10.1197/jamia.M2468 PMID:18096917

Chaudhry, B., Wang, J., Wu, S., Maglione, M., Mojica, W., & Roth, E. et al. (2006). Systematic review: impact of health information technology on quality, efficiency, and costs of medical care. *Annals of Internal Medicine*, *144*(10), 742–752. doi:10.7326/0003-4819-144-10-200605160-00125 PMID:16702590

Chen, H. (1990). *Theory-driven evaluations*. Newbury Part, California: Sage Publications.

Clegg, C., Axtell, C., Damodaran, L., Farbey, B., Hull, R., & Lloyd-Jones, R. et al. (1997). Information technology: a study of performance and the role of human and organizational factors. *Ergonomics*, *40*(9), 851–871. doi:10.1080/001401397187694

Coiera, E. (2004). Four rules for the reinvention of health care. *British Medical Journal*, *328*(7449), 1197–1199. doi:10.1136/bmj.328.7449.1197 PMID:15142933

Committee on Patient Safety and Health Information Technology; Institute of Medicine. (2011). *Health IT and Patient Safety: Building Safer Systems for Better Care*. Washington, DC, USA: National Academies Press.

Davidson, E. J. (2005). *Evaluation Methodology Basics*. Thousand Oaks: Sage Publications.

Deeble, J., & Lewis-Hughes, P. (1991). *Directions for pathology*. Melbourne: National Health Strategy.

Fayol, H. (1967). *General and Industrial Management*. London: Pitman.

Fernando, S., Georgiou, A., Holdgate, A., & Westbrook, J. (2009). Challenges associated with electronic ordering in the emergency department: A study of doctors' experiences. *Emergency Medicine Australasia*, *21*(5), 373–378. doi:10.1111/j.1742-6723.2009.01214.x PMID:19840086

Forsman, R. W. (1996). Why is the laboratory an afterthought for managed care organizations? *Clinical Chemistry, 42*(5), 813–816. PMID:8653920

Georgiou, A., Ampt, A., Creswick, N., Westbrook, J., & Braithwaite, J. (2009). Computerized provider order entry - what are health professionals concerned about? A qualitative study in an Australian hospital. *International Journal of Medical Informatics, 78*(1), 60–70. doi:10.1016/j.ijmedinf.2008.09.007 PMID:19010728

Georgiou, A., Greenfield, T., Callen, J., & Westbrook, J. (2009). Safety and efficiency considerations for the introduction of electronic ordering in a Blood Bank. *Archives of Pathology & Laboratory Medicine, 133*(6), 933–937. PMID:19492886

Georgiou, A., Lam, M., Allardice, J., Hart, G. K., & Westbrook, J. I. (2012). Troponin testing in the emergency department: a longitudinal study to assess the impact and sustainability of decision support strategies. *Journal of Clinical Pathology, 65*(6), 546–550. doi:10.1136/jclinpath-2011-200610 PMID:22412052

Georgiou, A., Lang, S., Alvaro, F., Whittaker, G., Westbrook, J. I., & Callen, J. (2007). Pathology's front line - a comparison of the experiences of electronic ordering in the Clinical Chemistry and Haematology departments. In J. Westbrook, E. Coiera, & J. Callen (Eds.), *Information Technology in Health Care; Socio-technical approaches* (pp. 121–132). Sydney, Australia: IOS Press.

Georgiou, A., Lang, S., Rosenfeld, D., & Westbrook, J. I. (2011). The Use of Computerized Provider Order Entry to Improve the Effectiveness and Efficiency of Coagulation Testing. *Archives of Pathology & Laboratory Medicine, 135*, 495–498. PMID:21466368

Georgiou, A., Morse, W., Timmins, W., Ray, S., & Westbrook, J. I. (2008). The use of performance metrics to monitor the impact of CPOE on pathology laboratory services. In S. K. Andersen, G. O. Klein, S. Schulz, J. Aarts & M. Cristina Mazzoleni (Eds.), *eHealth Beyond the Horizon - Get IT There; Proceedings of MIE2008* (pp. 291-296). Amsterdam: IOS Press.

Georgiou, A., Prgomet, M., Paoloni, R., Creswick, N., Hordern, A., Walter, S., & Westbrook, J. (2013). The Effect of Computerized Provider Order Entry Systems on Clinical Care and Work Processes in Emergency Departments: A Systematic Review of the Quantitative Literature. *Annals of Emergency Medicine, 61*(6), 644–653. doi:10.1016/j.annemergmed.2013.01.028 PMID:23548404

Georgiou, A., Prgomet, M., Toouli, G., Callen, J., & Westbrook, J. (2011). What do physicians tell laboratories when requesting tests? A multi-method examination of information supplied to the Microbiology laboratory before and after the introduction of electronic ordering. *International Journal of Medical Informatics, 80*(9), 646–654. doi:10.1016/j.ijmedinf.2011.06.003 PMID:21757400

Georgiou, A., Tariq, A., & Westbrook, J. I. (2013). The temporal landscape of residential aged care facilities-implications for context-sensitive health technology. In M.-C. Beuscart-Zéphir, M. W. M. Jaspers, & C. Kuziemsky (Eds.), *Context Sensitive Health Informatics: Human and Sociotechnical Approaches* (Vol. 194, pp. 69–74). Amsterdam, Netherlands: IOS Press.

Georgiou, A., Westbrook, J., & Braithwaite, J. (2010). Computerized provider order entry systems–Research imperatives and organizational challenges facing pathology services. *Journal of Pathology Informatics, 1*, 11. doi:10.4103/2153-3539.65431 PMID:20805962

Georgiou, A., Westbrook, J., & Braithwaite, J. (2010). What effect does electronic ordering have on the organisation dynamics of a hospital pathology service?. In C. Safran, H. Marin & S. Reti (Eds.), *Partnerships for Effective eHealth Soultions 13th World Congress on Medical and Health Informatics (Medinfo 2010)* (pp. 223-227). Cape Town, South Africa: IOS Press.

Georgiou, A., Westbrook, J., Braithwaite, J., & Iedema, R. (2005). Multiple perspectives on the impact of electronic ordering on hospital organisational and communication processes. *Health Information Management Journal, 34*(4), 130–134. PMID:18216417

Georgiou, A., & Westbrook, J. I. (2007). Computerised Physician Order Entry systems and their effect on pathology laboratories. *Hospital Information Technology Europe, 2007*(Autumn), 40–41.

Georgiou, A., Westbrook, J. I., & Braithwaite, J. (2011). Time matters - a theoretical and empirical examination of the temporal landscape of a hospital pathology service and the impact of e-health. *Social Science & Medicine, 72*, 1603–1610. doi:10.1016/j.socscimed.2011.03.020 PMID:21497430

Georgiou, A., Westbrook, J. I., & Braithwaite, J. (2012). An empirically-derived approach for investigating health information technology: the elementally entangled organisational communication (EEOC) framework. *BMC Medical Informatics and Decision Making, 12*(1), 68. doi:10.1186/1472-6947-12-68 PMID:22788698

Georgiou, A., Westbrook, J. I., Braithwaite, J., Iedema, R., Ray, S., & Forsyth, R. et al. (2007). When requests become orders - A formative investigation into the impact of a Computerized Physician Order Entry system on a pathology laboratory service. *International Journal of Medical Informatics, 76*(8), 583–591. doi:10.1016/j.ijmedinf.2006.04.002 PMID:16702022

Georgiou, A., Westbrook, J. I., Callen, J. L., & Braithwaite, J. (2008). Electronic test management systems and hospital pathology laboratory services. In N. Wickramasinghe & E. Geisler (Eds.), *Encyclopaedia of Healthcare Information Systems* (Vol. II, pp. 505–512). Hershey, PA: Medical Information Science Reference. doi:10.4018/978-1-59904-889-5.ch064

Georgiou, A., Williamson, M., Westbrook, J., & Ray, S. (2007). The impact of computerised physician order entry systems on pathology services: a systematic review. *International Journal of Medical Informatics, 76*(7), 514–529. doi:10.1016/j.ijmedinf.2006.02.004 PMID:16567121

Giddens, A. (1990). *The consequences of modernity*. Stanford, CA: Stanford University Press.

Gorman, P. N., Lavelle, M. B., & Ash, J. S. (2003). Order creation and communication in healthcare. *Methods of Information in Medicine, 42*(4), 376–384. PMID:14534637

Greenhalgh, T., & Russell, J. (2010). Why Do Evaluations of eHealth Programs Fail? An Alternative Set of Guiding Principles. *PLoS Medicine, 7*(11), e1000360. doi:10.1371/journal.pmed.1000360 PMID:21072245

Hawkins, R. C. (2007). Laboratory turnaround time. *The Clinical Biochemist. Reviews / Australian Association of Clinical Biochemists, 28,* 179–194. PMID:18392122

Jones, S. S., Rudin, R. S., Perry, T., & Shekelle, P. G. (2014). Health Information Technology: An Updated Systematic Review With a Focus on Meaningful Use. *Annals of Internal Medicine, 160*(1), 48–54. doi:10.7326/M13-1531 PMID:24573664

Kuziemsky, C., Borycki, E., Purkis, M., Black, F., Boyle, M., & Cloutier-Fisher, D. et al. (2009). An interdisciplinary team communication framework and its application to healthcare'e-teams' systems design. *BMC Medical Informatics and Decision Making, 9*(1), 43. doi:10.1186/1472-6947-9-43 PMID:19754966

Legg, M., & Cheong, I. (2004). *A Study of the Impact of the Use of General Practice Computer Systems on the Ordering of Pathology.* Retrieved from http://www.nhhrc.org.au/internet/main/publishing.nsf/Content/qupp-qupp-reports.htm

Mekhjian, H. S., Kumar, R. R., Kuehn, L., Bentley, T. D., Teater, P., & Thomas, A. et al. (2002). Immediate benefits realized following implementation of physician order entry at an academic medical center. *Journal of the American Medical Informatics Association, 9*(5), 529–539. doi:10.1197/jamia.M1038 PMID:12223505

Menou, M. J., & Taylor, R. D. (2006). A "grand challenge": Measuring information societies. *The Information Society, 22*(5), 261–267. doi:10.1080/01972240600903904

National Coalition of Public Pathology. (2012). *Encouraging Quality Pathology Ordering in Australia's Public Hospitals.* National Coalition of Public Pathology.

Organisation for Economic Co-operation Development. (2011). *OECD Guide to Measuring the Information Society 2011.* OECD.

Overhage, J. M., Tierney, W. M., Zhou, X.-H., & McDonald, C. J. (1997). A randomized trial of "corollary orders" to prevent errors of omission. *Journal of the American Medical Informatics Association, 4*(5), 364–375. doi:10.1136/jamia.1997.0040364 PMID:9292842

Pantanowitz, L., Henricks, W. H., & Beckwith, B. A. (2007). Medical laboratory informatics. *Clinics in Laboratory Medicine, 27*(4), 823–843. doi:10.1016/j.cll.2007.07.011 PMID:17950900

Peute, L., Aarts, J., Bakker, P., & Jaspers, M. (2009). Anatomy of a failure: A sociotechnical evaluation of a laboratory physician order entry system implementation. *International Journal of Medical Informatics.* PMID:19640778

Peute, L. W. P., & Jaspers, M. W. M. (2007). The significance of a usability evaluation of an emerging laboratory order entry system. *International Journal of Medical Informatics, 76*(2-3), 157–168. doi:10.1016/j.ijmedinf.2006.06.003 PMID:16854617

Poole, M. S. (2004). Central Issues in the study of change and innovation. In M. Poole & A. Van de Ven (Eds.), *Handbook of Organizational Change and Innovation* (pp. 3–31). New York: Oxford University Press.

Price, C. P. (2003). Application of the principles of evidence-based medicine to laboratory medicine. *Clinica Chimica Acta, 333*(2), 147–154. doi:10.1016/S0009-8981(03)00179-7 PMID:12849898

Putnam, L., Nicotera, A., & McPhee, R. (2009). Introduction - Communication Constitutes Organization. In L. Putnam & A. Nicotera (Eds.), *Building Theories of Organization - The Consitutive Role of Communication* (p. 222). New York: Routledge.

Sackett, D. L., Rosenberg, W. M., Gray, J. A., Haynes, R. B., & Richardson, W. S. (1996). Evidence based medicine: what it is and what it isn't. *British Medical Journal, 312*(7023), 71–72. doi:10.1136/bmj.312.7023.71 PMID:8555924

Scriven, M. (1991). *Evaluation Thesaurus* (4th ed.). Newbury, CA: Sage.

Sutcliffe, K. M., Lewton, E., & Rosenthal, M. M. (2004). Communication failures: an insidious contributor to medical mishaps. *Academic Medicine, 79*(2), 186. doi:10.1097/00001888-200402000-00019 PMID:14744724

The World Alliance For Patient Safety Drafting Group. (2009). Towards an International Classification for Patient Safety: the conceptual framework. *International Journal for Quality in Health Care, 21*(1), 2–8. doi:10.1093/intqhc/mzn054 PMID:19147595

van Walraven, C., & Raymond, M. (2003). Population-based study of repeat laboratory testing. *Clinical Chemistry, 49*(12), 1997–2005. doi:10.1373/clinchem.2003.021220 PMID:14633870

Wajcman, J. (2008). Life in the fast lane? Towards a sociology of technology and time. *The British Journal of Sociology, 59*(1), 59–77. doi:10.1111/j.1468-4446.2007.00182.x PMID:18321331

Westbrook, J. I., Braithwaite, J., Georgiou, A., Ampt, A., Creswick, N., Coiera, E., & Iedema, R. (2007). Multimethod evaluation of information and communication technologies in health in the context of wicked problems and sociotechnical theory. *Journal of the American Medical Informatics Association, 14*(6), 746–755. doi:10.1197/jamia.M2462 PMID:17712083

Westbrook, J. I., Georgiou, A., Dimos, A., & Germanos, T. (2006). Computerised pathology test order-entry reduces laboratory turnaround times and influences tests ordered by hospital clinicians: a controlled before and after study. *Journal of Clinical Pathology, 59*(May), 533–536. doi:10.1136/jcp.2005.029983 PMID:16461564

Westbrook, J. I., Georgiou, A., & Lam, M. (2009). Does computerised provider order entry reduce test turnaround times? A before-and-after study at four hospitals. In K.-P. Adlassnig, B. Blobel, J. Mantas, & I. Masic (Eds.), *Medical informatics in a united and healthy Europe: proceedings of MIE 2009* (pp. 527–531). Amsterdam: IOS Press.

Westbrook, J. I., Georgiou, A., & Rob, M. (2009). Test turnaround times and mortality rates 12 and 24 months after the introduction of a computerised provider order entry system. *Methods of Information in Medicine, 48*, 211–215. PMID:19283321

Westbrook, J. I., Georgiou, A., & Rob, M. I. (2008). Computerised order entry systems: sustained impact on laboratory efficiency and mortality rates?. In S. Andersen, G. Klein, S. Schulz, J. Aarts & M. Mazzoleni (Eds.), *eHealth Beyond the Horizon Get IT There; Proceedings of MIE 2008 IOS Press Amsterdam* (pp. 345-350). Goteborg, Sweden: IOS Press.

Whetton, S., & Georgiou, A. (2010). Conceptual challenges for advancing the socio-technical underpinnings of health informatics. *The Open Medical Informatics Journal, 4*, 221. doi:10.2174/1874325001004010221 PMID:21594009

ADDITIONAL READING

Aller, R., Georgiou, A., & Pantanowitz, L. (2012). Electronic Health Records. In L. Pantanowitz, J. M. Tuthill, & U. G. Balis (Eds.), *Pathology Informatics Theory and Practice* (pp. 217–230). Canada: American Society for Clinical Pathology.

Ash, J. S., Berg, M., & Coiera, E. (2004). Some unintended consequences of information technology in health care: the nature of patient care information system-related errors. *Journal of the American Medical Informatics Association*, *11*(2), 104–112. doi:10.1197/jamia.M1471 PMID:14633936

Barley, S. (1988). On technology, time, and social order: technically induced change in the temporal organization of radiological work. In F. Dubinskas (Ed.), *Making time: ethnographies of high-technology organizations* (pp. 123–169). Philadelphia: Temple University Press.

Bates, D. W., Boyle, D. L., Rittenberg, E., & Kuperman, G. J., Ma'Luf, N., Menkin, V.,... Tanasijevic, M. J. (1998). What proportion of common diagnostic tests appear redundant? *The American Journal of Medicine*, *104*(4), 361–368. doi:10.1016/S0002-9343(98)00063-1 PMID:9576410

Berg, M. (2001). Implementing information systems in health care organizations: myths and challenges. *International Journal of Medical Informatics*, *64*(2-3), 143–156. doi:10.1016/S1386-5056(01)00200-3 PMID:11734382

Berg, M., Aarts, J., & van der Lei, J. (2003). ICT in health care: sociotechnical approaches. *Methods of Information in Medicine*, *42*(4), 297–301. PMID:14534625

Callen, J. L., Braithwaite, J., & Westbrook, J. I. (2008). Contextual Implementation Model: A Framework for Assisting Clinical Information System Implementations. *Journal of the American Medical Informatics Association*, *15*(2), 255–262. doi:10.1197/jamia.M2468 PMID:18096917

Coiera, E. (2003). *Guide to Health Informatics* (2nd ed.). London: Oxford University Press. doi:10.1201/b13618

Coiera, E. (2004). Four rules for the reinvention of health care. *British Medical Journal*, *328*(7449), 1197–1199. doi:10.1136/bmj.328.7449.1197 PMID:15142933

Connelly, D., & Aller, R. (1997). Outcomes and informatics. *Archives of Pathology & Laboratory Medicine*, *121*(11), 1176–1182. PMID:9372745

Dighe, A. S., Soderberg, B. L., & Laposata, M. (2001). Narrative interpretations for clinical laboratory evaluations: an overview. *American Journal of Clinical Pathology*, *116*(8), S123–S128. PMID:11993697

Friedman, B. A., & Mitchell, W. (1991). Using the laboratory information system to achieve strategic advantage over the competitors of hospital-based clinical laboratories. *Clinics in Laboratory Medicine*, *11*(1), 187–202. PMID:2040141

Friedman, C. P. (2013). What informatics is and isn't. *Journal of the American Medical Informatics Association*, *20*(2), 224–226. doi:10.1136/amiajnl-2012-001206 PMID:23059730

Georgiou, A. (2001). Health informatics and evidence based medicine - more than a marriage of convenience? *Health Informatics Journal*, *7*(3-4), 127–130. doi:10.1177/146045820100700303

Georgiou, A. (2002). Data information and knowledge: the health informatics model and its role in evidence-based medicine. *Journal of Evaluation in Clinical Practice, 8*(2), 127–130. doi:10.1046/j.1365-2753.2002.00345.x PMID:12180361

Georgiou, A., Ampt, A., Creswick, N., Westbrook, J., & Braithwaite, J. (2009). Computerized provider order entry - what are health professionals concerned about? A qualitative study in an Australian hospital. *International Journal of Medical Informatics, 78*(1), 60–70. doi:10.1016/j.ijmedinf.2008.09.007 PMID:19010728

Georgiou, A., Callen, J., Westbrook, J., Prgomet, M., & Toouli, G. (2007). Information and communication processes in the microbiology laboratory - implications for Computerised Provider Order Entry. In K. Kuhn, J. Warren & L. Tze-Yun (Eds.), *12th World Congress on Health (Medical) Informatics Medinfo 2007* (Vol. 2, pp. 943-947). Amsterdam: IOS Press.

Georgiou, A., Greenfield, T., Callen, J., & Westbrook, J. (2009). Safety and efficiency considerations for the introduction of electronic ordering in a Blood Bank. *Archives of Pathology & Laboratory Medicine, 133*(6), 933–937. PMID:19492886

Georgiou, A., Lam, M., Allardice, J., Hart, G. K., & Westbrook, J. I. (2012). Troponin testing in the emergency department: a longitudinal study to assess the impact and sustainability of decision support strategies. *Journal of Clinical Pathology, 65*(6), 546–550. doi:10.1136/jclinpath-2011-200610 PMID:22412052

Georgiou, A., Lang, S., Rosenfeld, D., & Westbrook, J. I. (2011). The Use of Computerized Provider Order Entry to Improve the Effectiveness and Efficiency of Coagulation Testing. *Archives of Pathology & Laboratory Medicine, 135*, 495–498. PMID:21466368

Georgiou, A., Prgomet, M., Paoloni, R., Creswick, N., Hordern, A., Walter, S., & Westbrook, J. (2013). The Effect of Computerized Provider Order Entry Systems on Clinical Care and Work Processes in Emergency Departments: A Systematic Review of the Quantitative Literature. *Annals of Emergency Medicine, 61*(6), 644–653. doi:10.1016/j.annemergmed.2013.01.028 PMID:23548404

Georgiou, A., Westbrook, J., & Braithwaite, J. (2010). Computerized provider order entry systems–Research imperatives and organizational challenges facing pathology services. *Journal of Pathology Informatics, 1*, 11. doi:10.4103/2153-3539.65431 PMID:20805962

Georgiou, A., Westbrook, J. I., & Braithwaite, J. (2011). Time matters - a theoretical and empirical examination of the temporal landscape of a hospital pathology service and the impact of e-health. *Social Science & Medicine, 72*, 1603–1610. doi:10.1016/j.socscimed.2011.03.020 PMID:21497430

Georgiou, A., Westbrook, J. I., & Braithwaite, J. (2012). An empirically-derived approach for investigating Health Information Technology: the Elementally Entangled Organisational Communication (EEOC) framework. *BMC Medical Informatics and Decision Making, 12*(1), 68. doi:10.1186/1472-6947-12-68 PMID:22788698

Georgiou, A., Westbrook, J. I., Braithwaite, J., Iedema, R., Ray, S., & Forsyth, R. et al. (2007). When requests become orders - A formative investigation into the impact of a Computerized Physician Order Entry system on a pathology laboratory service. *International Journal of Medical Informatics, 76*(8), 583–591. doi:10.1016/j.ijmedinf.2006.04.002 PMID:16702022

Georgiou, A., Williamson, M., Westbrook, J., & Ray, S. (2007). The impact of computerised physician order entry systems on pathology services: a systematic review. *International Journal of Medical Informatics, 76*(7), 514–529. doi:10.1016/j.ijmedinf.2006.02.004 PMID:16567121

Kim, J. Y., Kamis, I. K., Singh, B., Batra, S., Dixon, R. H., & Dighe, A. S. (2011). Implementation of computerized add-on testing for hospitalized patients in a large academic medical center. *Clinical Chemistry and Laboratory Medicine, 49*(5), 845–850. doi:10.1515/CCLM.2011.140 PMID:21303296

Kuperman, G. J., Teich, J. M., Gandhi, T. K., & Bates, D. W. (2001). Patient safety and computerized medication ordering at Brigham and Women's Hospital. *Joint Commission Journal on Quality and Safety, 27*(10), 509–521. PMID:11593885

Leonardi, P. M., & Barley, S. R. (2008). Materiality and change: Challenges to building better theory about technology and organizing. *Information and Organization, 18*(3), 159–176. doi:10.1016/j.infoandorg.2008.03.001

Pantanowitz, L., Henricks, W. H., & Beckwith, B. A. (2007). Medical laboratory informatics. *Clinics in Laboratory Medicine, 27*(4), 823–843. doi:10.1016/j.cll.2007.07.011 PMID:17950900

Pantanowitz, L., Tuthill, J. M., & Balis, U. G. (Eds.). (2012). *Pathology Informatics - Theory & Practice*. Canada: American Society for Clinical Pathology.

Peute, L., Aarts, J., Bakker, P., & Jaspers, M. (2009). Anatomy of a failure: A sociotechnical evaluation of a laboratory physician order entry system implementation. *International Journal of Medical Informatics*. PMID:19640778

Peute, L. W. P., & Jaspers, M. W. M. (2007). The significance of a usability evaluation of an emerging laboratory order entry system. *International Journal of Medical Informatics, 76*(2-3), 157–168. doi:10.1016/j.ijmedinf.2006.06.003 PMID:16854617

Putnam, L., Nicotera, A., & McPhee, R. (2009). Introduction - Communication Constitutes Organization. In L. Putnam & A. Nicotera (Eds.), *Building Theories of Organization - The Consitutive Role of Communication* (p. 222). New York: Routledge.

Putnam, L., & Pacanowsky, M. E. (1983). *Communication and organizations, an interpretive approach* (Vol. 65). Sage Publications, Inc.

Westbrook, J. I., Georgiou, A., Dimos, A., & Germanos, T. (2006). Computerised pathology test order-entry reduces laboratory turnaround times and influences tests ordered by hospital clinicians: a controlled before and after study. *Journal of Clinical Pathology, 59*(May), 533–536. doi:10.1136/jcp.2005.029983 PMID:16461564

Westbrook, J. I., Georgiou, A., & Lam, M. (2009). Does computerised provider order entry reduce test turnaround times? A before-and-after study at four hospitals. In K.-P. Adlassnig, B. Blobel, J. Mantas, & I. Masic (Eds.), *Medical informatics in a united and healthy Europe: proceedings of MIE 2009* (pp. 527–531). Amsterdam: IOS Press.

Westbrook, J. I., Georgiou, A., & Rob, M. I. (2008). Computerised order entry systems: sustained impact on laboratory efficiency and mortality rates?. In S. Andersen, G. Klein, S. Schulz, J. Aarts & M. Mazzoleni (Eds.), *eHealth Beyond the Horizon Get IT There; Proceedings of MIE 2008 IOS Press Amsterdam* (pp. 345-350). Goteborg, Sweden: IOS Press.

Whetton, S., & Georgiou, A. (2010). Conceptual challenges for advancing the socio-technical underpinnings of health informatics. *The Open Medical Informatics Journal*, *4*, 221. doi:10.2174/1874325001004010221 PMID:21594009

KEY TERMS AND DEFINITIONS

Commercial System: System software purchased from a software developer (also referred to as an "off-the-shelf" system).

Computerised Provider Order Entry: Computer systems that allow physicians (or other authorised staff) to electronically issue orders, e.g., laboratory tests, medical imaging, diets, medications.

Electronic Decision Support System: Electronically-stored knowledge which can be used to aid health care decisions.

Electronic Medical Record (EMR): Computerised medical record which is found in an organisation that provides health care. The EMR encompasses tasks related to the storage, retrieval and modification of record.

Evaluation: To determine the merit, worth, or value of something, or the product of that process (Scriven, 1991).

Home-Grown System: Systems developed within the hospital or clinical setting in which they are used.

Impact: Change or (sometimes) lack of change caused by an evaluand (that which is being evaluated). Can also mean outcome or effect (Davidson, 2005).

Organisational Communication: A theoretical perspective which emphasises the essential (constitutive) role that communication processes play in the makeup of an organisation (Putnam et al., 2009).

Test Appropriateness: While there are many pathology tests that are conducted repeatedly in order to monitor a condition or treatment, when a repeat test is ordered within a brief time frame there is a high likelihood that it will be redundant and provide no additional information (National Coalition of Public Pathology, 2012; van Walraven & Raymond, 2003).

Turnaround Times (TAT): Can be defined as the time of physician order request to when the physician views the result (Total TAT), or the time a request and accompanying specimen arrive at the laboratory, to the time a result is dispatched (Laboratory TAT)(A Georgiou, M Williamson, et al., 2007; Hawkins, 2007).

This work was previously published in Laboratory Management Information Systems edited by Anastasius Moumtzoglou, Anastasia Kastania, and Stavros Archondakis, pages 50-66 copyright year 2015 by Medical Information Science Reference (an imprint of IGI Global).

Chapter 5
The Importance of Information and Communication Technologies in Establishing Healthcare Services with a Universal Coverage

Davuthan Günaydin
Namık Kemal University, Turkey

GamzeYıldız Şeren
Namık Kemal University, Turkey

Hakan Cavlak
Namık Kemal University, Turkey

Korhan Arun
Namık Kemal University, Turkey

ABSTRACT

One of the most important challenges faced by the healthcare system is the organization of healthcare services to cope with the increase in population and aging of citizens. Especially in developing countries, demographic movements of the population, regional disparities, political concerns, and increasing expectations of health services have led to a search for new ways to serve all of the population with healthcare services. With traditional methods, it is not possible to increase the supply of health services because of inadequate infrastructure and shortcomings in quantity and quality of healthcare staff. This new health system called e-health and uses all of the possibilities provided by information and communication technologies that aim to improve public health. In this chapter, the effects of e-health practices on the quality and accessibility of healthcare services are assessed and the extent of e-health practices in Turkey are evaluated.

INTRODUCTION

One of the most important problems occurring in offering healthcare services is that the organization of healthcare services becomes difficult due to increase in population and aging effect. Especially in the developing countries, such reasons as demographical waves in population, geographical distribution of population, regional development differences and political concerns and increase

DOI: 10.4018/978-1-4666-8756-1.ch005

in expectation from the healthcare services have lead developing countries into looking for ways of re-structuring the healthcare services to include everybody. In reality, these countries don't have an established healthcare services system and this structure is not possible due to increasing demand of healthcare services via traditional methods, inefficient health infrastructure, and lack of qualified healthcare staff and inefficient funds of these countries.

At this point, technological developments present new solutions offering to meet the mentioned inefficiencies. The use of information and communication technology, which is rapidly developing especially since the beginning of the 21th century in the field of healthcare services, helped eliminate many problems related to the offering of healthcare services and also enabled people living in the developing countries to reach healthcare services. Communication opportunities provided by these technologies have important functions in eliminating the disadvantages resulting from geographical distances, regional development differences and health infrastructure. Especially the increased use of mobile telephones and internet in the last decade resulted in the healthcare services being re-organized via using these technological infrastructures. This increase has also enabled governments and non-governmental organizations to reach disadvantaged regions and people living in these regions via using these opportunities of information and communication technologies.

The new understanding of healthcare services, referred to as e-health, aims to improve individual and public health by means of using all the opportunities provided by the information and communication technologies. Especially the applications of tele-medicine and m-health increase the quality of healthcare services in the developed countries and also these applications are presenting a role model to realize a universal healthcare system in the case of developing countries.

UNIVERSALISM IN HEALTHCARE SERVICES

The most important issue discussed in the field of healthcare services is whether it is possible to develop a system from which every person is able to benefit. Especially, in many of the developing countries, which do not have an established healthcare system, a significant rate of the population cannot reach the healthcare services or they have to pay for the use of healthcare services due to not having efficient social security. This situation causes the poor and disadvantaged people to be deprived of the healthcare services and also harms public consensus.

The main equity principle for the use of healthcare services is to enable all the citizens to access the healthcare services equally through the existent health institutes (public and private) of the country (NERA, 2009, p. 8). The concept of health is of equal importance for all people. The fact that people are poor or rich and they live in rural or urban area does not create a difference in their needs of health services. However, especially in the developing countries people living in urban areas with a high financial ability benefit from healthcare services much further compared to people living in the rural areas. People living in urban areas also know the procedure to reach the healthcare services better and so they can easily reach both public and private healthcare services. In fact, low cost investments on basic healthcare services made by governments can increase the general healthcare conditions and healthcare development of the country. However, especially in the developing countries, it has been seen that already limited health funds are used mostly for expensive technologies and urban areas (Akin &Ferranti, 1988, p.2).

The concept of globalization that became a slogan with the statement of "new world order" after 1980 lead nearly all countries to transform their economic and political structures with the prediction that nearly all of the countries cannot opt out of this process (Yaşgül, 2002, p. 211). This new order with the aim of unlimited and lawless capital flows and also creating a global market mentioned in the philosophy of "laissez faire" by eliminating all the obstacles of the free market economy imposes the thought that the government stays in the minimum level and the operation of economy should be left to the actors of free market.

It has been seen that the countries have a tendency in amending their practices of healthcare against this global imposition. Previously, eliminating the social risks in the national level was included in the content of health policies, however, today it comes forth as a concept supporting global capital. Social solidarity and assistance is defeated to personal interests and health expenses are regarded as an obstacle for the development of nation state (Pepe, 2006, pp. 136-137).

The nation states have a tendency in leaving less resources for the healthcare sector with the effect of globalization. However, it has been known that globalization increases the cost of health related goods and services, rather than decreasing it. Because, commercial agreements and audit practices of international organizations for patent and authors royalties increased significantly the prices of medicines. The increase in cost and price of pharmaceuticals affects both the underdeveloped countries and developed countries. Also it has been known that the dispute between the trade rights and health rights makes fundamental human rights of secondary importance. Also commercial buildings are in favor of the developed countries from the aspect of the health sector and medicine industry while it is to the detriment of underdeveloped and undeveloped countries. Because, it has been known that health policies of many countries are implemented in the name of protecting trade rights of the developed countries and multinational corporations, this situation puts the public health interests to jeopardy (Koivusalo, 2006, p. 20).

TECHNOLOGY AND HEALTHCARE SERVICES

Health technologies can be described as processes determining the use of medicines, medical equipment and medical and surgical procedures for healthcare services and also determining the offering of healthcare services within the scope of an organizational system (Garrdo, Zentner & Busse, 2008, pp. 55-57). This is a very comprehensive description and it states that not only the evaluation of medicine for the medical treatment, equipment or procedures but also the evaluation of health policies should be included within the health technologies.

Technological innovations cause many developments from offering the healthcare services to medical diagnosis and treatment equipment and from the structure of the organization to the qualification. Even, technology has become a basic factor determining the quality of the health services. But this also caused the increase in the health expenses after the II. World War. During 1960s and 1970s, the expenses made for healthcare services by the governments gained a sharp momentum (Docteur & Oxley, 2003, p. 44-48). Medical technology rapidly developing since 1980s brought about new treatment opportunities. These developments were also effective in changing the thoughts on reliance on healthcare services, efficiency, service quality and prestige. As a result, the institutions offering healthcare services remained under pressure on the issue of adapting to the new technologies (Erener & Yelkikan, 2006, p. 10).

Research studies on health policies indicate that efficient and ethical use of health technology is an important factor in terms of creating resources for health systems. Taking into account important developments in the health technology, the European Union attracts attention to Health Technology Assessment for the effective organization, distribution and use of the health technologies. According to the health technology assessment, such social, institutional, legal and ethical factors as security, effectiveness, cost and cost limitation criteria are not taken into account. This application is settled in many of the EU countries. Moreover, analysis methods are developed and practiced for the assessment of new technologies.

It is clear that there is a close relationship between the healthcare services sector and technological developments. According to the World Health Organization, technology is the most important factor in prevention, diagnosis and treatment of diseases. According to the World Bank, reliable information and effective communication play an important role in public health practices. The use of suitable technologies increases the quality in healthcare services and the individuals can keep up with their own health status with the help of information and communication technologies (WITSA, 2006, p. 2).

For the solution of the problems that the countries are experiencing, it is not possible to talk about a model to be adapted to all countries within the reforms necessary to realize in the field of healthcare services. However, it is taken into account that the information and communication technologies increased the access to the healthcare services and also the quality of services and contributed to take the expenses under control. In this respect, it is possible to improve the fields of public health, first aid, long-term care services, clinical care, medical training, nutrition and hygiene (WITSA, 2006, p. 3).

It has been stated that especially for many of the low and middle income countries where the access to healthcare services, the quality and cost of the service is a problem, the use of information and communication technology tools will be beneficial to establish a new healthcare services to which all people can easily reach (Lewis, Synowiec, Lagomarsinoa & Schweitze, 2012, p. 332).

E-HEALTH

The developments in the information and communication technologies cause changes in many fields such as economic, social, and cultural. The healthcare services also take its share from these developments and the healthcare services are increasingly integrated with information and communication technologies. This integration reinforces electronic information flow and support the management and provision of healthcare services. So, the costs and accessibility of the healthcare services can be monitored.

On the other hand, healthcare services supported by the information and communication technologies bring changes to the management and provision of healthcare services and also make easier the offering of healthcare services at a national and international level by means of personal and public health. By these means, the information flow is supported in a wide range from molecular genetics to humanitarian aid. This also makes possible the offering of decentralized healthcare service (WHO & IT, 2012, p. 18).

The use of information and communication technologies in the field of health-care services is called e-health. World Health Organization also describes e-health as using information and communication technologies for healthcare services (WHO & IT, 2012, p. 17). The European Union E-Health Research Area Action Plan also describes e-health as the effect of all functions of information and communication technology applications on the health sector (European Commission, 2007, p. 23).

E-health investments come into prominence in the offering of optimal health services for all citizens with its quality to integrate and combine all the actors from different positions, functions and factors in the healthcare service. Moreover, e-health investments also give chance to increase effectiveness and efficiency in all stages of healthcare services by means of information sharing.

Through the use of e-health systems, it is possible to communicate the information on health related issues to any place if and when requested by a party, and also protecting such values as privacy and secrecy. So, the quality, reliability, accessibility and the use of capacity of the health services will be increased along with the training of the providers of healthcare services. This situation will inevitably support the providers of healthcare services at all levels in diagnosing, treatment and prevention of the diseases. This also will give the opportunity to establish a new system which is reliable and accountable in the distribution and provision of medicines, vaccines and medical equipment (WHO & IT, 2012, p. 18).

It has been stated that the most important benefit of using information and communication technologies in healthcare services especially from the aspect of developing countries that do not have an established health system is that, this increases the access to healthcare services. In the World Health Assembly in 2005, it was stressed that e-health can be a solution for the development, security, quality and efficiency of healthcare services. On the other hand, it has been also stated that e-health proposes solutions against demographical changes, the threat of contagious disease, the increase in lifespan and the increase in health expenses depending on the developments in technology (Pijen, Wynchank, Covvey, & Ossebaard, 2012, p. 323).

In the EU countries, the understanding of regarding e-health as an indispensable part of the healthcare services has been increasingly widespread. E-health comes into prominence in the policies implemented to increase the health expenses and for the most efficient and effective offering of healthcare services within the Union. It has been evaluated that with the technology-based tools, the prevention, diagnosis, treatment, observation of diseases and management of life style will be possible (European Commission, 2007, p. 23).

Briefly, the reasons that make e-health important can be explained as reaching to patient history much easily, the patients' easier access to suggestions and easier access of patients to distance-consultation, tele-medicine applications and first aid services. E-health also enables the distance observation of the patients. On the other hand, e-health also gives the opportunity to provide better training possibilities to the health personnel, to store data and to manage patient records and also the transfer of accounts in this way (WHO, 2012b, p. 330). In general terms, the use of information and communication technologies in health sector is categorized under four main titles. These are communication systems, managerial systems, decision-support systems and information systems (King et al., 2010, p. 352).

In a research conducted by World Health Organization and International Telecommunication Union (WHO & IT, 2012, p. 19) it was determined that seven steps should be taken to establish health systems. The first step is leadership and management. Leadership and management is the stage of completing the leadership and managerial process required for establishment of international health system. In this process, the relationships, roles and responsibilities, administrative structure and mechanisms of governmental and non-governmental organizations and national, regional and local government institutions should be determined. Moreover, the preferred governance and leadership model should be determined. The next step is the determination of national e-health strategy and its framework and then comes the strategy and investment step in which the necessary investments are determined to process and maintain the system by these means. In this step, it is necessary to explain the investment components required to develop and support e-health environment.

The third step is services and practices. In this process, the targets of e-health service are determined. These targets should be realistic and in compliance with the needs of providers of health service and managers. The content of this step should include the accessibility of the shareholders, the share and use of health information and the methods to offer health services. In addition, the development of health information flow should be conducted and the method to offer health services by using electronic systems should be determined within this process.

The fourth step is the infrastructure of e-health. In this process, it is required to set an infrastructure system that will enable the sharing of health information that makes sense within the borders of geography and health sector. The system should also be supportive for the innovations and developments in the offering methods of health services and the information systems. The research studies indicate that the countries which significantly made a progress at an international level primarily set up an infrastructure of health systems that supports health information exchange. The infrastructure to be set up should support physical technology, software technologies and the share of health information in the health sector.

The fifth step is standards and collaboration. In order to ensure an effective system e-health standards and collaboration should comprise all the shareholders. This is especially required for information exchange and accurate collection of data. Without this factor, it is not possible to collect consistent health information. Due to data structure and inconsistency in terminology, some problems on misinterpretation and information exchange may arise.

The sixth step is regulations, policy and harmonization process. The regulations and policies of the country should be in line with the development of practice of e-health. Especially, political will and stability are indispensable for safe establishment and functioning of the system. Legal gaps especially require a faultless construct because they can cause malfunctions in information exchange and diagnoses and treatments. The final step is labor force. The labor force should design, develop, operate and support the national

e-health system in quality and in quantity. While the health personnel perform their duty they should perfectly use the tools of e-health as a part of their job. They should also collaborate with the experts of information technologies.

E-HEALTH APPLICATION TOOLS

The opportunities offered by information and communication technologies enable to carry out different e-health practices. In fact, e-health better building and management of the complex structure ranging from the planning of health systems to patient satisfaction in the direction of the opportunities provided by technological developments. In this context, it is possible to mention about various e-health applications. The most widespread of these applications are tele-medicine, electronic health records, hospital information systems and mobile health (m-health).

Tele-Medicine

Tele-medicine is one of the specific applications of e-health. The word "tele" means "distance" in Ancient Greek and "mederi" means to cure and heal in Latin language. The first example of the application was the transfer of electro-cardiogram data via using telephone lines in the beginning of 20th century (WHO, 2010, p. 9). In modern sense, the first use was realized in the beginning of 1960s. Closed circuit television system was used in the first practice and this practice was conducted between a local mental health and disorders hospital in the United States of America and the psychiatry institution which is in a distance of 180 km. In the same period, the necessity of continuous existence of doctors was eliminated with the help of a video-conference system set up in an airport. In the future periods, specific practices were carried out especially in America and Canada depending on the development of satellite technology. Today, thanks to the improved information and communication technologies, tele-medicine applications are becoming widespread (Işık & Güler, 2010, p. 2).

WHO describes tele-medicine as conducting diagnosis and treatment and preventing diseases via information exchange by means of information and communication technologies with all the health personnel and increasing the health quality of individuals and public by means of maintaining the continuous training of the providers of health services (Vittacca, Mazzü, & Scalvini, 2009, p. 92). In general, it can be stated that the aims of tele-medicine applications are to provide clinical support, to enable the individuals living far away from each other to overcome the geographical obstacles via communication and to improve the health outputs by means of using different kinds of information and communication technologies.

The recent technological developments and the increasing use of information and communication technologies have resulted in widespread use of tele-medicine. So, new opportunities for health services and their presentation have been created. Especially the use of digital systems rather than analog systems has brought about reductions in the cost of information and communication technologies and this has enabled the providers of health services to widely use tele-medicine applications. This situation also has lead to the ability to offer a much efficient service from the point of view of the organizations offering health systems (WHO, 2010, p. 9).

The application area of tele-medicine is comprised of tele-dermatology, tele-pathology and tele-radiology. Tele-medicine is examined under two categories according to the timing of information transfer and the interaction between the parties (Ouma & Herselman, 2009, p. 194). The first one of these is asynchronous applications that the data is registered in advance and then stored. This application includes the exchange of information that is previously registered in different times between two or more people. The patient or a health personnel can send information on medical status of his/her via electronic

mail to a doctor or a specialist and also can give information on diagnose and treatment via e-mail. In the second application, the individuals make the information exchange immediately and on a real-time basis by means of tele-conference or similar systems (WHO, 2010, p. 9).

Tele-medicine includes many applications as tele-nursing care at home, electronic information transfer to hospitals and specialists, tele-consultations among specialists and practitioners and online health services via call-centers (Vittacca et al., 2009, p. 92). Also this application enables doctors and nurses taking office in rural areas to continue their training and offices without taking into consideration time and distance factors. On the other hand, it eliminates the necessity for the health personnel and patients to travel to the long-distance hospitals and also prevent them from making great expenses (Ouma & Herselman, 2009, p. 194; Wootton et al., 2012, p. 341). Especially in the underdeveloped countries and regions with an insufficient health infrastructure, tele-medicine applications are the most significant links between the providers of health services and specialists and reference hospitals and regional health centers. Especially with the aim of observation of chronically ill patients, such equipment as heart monitoring devices, biometrical measuring tools of blood pressure and blood glucose are being increasingly used (WHO, 2010, p. 9).

Even though tele-medicine applications propose new solution offers for the countries without an established health system and underdeveloped regions, it has been seen that in practice, the developed countries have been using tele-medicine services much more compared with the developing countries. This can be evaluated as being due to the fact that developing countries do not have efficient funds, technology and political will to establish a tele-medicine infrastructure. The research studies (Alkmim et al., 2012, p. 374; Wootton et al., 2012, pp. 341-343) show that the tele-medicine applications are cost-effective, they increase the access to health services and improve health outputs. All the benefits can be obtained via such information and communication tools as computer, printer, digital electrocardiography, digital camera, webcam and internet and with less number of health personnel and less funds.

Electronic Health Records

It is a fact that information and communication technologies provide alternative solutions for the problems of health systems in the developing and developed countries. Electronic health records come into prominence especially with the benefits of increasing the quality of health services, reducing the costs and as the most significant one increase the accessibility of the services. This application increases the provision and quality of health services by means of watching disorders of individuals and providing optimal diagnose and treatment. This application gives the opportunity to record the data collected especially of chronic diseases as heart and diabetes and in mother-child health watching services on computer systems and so enables the use of the most suitable treatment method. In addition, the examination of the data in the system construct the infrastructure required to develop and apply much effective treatment methods for chronic and acute patients (WHO, 2012a, p. 9).

Many people do not keep their health records while moving or in case of emergency. This situation results in both lost time and over-usage of limited resources because the tests that were previously conducted will need to be conducted again. That is why information and communication systems by which individual health information of the patients are stored that are also available for the specialists independently from time and place can eliminate the problems of quality, cost and access. Moreover, the data base provided by the information and communication technologies is important in terms of reducing medical faults and providing the flow of statistical information (Ouma & Herselman, 2009, pp. 194-195).

Electronic health record systems have a complex structure. This complexity makes it necessary to realize the successful designs on the establishment of the infrastructure of the system. On the other hand, the training of the health personnel on the operation of the system is indispensable for the perfect functioning of the system. It has been concluded from the research data that the existence of these conditions is required for the system (Kwankam, 2012, p. 395). Especially, this system provides the communication between the patients and health personnel, increasing productivity of the health personnel, minimizing medical faults and enabling the health personnel to use the time efficiently. On the contrary, it is possible to mention about time consuming data entry processes, slow access to data and weak patient-doctor interaction (WHO, 2012a, p. 9).

Hospital Information Systems

There are several applications to follow a health system by using information and communication technologies, take information on the functioning of the system, to make evaluations and by these means to take medical and administrative decisions. Hospital information systems can be shown as an example of these systems. Information support is provided to all the doctors and hospital managers on the daily health services and all other processes. So, it is aimed to increase effectiveness of all the existent healthcare systems in the hospital, to reach the targets determined on the service quality and to increase patient satisfaction (Ouma & Herselman, 2009, p. 194). In addition, this system also enables to use the information within the e-health system by means of the storage, evaluation and updating of the information on patients.

Via hospital information system, much data compared to the past on health services can be immediately obtained to be used in the decision process. This situation, especially with the aim of increasing the productivity of resource provision, gives the opportunity to prevent from the damages given to the system by unexploited aid services and plans that are not in line with the needs. While it has been stated that the time of obtaining the data to be used in the decision process changes between 6 and 12 months, this time can be minimized to a few months thanks to the hospital information systems. This makes possible a functional organization and also re-organization. Moreover, risk priorities and local investing needs can be much healthy determined and the source use can be activated (WHO, 2012a, pp. 326-327).

M-Health

The concepts of m-health (mobile health) and e-health are closely related. E-health states the offering of the health services and the technologies that support to continue to the functions of health services (Ganesan, 2012, p. 2). M-health, as a part of e-health, aims to increase the effectiveness, accessibility and productivity of health services without using mobile phones, patient watching devices, personal digital devices and other wireless information and communication technology tools. Especially, the third and fourth generation communication opportunities of mobile phones are used in this system. Commonly, such complex applications as short message services, radio services, global positioning systems and bluetooth are important parts of the system. In a research conducted by the World Health Organization, it has been detected that the most commonly used applications are call-center, emergency case free of charge call center and mobile tele-medicine within the m-health system. The common characteristic of these services is that mostly voice communication areas of the mobile devices are used (WHO, 2011, p. 12).

Mobile electronic devices are used in many areas as clinical decision support systems, data storage, and health attitude change and chronicle disease management by health personnel and

individuals. The existent data and different m-health tools as telephone messages are used on the treatment of many diseases as HIV, eating disorder, asthma, hypertension and diabetes and significant successes have been gained. In addition, while the healthcare services and research on health are supported, the training of the health personnel also should be supported (Free et al., 2010, p. 2).

By this respect, m-health affects the health services from the aspect of demand and supply. In terms of supply, the access opportunities to the health services can be improved and the problem of limited source of health service providers can be overcome. On the other hand, structural obstacles and behavioral restrictions will be effective in terms of demand (Thirumurthy & Lester, 2012, p. 390). In a research conducted for the EU, it has been stated that m-health applications change the behaviors to receive health services of individuals and also these applications achieve fund savings at a tremendous rate (PWC, 2013, p. 4).

Via m-health, low-cost high-quality services can be offered, the need for hospitalization can be reduced and a much healthier environment can be created and an effective labor force base can be constituted. The socio-economic effects of m-health can be examined under four dimensions in general (PWC, 2013, p. 9):

1. The awareness can be raised and the frequency of diseases can be decreased by creating behavioral change to change social life style and so they can be enabled to live a much healthier life.
2. The diagnosis of chronic diseases can gain momentum to minimize the costs and to restrict the degree of disease.
3. To support patient mobility and to decrease the necessity of hospital visits, patient treatments and care services can be carried out remotely by using mobile communication technologies.

4. The clinical decision making process is strengthened by providing system and personnel for more information and analysis. So, the benefits of physical and health sources of man power are increased and a stronger health system can be constituted.

INTERNET

Internet is without doubt one of the most important social reform of today. With the other communication tools, internet substantially contributes to the development and provision of health services. The great increase in the number of internet users especially in the developed and developing countries comes into prominence as a method by which the countries intending to set up a global health systems can reach their targets (WHO, 2010, p. 9).

Internet is a healthy information link that provides health services, interactive applications, discussion forums, disease simulators, audio and video files, and support groups, web sites for the members, online medical examination, blogs and feed-back applications to the users at home or in office environments.

In the traditional health systems, the only way for the patients to obtain information on their health status is the meeting they make with the health specialists in the health institutions. However, with the advantages of internet technology, the individuals can access to all the information on diseases and can contact with the specialists. On the other hand, health personnel can conduct their researches and maintain the training via online contacts provided by internet technology. The medical representatives can introduce their products and the insurance companies can control fund movements and management (Ouma & Herselman, 2009, p. 195).

The fact that especially using Internet we can share folder or documents via e-mail or other ways makes internet technologies much effective compared to other information technologies. The health web-sites created with the help of web-based applications can enable the people intending to take information and recommendation on health services and treatments to reach these information and services. In this manner, internet facilitates the functioning and watching of local and regional public health applications. Moreover, the fact that internet gives the opportunity to audial and visual communication of patient- health personnel facilitates the realization of tele-medicine applications.

Previously conducted research studies (Perez, 2009, p. 278; WHO, 2012a, p. 326; Alkmim et al., 2012, p. 374) indicated that with the help of health networks established by using internet technologies, the rate of accession to the health services increased especially in the underdeveloped countries. In developed countries, it has been detected that the individuals use internet with the aim of taking decisions on their health status and learning the methods to treat themselves. In addition, the international humanitarian aid institutions offer health services by mobile internet networks to the regions that are disadvantaged to reach the health services.

MOBILE PHONES

Mobile phones have a privileged place among the applications within information and communication technologies as the applications developing fast. Especially in developing countries, the rates of smart phone usage have increased sharply recently. This makes mobile phones important within e-health applications. In the developing countries without a developed health system, sufficient number of health personnel and a favorable health infrastructure, mobile phones offer advantages from the aspect of individual and public health.

Mobile phones are transforming into "smart phones" that are performing many functions quickly. Examinations can be made with the censors placed to the devices adapted to work in harmony with the mobile internet applications and the results of these examinations to the health centers and the specialists (Alexios, Vasilis, Lilian, & Dimitris, 2013, p. 51). These sensors can be used in a wide range of analyses as vision, color blindness, mental health or skin analysis (Bourouisa, Zerdazia, Fehamband & Bouchachiac, 2013, p. 3). On the other hand, the patients can reach to the information on their health status via smart phones and can continue to their communication with the health service providers. Especially, the access of old or chronic patients to health services are much easier and cheaper with the easy to use smart phone applications (Vinay & Vishal, 2013, p. 59).

Smart phones are also commonly used to inform the individuals with the aim of developing public health. They are used in underdeveloped regions especially to inform the public on the causes of health problems, protection ways and treatment types. By using the facilities of smart phones as short message service, voice message or video message, the individuals are informed on health services. By this method, important steps were taken in the fight against HIV and tuberculosis in Africa (WHO, 2012a, pp. 326-327). People are motived to have HIV test made with the messages sent to their mobile phones and by this way the rate of people having this test made have been doubled. In addition, it is possible to collect information to conduct research, education and clinical practices via smart phones and especially in developing countries, tele-medicine applications are encouraged.

COMMON PROBLEMS IN E-HEALTH APPLICATIONS

The factors that play a role in the organization and offering of health services differ among countries. This situation is valid also for the reforms in the area of health services. Numerous justifications can be put forth, however, generally the factors shaping the health services of the countries can be ranged as history of the society, cultural background, the characteristics of diseases prevalent in the society, the economic status of the country and the welfare regime adopted by the country. At a more national level, the factors can be the competition between public and private sector, a view to the private services against general services, a view to the therapeutically services against the preventive services, productivity, equality, effectiveness and cost, and finance structure (Twaddle, 2002, p. 3).

E-health bursts into prominence as a complementary application alternative from the aspect of the countries searching for reforms in the field of health systems. However, the establishment and operation of the systems depend on certain conditions. The obstacles arising in the implementation of information and communication technologies in the field of health services can be categorized under three titles. These are technologic obstacles, social and human obstacles, political and legal obstacles (WITSA, 2006, p. 3-5).

Technological Obstacles

E-health services are complicated and they require the use of advanced technology tools. To obtain the desired results from the service, primarily the high-cost technology infrastructure should be established (Chetley, 2006, p. 21). On the other hand, industrial standards and managerial easiness should exist besides technological infrastructure. The fact that there is no adaptation between the norms and standards of health services sector and general industry prevent the extensive usage of advanced information technologies. The standards developed in the health services are evaluated under two basic categories: The first one is proprietary or consensus standards. Proprietary standard derives from the ownership of one seller of an efficient share of the market for a certain goods. Consensus standards are the standards developed among service providers, employers, the purchasers, medical communities and the committees comprising of government authorities. Administrative simplification is the establishment of the standards governing the sharing of the information used in health services by means of communication technologies (WITSA, 2006, p. 3).

Social and Human Obstacles

Social and human obstacles play an important role in the harmonization of health services industry with the information technologies. Principally, advanced information technologies require health services personnel having minimum skill to use computer. Moreover, the protection of privacy, provision of security and protection of the secrecy of information transferred to the computer environment are required for the system to obtained the desired level of success. Many patients believe that electronic recording and storing of their health status are dangerous from the aspect of personel security. They also believe that this situation will cause many illegal troubles such as misuse of the information. That is why the firms providing health information technologies are required to establish an information network to eliminate all the suspicions. This also obliges the firms providing information technologies and health service providers to develop systems in which the information is allowed to be seen only by the authorities (WITSA, 2006, p. 3).

On the other hand, the skills of health service personnel to use information and commnication technologies should be developed and they also should be encouraged on the favorableness to use electronic record systems rather than the traditional methods. Also, people offering information and communication technologies should develop user-friendly systems in which data entry and re-access to the data are effortless. Briefly, the health personnel should be "convinced"in the direction that the information technologies increase the quality of health services and direclty affect patient care (WITSA, 2006, p. 4).

Political and Legal Obstructs

Another factor preventing the use of information and communication technologies in health sector is political and legal obstructs. Operational and managerial responsibilites of health systems are considerably under the monopoly of governments. For this reason, the political will should be emphasized first and the regulations regarding the health servicess hould be adopted in a way that eliminates the discontents of individuals (WITSA, 2006, p. 3).

On the other hand, the frequency of malfunctioning of the devices used in e-health services burdens responsibilities on health service providers regarding health status of individuals. That's why the system should be supported with a perfect guidance service. The trust of all stakeholders should be gained and it should be confirmed that regional differences and such factors as religion, language, sex and etc do not affect the offering of the services. For the services offerred by the cooperation between public and private sector, the ethical values as profit motive, privacy and secrecy should be taken into account (WHO, 2010, p. 11).

E-HEALTH IN TURKEY

The first activities of e-health began within the scope of"Health Transformation Program" put into practice in 2003. The first concrete step was taken with "e-Transformation Turkey Project" published in 2004. Within this framework, Ministry of Health was allocated with the duty of creating an e-health study group. With the aim of establishing the base of e-health applications, this group has been responsible for studying to develop barcode systems on blood components, a model to be used for electronic patient records and content and structure standards, to improve theintegrated health information system, to determine the medical terminology to be used in coding the clinical data included in electronic patient records, to provide referances for the actions of determining the health information management standards, to publish the report in line with the related legal regulations on protecting secrecy and privacy, to design an education tree with the aim of determining and covering the needs of health informatics training, to model this design and to support the activites of curriculum programs in this area (DPT, 2004, pp. 9-21).

In "Information Society Strategy Action Plan" published in 2006, the tasks of establishing health information systems, blood bank data bases, online health services and conducting activities of tele-medicine systems were assigned to the Ministry of Health, private health institutions and other stakeholders (DPT, 2006, p. 25).

The most significant step taken for realization of national e-health system is the report prepared by International Telecommunication Union. In ac-cordance with this report, it was decided to set up an information sharing and communication platform with the name of Health-Net in which e-health ap-plications can be followed (Mandil, 2004, p. 23). E-health services implemented in Turkey are e-radiology, decision support systems, e-prescription, central physician appointment system and e-referral.

Health-Net

This application was carried into effect within the scope of Health Transformation Program. Within the framework of this project, National Health Data Standards and Health Coding Ref-erence Glossary were prepared in order to align the norms and standards. Also, it has been aimed to set up an online platform that is managing the services provided by tele-medicine applications and on the internet. By this way, the data collected in the health institutions can be opened up to the access of all the stakeholders and so it is aimed to increase the effectiveness and productivity of health services (www.e-sağlık.gov.tr).

By means of Health-Net, it is aimed to put Electronic Health Record into practice in which the data on health problems individuals are experiencing throughout their lives and also Na-tional Decision Support System that will enable the stakeholders to use this data to improve the health status of individual. Also, ethical values of the collected data will be protected to be used in health researches.

E-Radiology

By e-radiology put into practice within the scope of Health-Net, it is aimed to store and transfer the required radiological images in order to offer the health services effectively. By this means, it will be prevented to scan one patient more than once and also the health personnel will be protected to be exposed to over-radiation. With this purpose, it is planned to create a radiology data base to which the authorities can reach and the electronic data and radiological images in Health-Net will be uploaded. When the patients have been radiologically examinedfor one time, they can maintain their treatments in another hospital and they are enabled to use the results of this examination in another hospital (www.e-saglik.gov.tr).

Decision Support System

This system aims to enable the use of data obtained from various levels of health services benefiting from information and communication technolo-gies while taking decisions on planning and strat-egy. Also, with this system, the data is planned to reported to the related health personnel via Geographical Information System. By this means, a systematic evaluation of the data collected from various units can be conducted and this method may be effective in the fight against contagious diseases (www.e-saglik.gov.tr).

E-Prescription

By this application, the patients can make appointments by using web page or mobile phone in second and third level health services and oral and dental health centers. It is aimed with this system to prevent the patient queues and the effective use of the resources.

Central Physician Appointment System

This is an application where the patients, who want a medical examination in secondary and tertiary stages or oral and dental health centers, determine a date of examination simultaneously via phone or web. This system is expected to prevent queues of patients and provide effective use of resources.

E-Referral

This application has been put into practice instead of the manuel application to make the referrals of the patients who are not able to be treated in their neighboorhood. With this system, the referrals will be made much planned and controlled. This application entered into force in 1 March 2013 (www.sgk.gov.tr).

CONCLUSION

It's certain that the recent advances in information and communication technologies will affect the health sector too. The sector has been benefiting from information technologies especially for developing medical diagnosis and treatment opportunities for a long time. However, the utilization of information and communication technologies in order to extend health services was accelerated with the attempts to found a global health system. E-health applications provide a significant opportunity especially for the countries that have not developed health systems.

Information and communication technologies could provide significant opportunities for Turkey as a country that has had an intention to found a comprehensive health system, from which all the population could benefit, within the scope of Project of Medical Transformation since 2003. When we consider the lack of labor force and inequalities between different regions together with the inadequate medical infrastructure, e-health applications could be some rational solutions in order to cope with current problems. First of all, the cooperation between health sector and information technologies should be developed in order to provide the adaptation of new technologies into the health sector. Doctors and nurses should have the knowledge of these technologies and diagnosis and consultation practices should be extended through e-health applications especially in some regions where health services and medical labor force are not adequate.

REFERENCES

Akin, B. J., & Ferranti, D. (1998). *Financing health services in devoloping countries, an agenda for reform*. Washington, DC: The World Bank Policy Study, Second Printing.

Alexios, M., Vasilis, M., Lilian, M., & Dimitris, G. (2013). Smartphone sensor data as digital evidence. *Computers & Security, 38*, 51–75. doi:10.1016/j.cose.2013.03.007

Alkmim, M. B., Figueira, R. M., Marcolino, M. S., Cardoso, C. S., Abreu, M. P., & Cunha, L. R. et al. (2012). Improving patient access to specialized care: The tele health network of minas gerais, Brazil. *Bulletin of the World Health Organization, 90*(5), 373–378. doi:10.2471/BLT.11.099408 PMID:22589571

Bourouisa, A., Zerdazia, A., Fehamband, M., & Bouchachiac, A. (2013). M-Health: Skin disease analysis system using smarthphone's camera. *Procedia Computer Science, 19*, 1116–1120. doi:10.1016/j.procs.2013.06.157

Chetley, A., (2006). *Improving health, connecting people: the role of ICT's in the health sector of developing countries.* Global Observatory for eHealth Series.

Docteur, E., & Oxley, H. (2003). *Healthcare systems: Lesson from the reform experiece.* OECD Health Working Paper.

DPT. (2004). *e-Dönüşüm Türkiye projesi kısa dönem eylem planı 2003-2004.* DPT.

DPT. (2006). *Bilgi toplumu eylem planı 2003-2004.* DPT.

E-Sağlık. (n.d.). Retrieved from www.e-sağlık. gov.tr

Erener, M., & Yelkikan, N. (2003). Gelişmekte olan ülkelerin sağlık sistemlerinin yeniden yapılanması ve finansmanı: Türkiye deneyimi. *Kocaeli Üniversitesi Sosyal Bilimler Enstitüsü Dergisi, (6)*, 99-113.

Europen Commission. (2007). *Conceptual framwork, healt careand e-health investment context and challenges.* Retrieved 20.10.2013, from http://www.financing-ehealth.eu/downloads/ documents/Financing_eHealth_D1_3_concept_ and_context_web.pdf

Free, C., Phillips, G., Felix, L., Leandro,L., Patel, V., & Edwards, P. (2010). *The effectiveness of m-health technologies for improving health and health services: A systematic review.* BMC Research Notes, 3.250.

Ganesan, S. (2012). *Smartphone application for m-health and environmental monitoring systems.* (Unpublished doctoral dissertation). Arizona State University.

Garrido, M. V., Zentner, A., & Busse, R. (2008). *Health systems, health policy and health technology assessment. European Observatory on Health Systems and Policies, Observatory Studies Series, No 14.* Copenhagen: Publications WHO Regional Office for Europe.

Isık, A. H., & İnan, G. (2010). Tele tıpta mobil uygulama çalışması ve mobil iletişim teknolojilerinin analizi. *Bilişim Teknolojileri Dergisi, Cilt: 3. Sayı, 1*, 1–10.

Jones, B.WHO. (2012b). The bigger picture for e health. *Bulletin of the World Health Organization, 90*(5), 330–331. doi:10.2471/BLT.12.040512 PMID:22589565

Keeton, C.WHO. (2012a). Measuring the impact of e-health. *Bulletin of the World Health Organization, 90*(5), 326–327. doi:10.2471/BLT.12.020512 PMID:22589563

King, G., Heaney, D. J., Boddy, D., O'Donnell, C. A., Clark, J. S., & Mair, F. S. (2010). Exploring public perspectives on e-health: Findings from two citizen juries. *Health Expectations, 14*(4), 351–360. doi:10.1111/j.1369-7625.2010.00637.x PMID:21029283

Koivusalo, M. (2006). The impact of economic globalisationon health. *Theoretical Medicine and Bioethics, 27*(1), 13–34. doi:10.1007/s11017-005-5757-y PMID:16532301

Kwankam, S. Y. (2012). Successful partnerships for international collaboration in e-health: The need for organized national infrastructures. *Bulletin of the World Health Organization, 90*(5), 395–397. doi:10.2471/BLT.12.103770 PMID:22589576

Lewis, T., Synowiec, C., Lagomarsinoa, G., & Schweitze, J. (2012). E-Health in low- and middle-income countries: Findings from the center for health market innovations. *Bulletin of the World Health Organization, 90*(5), 332–340. doi:10.2471/BLT.11.099820 PMID:22589566

Mandil, S. (2004). *Review of and recommended improvements to Turkey e-health strategy*. Retrieved 17.10.2013, from http://www.e-saglik.gov.tr

McKinsey & Company. (2010). *mHealth: A new vision for healthcare*. Retrieved 29:10.2013, from http://mpedigree.net/mpedigreenet/images/docs/McKinsey_mHealth_Study_Cites_mPedigree.pdf

NERA. (2009). *Global principles for better healthcare: A guide for policy makers*. Retrieved 16.3.2013, from http://www.ifpma.org/site_docs/HealthCarePolicy%20Softbook_Rev03.pdf

Ouma, S., & Herselman, M. E. (2009). E-Health in rural areas: Case of developing countries. *International Journal of Biological and Medical Science, 4*, 194–201.

Pepe, H. U. (2006). Küreselleşme, Avrupa sağlık reformları ve hekimlere etkileri: Batı Avrupa'dan bir bakış açısı. *Toplum ve Hekim, Cilt 2 Sayı 2, 136-142.*

Perez, E. (2009). E-Health: How to make the right choice. *Nursing Forum, 44*(4), 277–282. doi:10.1111/j.1744-6198.2009.00153.x PMID:19954467

Pijen, J. G., Wynchank, S., Covvey, H. D., & Ossebaard, H. C. (2012). Improving the credibility of electronic health technologies. *Bulletin of the World Health Organization*, 90–323A.

PWC. (2013). *Socio-economic impact of mhealth: An assessment report for the European Union*. Retrieved 25.10.2013 from, http://www.gsma.com/connectedliving/wp-content/uploads/2013/06/Socio-economic_impact-of-mHealth_EU_14062013V2.pdf

Schiavo, R. (2008). The rise of e-health: Current trends and topics on online health communications. *Journal of Medical Marketing: Device, Diagnostic and Pharmaceutical Marketing, 8*(1), 9-18.

SGK. (n.d.). Retrieved from www.sgk.go.tr

Thirumurthy, H., & Lester, R. T. (2012). M-Health for health behaviour change in resource-limited settings: Applications to HIV care and beyond. *Bulletin of the World Health Organization, 90*(5), 390–392. doi:10.2471/BLT.11.099317 PMID:22589574

Twaddle, A. C. (2002). *Healthcare reform around the world*. Greenwood Publishing Group.

Vinay, K. V., & Vishal, K. (2013). Smartphone applications for medical students and professionals. *NUJHS, 3*(1), 59–63.

Vittacca, M., Mazzü, M., & Scalvini, S. (2009). Socio-technical and organizational challenge to wider e-health implemention. *Chronic Respiratory, 2009*(2), 91–97. doi:10.1177/1479972309102805

WHO. (2010). *Telemedicine, opportunities and developments in member states*. Global Observatory for eHealth Series, Volume 2.

WHO. (2011). *mHealth new horizons for health through mobile technologies*. Global Observatory for e-Health Series, Volume 3.

WHO. (2012c). *Management of patient information trends and challenges in member states*. Global Observatory for eHealth Series, Volume 6.

WHO & IT. (2012). *National e-health strategy toolkit*. Retrieved 15.10.2013 from, http://www.itu.int/dms_pub/itu-d/opb/str/D-STR-E_HEALTH.05-2012-PDF-E.pdf

WİTSA. (2006). *Health care and information and communications technologies: Challenges and opportunities*. Retrieved 15.10.2013 from, http://www.witsa.org/papers/WITSA-HIT-final.pdf

Woottom, R., Geissbuhler, A., Jethwani, K., Kovarik, C., Person, D. S., & Vladzymyrskyy, A. et al. (2012). Long-running telemedicine networks delivering humanitarian services: Experience, performance and scintific output. *Bulletin of the World Health Organization*, *2012*(5), 341–347. doi:10.2471/BLT.11.099143

Yaşgül, S. (2002). Küreselleşme iktisadi yönelimler ve politik karşıtlıklar. Om Yayın Evi.

KEY TERMS AND DEFINITIONS

Acceptability: All health facilities, goods, and services must be respectful of medical ethics and culturally appropriate, as well as sensitive to gender and life-cycle requirements.

Accessibility: Health facilities, goods, and services accessible to everyone, within the jurisdiction of the state party.

Decentralization: To increase the effectiveness and efficiency of the management of health services and planning to transfer to local governments.

Health Technologies: Any intervention that may be used to promote health, to prevent, diagnose or treat disease or for rehabilitation or long-term care. This includes the pharmaceuticals, devices, procedures, and organizational systems used in healthcare.

Health Transformation Program: A program that implemented by the Justice and Development Party in accordance with the principles of effectiveness and efficiency of the organization, financing, and delivery of programs in Turkey.

Tele-Consultations: Among specialists and practitioners to exchange information by means of information and communication technologies.

Universal Coverage: An approach that advocates healthcare and covering the whole population.

This work was previously published in the Handbook of Research on Developing Sustainable Value in Economics, Finance, and Marketing edited by Ulas Akkucuk, pages 446-462 copyright year 2015 by Business Science Reference (an imprint of IGI Global).

Chapter 6
Lean Six Sigma in Healthcare:
A Review of Theory and Practice

Mohamed Gamal Aboelmaged
Ain Shams University, Egypt

ABSTRACT

The chapter clarifies emerging aspects and trends of Lean Six Sigma (LSS) in healthcare through the systematic examination of 162 peer-reviewed articles in business, management, and healthcare disciplines that have been published over a ten-year period from 2004 to January 2014. Every article is analyzed using a scheme of six distinct dimensions including year of publication, journal, applications areas, tools and techniques, benefits and improvements, and research type. The chapter provides significant insights into the state of the art of LSS in healthcare research and clarifies confusion in the literature as to what constitutes LSS role in improving healthcare context.

INTRODUCTION

Implementing Lean Six Sigma (LSS) in non-manufacturing sector like healthcare is interesting and challenging topic. Healthcare service contains many complex systems and processes with various stakeholders that should operate under pressures of high clinical and administrative quality levels. LSS methodology has been gradually adopted in healthcare since early 2000s in order to reducing medical errors and improving quality of patient care and safety levels for patients and healthcare workers (Taner et al, 2007).

The pressures on healthcare services have increased dramatically in the last decade due to increasing financial pressures, ageing population, managerial sophistications, and operational and technological inefficiency (de Koning et al, 2006). Accordingly, many researchers and practitioners consider LSS as the magic cure of healthcare problems as it supports and sustains capacity, speed and accuracy of various healthcare processes such as improving MRI exam scheduling and increasing capacity in X-ray rooms (Taner et al, 2007), improving waiting time for the medical service (Ahmed et al., 2013; Roth et al (2010), reducing clinical and administrative errors (Gowen III et al., 2012), eliminating waste Elimination (Cima et al., 2011; de Bucourt et al., 2011), increasing satisfaction of patients and health employees (Bucci and Musitano, 2011; Chiarini, 2013), and reducing length of stay (Gayed et al., 2013; Mandahawi, 2011).

DOI: 10.4018/978-1-4666-8756-1.ch006

While there is an agreement on the historical development of Six Sigma methodology as presented in the Figure 1, it appears that there is a little consensus on the definition of the term. Six Sigma has been developed by Motorola in the 1980s as a result of linking finest elements of scientific management and continuous quality improvement initiatives. From a statistical perspective, Six Sigma can be considered as a metric of process measurement symbolized by the Greek letter σ that represents the amount of variation with a normal data distribution that targets quality level of 3.4 defects per million opportunities (DPMO) (Aboelmaged, 2011).

The focus of Six Sigma is not on counting the defects in processes, but rather the number of chances or opportunities in a process that could produce defects therefore causes of quality problems can be eliminated before they are transformed into defects (Antony, 2006). From a managerial perspective, Six Sigma can be considered as an improvement program for reducing variation (Andersson et al., 2006). From a strategic perspective, Six Sigma could be described as a business strategy to improve business profitability, effectiveness and efficiency of all operations to increase customer satisfaction (Kwak and Anbari, 2006).

The labeled concept Lean Six Sigma (LSS) is a combination of two complementary philosophies; Lean and Six Sigma. LSS is a business improvement methodology aiming at maximizing shareholders' value by enhancing costs, speed, quality, speed, and customer satisfaction. Although LSS has its origins in manufacturing organizations, it has been widely adopted by service organizations. What makes Lean Six Sigma different from previous quality methodologies is the adoption of structured quality roles and tools across organizational hierarchy instead of transferring quality issues to first administrative line or to specific quality department (Snee, 2004). According to George (2002), the key focus of LSS is on activities that cause the customer's critical-to-quality issues and create the longest time delays in any process. Working on these activities offer the greatest opportunity for improvement in cost, quality, capital, and lead time. Although the guiding theories of Lean and Six Sigma methodologies are different, they are complementary in nature since both seek to improve the process. Lean philosophy establishes the standards of eliminating waste and reducing cycle time in processes with little impact on process variation, while Six Sigma shows how these standards can be achieved with minimum variation through applying a problem-solving approach using statistical tools and techniques (Aboelmaged, 2010). In addition, lean standards covers the entire organization value chain, while Six Sigma concentrates more attentively on certain projects or processes within an organization.

Figure 1. Timeline of LSS (adapted from Heckert, 2013)

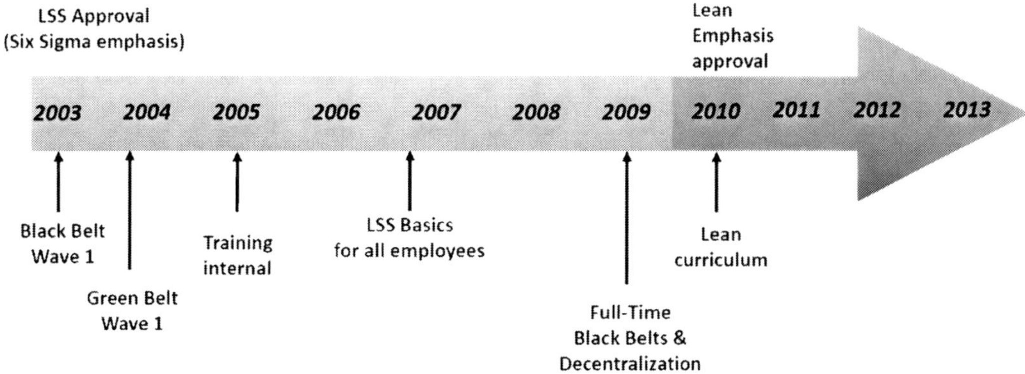

Such integration between Lean and Six Sigma as an improvement methodology brings many benefits to the organization including maximizing shareholder value and improve their satisfaction and cost, quality and speed of processes (Byrne et al., 2007).

Typically, LSS research efforts have been conducted in a wide range of manufacturing and service settings with scant literature on how LSS research is structured within specific setting or domain. Therefore, the purpose of this chapter is to investigate LSS research in healthcare context and present a comprehensive review of these studies. The review covers 162 journal articles published over 10 years between 2004 and January 2014. The paper is divided into four remaining sections. First, the research methodology used in the study is described. This is followed by the classification framework in the second section. Third, LSS in healthcare articles are analyzed and the classification results are reported. Finally, conclusions are presented and the implications for future research are presented.

RESEARCH METHODOLOGY

The structured review in this chapter focuses on papers that are published in peer-reviewed journals where academics and practitioners use to acquire and disseminate high quality research findings. Therefore, editorials, news reports, book reviews, viewpoints, conference papers, master and doctoral dissertations, textbooks, and unpublished working papers were excluded. The survey focused only on papers with 'Lean Six Sigma' and 'Healthcare', 'Hospital' or 'Medical' as a part of their titles or abstracts. Finally, to avoid never ending revision of the article, the January 2014 was selected as the cut-off date. These criteria should allow a quality and comprehensive set of papers on LSS in healthcare by different fields. This effort has been carried out over 22 months through extensive internet search, database search,

reference checking, etc. However, it is possible that there exist an article which is not surveyed in this paper.

Considering the diverse nature of LSS research, it would be difficult to classify the literature under any specific themes. As a result, different online databases were selected and searched to provide a comprehensive bibliography on LSS in healthcare. The literature contributions were primarily of articles from research databases including PubMed, Wiley Interscience, Science Direct, (Elsevier), EBSCO, Ingenta, Emerald, ProQuest, Inderscience, ASQ, Springer and IEEE-Xplore.

LSS IN HEALTHCARE: A CLASSIFICATION FRAMEWORK

The search yielded 162 articles on LSS in healthcare from 108 journals (for a full list of these articles see Appendix). Each article was carefully reviewed and classified from several perspectives. Although this research is not exhaustive, it serves as a comprehensive base for gaining robust insights into LSS in healthcare. The classification framework was based on the nature of LSS literature and the work of Glasgow et al. (2010) and De Koning et al. (2006). The articles were reviewed, analyzed and classified based on the following categories:

1. Year of publication
2. Publication journal
3. Major application areas
4. Key tools and methods
5. Improvements and benefits to healthcare context
6. Dominating research method

This framework provided guidelines for pursuing rigorous research on LSS in healthcare and clarify the confusion in the literature regarding what constitutes LSS theory and how does it integrate with improvement strategies in that context.

RESULTS AND ANALYSIS OF THE CLASSIFICATIONS

1. Distribution of LSS in Healthcare by Year of Publication

Figure 2 shows the distribution of 162 articles on LSS in healthcare published over the period from 2004 to January 2014. There appears to be scant research outputs before 2004. The publication trend has been improved in recent years and the number of articles has increased significantly in 2013 which indicates an increasing interest in LSS applications in healthcare.

2. Distribution of Articles by Journal

There were a total of 108 different journals from healthcare and business disciplines that published articles on LSS in healthcare (Figure 3).

3. Distribution of Articles by Area of Application

Figure 4 illustrate top areas of LSS application in healthcare. It is unavoidable to have an article that is relevant to more than one theme, so listing an article under more than one theme was allowed. For example, an article may address radiology department as an application and safety as a key

process for improvement. In such a case, a more weighted process is chosen to classify the article according to the author's judgment.

Twenty 20 areas of application were identified in the articles. The most heavily investigated area of application is *patient care* (19 articles) where quality of healthcare delivery in general is the key focus. The second largest area of LSS application in healthcare is *Laboratory* department (17 articles) where reliability of results, testing process, standards, reporting, waste elimination, turnaround time (TAT), and automation were of high LSS concern. Moreover, *Radiology* department (13 articles) was among the top three areas of LSS applications in healthcare. The main concern was improving imaging quality and processes, workflow, patient flow, procurement, examination time, satisfaction, waste elimination. Table 1 provides a list of author contributions within each area of LSS application in healthcare.

4. Distribution of Articles by LSS Tools and Methods

A great deal of literature on LSS in healthcare has focused on tools and techniques that can be employed by LSS teams to manage quality problems in healthcare. Examples of these tools and techniques include *DMAIC, DFSS, 5S, Pareto analysis, root cause analysis, process mapping* or

Figure 2. Distribution of articles on LSS in healthcare by year (2004 - January 2014)

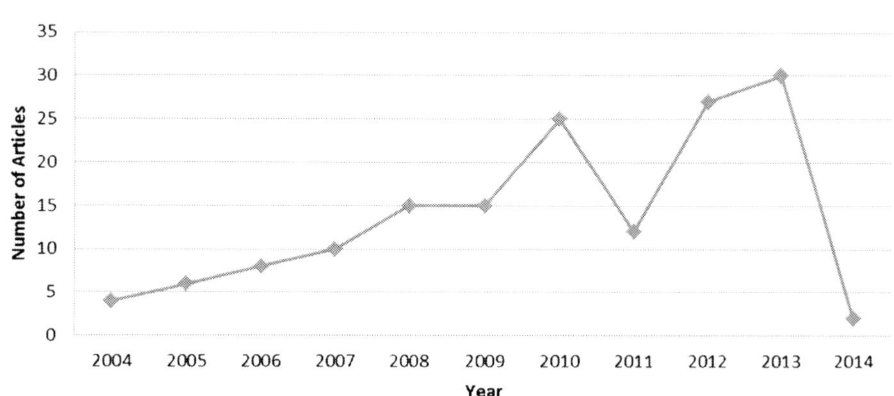

Figure 3. Distribution of articles on LSS in healthcare by journal

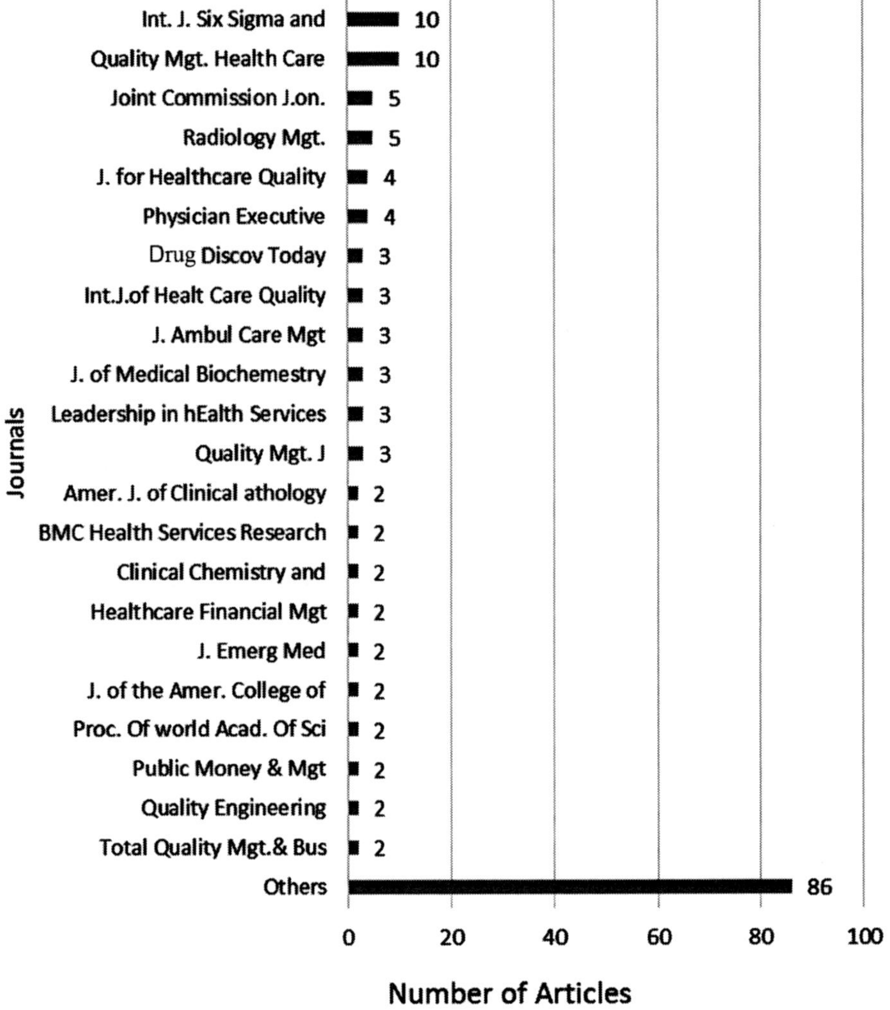

process flow chart, Gantt chart, affinity diagrams, run charts, histograms, quality function deployment (QFD), *suppliers-input-process-output-customer* (SIPOC), *Kano model, brainstorming, process capability analysis, benchmarking*, etc. Moreover, a LSS technique may utilize various tools. For example, *statistical process control* (*SPC*) is a technique that may utilize various tools including *control charts, histograms, root cause analysis*, etc.

Figure 5 shows that the largest part of LSS in healthcare literature deals with the theorization and application of *DMAIC* methodology (32 articles).

DMAIC is used to improve already existing processes and can be divided into five phases; define, measure, analyze, improve and control. Several studies have shown successful cases of *DMAIC* application in healthcare (see Table 2 for author contributions). The second largest LSS tools applied in healthcare is *5S principles* (27 articles). *5S principles* refer to five Japanese words that are used to organize and manage the workspace and workflow with intent of eliminating waste and reducing process inefficiencies. The *5S principles* are:

Figure 4. Distribution of articles by area of LSS application in healthcare

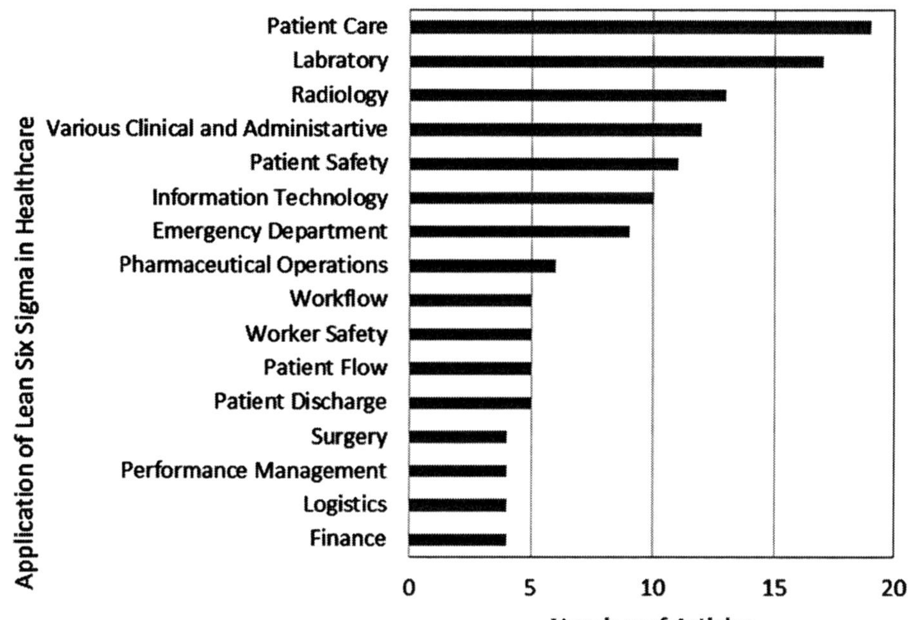

Figure 5. Distribution of articles by LSS tools and methods in healthcare

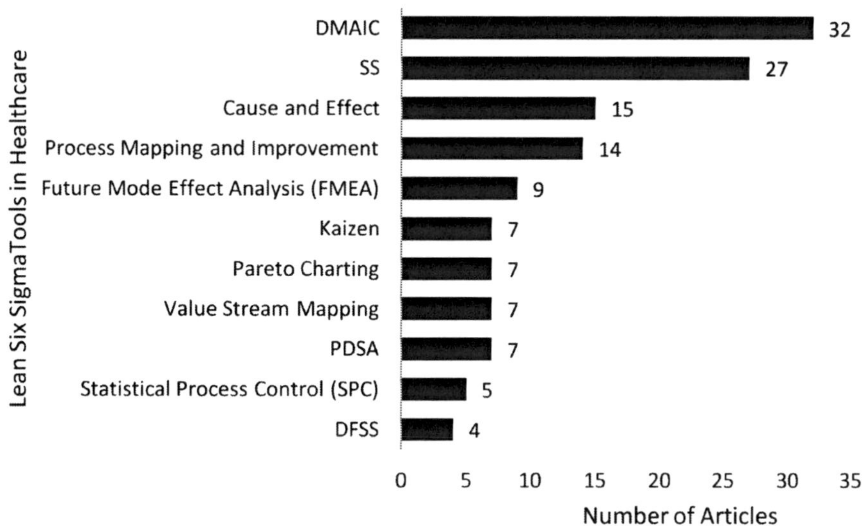

- **(Seiri) Sort:** Ensuring only important items are stored in the workspace and eliminating any other items that are not used in the process.

- **(Seiton) Straighten:** Focusing on "straightening" the work path for materials, tools and the work process through physically organizing the work area with the best locations for the needed items "ev-

Table 1. Author contribution to areas of LSS application in healthcare

Area of LSS Application in Healthcare	Authors
Patient Care	Aldarrab (2006); Black (2009); Dahl (2009); Fairbanks (2007); Farzianpour et al. (2012); Fillingham (2007); Garfield (2009); Glasgow et al. (2010); Hina-Syeda et al. (2013); Kim et al (2006); Lin et al (2013); Martin (2007); Mathieson (2006); Neufeld et al. (2013); Parks et al (2008); Veluswamy et al. (2010); Viau and Southern (2007); Young et al. (2004); Dahl (2009)
Laboratory	Blick (2013); Carlson et al. (2012); Cloete and Bester (2012); Das, B. (2011); Gijo et al (2013); Hassell et al. (2010); Llopis et al. (2011); Mayer et al (2011); Plebani and Lippi (2011); Stankovic (2004; 2008); Stankovic and DeLauro (2010); Stoiljković et al (2011); Sunyog (2004); Villa (2010); Pantanowitz et al (2008); Costello and Molloy (2009)
Radiology	Aakre et al (2010); Bashir et al (2012); Bucci and Musitano (2011); Coffin (2013); de Bucourt et al (2011); García-porres et al. (2013); McDonald and Kirk (2013); Waldron (2011); Yamamoto et al (2010); Bahensky et al (2005); Viau and Southern (2007); Chan et al. (2005); Roth et al (2010)
Various Clinical and Administrative Processes	Black (2009); Bullas et al. (2007); de Koning et al. (2006); Gamm et al (2007); Gremyr et al (2012); Gowen III et al. (2012); Jimmerson et al (2005); McJoynt et al. (2009); Taner et al. (2007); Schweikhart and Dembe (2009); Yusof et al. (2012); Van Den Heuvel et al. (2005)
Patient Safety	Buell (2010); Farzianpour et al. (2012); Gowen III et al. (2012); Karsten (2011); Martin (2007); McFadden et al. (2014); Niemeijer et al (2011); Schriefer and Leonard (2012); Shabot et al (2013); Stankovic (2004); Veluswamy et al. (2010)
Information Technology	Aleem (2013); Bhaskar et al. (2012); Holden and Hackbart (2012); Johnson et al. (2009); Stoiljković et al (2011); Pantanowitz et al (2008); Pate (2012); Villa (2010); Yusof et al. (2012); Zandi (2013)
Emergency Department	Aldarrab (2006); Dickson et al. (2009); Christianson et al (2005); Crane et al (2014); Eite et al. (2010); Mandahawiet al (2010); Mazzocato et al. (2012); Van den Heuvel et al. (2006); Zilm et al (2010)
Pharmaceutical operations	Al-Araidah et al (2010); Bi et al. (2013); Junker et al (2011); Noguera et al (2013); Sewing et al. (2008); Ullman and Boutellier (2008)
Patient Discharge	Allen et al. (2010); El-Banna (2012); Frings and Grant (2005); Niemeijer et al. (2010; 2012)
Patient Flow	Aakre et al (2010); Chan et al. (2005); Fairbanks (2007); Jimmerson et al (2005); Mathieson (2006)
Worker Safety	Baddour and Saleh, (2013); Carboneau et al (2010); Chassin (2013); Kaplan et al. (2009); Miles (2006)
Workflow	Bahensky et al (2005); Hassell et al. (2010); Holden and Hackbart (2012); Roth et al (2010); Sunyog (2004)
Surgery	Cima et al. (2011; 2013); Dickson (2013); Nicolay et al.(2012)
Performance Mgt.	Christianson et al (2005); Niemeijer et al (2011); Rajan et al. (2012); Robbins et al (2012)
Logistics	Al-Qatawneh et al. (2013); de Bucourt et al (2011); Jin, M. et al. (2008); Van Lent et al. (2012)
Finance	Caldwell (2006); Gitlow and Gitlow (2013); Mugdh and Pilla (2012); Tyson (2010)

ery item is in its place". Straighten involves removal of clutter and use of ergonomic principles to arrange required items in an efficient manner.

- **(Seiso) Sweep:** Keeping the workplace clean and neat. Cleanliness is a regular part of the daily work effort, not an extra effort initiated when the workplace gets too messy at the end of every shift or operation.
- **(Seiketsu) Standardize:** Applying consistent and standardized ways of working through which everyone knows their role and responsibility so that actions are taken the same right way every time.
- **(Shitsuke) Sustain:** Ensuring that the previous stated principles will be continually applied as a part of the culture of the institution and everyone's responsibility.

Table 2 illustrates a list of author contributions to each of LSS tools and methods in healthcare.

Table 2. Author contributions to LSS tools and methods in healthcare

LSS Tools	Authors
DMAIC	Al-Araidah et al (2010); Allen et al. (2010); Al-Qatawneh et al. (2013); Baddour and Saleh, (2013); Carboneau et al (2010); Chand (2011); Cheng and Chang (2012); Chiarini (2012); Cloete and Bester (2012); DuPree et al (2009); Elik (2013); Feng and Antony (2010); Feng and Manuel (2008); Gijo et al (2013); Gowen III et al. (2012); Hilton et al. (2008); Mandahawi (2011); Mandahawi et al (2010); Martinez et al. (2011); Mazzocato et al. (2012); McJoynt et al. (2009); Miles (2006); Mozammel and Mapa (2012); Niemeijer et al (2011); Niemeijer et al. (2010); Niemeijer et al. (2012); Paccagnella et al (2012); Pan et al. (2008); Robbins et al (2012); Taner (2013); Taner et al. (2007); Toledo et al (2013)
5S	Al-Araidah et al (2010); Bahensky et al (2005); Caldwell (2006); Chand (2011); Cheng and Chang (2012); Cima et al. (2011); de Bucourt et al (2011); Gayed et al (2013); Gowen III et al. (2012); Grove et al. (2010); Jin. et al. (2008); Junker et al (2011); Laureani et al (2013); Mathieson (2006); Niemeijer et al (2012); Niemeijer et al. (2010); Rajan et al. (2012); Roth et al (2010); Schattenkirk (2012); Stankovic (2008); Stankovic and DeLauro (2010); Taner (2013); Tyson (2010); Van den Heuvel et al. (2006); Viau and Southern (2007); Villa (2010); Yusof et al. (2012)
Cause and Effect	Allen et al. (2010); Chiarini (2012); El-Banna (2012); Gowen III et al. (2012); Gijo et al (2013); Hina-Syeda et al. (2013); Laureani et al (2013); Miles (2006); Schriefer and Leonard (2012); Seidl and Newhouse (2012); Taner (2013); Taner et al. (2007); Van den Heuvel et al. (2006); Viau and Southern (2007); Yu et al. (2008)
Process Mapping and Improvement	Allen et al. (2010); Christianson et al (2005); Deckard et al (2010); Feng and Antony (2010); Frings and Grant (2005); Gowen III et al. (2012); Lin et al (2013); Mazzocato et al. (2012); Schattenkirk (2012); Stankovic (2008); Stoiljković et al (2011); Taner (2013); Taner et al. (2007); Villa (2010)
Failure Mode Effect Analysis (FMEA)	Chiarini (2012); Cloete and Bester (2012); Hina-Syeda et al. (2013); Karsten (2011); Niu et al. (2010); Schriefer and Leonard (2012); Seidl and Newhouse (2012); Taner et al. (2007); Van den Heuvel et al. (2006)
PDSA	Feng and Antony (2010); Fischman (2010); Gowen III et al. (2012); Morrow (2012); Nicolay et al.(2012); Schriefer and Leonard (2012); Varkey and Kollengode (2011);
Value Stream Mapping	Chiarini (2012); Cima et al. (2011); Gowen III et al. (2012); Grove et al. (2010); McJoynt et al. (2009); Stankovic (2008); Yusof et al. (2012)
Pareto Charting	Allen et al. (2010); Chiarini (2012); Cloete and Bester (2012); Hina-Syeda et al. (2013); Mandahawi (2011); Taner et al. (2007); Van den Heuvel et al. (2006)
Kaizen	Bahensky et al (2005); Cloete and Bester (2012); Gowen III et al. (2012); Schattenkirk (2012); Stankovic (2008); Stoiljković et al (2011); van Leeuwen and Does (2010)
Statistical Process Control (SPC)	Allen et al. (2010); Gowen III et al. (2012); Nicolay et al.(2012); Taner et al. (2007); Van den Heuvel et al. (2006)
DFSS	Gremyr et al (2012); Junker et al (2011); Kaplan et al. (2009); Mandahawi et al (2010)
Ishikawa Diagram	Cloete and Bester (2012); Van den Heuvel et al. (2006)
Design of Experiment (DOE)	El-Banna (2012); Van den Heuvel et al. (2006)

5. Distribution of Articles by Improvements and Benefits to Healthcare Context

When LSS is implemented successfully in healthcare context, it will offer a disciplined approach for improving effectiveness and efficiency in a broad range of operations. The most cited benefit of LSS in healthcare is reducing *patient waiting time* (34 articles). Table 3 represents author contributions to LSS benefits in healthcare, while Figure 6 shows the rank of these benefits as their citation in the literature.

The literature has emphasized the key role of LSS in reducing *patient waiting time* in several healthcare departments such as pathology department (Gijo et al., 2013), emergency department (Mandahawi et al., 2010) and hospital registration (Yu and Yang, 2008). The second cited benefit of LSS in healthcare was

Figure 6. Distribution of articles by LSS benefits and improvement in healthcare

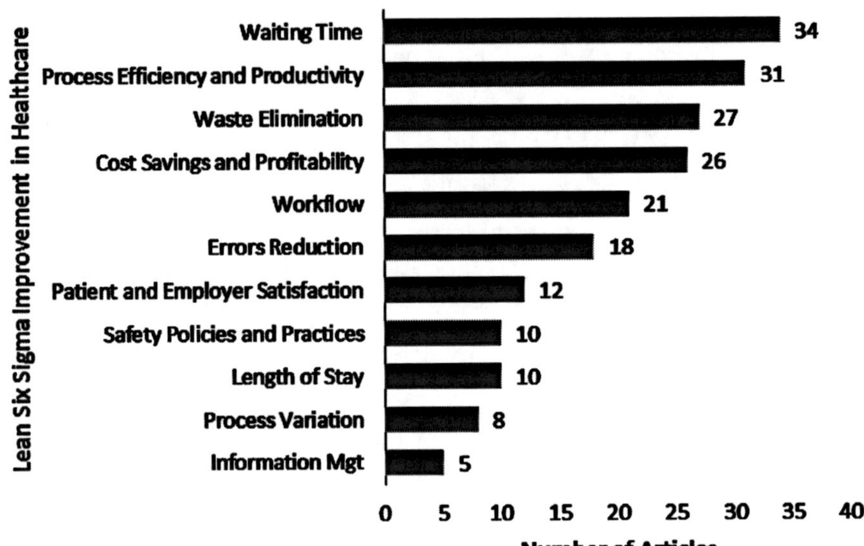

Table 3. Author contributions to LSS benefits and improvement in healthcare

Improvement	Authors
Waiting Time	Aakre et al (2010); Ahmed et al (2013); Al-Araidah et al (2010); Aleem (2013); Allen et al. (2010); Blick (2013); Chan et al. (2005); Christianson et al (2005); Cima et al. (2011); Costello and Molloy (2009); Das (2011); de Koning et al. (2006); Deckard et al (2010); Eite et al. (2010); El-Banna (2012); Fairbanks (2007); Fischman (2010); Gijo et al (2013); Hassell et al. (2010); Jimmerson et al (2005); Johnson et al. (2009); Lin et al (2013); Mandahawiet al (2010); Mathieson (2006); Mayer et al (2011); Mazzocato et al. (2012); Niemeijer et al. (2010); Paccagnella et al (2012); Roth et al (2010); Sunyog (2004); Van den Heuvel et al. (2006); Young et al. (2004); Yu et al. (2008); Zilm et al. (2010);
Process Efficiency and Productivity	Aakre et al (2010); Cheng and Chang (2012); Craven et al. (2006); Dahl (2009); Deckard et al (2010); Feng and Manuel (2008); Frings and Grant (2005); Garfield (2009); Gowen III et al. (2012); Gremyr et al (2012); Grove et al. (2010); Holden and Hackbart (2012); Junker et al (2011); Kovach et al. (2008); Langabeer et al (2009); Mandahawi (2011); Mazzocato et al. (2012); McJoynt et al. (2009); Mugdh and Pilla (2012); Niemeijer et al. (2012); Schriefer and Leonard (2012); Schweikhart and Dembe (2009); Sewing et al. (2008); Stankovic (2008); Stankovic and DeLauro (2010); Taner (2013); Tyson (2010); Ullman and Boutellier (2008); Yu et al. (2008); Yusof et al. (2012); Zilm et al. (2010)
Waste Elimination	Al-Araidah et al (2010); Bahensky et al (2005); Caldwell (2006); Chand (2011); Cheng and Chang (2012); Cima et al. (2011); de Bucourt et al (2011); Gayed et al (2013); Gowen III et al. (2012); Grove et al. (2010); Jin. et al. (2008); Junker et al (2011); Laureani et al (2013); Mathieson (2006); Niemeijer et al (2012); Niemeijer et al. (2010); Rajan et al. (2012); Roth et al (2010); Schattenkirk (2012); Stankovic (2008); Stankovic and DeLauro (2010); Taner (2013); Tyson (2010); Van den Heuvel et al. (2006); Viau and Southern (2007); Villa (2010); Yusof et al. (2012)
Cost Saving and Profitability	Bahensky et al (2005); Bucci and Musitano (2011); Caldwell (2006); Carboneau et al (2010); Carlson et al. (2012); Chiarini (2012); Christianson et al (2005); Cima et al. (2011); Dahl (2009); de Koning et al. (2006); El-Banna (2012); Feng and Antony (2010); Gayed et al (2013); Gitlow and Gitlow (2013); Gowen III et al. (2012); Impellizzeri et al (2009); Jimmerson et al (2005); Jin, M. et al. (2008); Kaplan et al. (2009); Kovach et al. (2008); Niemeijer et al (2012); Schweikhart and Dembe (2009); Sewing et al. (2008); Stankovic (2008); Sunyog (2004); Taner (2013)
Workflow	Bi et al. (2013); Crane et al (2014); Fairbanks (2007); Fischman (2010); García-porres et al. (2013); Holden and Hackbart (2012); Jin, M. et al. (2008); Johnson et al. (2009); Junker et al (2011); 9Kuo et al (2011); Mazzocato et al. (2012); McJoynt et al. (2009); Morrow (2012); Neufeld et al. (2013); Pantanowitz et al (2008); Parks et al (2008); Schriefer and Leonard (2012); Taner (2013); Taner et al. (2007); Toledo et al (2013); Villa (2010)

continued on following page

Table 3. Continued

Improvement	Authors
Clinical and Administrative Errors	Ahmed et al (2013); Chassin (2013); Cloete and Bester (2012); Costello and Molloy (2009); Das (2011); Elik (2013); Garfield (2009); Gowen III et al. (2012); Jimmerson et al (2005); Langabeer et al (2009); McJoynt et al. (2009); Noguera et al (2013); Paccagnella et al (2012); Pantanowitz et al (2008); Plebani and Lippi (2011); Stankovic (2004); Stankovic and DeLauro (2010); Van Den Heuvel et al. (2005);
Satisfaction of Patients and Employees	Bucci and Musitano (2011); Chiarini (2013); DuPree et al (2009); Eite et al. (2010); El-Banna (2012); Impellizzeri et al (2009); Kaplan et al. (2009); McDonald and Kirk (2013); McFadden et al. (2014); Mozammel and Mapa (2012); Stankovic (2008); Taner (2013)
Length of Stay	Ahmed et al (2013); Blick (2013); Gayed et al (2013); Mandahawi (2011); Mandahawiet al (2010); Niemeijer et al. (2010); Niemeijer et al. (2012); Toledo et al (2013); Van Den Heuvel et al. (2005); van Leeuwen and Does (2010)
Safety Policies and Practices	Baddour and Saleh, (2013); Carboneau et al (2010); Chassin (2013); Chiarini (2012); Christianson et al (2005); Deckard et al (2010); Farzianpour et al. (2012); Karsten (2011); Morrow (2012); Veluswamy et al. (2010)
Process Variation	Chand (2011); Cima et al. (2011); Gitlow and Gitlow (2013); Pan et al. (2008); Stankovic (2004); Stankovic (2008); Stuenkel and Faulkner (2009); Woodard (2005)
Information Management	Blick (2013); Costello and Molloy (2009); Mozammel and Mapa (2012); Yusof et al. (2012); Zandi (2013);

improving process efficiency and productivity (31 articles). Examples of include improve the efficiency of resident rounding process (Chand, 2011), operating room (Cima et al., 2011), internal medicine residency clinic (Fischman, 2010), laboratory department (Villa, 2010) and physician productivity in a clinical department (Feng and Antony, 2010). *Waste elimination* was among the top three benefits of LSS application in healthcare (27 articles). For example, Bahensky et al. (2005) reported that LSS has a positive impact on identification and elimination of non-value added activities in Radiology CT scanning.

Mozammel and Mapa (2012) applied LSS in nursing shift directors process improvement to create a baseline metric of the existing process, eliminate the non-value added tasks from the daily workload, and provide control methodologies for sustainability. They indicated that the greatest achievement has been the reduction in overall documentation from 39% to 26%. Jin et al. (2008) revealed that LSS applications in healthcare logistics center design and operation has resulted in better storage management, better use of space, an improved and cleaner workspace, more timely and efficient delivery of the right items with the right amount to the right patients and tracking and reducing waste. Other key benefits of LSS applications in healthcare include *cost saving, workflow, reduction of clinical and administrative errors, satisfaction of patients and employees, improving length of stay, enhancing safety policies and practices, process variation, and better management of healthcare information.*

6. Distribution of Articles by Research Method

The distribution of articles by research method is shown in Figure 7. About sixty-five percent of the articles (105 articles) were classified as empirical articles using either surveys or case studies, while about 35% of the articles (57 articles) were theoretical articles which usually employ extensive literature review to focus on the development of concepts, propositions, models, or theory building of LSS in healthcare. Also, it is clear that *case study* is the most dominant research method in LSS in healthcare articles (95 articles, 59%). Figure 8 shows the growing gap over the years between case study method and other research methods, particularly survey research. Case study method is used to document and analyze LSS application in a wide variety of hospitals, clinics, departments and processes such as emergency department (Dickson et al., 2009), healthcare logistics (Jin et al., 2008), cancer center (McJoynt et al., 2009), liver and knee MRI examinations (Ruth et al., 2010), patient care in a mammography center (Viau, 2007). On the contrary, survey research represents the least dominant research method in LSS in healthcare (10 articles, 6.2%) where typical wide perspective or superficial generalization are employed to a large number of respondents or cases.

Examples of LSS in healthcare survey research involve Farzianpour et al. (2012) who surveyed patient safety in inpatient wards in a university hospital. They suggested that the quality level of physical environment and safety training were medium while safety of patients' beds, health and management of incidents were at desirable quality level. Also, Gowen et al. (2012) surveyed six Sigma and lean management in US hospitals. They indicated that process improvement (PI) initiatives mediate the effect of medical error sources to enhance three hospital outcomes involving patient safety, operational effectiveness, and competitiveness.

Figure 7. Distribution of articles by empirical and theoretical LSS research in healthcare

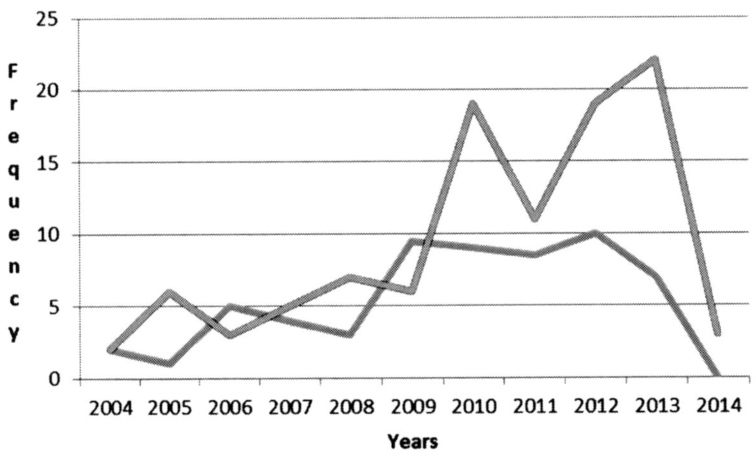

Figure 8. Distribution of LSS in healthcare articles by case, survey and review methods

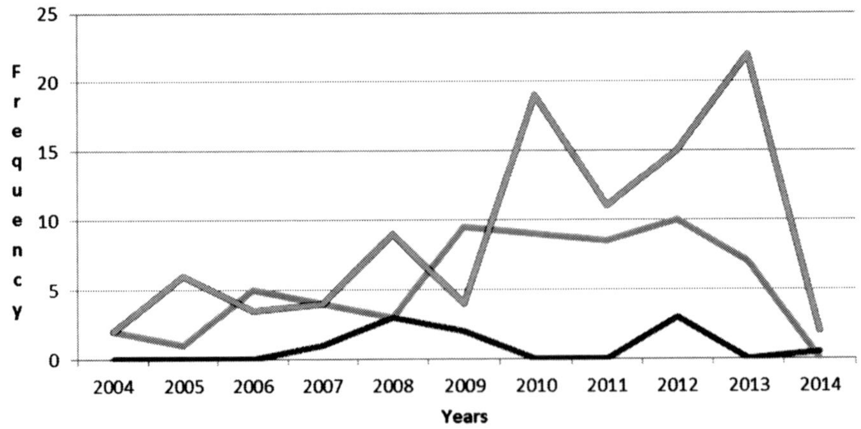

Hilton et al. (2008) applied survey research to examine factors critical to the success of LSS quality program in an Australian hospital. They indicated that there are gaps between what the respondents expect as being a necessary part of a quality program and the actual results in the hospital.

CONCLUSION AND IMPLICATIONS FOR FUTURE RESEARCH

Our conclusions are based on the analysis of 162 LSS in healthcare articles that were published in 108 journals over a ten-year period from 2004 to January 2014. Overall, we have observed that LSS research has attracted the attention of both practitioners and academics within the healthcare context reflecting an increasing trend over years. Clearly, LSS research is difficult to confine to specific healthcare discipline as it is scattered across various journals from different disciplines. However, the leading journals contributing to LSS in healthcare research represent multidisciplinary perspectives integrating quality, management and healthcare in general with less focus from clinical or medical journals on LSS. While processes related to *patient care* and *laboratory* quality dominate LSS application areas in healthcare, less emphasis has been given to issues related to processes involving healthcare safety, workflow, surgery and logistics. The review has observed that LSS in healthcare research is empirical in nature which fortifies the use of primary data. Case study was the dominant research method in LSS in healthcare and this is may be due to the nature of quality problems in general that need to be documented and examined over a period of time (Aboelmaged, 2010). In addition, the lack of LSS implementation across wide range of healthcare services and processes makes the use of survey methods impractical. In addition, empirical nature of LSS in healthcare research allow

for implementing various LSS tools and methods including DMAIC and 5S as expected. Nevertheless, little attention has been given to other tools such as *Kaizen, Ishikawa Diagram* and *Design of Experiment* (DOE). It is noteworthy that reducing *patient waiting time, improving process efficiency* and *waste elimination* are the greatest benefits of LSS application in healthcare. In contrast, reducing process variation and enhancing information management are barely perceived as among the key benefits of LSS applications in healthcare.

Although this review does not claim to be exhaustive, it does provide reasonable insights into the state of the art of LSS in healthcare research. There is very little room for clarifying the confusion in the literature as to what constitutes LSS theory and how does it integrate with improvement strategies in different contexts. We would argue that theoretical development is critical to enhance forthcoming LSS studies. Based on the literature review presented in this chapter, we identify below a number of research implications and directions for future research as follows:

- Mapping LSS research efforts in healthcare would encourage researchers and practitioners to propose standards for successful LSS projects in healthcare as well as designing LSS curriculum within healthcare context.
- Life cycle of LSS projects in healthcare is not well established. Therefore, documenting common phases in LSS life cycle within healthcare context and role of organizational factors that accelerate or hold up these phases.
- Distinguishing between clinical and administrative processes while examining LSS application in healthcare is also important.
- There is no doubt that LSS will grow rapidly in future covering various disciplines and domains. Hence, there is a need to

structure LSS application within each domain. Particularly, when there is a dominance of specific organizational culture model.

- There is a need for rigors research constructing LSS barriers based on user experience in such context.
- The link between LSS and other approaches such as reengineering and governance require further research efforts to underline the degree of integration and evolving tools and techniques that can be used.
- Researchers can benefit from integrating analytical and empirical research methods to provide deep insights into LSS research through applying triangulation approach and using multiple data sources.
- Researchers are also encouraged to compare findings of peer-reviewed articles with books and conference proceedings on LSS to inform managers and practitioners the current trends and challenges of LSS implementation.

Research on LSS is a never-ending process, however this chapter attempts to insinuate significant insights into the state of the art of LSS in healthcare research and clarify confusion in the literature as to what constitutes LSS role in improving healthcare context.

REFERENCES

Aboelmaged, M. G. (2010). Six Sigma quality: A structured review and implications for future research. *International Journal of Quality & Reliability Management, 27*(3), 269–318. doi:10.1108/02656711011023294

Aboelmaged, M. G. (2011). Reconstructing Six Sigma barriers in manufacturing and service organizations: The effects of organizational parameters. *International Journal of Quality & Reliability Management, 28*(5), 519–541. doi:10.1108/02656711111132562

Andersson, R., Eriksson, H., & Torstensson, H. (2006). Similarities and differences between TQM, six sigma and lean. *The TQM Magazine, 18*(3), 282–296. doi:10.1108/09544780610660004

Antony, J. (2006). Six Sigma for service processes. *Business Process Management Journal, 12*(2), 234–248. doi:10.1108/14637150610657558

Byrne, G., Lubowe, D., & Blitz, A. (2007). Using a lean Six Sigma approach to drive innovation. *Strategy and Leadership, 35*(2), 5–10. doi:10.1108/10878570710734480

De Koning, H., & Verver, J. P. S. (2006). Lean six sigma in healthcare. *Journal for Healthcare Quality, 28*(2), 4–11. doi:10.1111/j.1945-1474.2006.tb00596.x PMID:16749293

George, M. L. (2002). *Lean Six Sigma: Combining Six Sigma Quality with Lean Speed*. New York: McGraw-Hill.

Glasgow, J. M., Scott-Caziewell, J. R., & Kaboli, P. J. (2010). Guiding inpatient quality improvement: A systematic review of Lean and Six Sigma. *Joint Commission Journal of Quality Qual Patient Saf, 36*(12), 533–540. PMID:21222355

Heckert, L. (2013). *Lean Six Sigma at Alliant Energy*. Available at: http://www.alliantenergy.com/wcm/groups/wcm_internet/@int/@ae/documents/document/mdaw/mdmy/~edisp/032825.pdf

Kwak, Y. H., & Anbari, F. T. (2006). Benefits, obstacles, and future of Six Sigma approach. *Technovation*, *26*(5-6), 708–715. doi:10.1016/j.technovation.2004.10.003

Yamazaki, T., Ikeda, M., & Umemoto, K. (2011). Enhancement of healthcare quality using clinical-pathways activities. *Vine*, *41*(1), 63–75. doi:10.1108/03055721111115557

ADDITIONAL READING

Assarlind, M., Gremyr, I., & Bäckman, K. (2013). Multi-faceted views on a Lean Six Sigma application. *International Journal of Quality & Reliability Management*, *30*(4), 387–402. doi:10.1108/02656711311308385

Christenson, R. H., Snyder, S. R., Shaw, C. S., Derzon, J. H., Black, R. S., & Mass, D. et al. (2011). Laboratory medicine best practices: Systematic evidence review and evaluation methods for quality improvement. *Clinical Chemistry*, *57*(6), 816–825. doi:10.1373/clinchem.2010.157131 PMID:21515742

Psychogios, A., Atanasovski, J., & Tsironis, L. (2012). Lean Six Sigma in a service context. *International Journal of Quality & Reliability Management*, *29*(1), 122–139. doi:10.1108/02656711211190909

Ransom, S., Joshi, M., & Nash, D. (2004). *The Healthcare Quality Book: Vision, Strategy, and Tools*. Chicago: Health Administration Press.

KEY TERMS AND DEFINITIONS

5S Principles: An approach that is used to organize and manage the workspace and workflow aiming at eliminating waste and reducing process inefficiencies. The approach uses 5 Japanese words including (Seiri) Sort, (Seiton) Straighten, (Seiso) Sweep, (Seiketsu) Standardize and (Shitsuke) Sustain.

DMAIC: Is a step-by-step six sigma approach focusing on defining, measuring, analyzing, improving and controlling quality initiatives.

Lean Six Sigma: An approach focused on improving quality, reducing variation and eliminating waste in an organization.

Quality: A measure of excellence or a state of being free from defects, deficiencies, and significant variations.

Six Sigma: A metric of process measurement symbolized by the Greek letter σ that represents the amount of variation with a normal data distribution that targets quality level of 3.4 defects per million opportunities (DPMO).

This work was previously published in Lean Six Sigma Approaches in Manufacturing, Services, and Production edited by Edem G. Tetteh and Benedict M. Uzochukwu, pages 231-261 copyright year 2015 by Business Science Reference (an imprint of IGI Global).

APPENDIX

A Full List of Analyzed LSS in Healthcare Articles

160. Aakre, K.T., Valley T. B., & O'Connor, M. K. (2010). Quality initiatives: improving patient flow for a bone densitometry practice: results from a Mayo Clinic radiology quality initiative. *Radiographics*, 30(2), 309-315.

161. Ahmed, S., Manaf, N. H., & Islam, R. (2013). Effects of Lean Six Sigma application in healthcare services: a literature review. *Rev Environ Health*, 28(4), 189-194.

162. Al-Araidah, O., Momani, A., Khasawneh, M., & Momani, M. (2010). Lead-time reduction utilizing lean tools applied to healthcare: the inpatient pharmacy at a local hospital. *Journal for Healthcare Quality*, 32(1), 59–66.

163. Aldarrab, A. (2006). Application of lean six sigma for patients presenting with st-elevation myocardial infarction: the Hamilton health sciences experience. *Healthcare Quality*, 9(1), 56-61.

164. Aleem S. (2013). Translating 10 lessons from lean six sigma project in paper-based training site to electronic health record-based primary care practice: challenges and opportunities. *Qual Manag Health Care*, 22(3), 224-35.

165. Allen, T. T., Shih-Hsien, T., Swanson, K., & McClay, M. A. (2010). Improving the Hospital Discharge Process with Six Sigma Methods. *Quality Engineering* 22(1), 13-14.

166. Al-Qatawneh, L., Abdallah, A., & Zalloum, S. (2013). Reducing Stock-out Incidents at a Hospital Using Six Sigma. *Proceedings of World Academy of Science, Engineering and Technology* 77, 463-470.

167. Baddour, A. A., Saleh, & Hager A. (2013). Use Six Sigma Approach to Improve Healthcare Workers Safety, *International Journal of Pure and Applied Sciences and Technology*, 18(1), 54-71.

168. Bahensky, J. A., Roe, J., & Bolton, R. (2005), Lean sigma--will it work for healthcare? *J Healthc Inf Manag*. Winter, 19(1), 39-44.

169. Bashir, M. R., Dale, B. M., Gupta, R. T., Horvath, J. J., Boll, D. T., & Merkle, E. M. (2012). Gradient shimming during magnetic resonance imaging of the liver: comparison of a standard protocol versus a novel reduced protocol. *Invest Radiol*, 47(9), 524-539.

170. Bhaskar, R., Kapoor, A., & Vo, A. (2012). Pioneering the health care quality improvement in india using six sigma: a case study of a northern India hospital. *Journal of Cases on Information Technology*, 14(4), 41-55.

171. Bi, F. C., Frost, H. N., Ling, X., Perry, D. A., & Sakata, S. K. (2013). Driving external chemistry optimization via operations management principles. *Drug Discov Today*, pii: S1359-6446(13).

172. Black, J. (2009). Transforming the patient care environment with Lean Six Sigma and realistic evaluation. *J Healthc Qual*. 3, 29-35.

173. Blick, K. (2013). Providing critical laboratory results on time, every time to help reduce emergency department length of stay: how our laboratory achieved a six sigma level of performance. *American Journal of Clinical Pathology*. 140(2), 193-202.

174. Bonilla, C., Pawlicki, T., Perry, L., & Wesselink, B. (2008). Radiation oncology Lean Six Sigma project selection based on patient and staff input into a modified quality function deployment. *International Journal of Six Sigma and Competitive Advantage*, 4(3)196-208.

175. Bucci, R. V., & Musitano, A. (2011). A Lean Six Sigma journey in radiology. *Radiol Manage.* 33(3), 27-33.

176. Buell, J. M. (2010). Lean Six Sigma and patient safety: a recipe for success. *Healthc Exec.* 25(2), 26-38.

177. Bullas, S., & Bryant, J. (2007). Successful Systems Sustaining Change. *Studies in Health Technology and Informatics,* 129, 1199-1203.

178. Caldwell, C. (2006). Lean-Six Sigma: tools for rapid cycle cost reduction. *Healthc Financ Manage.* 60(10), 96-108.

179. Carboneau, C., Benge, E., Jaco, M., & Robinson, M. (2010). A Lean Six Sigma Team Increases Hand Hygiene Compliance and Reduces Hospital-Acquired MRSA Infections by 51%. *Journal for Healthcare Quality,* 32(4)61–70.

180. Carlson, R. O., Amirahmadi, F., & Hernandez, J. S. (2012). A primer on the cost of quality for improvement of laboratory and pathology specimen processes. *Am J Clin Pathol,* 138(3), 347-54.

181. Chan, W. P., Wen-Ta, C., Wan-Ming, C., Min-Fang, L., & Chu, B. (2005). Applying Six Sigma methodology to maximise magnetic resonance imaging capacity in a hospital. *International Journal of Healthcare Technology & Management,* 6 (3), 321-330.

182. Chand, D. (2011), Observational Study Using the Tools of Lean Six Sigma to Improve the Efficiency of the Resident Rounding Process. *Journal of Graduate Medical Education,* 3(2), 144-150.

183. Chassin, Mark (2013). Improving The Quality Of Health Care: What's Taking So Long?. *Health Affairs.* 32(10), 1761-1765.

184. Chen-Yang, C., & Pu-Yuan, C. (2012). Implementation of the Lean Six Sigma framework in non-profit organisations: A case study. *Total Quality Management & Business Excellence* 23(3/4), 431-441.

185. Chiarini, A. (2012). Risk management and cost reduction of cancer drugs using Lean Six Sigma tools. *Leadership in Health Services,* 25(4), 318 – 330.

186. Chiarini, A. (2013). Building a Six Sigma model for the Italian public healthcare sector using grounded theory. *International Journal of Services and Operations Management,* 14(4), 491-508.

187. Chiarini, A., & Bracci, E. (2013). Implementing Lean Six Sigma in healthcare: issues from Italy *Public Money & Management,* 33(5), 361-368.

188. Christianson, J., Warrick, L., Howard, R., & Vollum, J. (2005). Deploying Six Sigma in a Health Care System as a Work in Progress. *Joint Commission Journal on Quality and Patient Safety,* 31(11), 603-613.

189. Cima, R., Dankbar, E., & Lovely, J. (2013). Colorectal Surgery Surgical Site Infection Reduction Program: A National Surgical Quality Improvement Program–Driven Multidisciplinary Single-Institution Experience. *Journal of the American College of Surgeons,* 216(1), 23-33.

190. Cima, R., Brown, M., & Hebl, J. (2011). Use of Lean and Six Sigma Methodology to Improve Operating Room Efficiency in a High-Volume Tertiary-Care Academic Medical Center. *Journal of the American College of Surgeons,* 213(1), 83–92.

191. Cloete, B. C., & Bester, A. (2012) A Lean Six Sigma approach to the improvement of the selenium analysis method. *Onderstepoort J Vet Res,* 79(1), E1-E13.

192. Coffin, C. T. (2013). The continuous improvement process and ergonomics in ultrasound department. Radiol Manage, 35(1), 22-35.

193. Costello, C., Molloy, & O. (2009). A process model to support automated measurement and detection of out-of-bounds events in a hospital laboratory process. *Journal of Theoretical and Applied Electronic Commerce Research*, 4(2), 31-54.

194. Crane, P. W., Zhou, Y., Sun, Y., Lin, L., & Schneider, S. M. (2014). Entropy: A Conceptual Approach to Measuring Situation-level Workload Within Emergency Care and its Relationship to Emergency Department Crowding. *J Emerg Me*d., pii: S0736-4679(13)01106-2.

195. Craven, E., Clark, J., & Cramer, M. (2006). NewYork-Presbyterian Hospital uses Six Sigma to build a culture of quality and innovation. *Journal of Organizational Excellence*, 25(4), 11–19.

196. Dahl, O. J. (2009). Cost and efficiency lead to increased value for the patient and bottom line for the practice. *J Med Pract Manage.*, 25(2), 87-99.

197. Das, B. (2011). Validation Protocol: First Step of a Lean-Total Quality, Management Principle in a New Laboratory Set-up in a Tertiary Care Hospital in India. *Ind J Clin Biochem*, 26(3), 235–243.

198. De-Bucourt, M., Busse, R., & Guttler, F. (2011). Lean manufacturing and Toyota Production System terminology applied to the procurement of vascular stents in interventional radiology. *Insights Imaging*, 22, 415–423.

199. De-Koning, H., Verver, J., van den Heuvel, J., Bisgaard, S., & Does, R. (2006). Lean Six Sigma in Healthcare. *Journal for Healthcare Quality*, 28(2), 4–11.

200. Deckard, G. J., Borkowski, N., Diaz, D., Sanchez, C., & Boisette S. A. (2010). Improving timeliness and efficiency in the referral process for safety net providers: application of the Lean Six Sigma methodology. *J Ambul Care Manage.* 33(2), 124-130.

201. Delisle, D. (2013). Care transitions programs: a review of hospital-based programs targeted to reduce readmissions. *Professional Case Management* 18(6), 273-283.

202. DelliFraine, J., & Langabeer, J. (2009).An institutional perspective on quality initiatives: evidence beyond manufacturing. *International Journal of Information Systems and Change Management*, 4(1), 3-14.

203. DelliFraine, J. L, Langabeer, J. R., & Nembhard, I. M. (2010). Assessing the evidence of Six Sigma and Lean in the health care industry. *Qual Manag Health Care.* 19(3), 211-25.

204. Dickson, A. (2013). Utilizing a Lean Six Sigma Approach to Reduce Total Joint Arthroplasty Surgical Site Infections in a Community Hospital. *American Journal of Infection Control*, 41(6), S131-S132.

205. Dickson, E., Anguelov, Z., Vetterick, D., Eller, A., & Singh, S. (2009). Use of Lean in the Emergency Department: A Case Series of 4 Hospitals. *Annals of Emergency Medicine*, 54(4), 504-510.

206. DuPree, E., Martin, L., & Anderson, R. (2009). Improving Patient Satisfaction with Pain Management Using Six Sigma Tools. *Joint Commission Journal on Quality and Patient Safety*, 35(7), 343-350.

207. Eitel, D. R., Rudkin, S. E., Malvehy, M. A., Killeen, J. P., & Pines, J. M. (2010). Improving service quality by understanding emergency department flow: a White Paper and position statement prepared for the American Academy of Emergency Medicine. *J Emerg Med.*, 38(1), 70-9.

208. El-Banna., & Mahmoud, A. (2012). Improving Patients Discharge Process in Hospitals by using Six Sigma Approach, Improving Patients Discharge Process in Hospitals by using Six Sigma Approach. *Proceedings of World Academy of Science, Engineering and Technology,* 68, 112-121.

209. Elik, L. L. (2013). Learning and applying new quality improvement methods to the school health setting. NASN Sch Nurse., 28(6), 306-11.

210. Everett, L. Q., & Sitterding, M. C. (2013). Building a culture of innovation by maximizing the role of the RN. *Nurs Adm Q.*, 37(3), 194-202.

211. Fairbanks, C. B. (2007). Using Six Sigma and Lean methodologies to improve OR throughput. *AORN J.* 86(1), 73-82.

212. Farzianpour, F., Fouroshani, A., Dargaha, K., & Hosseini, H. (2012). Patient safety in inpatient wards: sample of a university hospital. *American Journal of Applied Sciences*, 9(12), 2004-2011.

213. Feng, M. & Manuel, C. (2008). Under the knife: a national survey of six sigma programs in US healthcare organizations. *International Journal of Health Care Quality Assurance*, 21(6), 535 – 547.

214. Feng, Q., & Antony, J. (2010). Integrating DEA into Six Sigma methodology for measuring health service efficiency. *The Journal of the Operational Research Society*, 61(7), 1112-1121.

56. Fillingham, D. (2007). Can lean save lives?. *Journal of Leadership in Health Services*, 20(4), 231-241.

58. Fischman, D. (2010). Applying Lean Six Sigma methodologies to improve efficiency, timeliness of care, and quality of care in an internal medicine residency clinic. *Qual Manag Health Care*, 19(3), 201-10.

215. Frings, G. W., & Grant, L. (2005). Who Moved My Sigma Effective Implementation of the Six Sigma Methodology to Hospitals. *Quality and Reliability Engineering International*, 21(3), 311-328.

216. Gamm, L., Kash, B., & Bolin, J. (2007). Organizational technologies for transforming care: measures and strategies for pursuit of IOM quality aims. *J Ambul Care Manage*, 30(4), 291-301.

217. García-porres, J., & Ortiz-posadas, M. R. (2013). Sigma Level Performance of the Innovated Process in the Imaging Department at a Mexican Health Institute. *Journal of Digital Imaging*, 26(2), 353-60.

218. Garfield, S., Barber, N., Walley, P., Willson, A., & Eliasson, L. (2009). Quality of medication use in primary care - mapping the problem, working to a solution: a systematic review of the literature. *BMC Medicine*, 7(50), 1-12.

219. Gayed, B., Black, S., Daggy, J., & Munshi, I. A. (2013). Redesigning a joint replacement program using Lean Six Sigma in a Veterans Affairs hospital. *JAMA Surg.*, 148(11), 1050-6.

220. Gijo, E., Antony, J., & Hernandez, J. (2013). Reducing patient waiting time in a pathology department using the Six Sigma methodology. *Leadership in Health Services*, 26(4), 253 – 267.

221. Gitlow, H. S., & Gitlow, A. L. (2013). Deming-Based Lean Six Sigma Management as an Answer to Escalating Hospital Costs. *The Quality Management Journal*, 20(3), 6-9.

222. Glasgow, J. M., Scott-Caziewell, J. R., & Kaboli, P. J. (2010). Guiding Inpatient Quality Improvement: A Systematic Review of Lean and Six Sigma. *Joint Commission Journal on Quality and Patient Safety*, 36(12), 533-540.

223. Gowen, C., Stock, G., & Mcfadden, C. (2008). Simultaneous implementation of Six Sigma and knowledge management in hospitals. *International Journal of Production Research,* 46(23), 6781-679.

224. Gowen, C. R., McFadden, K. L., & Settaluri, S. (2012). Contrasting continuous quality improvement, Six Sigma, and lean management for enhanced outcomes in US hospitals. *American Journal of Business*, 27(2), 133-153.

225. Gremyr, I., Gustavsson, S., & Gideberg, A. (2012). The medication process - a design for Six Sigma project. *International Journal of Six Sigma and Competitive Advantage* (7)1, 1-11.

226. Grove, A L., & Meredith, M. J. O. (2010). Lean implementation in primary care health visiting services in National Health Service UK. *Qual Saf Health Care*, 19(5), 9 – 13.

227. Hassell, L., Glass, C., Yip, C., & Eneff, P. (2010). The combined positive impact of Lean methodology and Ventana Symphony autostainer on histology lab workflow. *BMC Clinical Pathology*, 10(2), 1-9.

228. Hilton, R., Balla, M., & Sohal, A. S. (2008). Factors critical to the success of a Six-Sigma quality program in an Australian hospital. *Total Quality Management & Business Excellence*, 19(9) 887-896.

229. Hina-Syeda, H., Kimbrough, C., Murdoch, W., & Markova, T. (2013). Improving Immunization Rates Using Lean Six Sigma Processes: Alliance of Independent Academic Medical Centers National Initiative III Project. *The Ochsner Journal*, 13, 310–318.

230. Holden, R., & Hackbart, G. (2012). From group work to teamwork: A case study of "Lean" rapid process improvement in the ThedaCare Information Technology Department. *IIE Transactions on Healthcare Systems Engineering*, 2(3), 190-201.

231. Hurley, B. T., Taylor, J., Levett, C., & Huber, E. H (2008), Implementation of six sigma and lean methodology into the anticoagulation management process. *Journal of Thrombosis and Thrombolysis*, 25, 106-109.

232. Impellizzeri, F., Bizzini, M., Leunig, M. Maffiuletti, N., & Mannion, A. (2009). Money matters: exploiting the data from outcomes research for quality improvement. *Eur Spine J.*, 18, 348–359.

233. Jimmerson, C., Weber, D., & Sobek, II, D. (2005). Reducing Waste and Errors: Piloting Lean Principles at IHC. *Joint Commission Journal on Quality and Patient Safety*, 31(5), 249-257.

234. Jin, M., Switzer, M., & Agirbas, G. (2008). Six Sigma and Lean in healthcare logistics centre design and operation: a case at North Mississippi Health Services. *International Journal of Six Sigma and Competitive Advantage,* 4(3), 270-288.

235. Johnson, C. W., Chatterjee, M., & Kubala S. (2009). Efficient and effective compound management to support lead optimization. *J Biomol Screen.* 14(5), 523-30.

236. Junker, B., Maheshwari, G., & Ranheim, T. (2011). Design-for-Six-Sigma To Develop a Bioprocess Knowledge Management Framework. *PDA J Pharm Sci Technol.*, 65(2), 140-65.

237. Kaplan, S., Bisgaard, S., Truesdell, D., & Zetterholm, S. (2009). Design for Six Sigma In Healthcare: Developing an Employee Influenza Vaccination Process. *Journal for Healthcare Quality*, 31(3), 36–43.

238. Karsten, M (2011). Patient Safety: Commitment versus Compliance. *Nurse Leader*, 9(4), 47-49.

239. Kim, C., Spahlinger, D., Kin, J., & Billi J. (2006). Lean health care: What can hospitals learn from a world-class automaker?. *Journal of Hospital Medicine*, 1(3), 191–199.

240. Kollberg, B., Dahlgaard, J.. & Brehmer, P. O. (2007). Measuring lean initiatives in health care services: issues and findings. *International Journal of Productivity and Performance Management*, 56, 7 – 24.

241. Kovach, J., De La Torre, L., & Walker, D. (2008). Continuous improvement efforts in healthcare: a case study exploring the motivation, involvement and support necessary for success. *International Journal of Six Sigma and Competitive Advantage,* 4(3), 254-269.

242. Kuo, A. M. H., Borycki, A., & Kushniruk, A. (2011). A healthcare Lean Six Sigma system for postanesthesia care unit workflow improvement. *Qual Manage Health Care.* 20(1), 4-14.

243. Langabeer, J. R., DelliFraine, J. L., Heineke, J., & Abbass, I. (2009). Implementation of Lean and Six Sigma quality initiatives in hospitals: a goal theoretic perspective. *Operations Management Research*. 2, 13-27.

244. Laureani, A., Malcolm, B., & Jiju, A. (2013). Applications of Lean Six Sigma in an Irish hospital. *Leadership in Health Services*, 26 (4), 322 – 337.

245. Lin, S. Y., Gavney, D., Ishman, S. L., & Cady-Reh, J. (2013). Use of lean sigma principles in a tertiary care otolaryngology clinic to improve efficiency. *Laryngoscope*. 123(11), 2643-8.

246. Llopis, M., Trujillo, G., Llovet, M., & Tarres, E. (2011). Quality indicators and specifications for key analytical-extranalytical processes in the clinical laboratory. Five years' experience using the Six Sigma concept. *Clinical Chemistry and Laboratory Medicine*. 49(3), 463-470.

247. Mandahawi, N., Al-Shihabi, S., Abdallah, A., & Alfarah, Y. (2010). Reducing waiting time at an emergency department using design for Six Sigma and discrete event simulation. *International Journal of Six Sigma and Competitive Advantage*, 6(1-2), 91-104.

248. Mandahawi, N., Al-Araidah, O., Boran, A., & Khasawneh, M. (2011). Application of Lean Six Sigma tools to minimise length of stay for ophthalmology day case surgery. *International Journal of Six Sigma and Competitive Advantage*, 6(3), 156-172.

249. Mannon, M. (2014). Lean Healthcare and Quality Management: The Experience of ThedaCare. *Quality Management Journal*, 21(1), 4-7.

250. Martin, W. F. (2007). Quality Models: Selecting the Best Model to Deliver Results. *Physician Executive*. 33(3), 24-31.

251. Martinez, E., Chavez-Valdez, P., & Holt, N. (2011). Successful Implementation of a Perioperative Glycemic Control Protocol in Cardiac Surgery: Barrier Analysis and Intervention Using Lean Six Sigma. *Anesthesiology Research and Practice*, Article ID 565069.

252. Mathieson, S. (2006). Lean healthcare. Weight watchers. *Health Service Journal*, 116, 4-5.

253. Mayer, H., Brummer, J., & Brinkmann, T. (2011). Precise turnaround time measurement of laboratory processes using radiofrequency identification technology. *Clin Lab.*, 57(1-2), 75-81.

254. Mazzocato, P., Holden, R., & Brommels, M. (2012). How does lean work in emergency care? A case study of a lean-inspired intervention at the Astrid Lindgren Children's hospital, Stockholm, Sweden. *BMC Health Services Research*, 12(28), 1-13.

255. McDonald, A. P., & Kirk, R. (2013). Using lean Six Sigma to improve hospital based outpatient imaging satisfaction. *Radiol Manage.*, 35(1), 38-45.

256. McFadden, K., Lee, J., Gowen, C., & Sharp, B. (2014) Linking Quality Improvement Practices to Knowledge Management Capabilities. *Quality Management Journal*, 21(1), 34-55.

257. McJoynt, T., Hirzallah, M., & Satele, D. (2009). Building a Protocol Expressway: The Case of Mayo Clinic Cancer Center, *Journal of Clinical Oncology*, 27, 3855-3860.

258. Miles, E. N. (2006). Improvement in the incident reporting and investigation procedures using process excellence (DMAI2C) methodology, *Journal of Hazardous Materials*, 130(1-2), 169-181.

259. Morrow, R. (2012). Perioperative Quality and Improvement. *Anesthesiology Clinics*, 30(3), 555-563.

260. Mozammel, A., & Mapa, L. (2012). Application of Lean Six Sigma in Healthcare - Nursing Shift Directors Process Improvement. *Journal of Management & Engineering Integration*, 4(2), 58-65.

261. Mugdh, M., & Pilla, S. 2012. Revenue cycle optimization in health care institutions. A conceptual framework for change management. *Health Care Manag*, 31(1), 75-80.

262. Murphree, P., Vath, R. R., & Daigle, L. (2011). Sustaining Lean Six Sigma projects in health care. *Physician Exec.*, 37(1), 44-58.

263. Neufeld, N. J., Hoyer, E. H., Cabahug, P., González-Fernández, M., Mehta, M., Walker, N. C., Powers, R. L., & Mayer, R. S. (2013). A Lean Six Sigma quality improvement project to increase discharge paperwork completeness for admission to a comprehensive integrated inpatient rehabilitation program. *Am J Med Qual.*, 28(4), 301-317.

264. Nicolay, C. R., Purkayastha, S., Greenhalgh, A., Benn, J., Chaturvedi, S., Phillips, N., & Darzi, A. (2012). Systematic review of the application of quality improvement methodologies from the manufacturing industry to surgical healthcare. *British Journal of Surgery*, 99(3), 324–335.

265. Niemeijer, G. C., Flikweert, E., Trip, A., Does, R. J., Ahaus, K. T., Boot, A. F., & Wendt, K. W. (2012). The usefulness of lean six sigma to the development of a clinical pathway for hip fractures, Journal of Evaluation in Clinical Practice, 19(5), 909–914.

266. Niemeijer, G. C., Trip, A., de Jong, L, J., Wendt, K. W., & Does, R. J. (2012). Impact of 5 years of lean six sigma in a University Medical Center. Qual Manag Health Care, 21(4), 262-278.

267. Niemeijer, G., Does, R.. de Mast, J., Trip, A., & Huevel, J. V. D. (2011). Generic Project Definitions for Improvement of Health Care Delivery: A Case-Based Approach, *Quality Management Health Care*, 20 (2), 152–164.

268. Niemeijer, G., Trip, A., Ahaus, K., Does, R. J., & Wendt, K. W. (2010). Quality in Trauma Care: Improving the Discharge Procedure of Patients by Means of Lean Six Sigma, *The Journal of TRAUMA® Injury, Infection, and Critical Care*, 69(3), 614-619.

269. Niu, G., Lau, D., & Pecht, M. (2010). Computer Manufacturing Management Integrating Lean Six Sigma and Prognostic Health Management, *International Journal of Performability Engineering*, 6(5), 453-466.

270. Noguera, F., Megía, F., Riquelme, F., Balasch, I., Parisi, S., Solsona, M. D., & Poveda, A. J. L. (2013). Improving inpatient pharmacoterapeutic process by Lean Six Sigma methodology, *Rev Calid Asist.*, 28(6), 370-80.

112. Paccagnella, A., Mauri, A., & Spinella, N. (2012). Quality improvement for integrated management of patients with type 2 diabetes. *Qual Manag Health Care*, 21(3), 146-59.

114. Feng-Chuan, P., Mei, Y. S., & Shen, J. C. (2008). Reducing unplanned endotracheal extubation in hospital ICU through Six Sigma and HQIC. *International Journal of Six Sigma and Competitive Advantage*, 4(4), 382-394.

271. Pantanowitz, L., Hornish, M., & Goulart, R. A. (2008). Informatics applied to cytology. *Cytojournal*, 29(5), 16-24.

272. Parks, J. K., Klein, J., Frankel, H. L., Friese, R. S., & Shafi, S. (2008). Dissecting delays in trauma care using corporate lean six sigma methodology. *J Trauma*, 65(5), 1098-104.

273. Pate, C. (2012). Focusing Quality Improvement Efforts through Lean Six Methods in Health Information Technology. *International Journal of Reliable and Quality E-Healthcare*, 1(1), 21-23.

274. Plebani, M., & Lippi G. (2011). Closing the brain-to-brain loop in laboratory testing. *Clin Chem Lab Med.*, 49(7), 1131-3.

275. Pocha, C. (2010). Lean Six Sigma in health care and the challenge of implementation of Six Sigma methodologies at a Veterans Affairs Medical Center. *Qual Manag Health Care*, 19(4), 312-8.

276. Polk, J. D. (2011) Lean Six Sigma, innovation, and the change acceleration process can work together. *Physician Exec.*, 37(1), 38-42.

277. Proudlove, N., Moxham, C., & Boaden, R. (2008). Lessons for Lean in Healthcare from Using Six Sigma in the NHS. *Public Money & Management*, 28, 27-34.

278. Rajan, A., Sullivan, R., Bakker, S., & van Harten, W. H. (2012). Critical appraisal of translational research models for suitability in performance assessment of cancer centers. Oncologist, 17(12), e48-57.

279. Reijula, J., & Tommelein, I. (2012). Lean hospitals: a new challenge for facility designers, *Intelligent Buildings International*, 4(2), 126-143.

280. Robbins, J., Garman, A. N., Song, P. H., & McAlearney, A. S. (2012). How high-performance work systems drive health care value: an examination of leading process improvement strategies. *Qual Manag Health Care.*, 21(3), 188-202.

281. Roth, C., Boll, D., Wall, L., & Merkle, E. (2010). Evaluation Of MRI Acquisition Workflow With Lean Six Sigma Method: Case Study Of Liver And Knee Examinations, *American Journal of Roentgenology*, 195(2), 150-156.

282. Schattenkirk, D. (2012). Building sustainable internal capacity for quality within a healthcare environment, *TQM Journal*, 24(4), 374-382.

283. Schriefer, J., & Leonard, M. S. (2012). Patient safety and quality improvement: an overview of QI. *Pediatr Rev.* 33(8), 353-359.

284. Schweikhart, S., & Dembe, A. (2009). The Applicability of Lean and Six Sigma Techniques to Clinical and Translational Research, *J Investig Med.*, 57(7), 748–755.

285. Seidl, K. L., & Newhouse, R. P. (2012). The intersection of evidence-based practice with 5 quality improvement methodologies. *J Nurs Adm.* 42(6), 299-304.

286. Sewing, A., Winchester, T., Carnell, P., Hampton, D., & Keighley, W. (2008). Helping science to succeed: improving processes in R&D. *Drug Discov Today.* 13(5-6), 227-33.

287. Shabot, M. M., Monroe, D., Inurria, J., Garbade, D., & France, A. C. (2013). Memorial Hermann: high reliability from board to bedside. *Jt Comm J Qual Patient Saf.*, 39(6), 253-7.

288. Stankovic, A. K., & DeLauro, E. (2010). Quality improvements in the preanalytical phase: focus on urine specimen workflow. *MLO Med Lab Obs.*, 42(3), 20, 22, 24-7.

289. Stankovic, A. K. (2004). The laboratory is a key partner in assuring patient safety. *Clin Lab Med.*, 24(4), 1023-35.

290. Stankovic, A. (2008). Developing a Lean Consciousness for the Clinical Laboratory. Journal of Medical Biochemistry, 27(3), 354-361.

291. Stoiljkovic, V., Trajkovic, J., & Stoiljkovic, B. (2011). Lean Six Sigma Sample Analysis Process in a Microbiology Laboratory. *Journal of Medical Biochemistry.* 30(4), 346–353.

292. Stuenkel, K., & Faulkner, T., (2009). A community hospital's journey into Lean Six Sigma. Fr*ont Health Serv Manage.*, 26(1), 5-13.

293. Sunyog, M. (2004). Lean Management and Six-Sigma yield big gains in hospital's immediate response laboratory. Quality improvement techniques save more than $400,000. *Clin Leadersh Manag Rev.*, 18(5), 255-8.

294. Taner, M. (2013). Application of Six Sigma methodology to a cataract surgery unit. International Journal of Health Care Quality Assurance, 26(8), 768 – 785.

295. Taner, M., Sezen, B., & Antony, J. (2007). An overview of six sigma applications in healthcare industry", *International Journal of Health Care Quality Assurance*, 20(4), 329 – 340.

296. Toledo, A. H., Carroll, T., Arnold, E., Tulu, Z., Caffey, T., Kearns, L. E., & Gerber, D. A. (2013). Reducing liver transplant length of stay: a Lean Six Sigma approach. *Prog Transplant*, 23(4), 350-64.

297. Tyson, P. (2010). Preparing for the new landscape of payment reform. *Healthc Financ Manage*. 64(12), 42-8.

298. Ullman, F., & Boutellier R. (2008). A case study of lean drug discovery: from project driven research to innovation studios and process factories. *Drug Discov Today*, 13(11-12), 543-50.

299. Heuvel, V. D., Does, R. & de Koning, H. (2006). Lean Six Sigma in a hospital, *Int. J. Six Sigma and Competitive Advantage*, 2(4), 377-381.

300. Heuvel, V. D., Does, J., Ronald, J. M. M., & Verver, J, P, S. (2005). Six Sigma in healthcare: lessons learned from a hospital. *International Journal of Six Sigma and Competitive Advantage*. 1(4), 380-388.

301. van Leeuwen, K., & Does, R. (2010). Quality Quandaries: Lean Nursing. *Quality Engineering*, 23(1), 94-99.

302. Van Lent, W., Sanders, E., & Van Harten, W. (2012). Exploring improvements in patient logistics in Dutch hospitals with a survey, *BMC Health Services Research*, 12, 1-9.

303. Varkey, P., & Kollengode, A. (2011). A framework for healthcare quality improvement in India: the time is here and now!. *J Postgrad Med*. 57(3), 237-41.

304. Varkey, P., Reller, M., & Resar, R. (2007). Basics of Quality Improvement in Health Care. *Mayo Clinic Proceedings*, 82(6), 735–739.

305. Veluswamy, R., & Price, R. (2010). I've Fallen and I Can't Get Up: Reducing the Risk of Patient Falls. *Physician Executive*. 36(3), 50-3.

306. Vest, J., & Gamm, L. (2009). A critical review of the research literature on Six Sigma, Lean and StuderGroup's Hardwiring Excellence in the United States: the need to demonstrate and communicate the effectiveness of transformation strategies in healthcare. *Implementation Science*, 4(35), 1-9.

307. Viau, M., & Southern, B. (2007). Six Sigma and Lean concepts, a case study: patient centered care model for a mammography center. *Radiol Manage*,29(5), 19-28.

308. Villa, D. (2010). Automation, Lean, Six Sigma: Synergies for Improving Laboratory Efficiency. *Journal of Medical Biochemistry Journal of Medical Biochemistry*, 29(4), 339–348.

309. Waldron, D. (2011). Visit, revamp, and revitalize your business plan: Part 2. *Radiol Manage.*, 33(3), 16-20.

310. Waring, J., & Bishop, S. (2010). Lean healthcare: Rhetoric, ritual and resistance. *Social Science & Medicine*, 71(7), 1332–1340.

311. Woodard., & Tanisha, D. (2005). Addressing Variation in Hospital Quality: Is Six Sigma the Answer?. *Journal of Healthcare Management*. 50(4), 226-36.

312. Yamamoto, J. J., Malatestinic, B. L., & Angela, J. R. (2010). Facilitating process changes in meal delivery and radiological testing to improve inpatient insulin timing using Six Sigma method. *Qual Manage Health Care*, 19(3), 189-200.

313. Young, T., Brailsford, S., Connell, C., Davies, R., Harper, P., & Klein, J. H. (2004). Using industrial processes to improve patient care. *BMJ*, 17, 162–164.

314. Yu, Q., & Yang, Kai (2008). Hospital registration waiting time reduction through process redesign. *International Journal of Six Sigma and Competitive Advantage*, 4(3), 240-253.

315. Yusof, M., Khodambashi, S., & Mokhtar, A. (2012). Evaluation of the clinical process in a critical care information system using the Lean method: a case study. *BMC Medical Informatics and Decision Making*, 12, 1-14.

316. Zandi, F. (2013). Identification of e-Health reference architecture using a bi-objective medical informatics decision support framework: the optimal lean and six sigma alignment. *Journal of Decision Systems*, 22(3), 202-223.

317. Zilm F., Crane, J., Roche., & K. T. (2010). New directions in emergency service operations and planning. *J Ambul Care Manage*, 33(4), 296-306.

Chapter 7

Organizational Factors Influencing the Use of Clinical Decision Support for Improving Cancer Screening Within Community Health Centers

Timothy Jay Carney
University of North Carolina, USA

Anna M. McDaniel
Indiana University School of Informatics (IUPUI), USA & Indiana University School of Nursing, USA

Michael Weaver
Indiana University School of Nursing, USA

Josette Jones
Indiana University School of Informatics (IUPUI), USA

David A. Haggstrom
Indiana University School of Medicine, USA

ABSTRACT

Adoption of clinical decision support (CDS) systems leads to improved clinical performance through improved clinician decision making, adherence to evidence-based guidelines, medical error reduction, and more efficient information transfer and to reduction in health care disparities in under-resourced settings. However, little information on CDS use in the community health care (CHC) setting exists. This study examines if organizational, provider, or patient level factors can successfully predict the level of CDS use in the CHC setting with regard to breast, cervical, and colorectal cancer screening. This study relied upon 37 summary measures obtained from the 2005 Cancer Health Disparities Collaborative (HDCC) national survey of 44 randomly selected community health centers.

DOI: 10.4018/978-1-4666-8756-1.ch007

A multi-level framework was designed that employed an all-subsets linear regression to discover relationships between organizational/practice setting, provider, and patient characteristics and the outcome variable, a composite measure of community health center CDS intensity-of-use. Several organizational and provider level factors from our conceptual model were identified to be positively associated with CDS level of use in community health centers. The level of CDS use (e.g., computerized reminders, provider prompts at point-of-care) in support of breast, cervical, and colorectal cancer screening rate improvement in vulnerable populations is determined by both organizational/practice setting and provider factors. Such insights can better facilitate the increased uptake of CDS in CHCs that allows for improved patient tracking, disease management, and early detection in cancer prevention and control within vulnerable populations.

BACKGROUND

Organizational issues are frequently encountered barriers to the implementation and adoption of clinical decision support (CDS) systems in health care settings. According to the Agency for Healthcare Research and Quality (AHRQ), failure to understand organizational and cultural issues may affect the adoption and use of CDS systems (HHS, 2009). Implicit in the AHRQ statement is that CDS adoption and use can significantly impact the quality and performance of health care through the influence of select organizational factors. Recent research suggests that structural differences in the health care organization may explain greater performance variance than patient factors alone (Soban & Yano, 2005). In particular, organizational factors can serve as inhibitors or facilitators in the adoption and implementation of any new technology, such as a clinical decision support system or the conceptually similar clinical information system (CIS) (Weiner, Savitz, Bernard, & Pucci, 2004).

The Chronic Care Model (CCM) describes *clinical decision support* as a practice to promote clinical care that is consistent with scientific evidence and patient preferences, and it involves efforts to embed evidence-based guidelines into daily clinical practice, share evidence-based guidelines, and enhance provider decision making through proven provider education methods (Haggstrom, 2010; Sperl-Hillen et al., 2004). CCM defines a *clinical information system* as a set of tools and processes enabling the organization of patient and population data in order to facilitate efficient and effective care. CIS tools include encounter reminders, flowcharts, tracking lists of high-risk patients due to lack of screening adherence, follow-up, or other recommendations (Haggstrom, 2010; Sperl-Hillen et al., 2004). Henceforth, the authors will use the composite term CDS/IS or simply CDS as indicative of a combined concept of comprehensive capability in this area.

A close examination of CDS use in community health centers reveals that approximately 40% (or 3,160) of all 7,900 CHCs in the United States have some form of Electronic Health Record (EHR) in use today (Lardiere, 2010). The EHR will be an essential component in the eventual deployment of specialized clinical decision support systems supporting disease-specific target areas. Seventy percent of the community health centers with EHRs (2,212) also use some form of clinical decision support such as electronic dashboards, data repositories, tele-health technologies, kiosks, or other technologies (Lardiere, 2010). However, less than 28% of all 7,900 CHCs use some form of clinical decision support for practices such as cancer screening. These statistics are reinforced by the 2009 Commonwealth Fund National Survey of Federally Qualified Health Centers (Abrams et al., 2010). The survey of 1000 community health centers found that despite 40% of the community health centers having electronic medical record capability, the capacity for more advanced health information technology (e.g., electronically ordering prescriptions and tests, creating and maintaining patient registries, tracking patients and tests, and providing alerts or prompts) varied tremendously among centers (Abrams et al., 2010). Organizational factors, such as budget priorities and technology affordability, remain inhibiting factors to widespread CDS adoption and use (Lardiere, 2010, Abrams et al., 2010).

A number of incentives motivate health care organizations to adopt computerized clinical decision support (CDS), including cost savings, clinical performance improvement, improved clinician decision making, adherence to evidence-based guidelines, medical error reduction, and more efficient information transfer (Bates et al., 2001; Bates et al., 1999; Doebbeling, Chou, & Tierney, 2006; Reid et al., 2005). CDS has also been shown to have a positive impact on reducing health disparities (HHS, 2010). However, slower adoption of CDS within institutions that provide care to historically underserved populations could result in even greater health disparities (Shields et al., 2007).

The Bureau of Primary Health Care (BPHC), the part of the Health Resources and Services Administration (HRSA) that oversees federally funded health centers, employs collaboratives to reduce health disparities, improve quality of care in health centers, and reduce costs (HRSA, 2008). The model, then called the Collaborative Model for Achieving Breakthrough Improvement, was first implemented in 1996 by the Institute for Healthcare Improvement (IHI); it became widely known as the Breakthrough Series (BTS). BTS represented a way to "help healthcare organizations make breakthrough improvements in quality, while reducing costs" (HRSA, 2008). HRSA has employed the collaborative model since 1999 as a means of providing structure for health care organizations to learn from one another and to be exposed to recognized experts in the specific areas identified for improvement (HRSA, 2008).

The HRSA collaboratives have focused on a variety of areas, including health disparities (e.g. related to cancer, asthma, cardiovascular disease, depression, etc.), patient safety, obesity, tobacco cessation, organ donation, newborn screening, HIV/AIDS, and other areas (HRSA, June 2008). Several studies have highlighted the benefit of HRSA collaborative participation (Asch et al., 2005; Chin et al., 2004; Haggstrom, Clauser, & Taplin, 2008; Landon et al., 2004). The Health Disparities Cancer Collaborative (HDCC), in collaboration with the National Cancer Institute (NCI), was a quality improvement program designed to increase the cancer control activities of screening and follow-up among underserved populations. Over 45% of CHC patients receive Medicaid, Medicare, CHIP (Child Health Insurance Protection), or other forms of public insurance, and nearly 40% are uninsured (HRSA, June 2008). HDCC operated from 2003 to 2005 among community health centers supported by HRSA to serve financially, functionally, and culturally vulnerable populations (Harmon & Carlson, 1991; Iglehart, 2008).

A dearth of information on CDS adoption among CHCs exists. A 2010 systematic literature review of 105 peer-reviewed studies published between 2004 and 2009, along with eight key informant interviews, was conducted to examine the link between health information technology (IT) and quality outcomes in under-resourced settings (URSs) and their corresponding impact on disparities (Millery & Kukafka, 2010). Fifteen studies met the URS criteria, and 7 of the 15 studies did not focus specifically on the topic of URSs and found no evidence linking health IT and URS quality. Key informants' comments and recommendations regarding URSs were to (1) stress the need for health IT to be used as a tool and not an end in itself, (2) emphasize that URSs face competing priorities and great challenges to introducing new technology, and (3) encourage partnerships and collaboration as a means to implementing new technology. This research also identified four major gaps in evidence regarding health IT, quality, and URSs: (1) lack of research conducted in URSs related to barriers to implementing new technology; (2) effectiveness studies to examine external generalizability of the quality impact of health IT; (3) research to examine clinical quality improvement methods, particularly with respect to health IT; and (4) research in the largely untapped patient, organizational, and environmental levels of the health care system with regard to health IT.

This study addresses the fourth evidence gap, examining the relationship between health IT and under-resourced settings from a multi-level perspective. Specifically, it views CHCs from the perspectives of patient characteristics, provider characteristics, and organizational and/or practice setting factors and seeks to examine their influence on CDS utilization. The presumption is that at least some patient, provider, and/or organizational factors can be found to be associated the level of CDS use in these settings and should also be related to concrete measures of health care quality and performance. This hypothesis, specifically related to cancer screening practices, has yet to be tested within community health centers, where the focus is typically on access for poor and underserved populations in both rural and urban areas.

Methods

This study's research design was a retrospective cross-sectional cohort. Its ordinal ranked outcome variable was a measure of the intensity-of-use of a CDS system in a community health center. Employing data based on a 2005 Health Disparities Cancer Collaborative (HDCC) survey, we employed all-subsets linear regression models to identify CHC-related factors which were statistically significant in accounting for a CHCs CDS cancer-screening capabilities. Our aim was to identify what characteristics of a CHC contribute to an environment supportive of a multi-capable clinical decision support system.

Survey data and methods. The source of the study's data was a National Cancer Institute (NCI)/Health Resources and Services Administration (HRSA) Health Disparities Cancer Collaborative (HDCC) survey (Haggstrom et al., 2008; Haggstrom, Taplin, Monahan, & Clauser, 2012) that examined organizational structure, implementation level of Chronic Care Model (CCM) components, and such contextual factors as teamwork and leadership of federally funded HRSA community health centers (Sperl-Hillen et al., 2004; Taplin et al., 2008). According to Haggstrom the HDCC survey was "comprised of several domains that were measured with Likert scales divided into four response categories: strongly agree, agree, disagree, and strongly disagree. Chronic care model implementation and teamwork scales were assessed using factor analysis by specifying the principal component method of factor extraction, initial communalities of 1.0, varimax rotation, and scree plots (Haggstrom et al, 2008)." The specific sample data selected for our study consisted of two nonequivalent groups each containing 22 CHCs randomly selected from a representative sampling of CHCs from the U.S. population of CHCs. The characteristic distinguishing the two groups was participation in the HDCC, and the survey's data were as of 2005. The HDCC survey was intentionally biased to include a larger proportion CHCs previously designated as high performing or exemplar centers in an attempt minimize the impact of non-response and missing data that would limit the examination of key tests of association of among Chronic Care Model quality improvement domains given the sample size. This performance bias did not impact the CHC assignment to either of the two groups of community health centers based on HDCC participation.

The HDCC survey consisted of 99 unique questions with respondent categories for the community health center's director (CEO), chief financial officer (CFO), providers (physicians and nurses), general staff (e.g., lab and pharmacy workers) and chief informatics officer (CIO). Appendix A lists the survey items, properties, and mapping to the final list of 37 summary measures used in our modified Zapka framework (e.g., organizational practice and/or setting factor, provider characteristic, or patient characteristic). A reconciliation algorithm was applied to a question's multiple responses to create a single summary measure representing a consensus response for the CHC. The unit of analysis in the research was the facility and, as such, the goal was to obtain representative facility-level responses to each summary measure. This was intended as a minimally intrusive way to reduce varying responses to the same question to a single value.

Dependent measures of clinical decision support utilization. The dependent variable for our study's linear regression models was based on four possible CDS systems capabilities related to breast, cervical, and/or colorectal cancer screening in community health centers. These four measures were drawn directly from the list of HDCC survey items responded to by the chief informatics officer (CIO) regarding CHC health information technology practices and capability. Our rationale for the use of CDS in association with cancer screening improvement was consistent with the Zapka et al. description of clinical decision support and clinical information systems as organizational and/or practice variables that predict cancer screening performance (Zapka, Taplin, Solberg, & Manos, 2003). Given the slow uptake of CDS in CHCs we chose to examine (1) which organizational, provider, and/or patient factors would explain the *presence* of one or more of each of the four components of CDS individually (logistic regression), (2) the predictors of cumulative component *utilization* of CDS (linear regression), and (3) the extent to which CDS use was correlated with CHC facility-level cancer screening performance (Spearman's Rho Correlation). An additional virtual experiment was later added to examine simulated behavior

over time. The results of these various tests are presented in separate manuscripts. This study presents the second of these tests which examined the level of use of CDS where the number of components in use served as a measure of the *intensity* of CDS use within CHCs. Our CDS composite construct, as shown in Figure 1 under "Proximal Outcomes," are comprised of (1) the system's capacity to measure cancer screening need, (2) point-of-care user prompts, (3) computerized patient reminders (e.g., of appointments, screening tests due), and (4) system-generated correspondence to communicate test results to patients electronically.

A composite formed from these capabilities and measuring a CHC's CDS intensity-of-use functioned as our model's dependent variable. This composite, Y_i in the equation shown below, incorporates variables representing the four CDS cancer-screening capabilities, represented by X_{ij}, with $i = 1,..., 44$ denoting the CHC and $j = 1,..., 4$ the four capabilities:

$$Y_i = X_{i1} + X_{i2} + X_{i3} + X_{i4}$$

where

$X_{i1} = 1$ if CHC i has the capacity to measure cancer-screening need; 0 otherwise

$X_{i2} = 1$ if CHC i has point-of-care user prompts; 0 otherwise

$X_{i3} = 1$ if CHC i has computerized patient reminders; 0 otherwise

$X_{i4} = 1$ if CHC i has system-generated correspondence; 0 otherwise

Thus, a Y_i of 0 or 1 indicates that CHC i possesses no or one CDS cancer-screening capability, respectively. $Y_i = 2$, $Y_i = 3$, or $Y_i = 4$ indicate two, three, or four such capabilities, respectively. Intensity-of-use scores were calculated for 44 CHCs in the HDCC study as of the time covered by the survey.

Figure 1. Carney Study Conceptual Model

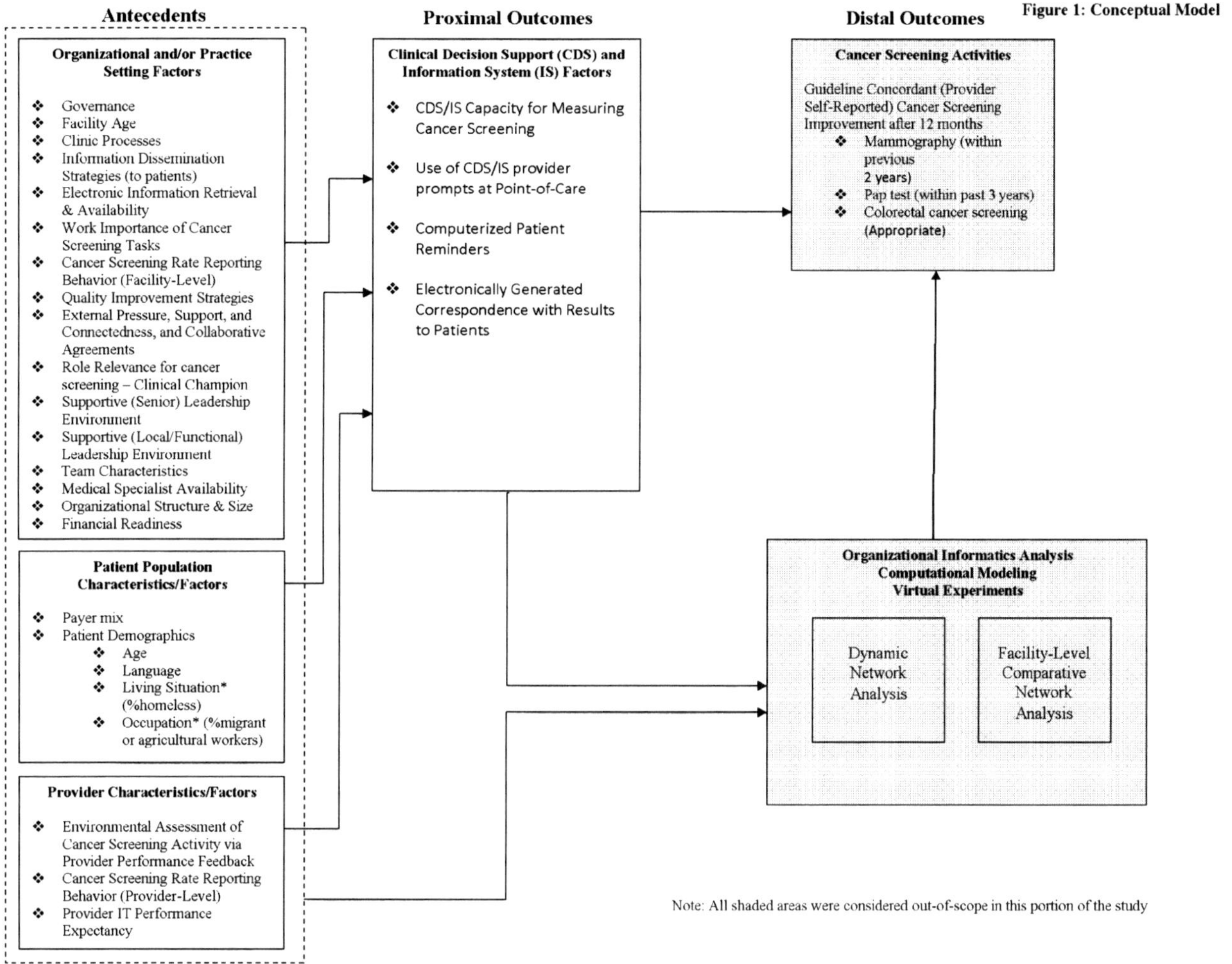

Independent measures of community health center characteristics. The Zapka et al. framework provided the basis for organizing the independent measures of our regression models. It describes how four distinct levels of influence, with each smaller unit operating as a sub-member of the next higher level, work together to influence screening behavior. These four levels of influence, given in order of increasing scope, are patient population level characteristics; provider characteristics; organizational and/or practice settings; and sectors of influence (e.g., federal and state policy). In both the Chronic Care Model and Zapka's framework, these levels are then mediated in the clinical micro-environment by proactive team membership, productive encounters, and activated patients to produce improved patient screening outcomes (Zapka, 2008; Zapka, Taplin, Solberg, & Manos, 2003; Zapka, Taplin, Solberg, & Manos, 2003).

Our study employed this framework to map each of the 99 survey items in the HDCC study into one of three primary categories: organizational and/or practice setting, provider, and patient. In its design, the HDCC survey developed by Haggstrom et al. did not directly employ the

Zapka et al. framework, and thus the current study's subject matter expert guided coding process, matching HDCC survey items to Zapka et al. constructs, represents a modified Zapka et al. framework. Nonetheless, the shared focus of the HDCC survey and of the Zapka et al. framework on multilevel factors and on cancer screening as the outcome of interest made the modified Zapka et al. conceptual approach ideally suited for this study.

Aspects of a CHCs organizational, provider, and patient characteristics were the independent variables of the study; these aspects are shown in Figure 1 under "Antecedents." The abbreviated names and explanations of the CHC organizational and/or practice setting factors are given in Table 1 and Appendix A details the conceptual and operation definitions for each variable. Linear regression models were then fitted, using these aspects, separately and in combination, to account for CHC level of CDS capability with regard to cancer screening. To provide for an adequate ratio of independent measures per observation for parameter estimation, a model reduction technique was employed that would yield the best subset of independent measures to account for the dependent measure (Good, 2011; Kutner, Nachtsheim, & Neter, 2004).

Statistical analysis. Linear regression was used to examine associations between organizational and/or practice setting, provider, and patient factors and the facility-level composite CDS intensity-of-use score, a measure of a CHCs CDS cancer-screening capability. Multicollinearity among the set of independent variables was examined, and distributions of study variables were described with appropriate measurement-level descriptive statistics, which were reported at the facility level. Missing and out-of-range values were identified. A Type I error rate of 0.05 was used to determine statistical significance. We examined conformance to statistical assumptions for each model and identified outlying and influential observations. All statistical testing in this study was conducted using SAS Version 9.2.

The study's unit of analysis was the community health center, of which 44 were selected for inclusion. With a 0.05 significance level and a maximum of 6 predictor variables, an effect size, or R^2, of 0.27 yields a power of 80%. All power estimates were calculated using PASS 11 (Hintze, 2011).

Based on an adjusted R^2 and an all-subsets linear regression, separate best subsets of predictors for CDS intensity-of-use were identified from among antecedents categorized as organizational and/or practice setting, provider, and patient.

Table 1. CHC organizational and/or practice setting factors

Name	Explanation
HRSA	HRSA Collaborative Experience
Facility Age 1	Facility Age Measured in No. Years Receiving BPHC Funding
Facility Age 2	Facility Age Measured in No. Years in Any Collaborative
Clinic Proc.	Clinic Processes
Information	Information Dissemination Strategies
EI	Electronic Information Retrieval & Availability
EHR	Electronic Health Record Function Capabilities
Screening	Work Importance of Cancer Screening Tasks
Reporting	Cancer Screening Rate Reporting Behavior (Facility Level)
Quality	Quality Improvement Strategies
Externals	External Pressure, Support, Connectedness, Collaborative Agreements
Delivery	For Cancer Screening (e.g., Role Responsibility, Overlap, Clinical Champions)
Support Senior	Supportive Senior Leadership Environment
Support Local	Supportive Local Leadership Environment
Team Char.	Team Characteristics
Specialist	Medical Specialist Availability
Structure/Size	Organizational Structure & Size
Financial 1	Financial Readiness-Total Budget
Financial 2	Financial Readiness-Cash Reserves

Models having the largest adjusted R^2 were selected as best (Kutner et al., 2004). Collaborative participation was included as a covariate in each multivariable organizational and/or practice setting model only when it was identified as a member of the best subset of predictors.

Results: Exploration of Explanatory and Outcome Variables

CDS intensity-of-use outcome variable. Table 2 presents the pertinent statistics of the composite measure of CDS intensity-of use (Y_i) and of the four capabilities on which it was based $(X_{i1}$ through $X_{i4})$. In total, 44 CHCs were selected for inclusion in the study. Of these, 22 were HDCC participants and 22 were not. Degree to which a health center used a clinic decision support system varied greatly depending on HDCC participation is evident in Figure 2.

Independent organizational and/or practice setting, provider, and patient variables. Table 3 presents the descriptive statistics for each of the 19 organizational and/or practice setting factors selected for the study.

One assumption explored was that the community health center was an under-resourced setting (URS), as presented in the 2010 review on Health IT and quality of health care (Millery & Kukafka, 2010). Therefore, we selected as

Table 2. Community health center CDS capabilities

Factors	N Valid	Missing	Mean	Std.Dev.	Range
Measuring cancer screening (Xi1)	42	2	0.4	0.5	0-1
POC provider prompts (Xi2)	41	3	0.73	0.45	0-1
Computerized patient reminders (Xi3)	41	3	0.73	0.45	0-1
Electronic correspondence (Xi4)	41	3	0.78	0.42	0-1
CDS intensity-of-use (Yi)	44	0	2.48	1.41	0-4

Figure 2. Community health center clinical decision support level of use by component

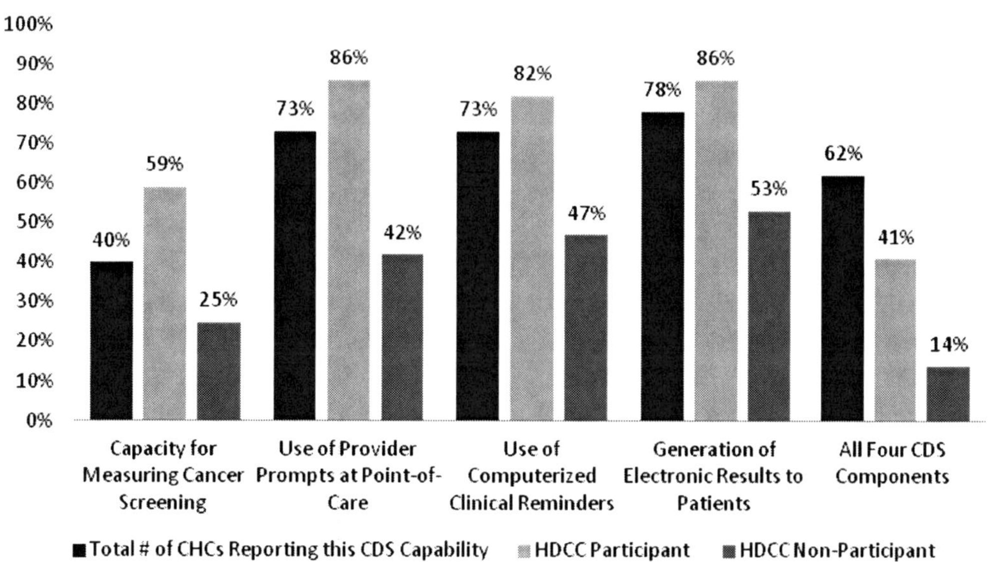

Table 3. CHC organizational and/or practice setting factors – statistical distribution characteristics

Factors	N Valid	Missing	Mean	Std. Dev.	Range
HRSA	44	0	2.66	1.12	0-3
Facility Age 1	36	8	23.44	10.58	7-50
Facility Age 2	34	10	19.56	10.43	3-36
Clinic Proc.	44	0	2.59	1.09	0-4
Information	44	0	15.98	5.04	0-23
EI	44	0	0.59	0.62	0-3
EHR	44	0	5.95	2.96	0-8
Screening	44	0	23.36	5.33	0-28
Reporting	44	0	3.8	2.1	0-6
Quality	44	0	30.82	10.19	0-43
Externals	44	0	1.82	2.13	0-8
Delivery	44	0	64.8	21.85	0-100
Support Senior	44	0	24.93	6.59	0-36
Support Local	44	0	12.61	3.92	0-16
Team Char.	44	0	33.7	10.16	0-44
Specialist	44	0	6.77	4.44	0-10
Structure/Size	44	0	48.11	55.36	12*-251
Financial 1	37	7	$11.6M	$9.83M	$1.98M-$45.61M
Financial 2	37	7	4.54	1.02	1-6

*Note: For Organizational Size, the smallest number of personnel was 12, and any "0" responses were treated as missing data.

one of our study's organizational/practice setting independent variables a summary measure of the level of cash reserves as an indicator of health center financial readiness for CDS adoption and implementation; this variable is referred to as "Finance 2" in Tables 1 and 3. Out of the 37 health centers reporting revenue and expense information only 6 CHCs (16%) reported operating at a deficit where expenses exceeded revenue. These results suggest either that the sample of 44 community health centers used in this study do not accurately represent the larger population of community health centers as a URS or that this measure for financial readiness was not exactly comparable to the measures used by Millery et al. Tables 4 and 5 present descriptive statistics of provider and patient variables respectively.

Organizational and/or practice setting factors. The results of the fitting the all-subsets linear regression models to the study data are shown in Table 6. The model indicated that the best subset of predictors within organizational and/or practice setting factors explained approximately 40% of CDS intensity-of-use ($F = 3.31, DF = 6, p = 0.013$) and included (1) the level of experience the CHC had with HRSA collaborative activities, (2) the health center age expressed in terms of how long it had been receiving BPHC funding, (3) the degree of importance providers placed in cancer screening activities, (4) the level of external connections the health center had in the form of support structures, collaborative agreements, and external drivers, (5) the cancer screening delivery system design (expressed as roles and responsibilities, clinical champions, etc.), and (6) the level of support health

Table 4. Patient factors – statistical distribution characteristics

Factors	N Valid	Missing	Mean	Std.Dev.	Range
Uninsured	37	7	37.38	17.79	5-77
Medicare	37	7	14.11	15.4	2-84
Medicaid	37	7	48.68	23.53	5-88
Insurance-Commercial	37	7	9.86	8.74	1-35
Self Pay	36	8	27.36	20.65	2-79
Language	37	7	22.14	23.99	1-95
Migrant	34	10	1.85	4.53	0-21
Homeless	30	14	1.97	2.77	0-10
Age	35	9	1.46	0.7	1-3

Table 5. Provider factors – statistical distribution characteristics

Factors	N Valid	Missing	Mean	Std. Dev.	Range
Environment assessment of cancer screening & follow-up activity	44	0	54.32	14.2	0-68
Cancer screening rate reporting behavior (provider level)	44	0	5.05	1.84	0-6
Provider IT performance expectancy	44	0	25.07	7	0-38

center staff received from its functional, that is clinical, leadership team. The model coefficients of the variables representing HRSA collaborative experience and level of external connections were positive and statistically significant, indicating that community health centers with more HRSA collaborative experience and greater external ties have higher intensity of CDS utilization.

Variables that were not independently associated with CDS intensity-of-use included facility age as a function of when the health center commenced receiving BPHC funding, work importance of cancer screening tasks, the delivery system design for cancer screening (e.g., role responsibility, overlap, and clinical champions), and supportive local (functional) leadership environment.

Provider factors. Of the three provider factors chosen for inclusion in the study, only two–(1) cancer screening rate reporting behavior at the provider level and (2) provider expectations of the health center information technology (IT) to address cancer-screening activities–were included in the overall linear regression model (See Table 6).

This best subset of provider predictors explained approximately 34% of CDS intensity-of-use (F = 10.48; DF = 2; p < 0.001).

The coefficient of the provider-level cancer screening rate reporting behavior was positive and significantly associated (p < 0.05), indicating an independent positive association with CDS intensity-of-use. The second provider-category variable included in the optimized regression model, provider IT performance expectancy, showed no independent statistically significant association with CDS intensity-of-use based on this sample of community health centers.

Patient factors. Patient factors included method of remuneration for service (e.g., patient uninsured and therefore nonpaying, Medicare, Medicaid, commercial insurance, and self pay) and patient demographics (e.g., language, migrant worker, homeless, and age). See Table 6 for the results of the model fit. The best subset of predictors within patient characteristics included the patient demographics (1) primary language of the patient population and (2) age. The R^2 for

Table 6. Results of linear regression

Category of Predictors	Conceptual Model Construct	R2	Parameter Estimate	Pr > |t|	Standardized Estimate
Organizational and/or Practice Setting Factors	Overall Model–Testing Global Null Beta=0^^ (F=3.31; DF=6; p=.013*)	0.41	N/A	N/A	N/A
	HRSA Collaborative Experience		0.6	0.02*	0.37
	Facility Age1–Year began receiving BPHC funding		0.03	0.1	0.27
	Work Importance of Cancer Screening Tasks		-0.3	0.09	-0.27
	External Pressure, Support, Connectedness, and Collaborative Agreements		0.2	0.04*	0.37
	Delivery System Design for Cancer Screening (e.g., Role Responsibility, Overlap, and Clinical Champions)		-0.03	0.09	-0.28
	Supportive Local (Functional) Leadership Environment		0.13	0.22	0.19
Patient Characteristics	Overall Model–Testing Global Null Beta=0^^ (F=3.10; DF=2; p=.059)	0.16	N/A	N/A	N/A
	Patient Demographics (Language)		0.02	0.05	0.35
	Patient Demographics (Age)		0.62	0.04**	0.37
Provider Characteristics	Overall Model–Testing Global Null Beta=0^^ (F=10.48; DF=2; p<0.001*)	0.34	N/A	N/A	N/A
	Cancer Screening Rate Reporting Behavior (Provider Level)		0.46	<.0001*	0.6
	Provider IT Performance Expectancy		-0.03	0.2	-0.17

* Statistically significant (p<.05)

**Test of global null not statistically significant, indicating that those individual p values should not be interpreted.

^^Global Null Test (Pr > F)

this set of predictors was 0.161, and the overall model was not statistically significant (F = 3.10; DF = 2; p = 0.059), indicating little or no association between patient characteristics and intensity of CDS use.

Discussion

Community health center factors contributing to CDS use. Experience with the Health Disparities Cancer Collaborative was associated with greater utilization of CDS. These findings corroborate the impact that team-based, collaborative quality-improvement activities have been found to have on improving the process of care within health care organizations (Chin et al., 2004; Haggstrom, Clauser, & Taplin, 2010; Haggstrom et al., 2008; Haggstrom et al., 2012; Landon, Hicks, & O'Malley, 2007; Taplin et al., 2008). External environmental forces in the form of (1) external pressures (e.g., Board of Director accountability for HRSA collaborative activities), (2) explicit or implied performance benchmarking as a member of the HRSA collaborative), (3) support (e.g., listings of community cancer resources, staff/resources needed to make use of community cancer resources), (4) connectedness, and (5) collaborative agreements (e.g., informal or formal contractual agreements with outside organizations) were associated with increased level of utilization of CDS systems in support of cancer screening activities. This finding was consistent with previous studies which found that external environmental factors (Shortell et al., 2005) and external communication (Kilsdonk, Peute, Knijnenburg, & Jaspers, 2011) may have an impact on health information technology utilization. External agreements or contracts may promote CDS use by providing more reliable support from outside organizations that, in turn, reduce the risks taken by community health centers investing in health information technology. This external support and interaction could also lead to a greater diffusion of technology and innovation, a greater sharing of best practices, and perhaps a greater level of shared accountability among multiple practices.

Based on this study's findings, provider-level cancer screening rate-reporting behavior appears to be associated with CDS intensity-of-use within community health centers. These findings are consistent with previous findings which reported that both the provider work environment and clinical task-related behaviors are associated with CDS use (Yarbrough & Smith, 2007; Zapka et al., 2005).

This study's results indicate that audit and feedback, expressed here as provider-level cancer screening reporting, is more likely to occur when a CDS system has also been implemented, even in the low-resource setting of a community health center. Previous literature suggests that provider audit and feedback, on specific clinical processes, is associated with positive, although incremental, improvements in health care quality (Jamtvedt, Young, Kristoffersen, O'Brien, & Oxman, 2006). Unlike Jatvedt et al., the current study did not find that audit and feedback is associated with improved clinical processes (or cancer screening) in these settings. However, other literature reported that audit and feedback are not uniformly effective in improving clinical practice. In one study conducted in a community primary care practice setting, office system changes, including audit and feedback, did not increase breast cancer screening. Providers were allowed to offer feedback on 12- to 18-month facility-level cancer screening performance, but this feedback alone did not significantly change breast cancer screening rates (Kinsinger, Harris, Qaqish, Strecher, & Kaluzny, 1998). Given these mixed results, audit and feedback may need to be applied in association with other strategies, such as clinical reminders, provider incentives, outreach, and cultivation of opinion leaders. It may also have to be tailored to organizational contextual variables such as structure, size, budget, etc.

CONCLUSION

The community health care system is a national network of clinics providing care in both urban and rural areas. Because of its focus on primary care and its mission to provide health care to vulnerable populations, the community health care setting is unique. Attempts of community health center leadership to promote clinical decision support systems face several challenges, not the least of which are limited resources and time (Millery & Kukafka, 2010). Because individuals operating in such pressured environments commonly face high cognitive demands (Nemeth, Connor, Klock, & Cook, 2006), this research seeks to provide a theory-driven foundation for future CDS adoption, implementation, and use studies in these settings.

Therefore, it identified measures at multiple levels, in both organizational and provider categories, that were associated with intensity of CDS use within community health centers. HDCC experience showed a positive association with the CDS intensity-of-use outcome, while current HDCC membership/participation did not. These findings suggest that cumulative exposure to collaborative activities rather than any single quality-improvement collaborative is more influential in the adoption and ultimate use of certain types of health information technology.

No patient characteristics were found to have an association with the intensity-of-use of CDS systems within community health centers. This negative finding regarding patient characteristics is consistent with several other studies that confirm the relative importance of organizational structure and processes to an overall health information technology implementation strategy (Burke, Menachemi, & Brooks, 2005; Millery & Kukafka, 2010; Shortell et al., 2005).

Study Limitations

This secondary analysis used a relatively small (N = 44) sample of the community health centers in the U.S. and as a result may not fully explain the high level of variability of CDS use among CHCs. Future studies may be needed to more precisely examine this in both national and international settings. Community health centers have participated in many different types of collaboratives than the one described here. One type consists of global technology collaboratives aimed exclusively at increasing the uptake of health information technology within community health centers (Lardiere, 2010). These types of collaboratives are not typically disease focused; rather, they are primarily concern with the overall uptake of any given form of health information technology. The current study did not examine the potential influence that such activities would have on outcomes, as the HDCC survey predated the latest technology-focused collaborative effort. Further studies might be needed to further examine the convergence of multiple collaboratives, where each has some relevance to the outcomes of interest in the other, with the understanding that the community health center, like many health care organizations, is a multifaceted, dynamic, and complex environment with many different interests. Finally, we exercised a subtle but necessary distinction between CDS adoption and CDS utilization throughout this study. We operationally defined a CDS adoption study as an examination of transition that might examine readiness for change, as well as, pre and post CDS practices. Our secondary data did not provide such data and as a result we limited our investigation to what CHCs had at the time of the survey. Future studies may be needed that examine stages of CDS adoption, CDS implementation issues, and ultimately CDS use and impact on cancer quality health outcomes.

Research Contribution

The purpose of this study was to identify a set of factors that may be associated with the use of clinical decision support used in support of cancer screening activities. This study is important because (1) clinical decision support has oftentimes been shown to be effective in improving clinical outcomes and (2) the overall uptake of clinical decision support in U.S. health care organizations remains fairly low. This study focused on identifying factors associated with the level, or intensity-of-use, of clinical decision support used to support cancer screenings. Sets of organizational and/or practice setting factors, patient characteristics, and provider characteristics were linked with a previously developed theoretical framework by Jane Zapka (Zapka et al., 2003). Previous studies have shown that CDS is effective in improving clinical outcomes and health care facility performance (Kilsdonk et al., 2011; Saleem et al., 2005; Shortell et al., 2005). The value added goal of this study was to provide a foundation to support future research and intervention strategies aimed at increasing CDS uptake and use in support of cancer screening through changes in organizational factors and/or provider practices, especially among community health centers serving vulnerable populations. This study contributes to existing literature by providing support for an evidence-based approach toward increasing cancer-screening-specific CDS levels within community health and health care settings.

Competing Interests

The authors declare that they have no competing interests.

Authors' Contributions

TJC and MW performed the statistical analyses. TJC, DH, and MW interpreted the data and drafted the manuscript. TJC, DH and MW conceived of the study and participated in its design and execution. TJC, AM, and JJ participated in the conceptual model development, design, and literature review. All authors read and approved the final manuscript. This work represents the opinion of the authors and cannot be construed to represent the opinion of the U.S. Federal Government.

Authors' Information

Timothy Jay Carney is an Assistant Professor at the Gillings School of Global Public Health, University of North Carolina at Chapel Hill, Department of Health Policy and Management. *Timothy Jay Carney* holds a doctoral degree in Health Informatics from Indiana University. *Timothy Jay Carney* is also a graduate of the Centers for Disease Control and Prevention Public Health Informatics Fellowship training program and worked at the CDC as an Informatics Specialist for nine years. *Timothy Jay Carney*'s current research focuses on applied public health informatics, intelligent organizational design, systems science methodologies, social and organizational network analysis, and computational modeling and simulation to impact on public health practice, cancer prevention and control, and health disparities.

ACKNOWLEDGMENT

This research was supported by the Indiana University (IUPUI) School of Nursing Training in Research for Behavioral Oncology and Cancer Control Program (TRBOCC) - National Cancer Institute Pre-Doctoral Fellowship R25-CA117865-04 The manuscript development was supported by University of North Carolina Gillings School of Public Health and Lineberger Comprehensive Cancer Center Cancer Health Disparities Training Fellowship T32CA128582 and editing services funded by the Carolina Community Network Center to Reduce Cancer Health Disparities (CCN II) Fellowship 3U54CA153602 Dr. Stephen H. Taplin and Dr. Stephen B. Clauser of the National Cancer Institute informed this research endeavor in many ways including allowing access to their original data set, providing the foundation for this research agenda through their previous findings, and demonstrating a willingness to shape the future direction of this overall research project.

REFERENCES

Abrams, M. K., Beal, A. C., Doty, M. M., Hernandez, S. E., & Stremikis, K. (2010). *Enhancing the capacity of community health centers to achieve high performance*. Retrieved from http://www.issuelab.org/permalink/resource/9153

Asch, S., Baker, D., Keesey, J. W., Broder, M., Schonlau, M., & Rosen, M. et al. (2005). Does the collaborative model improve care for chronic heart failure? *Medical Care, 43*, 667–675. doi:10.1097/01.mlr.0000167182.72251.a1 PMID:15970781

Bates, D., Cohen, M., Leape, L., Overhage, J., Shabot, M., & Sheridan, T. (2001). Reducing the frequency of errors in medicine using information technology. *Journal of the American Medical Informatics Association, 8*(4). doi:10.1136/jamia.2001.0080299 PMID:11418536

Bates, D. W., Pappius, E., Kuperman, G. J., Sittig, D., Burstin, H., & Fairchild, D. et al. (1999). Using information systems to measure and improve quality. *International Journal of Medical Informatics, 53*(2-3). doi:10.1016/S1386-5056(98)00152-X PMID:10193881

Burke, D., Menachemi, N., & Brooks, R. G. (2005). Diffusion of information technology supporting the institute of medicine's quality chasm care aims. *Journal for Healthcare Quality, 27*(1). doi:10.1111/j.1945-1474.2005.tb00542.x PMID:16416889

Chin, M. H., Cook, S., Drum, M. L., Jin, L., Guillen, M., & Humikowski, C. A. et al. (2004). Improving diabetes care in midwest community health centers with the health disparities collaborative. *Diabetes Care, 27*, 2–8. doi:10.2337/diacare.27.1.2 PMID:14693957

Doebbeling, B. N., Chou, A. F., & Tierney, W. M. (2006). Priorities and strategies for the implementation of integrated informatics and communications technology to improve evidence-based practice. *Journal of General Internal Medicine, 21*(2), S50–S57. doi:10.1007/s11606-006-0275-9 PMID:16637961

Good, P. I. (2011). *Analyzing the large numbers of variables in biomedical and satellite imagery.* Hoboken, NJ: Wiley. doi:10.1002/9780470937273

Haggstrom, D., Clauser, S., & Taplin, S. (2010). The health disparities cancer collaborative: A case study of practice registry measurement in a quality improvement collaborative. *Implementation Science; IS, 5*(1), 42. doi:10.1186/1748-5908-5-42 PMID:20525355

Haggstrom, D. A., S. C., Monahan, P., & Taplin-Haggstrom, S. H. (2010). Chronic care model implementation for cancer care processes in community health centers. *Medical Care, 15*.

Haggstrom, D. A., Clauser, S. B., & Taplin, S. H. (2008). Implementation of the chronic care model in the HRSA health disparities cancer collaborative. In *Proceedings of the Presentation at Society of General Internal Medicine National Meeting,* Pittsburgh, PA.

Haggstrom, D. A., Taplin, S. H., Monahan, P., & Clauser, S. (2012). Chronic care model implementation for cancer screening and follow-up in community health centers. *Journal of Health Care for the Poor and Underserved, 23*(3), 49–66. doi:10.1353/hpu.2012.0131 PMID:22864487

Harmon, R. G., & Carlson, R. H. (1991). HRSA's role in primary care and public health in the 1990s. Public Health Rports (Washington, D.C.: 1974), 106(1).

HHS. U. S. D. o. H. a. H. S.-. (2010). Understanding the impact of health IT in underserved communities and those with health disparities. Washington, DC: University of Chicago NORC.

Hintze, J. (2011). *PASS 11. NCSS, LLC.* Kaysville, UT. Retrieved from www.ncss.com

HRSA. H. R. a. S. A. (2008). Health centers: America's primary care safety net reflections on success, 2002-2007. Rockville, MD.

Iglehart, J. K. (2008). Spreading the safety net--obstacles to the expansion of community health centers. *The New England Journal of Medicine, 358*(13), 1321–1323. doi:10.1056/NEJMp0801332 PMID:18367733

Jamtvedt, G., Young, J. M., Kristoffersen, D. T., O'Brien, M. A., & Oxman, A. D. (2006). Does telling people what they have been doing change what they do? A systematic review of the effects of audit and feedback. *Quality & Safety in Health Care, 15*(6), 433–436. doi:10.1136/qshc.2006.018549 PMID:17142594

Kilsdonk, E., Peute, L. W., Knijnenburg, S. L., & Jaspers, M. W. (2011). Factors known to influence acceptance of clinical decision support systems. *Studies in Health Technology and Informatics, 169*, 150–154. PMID:21893732

Kinsinger, L. S., Harris, R., Qaqish, B., Strecher, V., & Kaluzny, A. (1998). Using an office system intervention to increase breast cancer screening. *Journal of General Internal Medicine, 13*(8), 507–514. doi:10.1046/j.1525-1497.1998.00160.x PMID:9734786

Kutner, M. H., Nachtsheim, C., & Neter, J. (2004). *Applied linear regression models.* Boston, MA: McGraw-Hill/Irwin.

Landon, B. E., Hicks, L. S., & O'Malley, A. J. (2007). Improving the management of chronic disease at community health centers. [see comment]. *The New England Journal of Medicine, 356,* 921–934. doi:10.1056/NEJMsa062860 PMID:17329699

Landon, B. E., Wilson, I. B., McInnes, K., Landrum, M. B., Hirschhorn, L., & Marsden, P. V. et al. (2004). Effects of a quality improvement collaborative on the outcome of care of patients with HIV infection: the EQHIV study. *Annals of Internal Medicine, 140,* 887–896. doi:10.7326/0003-4819-140-11-200406010-00010 PMID:15172903

Lardiere, M. R. (2010). *Assessment of Community Health Center EHR Capability, National Association of Community Health Centers, director of health information technology.*

Lardiere, M. R. (2010). National Association of Community Health Centers, Director of Health Information Technology. *Assessment of Community Health Center EHR Capability.*

Millery, M., & Kukafka, R. (2010). Health information technology and quality of health care: Strategies for reducing disparities in underresourced settings. [Supplement]. *Medical Care Research and Review,* 67. PMID:20675348

Nemeth, C., Connor, M., Klock, P., & Cook, R. (2006). Discovering healthcare cognition: The use of cognitive artifacts to reveal cognitive work. *Organization Studies, 27*(7), 1011–1035. doi:10.1177/0170840606065708

Reid, P. P., Compton, W. D., Grossman, J. H., & Fanjiang, G. National Academy of, E., Institute of, M., & National Academies, P. (2005). Building a better delivery system: A new engineering/health care partnership. Washington, DC: National Academies Press.

Saleem, J. J., Patterson, E. S., Militello, L., Render, M. L., Orshansky, G., & Asch, S. M. (2005). Exploring barriers and facilitators to the use of computerized clinical reminders. *Journal of the American Medical Informatics Association, 12*(4), 438. doi:10.1197/jamia. M1777 PMID:15802482

Shields, A. E., Shin, P., Leu, M. G., Levy, D. E., Betancourt, R. M., Hawkins, D., & Proser, M. (2007). Adoption of health information technology in community health centers: Results of a national survey. *Health Affairs (Project Hope), 26*(5). doi:10.1377/hlthaff.26.5.1373 PMID:17848448

Shortell, S., Schmittdiel, J., Wang, M., Li, R., Gillies, R., & Casalino, L. et al. (2005). An empirical assessment of high-performing medical groups: Results from a national study. *Medical Care Research and Review, 62*(4), 407–434. doi:10.1177/1077558705277389 PMID:16049132

Soban, L. M., & Yano, E. M. (2005). The impact of primary care resources on prevention practices. *The Journal of Ambulatory Care Management, 28*(3). doi:10.1097/00004479-200507000-00007 PMID:15968216

Sperl-Hillen, J. M., Solberg, L. I., Hroscikoski, M. C., Crain, A. L., Engebretson, K. I., & O'Connor, P. J. (2004). Do all components of the chronic care model contribute equally to quality improvement? *Joint Commission Journal on Quality and Safety, 30*(6), 303–309. PMID:15208979

Taplin, S. H., Haggstrom, D., Jacobs, T., Determan, A., Granger, J., & Montalvo, W. et al. (2008). Implementing colorectal cancer screening in community health centers: Addressing cancer health disparities through a regional cancer collaborative. *Medical Care, 46*, S74–S83. doi:10.1097/MLR.0b013e31817fdf68 PMID:18725837

U.S. Department of Health and Human Services. A. f. H. R. a. Q.-A. (2009). Best practices transforming quality, safety, and efficiency. *Key topics: Clinical decision support*. Retrieved from http://healthit.ahrq.gov/portal/server.pt?open=512&objID=650&parentname=CommunityPage&parentid=1&mode=2&in_hi_userid=3882&cached=true

Weiner, B. J., Savitz, L. A., Bernard, S., & Pucci, L. G. (2004). How do integrated delivery systems adopt and implement clinical information systems? *Health Care Management Review, 29*(1). doi:10.1097/00004010-200401000-00007 PMID:14992484

Yarbrough, A., & Smith, T. (2007). Technology acceptance among physicians. *Medical Care Research and Review, 64*(6), 650–672. doi:10.1177/1077558707305942 PMID:17717378

Zapka, J. (2008). Innovative provider- and health system-directed approaches to improving colorectal cancer screening delivery. *Medical Care, 46*(9), 62–67. doi:10.1097/MLR.0b013e31817fdf57 PMID:18725835

Zapka, J. G., Puleo, E., Taplin, S., Solberg, L. I., Mouchawar, J., & Somkin, C. et al. (2005). Breast and cervical cancer screening: clinicians' views on health plan guidelines and implementation efforts. *Journal of the National Cancer Institute. Monographs, 35*, 46–54. doi:10.1093/jncimonographs/lgi037 PMID:16287885

Zapka, J. G., Taplin, S. H., Solberg, L. I., & Manos, M. M. (2003). Commentary - a framework for improving the quality of cancer care: the case of breast and cervical cancer screening. *Cancer Epidemiology, Biomarkers & Prevention: A Publication of the American Association for Cancer Research, 12*(1), 4.

Zapka, J. G., Taplin, S. H., Solberg, L. I., & Manos, M. M. (2003). A framework for improving the quality of cancer care: The case of breast and cervical cancer screening. *Cancer Epidemiology, Biomarkers & Prevention, 12*, 4–13. PMID:12540497

This work was previously published in the International Journal of Healthcare Information Systems and Informatics (IJHISI), 9(1); edited by Joseph Tan, pages 1-29 copyright year 2014 by IGI Publishing (an imprint of IGI Global).

APPENDIX

Survey Item Descriptions

Table 7. Summary measure conceptual definitions

Summary Measure	Summary Measure Conceptual Definition
Governance Strategy based upon HRSA Collaborative Experience	Overall Community Health Center Management Strategy, Policies, Procedures, etc.
Facility Age	Year community center was formed
Clinic Processes	Community Health Center Clinical Operations
Information Dissemination Strategies (to patients)	Strategies employed to support patient decision making and informed choices and change behavior relative to cancer screening
Electronic Information Retrieval & Availability	Computer and internet access at the clinical for use in patient care
Electronic Health Record Capabilities	Core functions performed by the Electronic Health Record (EHR)
Work Importance of Cancer Screening Tasks	An individual's tendency or orientations to value of the work (specific cancer screening tasks) in general
Quality Improvement Strategies	Institute of Medicine's (IOMs) definition of quality of care as "the degree to which health care services for individuals and populations increase the likelihood of desired health outcomes and are consistent with current professional knowledge." A quality measure is a mechanism that enables the user to quantify the quality of a selected aspect of care by comparing it to a criterion. A subtype of a quality measure is a clinical performance measure. Specifically, a clinical performance measure is a mechanism for assessing the degree to which a provider competently and safely delivers clinical services that are appropriate for the patient in the optimal time period. Quality measures can be used for both quality improvement within an institution or system of care (internal quality improvement) or across institutions or systems of care (external quality improvement). Using measures for internal quality improvement involves three basic steps: identifying problems or opportunities for improvement, selecting appropriate measures and using them to obtain a baseline assessment of current practices, and using them to reassess or monitor the effect of improvement efforts on measure performance. Baseline quality measure results can be used to better understand a quality problem, provide motivation for change, and establish a basis for comparison across institutional units or over time. Baseline results also enable the user to prioritize areas for quality improvement. Results from repeated measurements of clinical performance can be used by internal quality improvement programs to assess whether performance has changed after improvement efforts have been implemented.
External Pressure, Support, and Connectedness via Collaborative Agreements	*According to Iacovou et al. (1995), external pressure refers to influences from the organizational environment. Grandon and Pearson (2003) suggested five external pressure elements in ERP which are competition, social factors, dependency on other firms already using ERP, the industry,* *and government.*
Cancer Screening Rate Reporting Behavior (Facility Level)	The way that a situation is categorized or defined by formal reporting at the facility level. Assessment of over-arching goals (meeting clinical guidelines for colorectal, breast, and cervical cancer screening) will impact how the situation (cancer screening) is perceived.
Delivery System Design for Cancer Screening (e.g., Role Responsibility, Overlap, and Clinical Champions) *(The inclusion of this measure will depend on whether or not there is sufficient variability, as obtained in a frequency distribution, of the population)*	*Role Relevance*: The belief that the situation or action is relevant to the individual's role. For example, a person's belief about being clinically responsible is a significant contribution to how the individual carries out the relevant behavior.

continued on following page

Table 7. Continued

Summary Measure	Summary Measure Conceptual Definition
Supportive Leadership Environment	*Supportive Leadership* Environment: The degree to which the environment is perceived as supportive, including organizational leaders, the physical structure, and even "help".
Supportive Local (Functional) Leadership	*Supportive Local (Functional) Leadership* Environment: The degree to which the environment is perceived as supportive, including organizational leaders, the physical structure and even "help" specifically related to clinical function.
Team Characteristics	Team: Group of individuals responsible for both delivering and improving the quality of care in the clinic, including both clinicians and non-clinicians. (2009 Haggstrom et al.)
Medical Specialist Availability	*A Board Certified Physician specifically trained to conduct colorectal cancer screening.*
Organizational Structure/Size	Organizational Size: Likely surrogate for total and slack resources; ability to obtain and sustain technical expertise, organizational structure.
Financial Readiness	Organizational readiness refers to the level of financial and technical resources of the firm (Kuan & Chau, 2001). There are two dimensions to organizational readiness: financial and technical. Financial readiness refers to the financial resources available to pay for new technological innovation costs, implementation of any subsequent enhancements, and ongoing expenses during usage. Iacovou et al. (1995).
Payer mix	Payer mix represents the percentage of revenue coming from private insurance versus government insurance versus self-paying individuals.
Patient Demographics	Percentage of patient population 50 years of age or older
Environmental Assessment of Cancer Screening and Follow-up Activities	The way that a situation is categorized or defined by the person (provider). Assessment of over-arching goals (meeting clinical guidelines for colorectal, breast, and cervical cancer screening) will impact how the situation (cancer screening) is perceived.
Cancer Screening Rate Reporting Behavior (Provider-Level)	The way that a situation is categorized or defined by formal reporting at the provider-level. Assessment of over-arching goals (meeting clinical guidelines for colorectal, breast, and cervical cancer screening) will impact how the situation (cancer screening) is perceived.
Provider IT Performance Expectancy	*Provider IT Performance Expectancy* is defined as the degree to which an individual provider believes that using IT will help him or her to attain gains in job performance
IS & CDS Capacity for Measuring Cancer Screening	***Clinical Decision Support (CDS)–Promote clinical care that is consistent with scientific evidence and patient preferences*** Embed evidence-based guidelines into daily clinical practice Share evidence-based guidelines and information with patients to encourage their participation Use proven provider education methods Integrate specialist expertise and primary care ***Clinical Information Systems (IS)–Organize patient and population data to facilitate efficient and effective care*** Provide timely reminders for providers and patients Identify relevant subpopulations for proactive care Facilitate individual patient care planning Share information with patients and providers to coordinate care Monitor performance of practice team and care system
Use of IS & CDS provider prompts at Point-of-Care	Same as above for CDS & IS
Computerized Patient Reminders	Same as above for CDS & IS
Generated Correspondence with Results to Patients	Same as above for CDS & IS
Composite CDS Practices Scores	Level of or "intensity of use of CDS
Cancer Screening Improvement Scores	Guideline concordant care for Colorectal, Breast, and Cervical Cancer

Table 8. Organizational and/or practice setting operational definitions

Summary Measure Name	Operational Definition (HDCC Survey Mappings)	Item Scales
Governance Strategy based upon HRSA Collaborative Experience	Question Set {1, 2, 74}	
	Question 1	1=yes; 0=no
	Did you ever participate in any HRSA Health Disparities Collaborative prior to 2006?	Range: 0 to 1
	Question 2	1=yes; 0=no
	Did you participate in the HRSA Health Disparities Cancer Collaborative anytime from 2002 through 2004?	Range: 0 to 1
	Question 74	1=yes; 0=no
	Has your health center ever participated in any HRSA Collaborative?	Range: 0 to 1
		Total range for governance Y/N questions = 0 to 3
Facility Age	Question Set {72, 73}	Numerical entry (data expressed as year)
	Question 72	
	In what year did your organization open as a health center?	Facility Age(1) With date of survey as reference point (2006) 2006–year = Facility Age(1) Range: 00 to 99 Facility Age(2) Numerical entry (data expressed as year)
	Question 73	
	In what year did your health center begin receiving Bureau of Primary Health Care (BPHC) funding?	Facility Age(2) With date of survey as reference point (2006) 2006 – year = Facility Age(2) Range: 00 to 99
Clinic Processes	Question Set {5a, 5b, 5c, 6}	
	Question 5a, 5b, 5c	1=yes; 0=no
	Does your health center have clinical guidelines available to health care providers (physicians, physician assistants, nurse practitioners) for cancer screening Question Set includes: In writing in the room where they see patients? On-line in the room where they patients? On-line at some other location than where they routinely see patients?	Range: 0 to 3
	Response Set	1=yes; 0=no
	yes=1 no=0	Range: 0 to 1
	Question 6	
	Are individuals working at your health center instructed to document discussions about cancer screening?	Total range for clinic processes = 0 to 4

continued on following page

Table 8. Continued

Summary Measure Name	Operational Definition (HDCC Survey Mappings)	Item Scales
Information Dissemination Strategies (to patients)	Question Set {17,18,19,20,21,22,23,24}	4-Item Likert Scale (Items 3a-10a)
	Question 17	0=not at all; 1=Rarely; 2=Sometimes; 3=Often
	How often does your health center connect patients with available community resources for cancer screening?	Range: 0 to 3
	Question 18	
	The available community resources for cancer screening are adequate for your health center's patient population	Range: 0 to 3
	Question 19	
	How often do you or the health center staff provide patients with educational materials about cancer screening, such as pamphlets or brochures?	Range: 0 to 3
	Question 20	
	How often do you or the health center staff provide patients with written or online directories that provide guidance to cancer resources?	Range: 0 to 3
	Question 21	
	During acute care visits, how often are cancer screening guidelines discussed with eligible patients by you?	Range: 0 to 3
	Question 22	
	During acute care visits, how often are cancer screening guidelines discussed with eligible patients by others who work in the clinic?	Range: 0 to 3
	Question 23	
	During non-acute care visits, how often are cancer screening guidelines discussed with eligible patients by you?	Range: 0 to 3
	Question 24	
	During non-acute care visits, how often are cancer screening guidelines discussed with eligible patients by others who work in the clinic?	Range: 0 to 3
		Note: Often and Routinely are considered synonymous in this question response set. Total range for Information Dissemination 0 to 24
Electronic Information Retrieval &	Question Set {47,48,49}	
	Question 47	1=yes; 0=no
Availability	Is there a computer with Internet access available at your clinic to use for patient care? Question 48 Is there a computer with Internet access available at the point of care (e.g., exam room)?	Range: 0 to 1 1=yes; 0=no Range: 0 to 1
	Question 49	1=yes; 0=no
	Is there a computer with Internet access available at a work station, away from the point of care?	Range: 0 to 1 Total range for Computer Access is 0 to 3

continued on following page

Table 8. Continued

Summary Measure Name	Operational Definition (HDCC Survey Mappings)	Item Scales
Electronic Health Record Capabilities	Question 41a-f	1=yes; 0=no
	Indicate whether each piece of information listed is available in the clinic's computer system or electronic medical/health record (EHR) Mammography results Pap test results Fecal occult blood test results Results of procedures for breast cancer detection, including biopsy Results of gynecologic procedures for cervical cancer detection, including colposcopy Results of lower endoscopy procedures for colorectal cancer detection	Range: 0 to 6
Work Importance of Cancer Screening Tasks	Questions (3a-10a):	3-Item Likert Scale
	DESCRIBE YOUR LEVEL OF AGREEMENT OR DISAGREEMENT WITH THE FOLLOWING STATEMENTS in terms of the response set below:	(Items 7a-13a) 1=strongly disagree; 2=disagree; 3=agree; 4=strongly agree
	Providing formal assessment of patient self-management goal-setting (i.e., tracking whether patients meet their specified goals) for cancer screening and follow-up… Initiating or maintaining programs to increase patient shared decision-making skills for cancer screening and follow-up… Providing clinical guidelines to patients for cancer screening and follow-up… Providing clinical guidelines to individual health care providers (physicians, physician assistants, nurse practitioners) through reminders for cancer screening and follow-up… Changing responsibilities of health care providers and staff in the clinic to enable them to function more like a team to deliver cancer screening and follow-up… Designing the appointment system to facilitate the scheduling of cancer screening and follow-up at any related facility where screening occurs… Providing written feedback reports or data to health care providers (physicians, physician assistants, nurse practitioners) regarding their performance of cancer screening and follow-up… Providing written feedback reports or data to local clinic teams regarding their performance of cancer screening and follow-up… Response Set: Is a useful activity	Range: 8 to 32

continued on following page

Table 8. Continued

Summary Measure Name	Operational Definition (HDCC Survey Mappings)	Item Scales
Quality Improvement Strategies	Question Set {3,4a,4b,4c,4d,,25,26, 27a,27b,27c,27d,27e,27f,27g}	
	Question 3	1=yes; 0=no
	Have you ever participated, either formally or informally, in quality improvement activities at your health center?	Range: 0 to 1
	Question 4a-d How often do members of your health center engage in the following activities to improve cancer screening and follow-up?	3-Item Likert Scale 1=not at all; 2=rarely; 3=sometimes; 4=often
	Response Set Conference calls with experts outside your health center E-mail (listserv) discussions with experts outside your health center Visits from/to other health centers Ongoing measurement of clinical performance at your center	Range: 3 to 16
	Question 25a-d In the last 12 months, did your health center use measures of either patient satisfaction or clinical performance to do any of the following?	3-Item Likert Scale 0=used neither; 1=yes but only patient satisfaction or performance; 2=yes to both
	Response Set: Pay health care provider bonuses Adjust salary or base pay Implement a quality improvement initiative Have general discussions at practice meetings	Range: 0 to 8
	Question 26 In the past 12 months, did your health center compare its data on quality of care to data from other centers?	1=yes; 0=no
	Question 27a-g How much does your health center use each of the following strategies to ensure high quality care is delivered to primary care patients?	Range: 0 to 1
	Response Set Health care providers' informal monitoring of each others' practice patterns Chart reviews Health care provider peer review of selected cases Discussion of clinical guidelines at health center or team meetings Statistical reports of practice patterns Morbidity or mortality conferences External medical record audits (e.g., by representatives of the state or a health plan)	3-Item Likert Scale 1=not at all; 2=a little; 3=some; 4=a lot Range: 7 to 28 Total range for Quality Improvement Strategies is 11 to 53

continued on following page

Table 8. Continued

Summary Measure Name	Operational Definition (HDCC Survey Mappings)	Item Scales
External Pressure, Support, and Connectedness via Collaborative Agreements	Question Set {28,29,30,75,76}	
	Questions 28	1=yes; 0=no
	Does your organization make a list available of identified community cancer resources in an accessible format?	Range: 0 to 1
	Question 29	1=yes; 0=no
	Does your organization have staff or resources allocated to ensure health care providers and patients make use of community cancer resources?	Range: 0 to 1
	Question 30a-g	1=yes; 0=no
	Have you set up informal or contractual agreements with the following organizations? Response Set: Public health department Radiology department Gastroenterology practice Community oncology practice Cancer center Academic medical center Cancer survivorship support group	Range: 0 to 7
	Question 75	1=yes; 0=no
	Does the health center's Board of Directors receive updates on your center's Collaborative activities?	Range: 0 to 1
	Question 76	1=yes; 0=no
	Does your health center have a formal or informal relationship with any hospitals (e.g., referrals for specialty care; training or residency programs; quality improvement data sharing)?	Range: 0 to 1 Total range for external pressure is 0 to 11
Cancer Screening Rate Reporting Behavior (Facility Level)	Question Set {35a, 36a, 37a, 38a. 39a, 40a}	
	In the past 12 months, did you receive any reports from your health center about rates of clinical services, screening for colorectal, breast, and cervical cancer screening, test results, or discussion with patients	1=yes; 0=no
	Response Set At the health care facility (clinic) level Note: additional question frequency in months not currently included in this analysis	Range: 0 to 1 Total range for cancer screening reporting behavior is 0 to 6

continued on following page

Table 8. Continued

Summary Measure Name	Operational Definition (HDCC Survey Mappings)	Item Scales
Delivery System Design for Cancer Screening (e.g., Role Responsibility, Overlap, and Clinical Champions) *(The inclusion of this measure will depend on whether or not there is sufficient variability, as obtained in a frequency distribution, of the population)*	Question Set {43,44,45,46}	
	Question 43a-f Mark all members of the local clinic who participate in performing Breast Cancer Screening activity (e.g., mammography). Mark the consultant if that is a person who performs the activity. Mark "no one" if neither a consultant nor anyone in the local clinic performs the activity.	0=no one assigned to task; 1=one person assigned to the task…5=five people assigned to the task (see types below)
	Response Set: Generates a list of patients due for screening Actively contacts patients if due for screening Discusses decision to screen with patients Schedules screening mammogram Actively contacts patients with abnormal screening results within 30 days Arranges breast procedure if necessary (including biopsy)	physician other provider (NP, PA) nurse other staff (office, lab) GI consultant
	Question 44a-g Mark all members of the local clinic who participate in performing Cervical Cancer Screening activity (e.g., Pap test). Mark the consultant if that is a person who performs the activity. Mark "no one" if neither a consultant nor any one in the local clinic performs the activity.	Range 0 to 30
	Response Set: Generates a list of patients due for screening Actively contacts patients if due for screening Discusses decision to screen with patients Schedules Pap test Performs Pap test Actively contacts patients with abnormal screening results within 30 days Arranges gynecologic procedure, if necessary (including colposcopy)	0=no one assigned to task; 1=one personal assigned to the task…5=five people assigned to the task (see types below) physician other provider (NP,PA) nurse other staff (office, lab) GI consultant
	Question 45a-h Mark all members of the local clinic who participate in performing Colorectal Cancer Screening activity. Mark the consultant if that is a person who performs the activity. Mark "no one" if neither a consultant nor anyone in the local clinic performs the activity.	Range 0 to 35
	Response Set: Generates a list of patients due for screening Actively contacts patients if due for screening Discusses screening options with patients Distributes fecal occult blood tests (stool cards) Enters fecal occult blood test results (stool cards) into tracking database. Schedules screening lower endoscopy Actively contacts patients with abnormal screening results within 30 days Schedules diagnostic lower endoscopy	0=no one assigned to task; 1=one personal assigned to the task…5=five people assigned to the task (see types below) physician other provider (NP, PA) nurse other staff (office, lab) GI consultant
	Question 46 For all screening tests - Arranges referral for treatment if cancer detected	0=no one assigned to task; 1=one personal assigned to the task…5=five people assigned to the task (see types below) physician other provider (NP, PA) nurse other staff (office, lab) GI consultant Range 0 to 5 Total score for division of responsibilities or role relevance will range from 0 to 110

continued on following page

Table 8. Continued

Summary Measure Name	Operational Definition (HDCC Survey Mappings)	Item Scales
Supportive Leadership Environment	Question 51 Please describe your level of agreement or disagreement with the following statements about senior leadership overall.	3-Item Likert Scale 1=strongly disagree; 2=disagree; 3=agree; 4=strongly agree
	Response Set: Has demonstrated an ability to manage the changes (e.g., organizational, technological) needed to improve the quality of care and services. Always listens to the concerns of other members of the organization Provides needed feedback to members of the organization Helps members of the organization work well together Provides members of the organization with a clear expectation of their roles Makes sure people have the skills and knowledge to work in teams Makes sure a local clinic team that does a good job gets special rewards or recognition Strongly supports our work Regularly reviews our progress in making change Sees success in improving the quality of care as a high priority for the organization	Range: 10 to 30 Higher score = better leadership
Supportive Local (Functional) Leadership	Question 53 Please describe your level of agreement or disagreement with the following statements about functional (clinical) leadership overall.	3-Item Likert Scale 1=strongly disagree; 2=disagree; 3=agree; 4=strongly agree
	Response Set: Possesses the functional expertise necessary for leading the local clinic team successfully Always listens to the concerns of other local clinic team members Provides needed feedback to other local clinic team members Helps local clinic team members work well together Provides local clinic team members with a clear expectation of their roles on this team	Range: 5 to 20 Higher score = better leadership
Team Characteristics	Question 55 Please describe your level of agreement or disagreement with the following statements about team characteristics overall.	3-Item Likert Scale 1=strongly disagree; 2=disagree; 3=agree; 4=strongly agree
	Response Set: The number of people on my local clinic team is about right for the work to be accomplished The members of the local clinic team work together well as a team Members of my local clinic team vary widely in their knowledge, skills, and abilities Members of my local clinic team have skills and abilities that complement each other I generally prefer to work as part of a team Our local clinic team gets the information we need to plan our work Our local clinic team has the authority to manage its work pretty much the way members want to There is a great deal of room for initiative and judgment in the work that we do The participants on our local clinic team have substantial influence in managing care and influencing others to make improvements in care When our local clinic team does not know something it needs to know to do its work, there are people available to teach or help There are one or more well-respected members of our staff that support our work with their time, and verbal encouragement Our local clinic team is able to identify measures that were tracked on a regular basis to assess our work My skills, training, and experience are fully utilized	Range: 13 to 52

continued on following page

Table 8. Continued

Summary Measure Name	Operational Definition (HDCC Survey Mappings)	Item Scales
Medical Specialist Availability	Question 79 Which of the following categories best describes the availability of each of the specialists listed below to patients at your health center involved in cancer screening?	0=not available; 1=available
	Response Set: Gastroenterologist Gynecologist Oncologist General Surgeon Breast Cancer Surgeon Gynecologic Surgeon Colorectal Cancer Surgeon Radiologist – general Radiologist – interventional Radiologist with training in breast imaging	Range: 0 to 10 Specialist score = greater the score the more specialists available
Organizational Structure/Size	Question 80a-g How many of the following are employed by your health center?	Numerical entry
	Response Sets: Number of People: Physicians Nurse Practitioners Physician Assistants Registered Nurses Licensed Practical Nurses Laboratory personnel Scheduler/reception	Range: 0 to 9999 for each type
Financial Readiness	Question Set {85,93}	
	Question 85 What is your health center's annual operating budget (for the most recent fiscal year)? (in US dollars) Note: Assume fiscal year 2006 unless otherwise stated	Financial Readiness(1) Numerical entry (dollar figure) Range: 0 to N for each type
	Question 94 For your health center's most recent fiscal year, please circle the number of the phrase below that best reflects your center's financial situation.	Financial Readiness(2)
	Response Set: Operating expenses exceeded operating revenue by $\geq 25\% = 1$ Operating expenses exceeded operating revenue by 11-23% = 2 Operating expenses exceeded operating revenues by 1-10% = 3 Broke even = 4 Operating revenue exceeded operating expenses by 1-10% = 5 Operating revenue exceeded operating expenses by 11-23% = 6 Operating revenue exceeded operating expenses by $\geq 25\% = 7$	Range: 1 to 7 Where 1 is considered less "ideal" extreme and 7 is considered more "ideal" extreme

Table 9. Patient characteristics summary measure operational definitions

Summary Measure Name	Operational Definition (HDCC Survey Mappings)	Item Scales
Payer mix	Question Set {86,89a,89b,89c,89d}	
	Question 86 Approximately what proportion of your health center patients are uninsured?	Range: 0 to 100%
	Response Set % Uninsured 0–100%	
	Question 89a-d What percentage of your patient revenue comes from each of the following sources?	Range: 0 to 100% for each member of the response set
	Response Set: Medicare Medicaid Commercial Self-Pay	
Patient Demographics	Question Set {95,96,97,98,99}	
	Patient Demographics(1)	
	Question 95 What percentage of patients seen at your health center in the past 12 months speak a language other than English as their primary language?	Range: 0 to 100%
	Response Set 0 to 100%	
	Patient Demographics(2)	
	Question 96 What percentage of patients seen at your health center in the past 12 months are Migrant or seasonal agricultural workers?	Range: 0 to 100%
	Response Set 0 to 100%	
	Question 97 What percentage of patients seen at your health center in the past 12 months are Homeless?	Range: 0 to 100%
	Response Set 0 to 100%	
	Patient Demographics(3)	
	Question 99 Approximately what percentage of your patients seen in the past 12 months are 50 years of age of older?	Range: 1 to 4
	Response Set 1=Less than 25% 2=25-39% 3=50-73% 4=75-100% Note: Could be used as exclusion criteria, for example, exclude centers where less than 25% are eligible for CRC screening.	

Table 10. Provider characteristics summary measure operational definitions

Summary Measure Name	Operational Definition (HDCC Survey Mappings)	Item Scales
Environmental Assessment of Cancer Screening and Follow-up Activities	Questions (7b, c, & d-13b, c, & d): DESCRIBE YOUR LEVEL OF AGREEMENT OR DISAGREEMENT WITH THE FOLLOWING STATEMENTS in terms of the Question Set below:	3-Item Likert Scale 1=strongly disagree; 2=disagree; 3=agree; 4=strongly agree
	Providing formal assessment of patient self-management goal-setting (i.e., tracking whether patients meet their specified goals) for cancer screening and follow-up… Initiating or maintaining programs to increase patient shared decision-making skills for cancer screening and follow-up… Providing clinical guidelines to patients for cancer screening and follow-up… Providing clinical guidelines to individual health care providers (physicians, physician assistants, nurse practitioners) through reminders for cancer screening and follow-up… Changing responsibilities of health care providers and staff in the clinic to enable them to function more like a team to deliver cancer screening and follow-up… Designing the appointment system to facilitate the scheduling of cancer screening and follow-up at any related facility where screening occurs… Providing written feedback reports or data to health care providers (physicians, physician assistants, nurse practitioners) regarding their performance of cancer screening and follow-up… Providing written feedback reports or data to local clinic teams regarding their performance of cancer screening and follow-up… Response Set for items 7b,c,d-13b,c,d is an activity about which our health center has educated health care providers and staff has been supported by adequate resources from our health center. has been implemented in our health center	Total Range for Environmental Assessment: 22 to 88
Cancer Screening Rate Reporting Behavior (Provider-Level)	Question Set {35b,36b,37b,38b,39b,40b}	
	Question 35b to 40b In the past 12 months, did you receive any reports from your health center about rates of screening for colorectal, breast, and cervical cancer screening	1=yes; 0=no
	Response Set At the health care provider/individual level Note: additional question frequency in months not currently included in this analysis Response Set	Range: 0 to 1 Total Range for Cancer Screening Reporting Behavior (provider level) = 0 to 6
Provider IT Performance Expectancy	Question 42a-k Please describe your level of agreement or disagreement with the following statements about the information system in place at your health center:	3-Item Likert Scale 1=strongly disagree; 2=disagree; 3=agree; 4=strongly agree
	The center's information system is adequate to accommodate the size of the population eligible for cancer screening. The information system provides timely data on cancer screening and follow-up The center continually tries to improve the timeliness of its data on cancer screening and follow-up The center continually tries to improve the accuracy of its data on cancer screening and follow-up The information system accurately documents cancer screening among the health center's patients The information system accurately documents whether appropriate evaluation takes place after an abnormal screening result The information system accurately documents whether appropriate treatment takes place after cancer detection The data gathered in the information system is used by leadership to change the health center's activities related to cancer screening. The data gathered in the information system is used by health care providers to change their behavior. I use the data gathered in the information system to change my behavior. The data gathered in the information system is used by health care providers to change their behavior related to cancer screening	Range: 11 to 44

Table 11. Outcome summary measure operational definitions

Summary Measure Name	Operational Definition (HDCC Survey Mappings)	Item Scales
IS & CDS Capacity for Measuring Cancer Screening	Question 31 Does your health center's computer system have any capacity to measure cancer screening activities?	1=yes; 0=no Range: 0 to 1
Use of IS & CDS provider prompts at Point-of-Care	Question 32 Our health center is using an information system (not necessarily computerized) to send prompts to health care providers (physicians, physician assistants, nurse practitioners) at the time of the patient encounter about whether their patients are eligible for cancer screening.	1=yes; 0=no Range: 0 to 1
Computerized Patient Reminders	Question 33 Our health center is using an information system to send correspondence or reminders to patients eligible for cancer screening.	1=yes; 0=no Range: 0 to 1
Generated Correspondence with Results to Patients	Question 34 Our health center is using an information system to send correspondence to patients about screening test results.	1=yes; 0=no Range: 0 to 1
Composite CDS Practices Scores	Question Set {31,32,33,34}	1=yes; 0=no Range: 0 to 4
Cancer Screening Improvement Scores	Question 16 In the past 12 months, our health center has been able to improve the rate of:	1=yes; 0=no Range: 0 to 3
	Response Set: Screening Mammography within the past 2 years Pap test within the past 3 years Appropriate screening for colorectal cancer	Note: agreement in any sense constitutes a yes=1, disagreement in any sense constitutes a no=0. The greater the score the greater the increase in overall cancer screening (self-reported) rates. Hence, colorectal, breast, and cervical cancer screening (self-reported) rates are treated here as a composite score

List of Abbreviations

AHRQ: Agency for Healthcare Research and Quality
BPHC: Bureau of Primary Health Care
BTS: Breakthrough Series
CCM: Chronic care model
CDS: Clinical decision support
CHC: Community health center
CHIP: Child health insurance protection
CIS: Clinical information system
EHR: Electronic health record
HDCC: Health Disparities Cancer Collaborative
HIT: Health Information Technology
HRSA: Health Resources and Services Administration
ICI: Institute of Healthcare Improvement
IT: Information Technology
NCI: National Cancer Institute
POC: Point-of-Care
URS: Under-resourced setting

Chapter 8
Principles of Information Accountability:
An eHealth Perspective

Randike Gajanayake
Queensland University of Technology, Australia

Tony Sahama
Queensland University of Technology, Australia

Renato Iannella
Semantic Identity, Australia

ABSTRACT

Information accountability is seen as a mode of usage control on the Web. Due to its many dimensions, information accountability has been expressed in various ways by computer scientists to address security and privacy in recent times. Information accountability is focused on how users participate in a system and the underlying policies that govern the participation. Healthcare is a domain in which the principles of information accountability can be utilised well. Modern health information systems are Internet based and the discipline is called eHealth. In this paper, the authors identify and discuss the goals of accountability systems and present the principles of information accountability. They characterise those principles in eHealth and discuss them contextually. They identify the current impediments to eHealth in terms of information privacy issues of eHealth consumers together with information usage requirements of healthcare providers and show how information accountability can be used in a healthcare context to address these needs. The challenges of implementing information accountability in eHealth are also discussed in terms of our efforts thus far.

INTRODUCTION

Information accountability (IA) is a solution for usage control on the decentralised Web (Feigenbaum, Hendler, Jaggard, Weitzner, & Wright,

2011; Weitzner et al., 2008). IA is about holding the information users answerable for their actions and the ramifications of those actions. Weitzner et al. (2008) propose a transparent and accountable audit process that gives the users incentives to

DOI: 10.4018/978-1-4666-8756-1.ch008

abide by the policies put in place and the ability to determine whether a particular use of information is policy compliant. Though the concept is not new, IA is comparatively new to computer science and information and communication technology (ICT) and has been interpreted in various dimensions by computer scientists. These approaches have been carefully systematised by Feigenbaum et al. (2012) who state that the term "accountability" is far broader than just anonymity, identification or exposure and that it allows actions to be tied to consequences and violations to be tied to punishment. The approaches considered by Feigenbaum et al. (2012) define IA in a general context. However, being a multidimensional concept, IA needs to be contextualised for its applicability to be better understood. The lack of contextual definitions of its underlying principles makes it difficult to apply in complex domains. Information systems that utilise the principles of IA are called accountability systems. Current technological advancements eliminate the technical barriers previously present in implementing this type of systems, but the success of any accountability system depends on how the underlying policies are formulated, which in turn depends on the context in which the systems are implemented.

IA can address several issues in a vast array of disciplines. Usage control is one area of interest to computer scientists, through which, the information privacy conundrum can be addressed. Information privacy has been and still is a major obstacle to adoption and trust of information systems; for example in healthcare. Several factors can be considered when dealing with information privacy: the type of policies; the nature of participants and their requirements; data ownership; data provenance; and the nature of the information such as sensitivity and availability. These aspects differ significantly with context. In terms of information management through electronic media such as the Internet, privacy can be defined as the degree of control given to the subject of the information (Westin, 1967). Within a given context, the

policies differ in terms of user requirements and other external factors such as government regulations and organisational policies. The nature of the information is also a significant reason why information privacy becomes a critical factor for information systems. This is clearly evident in domains such as healthcare (Rindfleisch, 1997).

In this paper, we introduce IA to eHealth as a means of addressing information privacy. To this end, we formulate a series of principles for IA drawn from prior research in computer science. We contextualise them to eHealth and lay foundations for IA to be utilised in eHealth as a means of adequate information privacy management.

In what follows, first we identify the problem addressed in the article and give an introduction of information accountability. Then, accountable systems are discussed in terms of their goals and objectives. The principles of IA are discussed followed by a discussion of IA in healthcare including the need for its implementation in eHealth. Next, the principles of IA in eHealth are discussed with the use of the case scenario. Finally, our efforts in the domain are discussed under a section entitled implementation challenges and the article is concluded with some closing remarks.

PROBLEM STATEMENT

Information privacy concerns are usually coupled with information security, which mainly involves unauthorised access to information by external entities. But, addressing data breaches by authorised users pose the biggest challenge and it is a significant aspect for eHealth systems. Some even claim that privacy threats are internal factors and not external (Kierkegaard, 2011). Therefore, patients have an expectation of confidentiality in their dealings with any qualified clinician or healthcare professional (Croll, 2011).

In eHealth, the definition of privacy encompasses confidentiality, integrity, availability and accountability (Ishikawa, 2000). The protection of patient privacy has been governed by the *Hippocratic Oath* (Lasagna, 2001) where the patient-physician relationship remained a cooperative one. However, with the adoption of technology in healthcare, there is a shift in this relationship towards a more regulation and policy driven one (Parks, Chu, & Xu, 2011).

Requirements in eHealth can be divided into two: information requirements of healthcare professionals and information privacy requirements of eHealth consumers. These can be identified as competing concerns; preventing healthcare professionals from accessing information in favour of information privacy is not an adequate solution, and neither is the reverse. Whilst information privacy is seen as a critical impediment for eHealth success (Croll, 2011; Parks, et al., 2011; Raychaudhuri & Ray, 2010), the lack of adequate information is a crucial hindrance for the delivery of healthcare (Lehnbom, McLachlan, & Jo-anne, 2012; Williams, 2007). Without timely-access to complete patient records, healthcare providers are faced with a challenge not dissimilar to completing a jigsaw puzzle with half the pieces missing; it becomes an impossible task unless the quality is reduced. Therefore, information privacy concerns should not come in the way of effective data collection in eHealth (Raychaudhuri & Ray, 2010). A balance of these requirements is required for successfully implementing eHealth systems. Current approaches are limited in achieving this balance when addressing each requirement. As a solution to this conundrum, we propose the use of the IA in eHealth. In terms of IA as a measure for privacy management in eHealth, we observe a gap in the current knowledge. Principally, information accountability has not been defined in eHealth and its underlying principles are unclear. Therefore, it is imperative that the principles of IA in eHealth are discussed to lay the foundations for successful eHealth systems to be implemented with IA capabilities.

WHAT IS INFORMATION ACCOUNTABILITY?

Responsibility and accountability are used interchangeably by many people (Boyd, 2003). They are like the two sides of the same coin. Responsibility involves what is required from an employee, i.e. duties. Accountability is when someone is held answerable for their actions and their outcomes. In other words, responsibility operates up to the point of making a decision and accountability focuses on the ramifications after the decision is made (Boyd, 2003; Eriksen, 2002). According to Emanuel et al. (1996), "Accountability entails the procedures and processes by which one party justifies and takes responsibility for its activities". In essence, when focusing on information accountability, the user of the information is held liable to explain, justify or answer for their use of information, when requested by the party to whom the information belongs. The significance of information accountability in information intensive domains is highlighted from the statement below.

Information is widely available and the use of that information needs to be controlled. Rather than enforcing rigid up-front control over the use of information, there is a need to accommodate fair use. The control over the use of information is imperfect and exceptions are possible, but violators can be identified and held accountable (Weitzner, et al., 2008).

When investigating information accountability, transparency is one of the most important aspects that also need to be taken into account. Transparency and accountability will be critical in helping the society to manage the privacy risks that accumulate from the explosive progress in communication, storage and search technology (Weitzner et al., 2006). The subjects of information must have the privilege to observe how their information is used and by whom. Transparency can be defined differently in two contexts. In business ethics and information ethics, it's likely that transparency refers to the visibility of information. In computer science and ICT, it is more likely to refer to the invisibility of information (Turilli & Floridi, 2009). Despite the contradicting definitions in different contexts, here transparency refers to the visibility of the information held about a consumer and the use of that information such that all actions can be traced back to an individual, organisation or process. As Weitzner et al. (2008) states, "transparency and accountability makes bad acts visible to all concerned", hence referring to the visibility of information usage: clarifying our distinction.

According to Ferreira et al. (2003) the lack of success, in terms of utilisation of ICT, in large information-dependent areas such as hospitals is due to its deficient usability and poor security. Unlike paper-based systems, that have evolved through many years, where accountability processes are well understood, digital systems have very different and complex processes. The need for transparency and accountability is ever more important in information systems which are becoming ever more complex and decentralised (Weitzner, et al., 2006).

A serious concern for accountability systems is the lack of formal foundations. Formalising IA has been widely explored by several prominent researchers, especially in the information privacy domain (Feigenbaum, Hendler, et al., 2011; Feigenbaum, Jaggard, & Wright, 2011; Jagadeesan, Jeffrey, Pitcher, & Riely, 2009; Sloan & Warner, 2010; Weitzner, et al., 2008). It is accepted that a purely preventive approach to security and privacy is inadequate (Feigenbaum, Hendler, et al., 2011; Kagal & Abelson, 2010). Feigenbaum et al. (2012) investigate some existing frameworks for accountability and explore whether deterrence is a better term than accountability and puts forth a formal model for accountability in terms of punishment (Feigenbaum, Jaggard, et al., 2011). Jagadeesan

et al. (2009) present formal foundations for IA in terms of the privacy policies which define appropriate sharing of information among agents and provides algorithms that can be used by an auditor to check for compliance with rules. In their approach they focus on *after-the-fact* verification with recorded audit logs capable of detecting 'untrusted' access of information and assign blame when the privacy contract is violated. They rely on a principle underlying the accountability concept that the fear of being caught will deter users from misusing information. A solution to the question of compliance of privacy policies was proposed by Weitzner et al. (2008) by tracking all transactions and making them transparent. They assume the existence of appropriate policy rules (with a formal representation); policy-aware transaction logs; and a policy-reasoning capability that would enable accountability systems to hold information users accountable for their actions.

Sloan et al. (2010) address IA in a broader scope than what has been done by Weitzner et al. (2008) and consider both social policies and technical aspects. They point out that automated checking for compliance of privacy policy is a necessity for accountability systems and without the adequate foundations in both formal models and public policy issues; they are unlikely to do so. Many of these approaches to accountability assume that the appropriate policies exist and both the requirements and domain constraints are captured by them. Sloan et al. (2010) believe that policies required to develop accountability systems are informational norms and state that a proper balance between privacy requirements and competing concerns is necessary to sustain the architectural and social aspects introduced by Weitzner et al. (2008). It should be highlighted that the above mentioned policies and the informational norms are all dependent on the context.

Trust is another aspect related to accountability in terms of human interactions (Friedman & Grudin, 1998; Friedman et al., 1999). Due to the interactions people have through electronic media, trust and accountability play a significant role in how people perceive different aspects of their interactions. Systems that utilise information accountability thus must incorporate many aspects that are not present in current applications. These systems therefore inherit specific characteristics and goals towards information security, information privacy, trust and adoption.

ACCOUNTABILITY SYSTEMS

A common measure for managing access to information by authorised users is access control. In computer science, access control and accountability are closely related. Access control is about imposing restrictions on users to prevent unauthorised access. These approaches have proven to be successful in the past and in current information systems but bring with them inherent drawbacks. One such drawback is the hindrance to legitimate information accesses. However, as mentioned earlier, a purely preventive approach to information security and information privacy is inadequate (Feigenbaum, et al., 2012; Kagal & Abelson,

2010). Information accountability, on the other hand, is about deterrence. But the *after-the-fact* aspect of accountability may raise concerns over information abuse. This means that a violation must occur for it to be acted upon. It is argued that with accountability mechanisms in place, the *online* world would be more like the *offline* world where potential violators are deterred by the prospect of negative consequences (Feigenbaum, 2010). To this end, we identify certain goals for accountability systems and are shown in Figure 1.

The goals of accountability systems can be represented in a waterfall model. Accountability systems aim at reaching specific goals in terms of how information is manipulated. The first is to be non-restrictive by aiming to provide information to legitimate users without rigid access restrictions. However, to avoid misuse, appropriate use of information is implemented through deterrence rather than restriction. A fear of being caught is delivered with the presence of accountability mechanisms that are made known to the users. Incentives are given to the users to follow procedures and enforce appropriate use. By implementing the first two goals, accountability

Figure 1. Goals of accountability systems

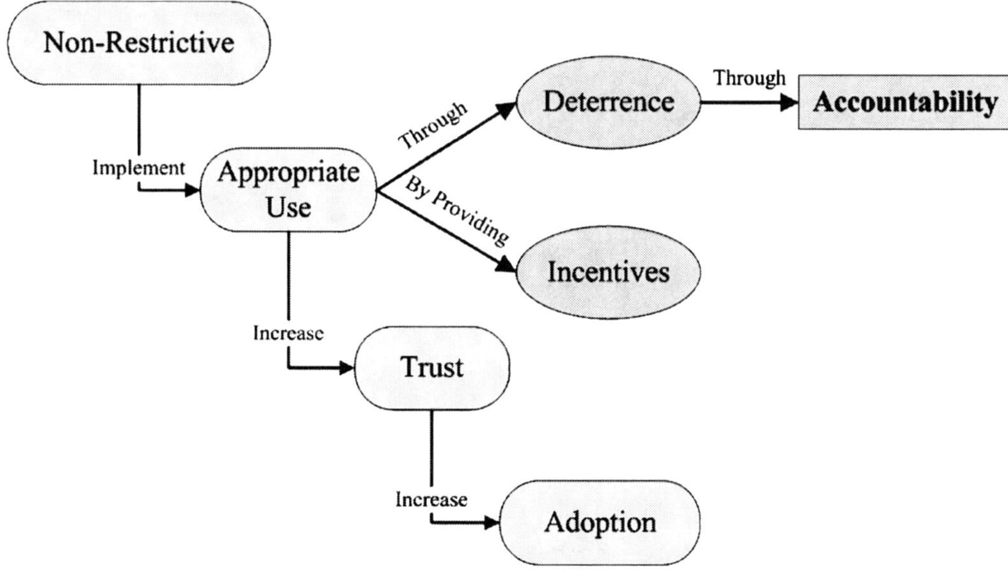

systems aim to increasing consumer trust which in turn achieve high adoption.

Creating proper incentives that would make consumers follow rules is an important aspect of accountability systems (Sloan & Warner, 2010). For example, the fear of getting caught for intentional misuse of information is an incentive to follow system rules. A strong assurance of information privacy should be given to consumers as an incentive to prevent them from withholding information or enforcing rigid restrictions on data, which is the obvious cause of action to secure their information from being unnecessarily or wrongfully disclosed.

PRINCIPLES OF INFORMATION ACCOUNTABILITY

Information accountability is built on several key principles. Accountability systems must adhere to these principles in order to achieve the expected goals. A conceptual map of the principles of IA and related attributes are shown in Figure 2.

Participation of users in an accountability system is a fundamental principle of IA. Users participate in information systems activities to fulfil a purpose. A user's purpose or intention to participate can be either to fulfil a *requirement*; because of a *responsibility*; or because of other *motivations*, for example gathering demographic data for research purposes. Capturing the actual intention of an information user is of great importance to accountability systems; it helps in defining usage policies for data objects and users within the system. A user's role within an organisation requires the fulfilment of certain tasks by manipulating information. Hence, a user is said to have certain *goals* of strategic interest (Bresciani, Perini, Giorgini, Giunchiglia, & Mylopoulos, 2004). The users perform various tasks to fulfil these goals. It is the aim of accountability systems

Figure 2. Principles of information accountability

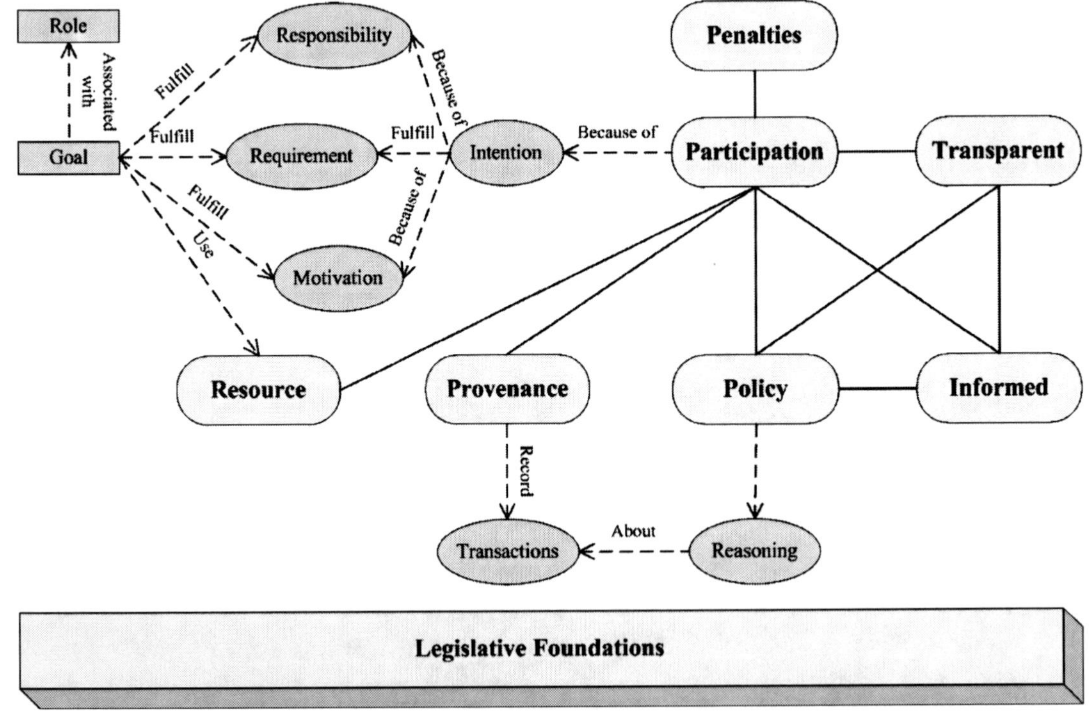

to manage the way these tasks are performed within the system to promote appropriate use of information. Therefore, accountability systems must have the capability to monitor user interactions with the system.

The definition of a resource is a fundamental principle of IA. In the digital arena, resources are digital assets or information artefacts. Their clear definition is vital for accountability systems because the nature of the resource brings with it usage constraints for users and information owners. We can couple three types of actors to information resources, the subject of the information, the owner of the information and the consumer of the information. Each of these actors will have inherently different roles to play within the system.

As highlighted earlier, transparency is a principle of IA that is of utmost importance. All *relevant* users must have the capability to observe how information is used and by whom. Transparency allows for the actions performed by data consumers to be traced back to an individual or process. According to Weitzner et al. (2006), transparency and accountability will be critical in helping the society to manage the privacy risks that accrue from the explosive progress in communication, storage and search technology.

Provenance of electronic data deals with the history or a record of transactions performed on a data object. A record of such would enable computer systems to reason over the life cycle of a data object. It helps develop many factors of quality information use including transparency and accountability (Cheney, Chong, Foster, Seltzer, & Vansummeren, 2009). However, Moreau et al. (2008) point out that electronic data does not have the necessary historical information that would help end-users, reviewers or regulators make the necessary verifications. In computer systems, a data's provenance is represented by process documentation, says Kifor et al. (2006). The availability of computer based provenance aware systems enable the users to decide whether they trust the electronic data in a computer based

information system. Provenance can provide facts about the authenticity of a data object and plays an even bigger role in IA and accountability systems. Guaranteeing the provenance of information on accountability is one of the most important questions that need to be addressed when developing accountability systems. When holding someone accountable, the trustworthiness of the data about the inappropriate transaction(s) or the evidence is crucial.

In IA, provenance is facilitated using appropriate *transaction logs*, which are also an essential component in current information systems (Lampson, 2009). These transaction logs are meant to be policy aware such that the system is capable of identifying inappropriate use of data or a breach of policy. Provenance data can be stored in transaction logs in a format that can facilitate *policy reasoning* within the system to give the users the capability to reason about misuse and against claims of misuse. The reasoning process includes inquiries about potential misuse of data by the subjects or owners of the data and justifications about the usage by data consumers.

Data consumers also have a right to be informed of the underlying policies and the ramifications of breach of policies, especially when the system facilitates a tracking process that monitors the transactions by every user. Therefore, users of an accountability system should be well informed; i.e. a notification process where users are informed about underlying policies before an action occurs must be put in place. For example, a user will be notified whether he is authorised to access/use a particular set of data he is trying to access, and the ramifications if he proceeds regardless of the warning. This will also help in facilitating non-repudiation, which is a significant aspect of information security.

In the case where an inappropriate use of information has taken place, the ramification of that occurrence towards the information user needs to be well defined in terms of appropriate penalties or negative consequences. In accountability systems inapt participation is entailed by negative consequences. A sense of awareness of these ramifications has to be delivered to the data consumers in the form of financial, professional, social or legal penalty. This awareness of the consequences is meant to deter users from inappropriate use of information in accountability systems. It will also give the victim or the claimant a sense of one's rights in terms of the use of their information by another. Furthermore, it will aid in increasing consumer trust in the system.

It is important to understand that the principles presented above must all be governed within an appropriate legislative framework. The legal foundations are a critical aspect of accountability systems. For example, if clear definitions of the penalties for violations are not given, the threat of negative consequences that deter users from misusing information will not be conveyed adequately; thus failing to provide the necessary incentives for users to abide by the rules.

INFORMATION ACCOUNTABILITY IN HEALTHCARE

Accountability relating to healthcare information manipulation arises mainly as a result of information privacy concerns. According to Emanuel et al. (1996), it is important to clearly identify the different parties in healthcare that can be held accountable; the issues for which a party can be held accountable; and the appropriate mechanisms for accountability in healthcare in order to understand the concept in healthcare. The components of accountability, Emanuel et al. (1996) say, are who, what and how. "*Who*" relate to the different parties that can be held accountable and the parties that can hold others accountable. '*How*' are the mechanisms for holding someone accountable. '*What*', as they define it, are the domains in which someone is held accountable. Another important component that has to be but was not considered

in their approach is the reason or the significance of why hold someone accountable for their actions, or the '*Why*' in accountability. Emanuel et al. (1996) delineate three models of accountability: professional accountability, economic accountability, and political accountability. They continue to say that one model of accountability is simply not enough in a complicated domain as healthcare. The models of accountability should not be confused with the different facets of the healthcare system.

According to Ferreira et al. (2003) the accountability information should be made usable by many stakeholders, each one having a different purpose and, therefore, different access to the information. The Joint Group of the General Practitioners' Committee and the Royal College of General Practitioners, as cited by Ferreira et al. (2003), says that in healthcare, this would allow a patient to review some of the actions associated with their electronic patient record. Healthcare professionals and auditors would be able to browse summary events as part of their normal work and to search further in extraordinary cases. They state that the main objective of accountability systems is to provide a means to verify, analyse and investigate users' actions. More importantly, its presence tends to ensure procedures are correctly followed, which is in accordance with the goals discussed above.

The Need For Information Accountability In Healthcare

Accountability can address a wide range of aspects of healthcare such as medical negligence, unethical practice, pharmaceutical abuse, and technology induced errors etc. In terms of usage control, information accountability mechanisms in healthcare allow to ensure that patient health information is not misused by care providers or other stakeholders. In other words, information is used for the purpose for which they have been collected and only for the benefit of the patient and other legitimate purposes. If we are to achieve information accountability in healthcare, the aforementioned purposes have to be comprehensively defined. This is a process that must be carried out with the required (domain) knowledge and expertise to determine the relationships (mapping) between data in electronic health records (EHR) and purposes. This mapping will identify which data element in an EHR is linked to which defined purpose(s). A healthcare professional that is authorised to access a particular data element can access and use it for only the linked purpose(s). But to facilitate unrestricted access, healthcare professionals may need access to data that they are not authorised to access. However, they will be required to provide justifications for their actions.

As brought to notice earlier, data ownership is a critical factor that needs to be properly understood if data usage control is to be achieved. In the healthcare domain it is difficult to determine who owns health information. It is clear that patients are the subjects of health information; however, patients are not always medical professionals. Therefore, it is impossible to give them complete control of their health information where the information is intended to be used in clinical decision making. As a result, information privacy policies of a patient should also accompany policies from a professional healthcare entity such as a trusted medical practitioner or a central health authority such that a balance between the patient's privacy requirements and the requirements of the healthcare providers (competing concerns), is reached. We note that the healthcare domain demands that while fulfilling these requirements of stakeholders, under no circumstances must the health of the patient be compromised. Clear procedures for overriding usage policies in emergency situations should be defined to this extent. The nature of the healthcare domain demands the implementation of a *break-the-glass* approach in such situations (National E-Health Transition Authority, 2011a).

MOTIVATING CASE SCENARIO

The case scenario depicted in Figure 3 illustrates how different eHealth stakeholders may behave in a care delivery scenario. The case scenario is designed to capture and illustrate how the policy formulation and manipulation protocols fulfil the information privacy and information access requirements. The activities presented in this scenario can be generalised into any other eHealth scenario.

Patient X has a comprehensive electronic health record managed by a central health authority in his home state called *StateHealth*. StateHealth is responsible for securely storing EHRs of residents in its state. StateHealth is also responsible for managing its healthcare professionals; including physicians, nurses, lab technicians and other relevant staff. StateHealth defines health policies and intended purposes for the data collected and stored in EHRs. These policies fulfil requirements of healthcare professionals and StateHealth itself. Patient X is also capable of setting his own policies on the data in his EHR. These policies mostly consist of his privacy requirements. Patient X maintains a list of trusted healthcare professionals, in an access control list (depicted as ACL in Figure 3), who can access all or parts of his EHR depending on the policy Patient X and StateHealth has defined for them. All healthcare professionals are required to specify the purpose for which they require access to a set of data before access is granted.

After noticing a skin rash, Patient X visits his trusted dermatologist Dr. S for a check up. After the preliminary examination, Dr. S thinks that Patient X's skin condition could be linked to a known sexually transmitted disease (STD). Patient X does not have a sexual health specialist in his list of trusted health professionals. However, Dr. S wants to share Patient X's details with a sexual health specialist, Dr. B, in order to get a specialists' opinion on the situation. Dr. B has a

Figure 3. Motivating healthcare scenario

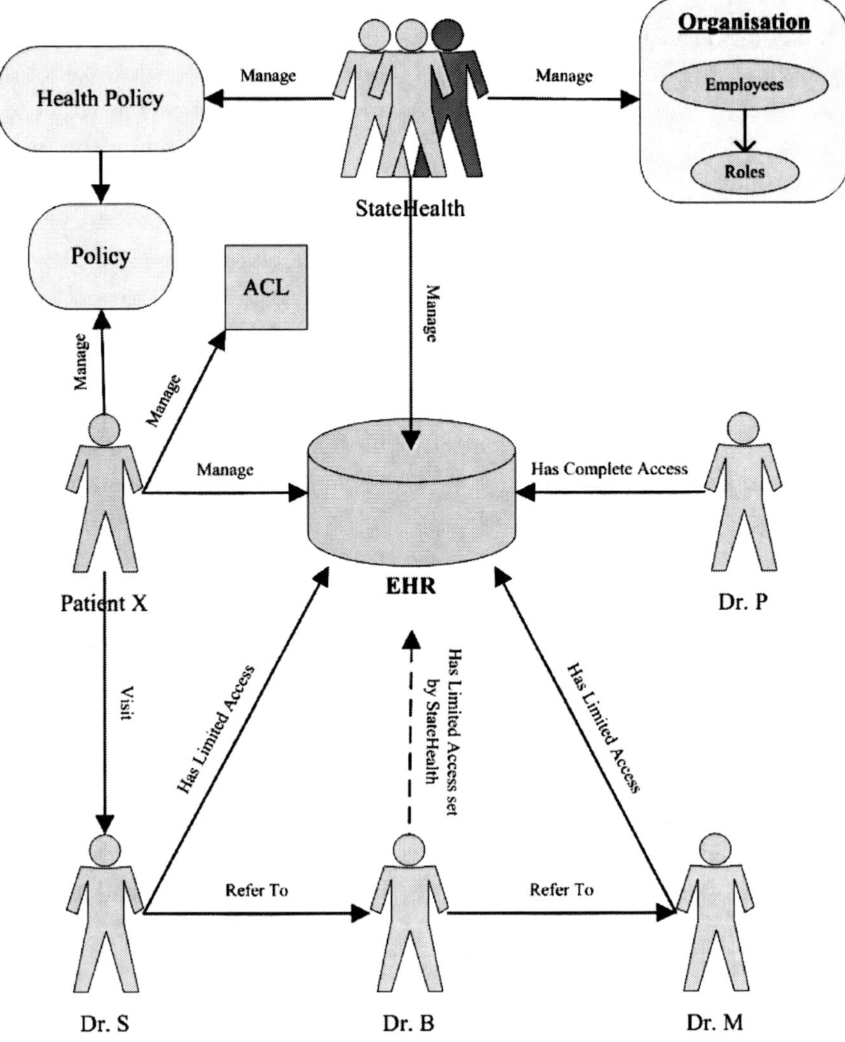

default access level set by StateHealth as a sexual health specialist. Since Dr. S is in Patient X's list of trusted health professionals, she can initiate a request to share Patient X's (relevant) details with other health professionals. Patient X, however, is notified of this action by Dr. S. After Dr. B receives (and accepts) this request, he initiates a usage request to use the data for diagnostic purposes. Patient X also has a history of mental illness and does not want anyone else other than his GP (Dr. P) and a trusted mental health specialist, who has treated him before (Dr. M), to know about it. Dr. B suspects that Patient X's skin condition could be stress related and tries to access his mental health record. At this point, because Dr. B is not authorised to access Patient X's mental health details, he is warned by the EHR system of this fact and Dr. B refers Patient X to Dr. M. Dr. M as Patient X's trusted mental health professional, investigates Patient X's condition and makes a diagnosis. Dr. M may or may not include Dr. B as a specialist in the diagnostic decision making process. After Patient X's illness has been diagnosed and a treatment plan is decided, his EHR is updated by the treating physician(s). Depending on the policy StateHealth has set on EHR updates; Dr. S, Dr. B, Dr. M or Dr. P will make relevant updates to the EHR. After or during this episode of care Patient X may decide to add Dr. B as a trusted healthcare professional in his EHR. We assume that certain medical conditions have relationships between them that give rise to the fact that a particular health professional e.g. a dermatologist who has access to a patient's dermatology details by default (set by StateHealth) may also have default access to the patient's sexual health details. In our scenario, Dr. S has default access to dermatology details and sexual health details of her patients and Dr. B's access may also be set likewise because of the relationship between skin conditions and STDs.

PRINCIPLES OF INFORMATION ACCOUNTABILITY IN EHEALTH

Participation

In healthcare, it is important that a careful balance is reached between responsibility and accountability (Emanuel & Emanuel, 1996), the reason being that healthcare decision making is driven by specialised knowledge and expertise, which is only possessed by healthcare professionals. Therefore, if accountability measures are put in place to govern how healthcare professionals should participate in healthcare activities, the aforementioned balance is critical. Accountability begins where responsibility ends. Accountability in the healthcare setting encompasses a magnitude of issues including the overall risks involved in providing healthcare; expected quality of life of patients; and also professional negligence. In the context of IA, however, after making a decision that was driven by the specialised knowledge and expertise, the decision maker is accountable for the ramifications of that decision imposed on the subject, i.e. the patient concerned. Therefore, adequate policies must exist that satisfies the information needs of the decision makers if they are to be held accountable after-the-fact, which could be set by a governing healthcare authority.

Each participant in a healthcare scenario can be categorised into roles within the healthcare domain. These roles can be thought to carry out professional tasks to fulfil their responsibilities, requirements and motivations as seen in Figure 2. Hence, the information access requirements must be adequately satisfied. Policies should be developed that address the different capabilities of roles within the industry. In our healthcare scenario, Patient X has three main rights: the right to decide whether or not to undergo medical treatment, after receiving a reasonable explanation of what the treatment involves and the risks associated with the treatment; the right to be treated with reasonable care and skill by a healthcare provider; and the right to confidentiality of information about medical conditions and treatment[1]. Therefore, Dr. S, Dr. B and Dr. M have a responsibility towards Patient X to make the appropriate communications with him and make decisions regarding his health.

Transparency

As discussed previously, transparency is a fundamental principle of IA (Weitzner, et al., 2006). In the eHealth scenario, Patient X, as the subject of the information, has the right to view what is contained in his EHR; who has access to it; and what they do with the data they retrieve. This gives Patient X the confidence to disclose his sensitive health information in the EHR system. StateHealth is responsible for providing this capability to Patient X and all who are registered with them and own an EHR. This transparency can be facilitated through transaction logs that record all transactions of users of the system. Transparency also covers the capability of the patients to make enquiries about any suspicious activities by information users; in this case, about any potentially suspicious actions performed by Dr. S, Dr. B, Dr. M, or Dr. P and also by StateHealth itself.

Policies

Patients have a fundamental right to confidentiality of information about medical conditions and treatment (Croll, 2011). This should allow patients to set their own privacy policies within a healthcare information system that manages his medical information. However, in a domain such as healthcare it is not always possible to allow every such policy set by the patient to be operationalised. As stated earlier, healthcare is a highly specialised area that requires domain specific knowledge when making a decision. Therefore, the policies that govern the control of information within EHRs need to also encompass policies formulated with a healthcare perspective. In our case scenario, Patient X defines privacy policies and relevant access rights for the health professionals in his list of trusted healthcare professionals. StateHealth will also set access policies for the health professionals depending on the role they play in the organisation. For example, Dr. S will be assigned the role of a dermatologist; Dr. P will be assigned a role of a general practitioner and so on. These two policies will then have to be combined to set the final operational policy in the system. In this process, Patient X will be notified of any changes made and the final state of the policy; keeping in accordance with the principle of being informed.

Provenance

Data provenance is a subject vital to any informatics domain (Moreau, et al., 2008). Here we will briefly discuss what role provenance plays in an eHealth environment. Unlike traditional information systems with network connections to known locations, Web based systems can interact with users from anywhere in the world. Tracing the transactions to their sources is therefore important to maintain authenticity of data and for identity purposes. The open architecture of the Web, meaning that the specifications of the Web services are public, raises concerns over the legitimacy of the

data being recorded and updated. In an eHealth environment this is a significant issue since the data retrieved from eHealth systems are used for diagnosis purposes to treat patients; and if not accurate, could lead to adverse effects. Hence, provenance plays a significant role in any health related information system. Groth et al. (2012) point out the significance of provenance and presented requirement for provenance on the Web using three hypothetical scenarios. They identified three major provenance dimensions: content, management and use. They raise the issues of reusability of the content of provenance data. This can be directly related to interoperability issues that are of concern in the health informatics domain. Once provenance data is correctly stored in systems, the management of data becomes an issue.

To what extent should provenance data be exposed to actors in the system? Besides providing evidence about the history (e.g. origin, authenticity, creators etc) of a data element, provenance can also provide insights into the life cycle of a data element. In accountability systems, this relates to making justifications about information use by a consumer with the use of appropriate transaction logs stored with provenance data. Revisiting the our eHealth scenario, if Dr. B has viewed Patient X's mental health records despite being warned not to do so, a notification would have been sent to Patient X informing him that Dr. B's action could be of intentional misuse of his health information. At this point, Patient X is able to lodge an enquiry requesting a justification from Dr. B as to why he accessed his mental health records. Under the conditions that users of the systems fall under, Dr. B would then have to provide a justification for his actions. This relates to the requirement that patients should be capable of observing how their information is being used.

Informed

In order to prevent unintentional misuse of information by users and to deliver the appropriate incentives (Feigenbaum, Hendler, et al., 2011), a notification process need to be put in place. As a results, the system users are aware of the policies in place within the system; their rights and capabilities; and the ramifications of breach of policies. These notifications together with the provenance and transparency can also facilitate non-repudiation within the system. They will also give the patients the confidence they need to disclose their sensitive information. However, because healthcare is highly specialised, patients cannot be given the ability to enquire about every transaction and request a justification from the healthcare professionals; this may hinder the healthcare professionals' professional activities. The system itself should be able to identify possible misuse of data and the patients are given the option to request a justification for those actions only.

Penalties and Legislative support

Legislative support is imperative for accountability systems (Sloan & Warner, 2010). In healthcare, information and privacy are governed by appropriate legislation. Several efforts in this regards are made around the world; for example, the Australian Law Reform Commission (ALRC) took on the task to review the *Privacy Act 1988 (Cth)* to inquire the extent to which it continued to provide an effective framework for the protection of privacy in Australia. In their report, the ALRC made recommendations towards the legislation focused on healthcare information and privacy in Australia (Australian Law Reform Commission, 2008). In a health information system governed by IA principles, the issues concerning information privacy and security as well as the appropriate methods of accountability in terms of penalties should be addressed by appropriate legislative constructs. In Australia, the operation of eHealth is subject to several Commonwealth, State and Territory privacy and information protection legislation (Australian Government Department of Health and Ageing, 2004; Australian Law Reform

Commission, 2008; Office of Legislative Drafting and Publishing, 2010) and an individual's ability to control who can access their information in certain circumstances are addressed in them (National E-Health Transition Authority, 2011b). Even though there is much attention to the information security and privacy issues in healthcare in a legal perspective, for accountability systems to successfully reach their goals in the eHealth domain, all aspects of IA principles discussed above must be completely and sufficiently covered by proper legislation, especially the aspects of appropriate penalties.

IMPLEMENTATION CHALLENGES

Three related aspects can be identified as implementation challenges of IA in eHealth: technological, social and legal. Figure 4 illustrates these aspects and the relationships between them. Together, these three aspects form an informa-

Figure 4. Information accountability framework for eHealth (Gajanayake, Sahama, Iannella, & Lane, 2013)

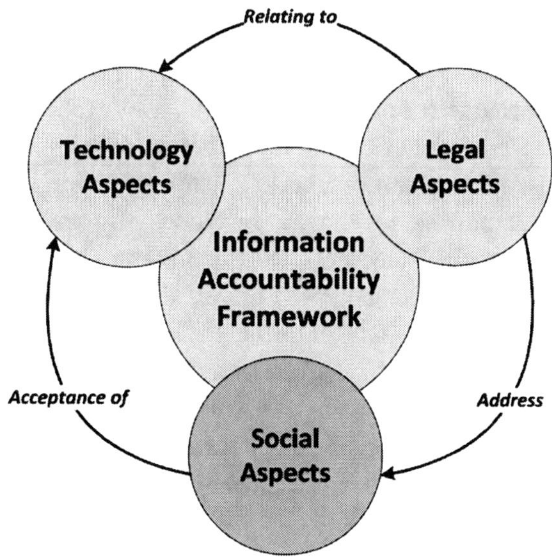

tion accountability framework for eHealth. Our investigation related to each aspect to date can be summarised as follows.

Technical aspects

The policy formulation and operation processes, which were described in our case scenario, were demonstrated using a novel access control model (Gajanayake, Iannella, & Sahama, 2012b) and an eHealth technical architecture (Gajanayake, Iannella, & Sahama, 2012a). As a novel solution to the policy representation problem, we adopted a model based on the Open Digital Rights Language (ODRL); an open-standard DRM technology capable of representing a wide range of policy-based information. Contrasting with current approaches, in our model, we assign usage policies to users instead of assigning them to assets (i.e., EHR data items). This allows eHealth consumers to assign a wide range of usage policies to their preferred healthcare professionals, which eliminates the problem of having to use a single sensitivity level for each data element in the EHR, which realistically would have different sensitivities for different consumers.

Social aspects

Favourable consumer perspectives are critical to eHealth success. In order to measure the impact the characteristics of IA in eHealth, we developed two empirical research models, each focused on eHealth consumers and healthcare professionals, by capturing previously developed technology acceptance constructs and incorporated an IA context to the models. Each model was tested using survey data collected from Universities around Queensland, Australia. Our preliminary results suggest that IA constructs have a significant effect on perceived system adoption and that the system would be accepted by both consumers and healthcare professionals. However, given the limitations in survey cohorts, we expect to further validate these models with a wide range of user groups in the future.

Legal Aspects

Legal aspects become crucial in the implementation phase of a system designed with IA characteristics where they rely on appropriate legislation for the governance and regulatory mechanisms. We conducted a case study of the Australian eHealth system and identified that in its current state, the Australian legal foundations are inadequate for implementing the regulatory mechanisms necessary for such systems to function as intended (Gajanayake, Lane, Iannella, & Sahama, 2012). In order for systems to operate effectively, issues such as mandatory data breach notification; information ownership; information access and use; and methods of accountability (penalties for misuse) must be addressed.

CLOSING REMARKS

In this article, we made the argument that IA is a viable solution to the information privacy conundrum in eHealth and that it should be defined in context. We presented the principles of IA that accountability systems should adhere in order to reach their intended goals. Information accountability is focused around how users participate in the system and the policies associated with the use of data. Data in an EHR and the actions users perform on data should have a clear record of provenance in the form of a policy-aware transaction log in order for accountability to be achieved. Accountability systems have an inherent drawback. This is the fact that actions are taken for misuse of data after the incident has occurred. This *after-the-fact* issue would be reason enough for concerns for information privacy. But the concept behind IA is that information users will be aware of the consequences of their actions and will deter from misusing data due to the fear of negative consequences, more like in the *offline* society we live in; it is a matter of facilitating this awareness (informed) and a sense of responsibility (participation) in the consumers through the IA principles.

The audit logs contained in accountability systems, which are openly available for consumers, may become the focus of legal issues. In most of these cases the healthcare professionals are blamed for misconduct or negligence. The presence of this type of audit logs may contribute to, for example, the insurability of a health professional who might agree to use such systems. Therefore, health professionals may not accept these accountability mechanisms as a practicable solution. This however, can be addressed through proper policies supported by legislation, which plays a major role in accountability systems.

It is important to understand that filling the *analog* and *digital holes* present in any information system is next to impossible[2]. In our case scenario we are dealing with the visibility of health information to the appropriate user. Once a person obtains the required data, the prevention of him using it outside the system boundaries remain an open question and cannot be control by policies enforced within computer systems.

We also identify some future directions towards making accountability systems a reality in eHealth. Issues such as designing methods for semantic reasoning of information use and justifications in the eHealth domain; development of ontologies that capture medical knowledge coupled with dynamic usage policies; legal issues; and consumer awareness and engagement remain yet to be addressed.

ACKNOWLEDGMENT

NICTA is funded by the Australian Government as represented by the Department of Broadband, Communications and the Digital Economy and the Australian Research Council through the ICT Centre of Excellence program.

REFERENCES

Australian Government Department of Health and Ageing. (2004). Submission to the office of the privacy commissioner review of the private sector provisions of the Privacy Act 1988.

Australian Law Reform Commission. (2008). For your information. Australian Privacy Law and Practice (No. 108).

Boyd, J. (2003). []. McMurry Inc.]. *Accountability*, *69*, 599.

Bresciani, P., Perini, A., Giorgini, P., Giunchiglia, F., & Mylopoulos, J. (2004). Tropos: An agent-oriented software development methodology. *Autonomous Agents and Multi-Agent Systems*, *8*(3), 203–236. doi:10.1023/B:AGNT.0000018806.20944.ef

Cheney, J., Chong, S., Foster, N., Seltzer, M., & Vansummeren, S. (2009). Provenance: A future history. In *Proceeding of the 24th ACM SIGPLAN Conference Companion on Object Oriented Programming Systems Languages and Applications*. doi:10.1145/1639950.1640064

Croll, P. R. (2011). Determining the privacy policy deficiencies of health ICT applications through semi-formal modelling. *International Journal of Medical Informatics*, *80*(2), e32–e38. doi:10.1016/j.ijmedinf.2010.10.006 PMID:21075675

Emanuel, E. J., & Emanuel, L. L. (1996). What Is accountability in health care? *Annals of Internal Medicine, 124*(2), 229–239. doi:10.7326/0003-4819-124-2-199601150-00007 PMID:8533999

Eriksen, S. (2002). Designing for accountability. In *Proceedings of the Second Nordic Conference on Human-Computer Interaction.* doi:10.1145/572020.572041

Feigenbaum, J. (2010). Accountability as a driver of innovative privacy solutions. Paper presented at the Privacy and Innovation Symposium.

Feigenbaum, J., Hendler, J., Jaggard, A. D., Weitzner, D. J., & Wright, R. N. (2011, June 11-17). Accountability and deterrence in online life. Paper presented at the WebSci Conference 11, Koblenz, Germany. doi:10.1145/2527031.2527043

Feigenbaum, J., Jaggard, A. D., & Wright, R. (2011). Towards a formal model of accountability. Paper presented at the New Security Paradigms Workshop.

Feigenbaum, J., Jaggard, A. D., Wright, R. N., & Xiao, H. (2012). *Systematizing "accountability" in computer science.* Yale University.

Ferreira, A., Shiu, S., & Baldwin, A. (2003, 26-27 June 2003). Towards accountability for electronic patient records. In *Proceedings on the 16th IEEE Symposium of the Computer-Based Medical Systems.* doi:10.1109/CBMS.2003.1212787

Friedman, B., & Grudin, J. (1998). Trust and accountability: Preserving human values in interactional experience. Paper presented at the CHI 98 Conference Summary on Human Factors in Computing Systems. doi:10.1145/286498.286699

Friedman, B., Thomas, J. C., Grudin, J., Nass, C., Nissenbaum, H., Schlager, M., et al. (1999). Trust me, I'm accountable: Trust and accountability online. Paper presented at the CHI'99 Extended Abstracts on Human Factors in Computing Systems. doi:10.1145/632716.632766

Gajanayake, R., Iannella, R., & Sahama, T. (2012a). An information accountability framework for shared e-health policies. Paper presented at the WWW2012 Workshop on Data Usage Management on the Web, Lyon, France.

Gajanayake, R., Iannella, R., & Sahama, T. (2012b). Privacy oriented access control for electronic health records. Paper presented at the WWW2012 workshop on Data Usage Management on the Web, Lyon, France.

Gajanayake, R., Lane, B., Iannella, R., & Sahama, T. (2012). Legal issues related to Accountable-eHealth systems in Australia. In *Proceedings of the 1st Australian eHealth Informatics and Security Conference.*

Gajanayake, R., Sahama, T. R., Iannella, R., & Lane, B. (2013). Designing an information accountability framework for eHealth. e-Health Technical Committee Newsletter, 2(2).

Groth, P., Gil, Y., Cheney, J., & Miles, S. (2012). Requirements for provenance on the web. *The International Journal of Digital Curation, 7*(1), 39–56. doi:10.2218/ijdc.v7i1.213

Ishikawa, K. (2000). Health data use and protection policy; based on differences by cultural and social environment. *International Journal of Medical Informatics, 60*(2), 119–125. doi:10.1016/S1386-5056(00)00111-8 PMID:11154962

Jagadeesan, R., Jeffrey, A., Pitcher, C., & Riely, J. (2009). Towards a theory of accountability and audit computer security. In M. Backes & P. Ning (Eds.), ESORICS 2009 (Vol. 5789, pp. 152-167). Springer Berlin / Heidelberg.

Kagal, L., & Abelson, H. (2010). Access control is an inadequate framework for privacy protection. Paper presented at the W3C Privacy Workshop.

Kierkegaard, P. (2011). Electronic health record: Wiring Europe's healthcare. Computer Law &. *Security Review, 27*(5), 503–515. doi:10.1016/j.clsr.2011.07.013

Kifor, T., Varga, L. Z., Vazquez-Salceda, J., Alvarez, S., Willmott, S., Miles, S., & Moreau, L. (2006). Provenance in agent-mediated healthcare systems. *IEEE Intelligent Systems*, *21*(6), 38–46. doi:10.1109/MIS.2006.119

Lampson, B. (2009). Privacy and security: Usable security: how to get it. *Communications of the ACM*, *52*(11), 25–27. doi:10.1145/1592761.1592773

Lasagna, L. (2001). Hippocratic oath: Modern version; 1964. Washington, DC: Public Broadcasting System (Nova Online).

Lehnbom, E. C., McLachlan, A., & Jo-anne, E. B. (2012). A qualitative study of Australians' opinions about personally controlled electronic health records. Paper presented at the Health Informatics: Building a Healthcare Future Through Trusted Information-Selected Papers from the 20th Australian National Health Informatics Conference (Hic 2012).

Moreau, L., Groth, P., Miles, S., Vazquez-Salceda, J., Ibbotson, J., & Jiang, S. et al. (2008). The provenance of electronic data. *Communications of the ACM*, *51*(4), 52–58. doi:10.1145/1330311.1330323

National E-Health Transition Authority. (2011a). Concept of operations: Relating to the introduction of a personally controlled electronic health record (PCEHR) system. Retrieved September 20, 2012, from http://www.yourhealth.gov.au/internet/yourhealth/publishing.nsf/Content/PCEHRS-Intro-toc#.T9BeK8VIuSo

National E-Health Transition Authority. (2011b). NEHTA BluePrint. Retrieved September 20, 2012, from http://www.nehta.gov.au/connecting-australia/ehealth-architecture

Office of Legislative Drafting and Publishing. (2010). Healthcare identifiers act.

Parks, R., Chu, C.-H., & Xu, H. (2011). Healthcare information privacy research: Iusses, gaps and what next? Paper presented at the Americas Conference on Information Systems. Retrieved from http://aisel.aisnet.org/cgi/viewcontent.cgi?article=1177&context=amcis2011_submissions

Raychaudhuri, K., & Ray, P. (2010). Privacy challenges in the use of eHealth systems for public health management. [IJEHMC]. *International Journal of E-Health and Medical Communications*, *1*(2), 12–23. doi:10.4018/jehmc.2010040102

Rindfleisch, T. C. (1997). Privacy, information technology, and health care. *Communications of the ACM*, *40*(8), 92–100. doi:10.1145/257874.257896

Sloan, R. H., & Warner, R. (2010). Developing foundations for accountability systems: Informational norms and context-sensitive judgments. In *Proceedings of the Annual Computer Security Applications Conference, Workshop on Governance of Technology, Information, and Policies*, 2010. doi:10.1145/1920320.1920324

Turilli, M., & Floridi, L. (2009). The ethics of information transparency. [. Ethics and Information Technology, 11(2), 105-112.10.1007/s10676-009-9187-9]

Weitzner, D. J., Abelson, H., Berners-Lee, T., Feigenbaum, J., Hendler, J., & Sussman, G. J. (2008). Information accountability. *Communications of the ACM*, *51*(6), 82–87. doi:10.1145/1349026.1349043

Weitzner, D. J., Abelson, H., Berners-lee, T., Hanson, C., Hendler, J., Kagal, L., et al. (2006). Transparent accountable data mining: New strategies for privacy protection.

Westin, A. (1967). *Privacy and freedom*. New York Atheneum.

Williams, P. A. (2007). Medical insecurity: When one size does not fit all. Paper presented at the 5th Australian Information Security Management Conference.

ENDNOTES

[1] Legal Services Commission of South Australia. (2012). Law Handbook Online. http://www.lawhandbook.sa.gov.au/ Retrieved 23 May, 2012

[2] Sandhu, R. (2012) *Grand Challenges in Data Usage Control*. Keynote speech at the WWW 2012 Workshop on Data Usage Management on the Web (DUMW), April 16, Lyon, France.

Chapter 9
Reach to Mobile Platforms and Availability:
A Planning Tutorial

Rex A Buddenberg
Naval Postgraduate School, USA

ABSTRACT

This chapter is practical system planning tutorial for internetworks that include radio-WANs. Author is retired USCG officer with both operational and program planning experience. In second career, author taught 'plowshares into swords internetworking' at the graduate level. The coaching herein reflects operational, planning, and academic experiences. Considering mobile communications requires adjusting some assumptions and working knowledge from a wholly wired internetwork. The advent of radio – the necessary means to mobile – entails changes in topology, capacity and nature of the media (shared). Further, the extension of the internetwork to mobile usually means rather overt embracing of mission critical applications.

INTRODUCTION

It was a dark, stormy and windy night. The weather service had forecast the 100 knot windstorm correctly and the fishing fleet had all scampered for port and were getting safely tied up. Except for one trawler, with a crew of three, who, as it turned out, pushed luck about an hour too far. As the wind built the Coast Guard established a communications watch, which meant radioing the fishing boat crew every half hour. Further, as the storm built, most of the crews at the lifeboat stations and air station had returned to duty, whether expressly called or not.

As the storm built further, trees started falling and electrical power went out for large swathes of the Oregon coast. The fishing boat was making maddeningly slow progress toward Cape Arago and safety in its lee.

As the windstorm peaked, the fishing boat skipper called the Coast Guard and said that he could make no further progress into the wind and

DOI: 10.4018/978-1-4666-8756-1.ch009

had turned around. Heading downwind meant out to sea and in the Pacific that means a really long ways to the next landfall. This electrified the Coast Guard: Coos Bay lifeboat station launched two motor lifeboats and North Bend Air Station launched a helicopter.

The search ended up being fruitless – the fishing vessel was never seen or heard from again. The helicopter only found the two motor lifeboats on scene. After a first search, hampered by darkness and the storm, we decided to recall forces and prepare for a thorough first-light search which was about five hours hence.

On the way back to the air station, the helicopter's engine failed and the pilot auto-rotated into the Pacific Ocean just offshore. The three-man crew exited the aircraft safely but the copilot drowned. The other two crew were washed up on the beach shortly before sunrise.

When the helicopter's engine failed, the pilot radioed a Mayday. Ten miles away, in the operations center (where the author was standing), we did not hear it. The communications system had failed.

Incident Evaluation

As this author unraveled the communications system problems, three stages of events showed.

The third, but immediate observation was that the existing equipment had been maintained properly. Indeed, the immediate failure cause was grid power failure and once electrical power returned, the communications system returned.

The second stage was that the system was inadequately provisioned with backups, especially backup power but also alternate routes. The principles of high availability engineering had not been observed.

But the engineers who deployed the system are not really to blame: the program sponsor had never specified a required level of availability. The first or root problem: the system was never acknowledged as mission critical. The requirements statement simply had no stated availability requirement.

Attending funerals is a graphic and convincing way to learn availability lessons but it's not the recommended approach. This chapter turns the problem around and addresses it in the above logical, albeit not chronological, order.

IMPACTS OF REACH TO MOBILE PLATFORMS

Considering mobile communications requires adjusting some assumptions and working knowledge from a wholly wired internetwork. The advent of radio – the necessary means to mobile – entails changes in topology, capacity and nature of the media (shared). Further, the extension of the internetwork to mobile usually means rather overt embracing of mission critical applications.

- **Topology**. The 'traditional' internet is made up of backbone wide area networks (hereafter terrestrial-WAN) and local area networks (LAN. Both wired and wireless LAN fall in this category). The terrestrial-WAN is largely made up of point-to-point cabling (predominately fiber optic) and can be described as interconnecting a fabric of routers. There are no end systems in this fabric – it's all router-to-router interconnect. The connectionless, stateless nature of Internet Protocol affords this terrestrial-WAN a great deal of modularity – new links can be added transparently and capacity mismatches from one hop to the next are not important to route-ability and hence interoperability. The routing protocols and supporting 'hello' messages find these new links and add them to the routing table. All of this is transparent to the user and allows the terrestrial WAN to grow in capacity and number of links.

As depicted in Figure 1, LANs are the reach from the last router to end systems and are the part of the infrastructure visible to the user. LANs, of course, come in wired and wireless variations.

Figure 1. Radio Network as LAN at fringe of Internet

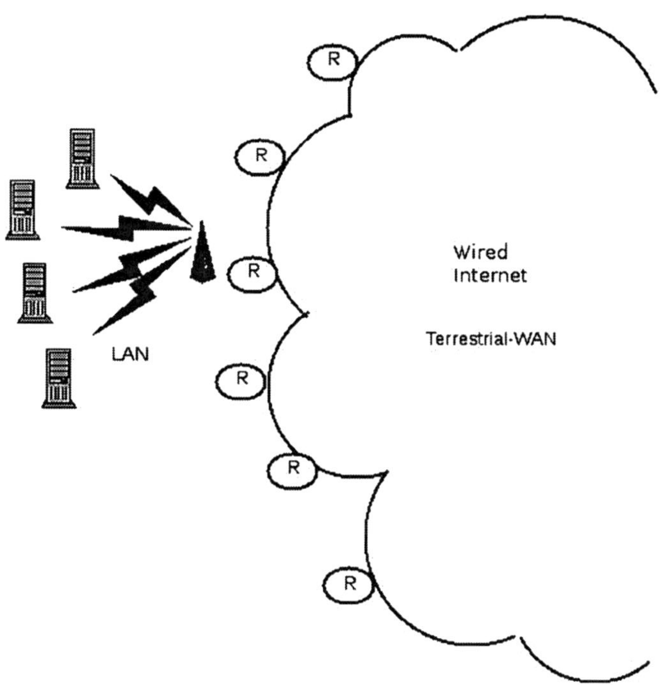

This classical topology has been 'stretched' with the advent of WiFi (Brittanica-WiFi). But WiFi remains a LAN technology. WiFi is effective for the LAN task: reach from last router to end system. Topologically, the cellular telephone system is similar – the technology reaching from the tower to the user fits the LAN definition: reach to end system.

But consider the case of a mobile platform such as an ambulance, fire truck, ship, or airplane, and in the foreseeable future the family sedan, where there are many end users in the platform, not just one. An 'instrumented ambulance' provides an excellent representative use case. There may be several end systems attached to a casualty in the ambulance (e.g. monitoring vital signs), an end system for the emergency medical technician wishing to talk with a doctor at the emergency room, a radio-navigation receiver gaining and relaying the vehicle's position, etc. The list can be long and with the internet, it can be open-ended. New applications can be incrementally added as can new instruments (end systems). The topology observation here is that the LAN is within the mobile platform.

The topology difference is that we now need a radio-WAN to interconnect the router in the vehicle and a point on the terrestrial-WAN. See Figure 2. The radio-WAN needs to get the router-router interconnect problem right. (The topology significance does not change if there happen to be multiple routers inside the radio-WAN cloud).

Both WiFi and older (i.e. '3G' and older) cell phone radio technologies can be pressed into this role. But neither will scale well; for example, multiple ambulances. Older cell phone technologies, despite the fact that they use radio, are point-to-point so each mobile platform-to-terrestrial-WAN connection requires a separate channel. And WiFi, while well-suited to the LAN role, is unstable in the radio-WAN role because of its contention-oriented Media Access Controller (MAC). Thus we need the radio-WAN and we need to consider its special constraints, design considerations and characteristics.

Figure 2. Radio-WAN interior of internetwork

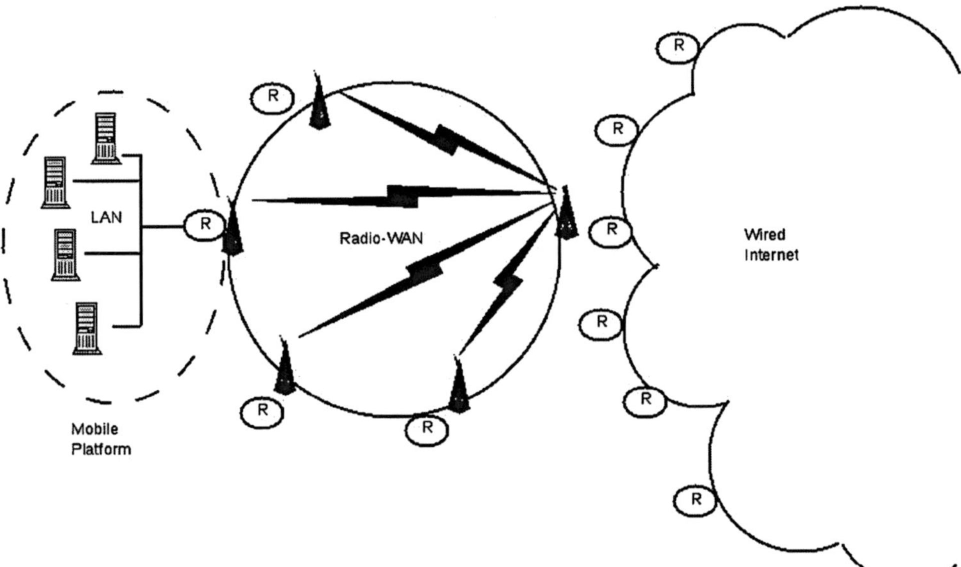

- **Shared Media:** Most of the internet 'plumbing', and almost all of it in the terrestrial-WAN backbone, is point-to-point. But radio is shared. This fact has one important constraint and enables one important concept. The constraint of shared media, is that you must have some way to share it. If every node offering traffic simply shouts it out, the system will jam itself and fail. In naturally point-to-point technologies (like fiber optic) the WAN protocols do not contain a media access protocol (MAC) at all because there are only two parties on the line. But with the radio 'party line' a means for sharing is necessary. Two protocol categories have evolved over the past century (long predating the internet): contention and contention-free. Both have uses – at the fringe of the internet, Figure 1, both are usable – but in the radio-WAN, contention-free is the appropriate choice.

Contention-free protocols (known in pre-internet radio as 'directed network') consist of a net controller (known as the base station or BS in the standards) that controls the network by allocating time slices for each of the subscriber stations (SS) to use. The basic rule is transmit in your time slice but not anyone else's. This means that the BS needs to 'hear' each SS but there is no requirement that the SS's be able to hear each other. A contention-free protocol will not jam – it is stable under overload. This stability under load is critical (as will become obvious when we discuss capacity, below).

There are two secondary benefits of contention-free protocols. One is bandwidth efficiency – most of the communications capacity is used for passing data, not fighting frames onto the network segment. The other major secondary benefit is susceptibility to control. This includes both fault management and configuration management. It is feasible to 'favor' some SS over others, but the basic benefit here is near-determinism – each SS that is recognized in a network segment will get a chance to transmit something every frame.

- **State of the Technology:** During the 1990s, these discussions were largely academic. But starting around 2002, multi-vendor protocols based on open standards started to appear. The best known of these protocols are IEEE 802.16 (WiMAX) and TIA LTE ('4G').

- **Frequency Reuse:** Many radio systems economize their use of scarce spectrum by building many smaller-footprint spots rather than a single high-site one. Existing Land Mobile Radio systems tend to fall in the second category – a small number of sites serves an entire city or county. But a larger number of smaller sites gets greater total capacity due to the frequency reuse – Cell A and its BS and SSs may be well out of range of Cell F and its associated nodes so both can use the same frequency without interfering. Additionally, more of the high availability and capacity burden is shifted to the terrestrial-WAN by increasing the number of radio base stations and decreasing their radius.

- **Multicast:** The other aspect of the shared media is that multicast has a much larger payoff than it does in an all-wired internet. Definition: multicast is delivery of data to more than one destination for the price of a single transit over the media. There are two reasons worth considering: nature of the data and conservation of (radio-WAN) capacity.

- **Nature of the Data:** Using the instrumented ambulance example use case shows that some of the data from end systems in the ambulance needs to go more than one place. For example, both the doctor in the emergency room and the (911) dispatcher would want to know the ambulance's position. In general, emergency services as a whole has a much higher incidence of data that is multicast in nature than we are used to in the internet to date. Multicast data becomes even more pronounced as applications like those known as Common Operational Picture enter the emergency

services world (they've been around in the military since WWII). And as 'self driving' features appear in automobiles, the incidence of multicast data increases here too – the position of my car needs to be transmitted to several other cars in order to keep them from colliding.

- **Capacity Conservation:** As illustrated in next section below, the radio-WAN is very capacity-limited compared to the terrestrial-WAN. Multicast applications that conserve capacity in an over-provisioned internet just don't sound attractive. So while the protocols (multicast IP at the center) for multicast exist and they are implemented in most routers, the industry uptake has been poor simply because there hasn't been much payoff. Few applications use multicast.

- **Capacity:** Both terrestrial-WANs and wired LANs can be provisioned at 10s of gigabits/second of capacity. Indeed, the internet has simply been ignoring Quality of Service issues because it can routinely overprovision by adding more fiber, upgrading the capacity of existing fiber, add more LANs, etc. If there is no congestion, no QoS control mechanism can possibly improve the situation. But the radio-WAN is limited in capacity.

Radio technology of any stripe uses spectrum to communicate. And there is only so much of it. Furthermore, because the radio medium is shared, the spectrum must be pro-rated across all the users of a channel. Some practical numbers should help reader perspective.

- **Narrowband:** Voice radio channels have historically been allocated in slices ranging up to 25KHz is width. Wired telephone (Plain Old Telephone Service (POTS) or POTS in the lingo) allocates 3KHz of bandwidth which allows transmission of human voice from 0-3000 Hz. If this voice is digitized and then compressed, it requires around 2Kbits/sec (with wide variances). If you hook a modem up to a POTS telephone line, you can usually get somewhere between 10 and 30kbits/sec, point-to-point.

- **Broadband:** Uses time slicing rather than frequency division multiplexing to share the medium. So broadband allocations are broader: in the nature of 6MHz (M = mega = million while K = kilo = thousand). In practical terms you will get Mbits of data per subscriber across a radio-WAN. What is important is not whether this is one or two Mbits but the fact that this is four orders of magnitude less than what is available every day in the terrestrial-WAN and the in-platform LANs. Four orders of magnitude may not immediately sound like a lot, but consider it this way: you can get 10,000 radio-WANs worth of capacity through a single terrestrial-WAN link.

In a topology where the wireless LAN is at the fringe of the internet all the reuse tricks (e.g. add more hotspots) are available to us. Typically a single end system is unlikely to use the entire capacity of a network segment. But in the Figure 1 topology, the multitude of end systems on the LAN side of a vehicle's router may very well saturate the capacity of the radio-WAN.

Understanding this capacity limitation does not in any way invalidate internet technology and an extend-the-internet approach. The same constraints would exist with some other technological approach. But the constraints should color both infrastructure design decisions and application development decisions – it makes things a bit different than what we've become used to.

AVAILABILITY

When we extend the internet to mobile platforms, we can expect the incidence of mission critical applications that run over it to increase. Indeed, this is a natural evolution: the tolerance for downtime in the internet tends to decrease over time as its use becomes more important and ubiquitous. The principles outlined below are equally applicable to all parts of the internet, indeed to any system. But internet reach to mobile platforms usually implies some high-availability requirements that need to be faced directly.

- **Definition of Availability (Ao):** Also denoted as Ao for *operational availability* (Wikipedia-Ao) the Availability is defined as the up-time divided by the total-time:

Ao = uptime / total time.

Sin #1: The most important shortcoming in communications acquisition programs is that they fail to state the required availability. At all. This guarantees a single-threaded, low-bidder result that will fail when you need it worst. In a single-threaded system components lack backups so equipment failure equals system failure. In author's experience if the availability requirement is stated, it's usually right, or close enough.

The above equation is simply the expression of the definition; it needs some help to be practically useful. Consider that total time = up time + down time. Or up-time = total-time – down-time. This allows us to substitute for a value that have operational meaning:

Ao = (total-time – down-time) / total-time

By considering how much downtime you can tolerate, you can easily calculate the Ao value required.

- **Workshop:** Usually total time is measured in a calendar quarter or year (Coast Guard radio-navigation systems used calendar quarter but it won't really matter much). So start with 130,000 minutes in a quarter. If you can tolerate a downtime of a half day, then you will get about two nines (0.995). If your tolerance for down time is in minutes rather than hours, you will get four to five nines (0.9997). How much down time can you stand? It is not proper to look at what the vendor advertises – spec-sheet requirements-writing is wrong. Look at your needs.
- **Effect:** Somewhere between Ao = two nines and Ao = four nines, your communications system needs cross a threshold where you must acquire a multiple-threaded system – nobody can repair equipment that fast (the reliability engineering texts refer to this as a 'repairable system'). In a multiply-threaded system, component failure is decoupled from system failure. In addition to increasing the Ao numbers, repairs can be effected on the failed equipment without impairing present operations. So this exercise is critical to capitalization costing – dual threading will double your equipment costs. In author's experience, availability is the easiest requirement to quantify and the easiest to defend in a budget – do it first.

Once we have determined the operational Ao requirement, we can proceed to the systems engineering aspects – how we go about obtaining the Ao requirement needed. There are three principles of high availability engineering; we need only apply them:

1. **Elimination of Single Points of Failure:** This is a slightly more elegant way of saying what most readers will have a gut feel for: add redundancy. When applying this principle to communications systems, this usually boils down to redundant communications paths (alternate routes) and backup power. These redundancies are technologically agnostic – you'd need to have them regardless of the technology choices you make. And these requirements drive your capitalization costs.

Arithmetic tutorial. Availability of a component is an instantaneous probability. So Ao of 0.999 for, say, a router, means that it will be available for all except 0.001 instants. Two routers mounted in parallel have a probability of down time of $0.001 * 0.001$ or 0.000001. This means that the pair of routers have a collective availability of $1 - 0.000001$ or Ao = 0.999999. This arithmetic depends of the assumption of independence of mode of failure – whatever causes one component to fail will not also cause the second to also fail. And system failure only occurs when both routers are down.

The common illustration of common-cause failures is in alternate routes – if they both travel through the same conduit then a single backhoe strike can break both of them. You have not eliminated the single points of failure until the alternate routes take diverse paths. In a reach-to-mobile-platforms environment, the need for extensive, distributed coverage tends to make this problem easier – both the terrestrial-WAN segment routes and the interconnecting routers will tend to be diverse anyway. The critical item in such situations is grid electrical power which tends to remain quite centralized.

The qualitative observation here is that as soon as you require dual-threaded infrastructure for Ao reasons, you decouple component failure from system failure. So a specified availability of three or four nines will often be 'good enough'. If it's not, through experience (and fault maintenance logs, see below), you can add more threads later.

The side effect to observe here is that meeting the Ao requirements often tends to mean over-provisioning the system – you have more capacity than is needed. This will be true in the terrestrial-WAN (and LAN) portions of the internetwork but not in the radio-WAN.

2. **Reliable Crossover:** This principle is best illustrated by the inverse – a backup comms channel is useless unless you can get to it. The 'gotcha' in redundant systems is that the crossover switch itself becomes a single point of failure. Here internet technology shines: the connectionless, stateless nature of Internet Protocol solves the problem by protocol design. Said in a slightly earthier way, routers do reliable crossover all day, every day.

Observance of this principle shows up a couple of 'don'ts'. Routing does solve the reliable crossover problem. But layer 2 bridging does not – the spanning tree algorithm identifies alternate routes and then refuses to use them to avoid frame ringing. Similarly layer 7 gateways do not demonstrate reliable crossover either; these should only be used for integration of necessary legacy (such as legacy narrowband voice radio, called Land Mobile Radio in the emergency services world. This solution is properly known as a Voice over IP Layer 7 gateway (Cisco-VOIP)).

3. **Prompt Notification of Failures on Occurrence:** If the first two principles are observed, then the user may never see a failure (exactly what we need). But somebody does need to find failed equipment in order to direct maintenance. For this purpose, all equipment should be equipped with Simple Network Management Protocol (SNMP) agents. The standards language is 'fault management' and fault management is sufficient reason.

SNMP does many useful things beyond fault management. The standards language refers to capacity, accounting, performance and security management as well. But for our purposes these are secondary benefits – fault management is head/shoulders more important.

Comprehensive. Failure notification applies to more than just the internetwork infrastructure. In one direction it applies to end systems – the handset in the EMT's hands and the applications embedded therein should have management agents and be within the management domain. In another direction fault management applies to equipment like air conditioners in the tower huts of a radio system – not normally considered part of the internetwork but critical to its continuing operation.

Ownership of various parts of the infrastructure should be irrelevant to fault management. It's highly likely that applications and the end systems they are installed in will be owned by a different entity than, say, the wired internet foundation. What is important is that one management entity have fault visibility throughout the system. This might be obtained by a contractual agreement to allow a 'look over the shoulder' of an ISPs management database. Early triage of faults is critical to fast restoration.

• **Compensation:** Investment in high availability sounds like a tall order, and it's not trivial. But by the time you have a fully redundant, fault monitored system you can usually relax the maintenance philosophy. Many systems which need high availability but were not engineered as such to start with try to increase availability by implementing 24-hour, on-call maintenance. This ad hoc approach is expensive (whether you use it or not). If you have observed the principles above, you can often relax the maintenance to next-working-day which represents a significant savings.

SECURITY: AUTHENTICITY AND CONFIDENTIALITY

The security concerns in information systems over the internet have existed as long as the internet has. But security over radio has existed for the century that radio existed. There are many examples of insecurities with technologies such as WiFi and cellular telephone – they make the existing internet security problems more acute. Unfortunately the reactions to these insecurities have tended to fall into two categories:

- The security problems are simply ignored at planning time. Then we try to apply duct tape.
- Non-sequiturs. The remedies applied (i.e. the duct tape above) are loosely related to the problem if at all.

This time, before we analyze requirements, it is probably useful to analyze some of the solutions and tools first.

The internet provides a modular differentiation between infrastructure and application that does not exist with the old telephone system or older voice-only radio systems (such as emergency services' Land Mobile Radio). Unrecognized, we will routinely try to provide infrastructure solutions to applications problems. A variant on this theme is the psychological difference between computer centric and network centric world views. Operating system distributions for computers are perfect examples of computer-centric in operation – most of the security measures in the typical distribution are designed to protect the operating system, not the network.

The muddle of security is made worse by other diversions. For example, in the early days of WiFi, the technology came with a rather weak encryption scheme known as Wireless Encryption Protocol. There was much ink spilled in the press about the ability to break the crypto (which was true) but the discussion missed the point that the

object protected was not much worth the effort anyway. The real security need – protection of the data – was not addressed at all. Further, if the WiFi network segment is at the fringe of an internetwork that requires public access then you don't want to turn it on anyway!

- **Scope Analysis:** The missing part of the discussion seems to be scope of the security protection. Exactly what is it that we need to be protecting? And over what parts of the information system? The problem is susceptible to easy analysis and the most important tool, the ISO Reference Model, already exists and is well understood – every introductory text on internetworking has an explanation. To analyze scope of security, we need only determine what layer of the ISO Reference Model a security implementation resides. Another way of asking exactly the same question is to determine the object that is being secured (frame, datagram, connection, message). This time, for illustration and sorting purposes, we will look at some existing security tools, then work up to requirements.

For example, layer 2 solutions (like Wireless Encryption Protocol, WEP) secure frames. A frame only surrounds a piece of data for a single hop so frame encryption only provides protection over a single network segment; the protection does not pass through any routers because the frame structure is only valid for that one hop. Protecting frames = layer 2 protection = one hop of scope.

Another example is virtual private network (VPN). A VPN protects IP datagrams from VPN port to VPN port which makes this protection a layer 3 solution. A VPN tunnels out a protected enclave within the internet in the large. A VPN provides no protection beyond that enclave (such as within end systems). VPNs are very useful for their infrastructure protection purposes, but they leave the data unprotected outside their scope.

The third example worth mentioning is transport level security (often recognized by the WWW labeling of 'https:'; labels include Secure Sockets Layer and Transport Level Security). Here the object being secured is a connection. As in TCP connection. Which makes the protection a layer 4/5 one. The scope of this protection is from the TCP 'socket' on one computer to the socket on the other. This provides pretty complete protection over the internet but none at all within the operating systems in each end system beyond the socket. So any malware within either end system's operating system (e.g. key loggers) see the data in unprotected form.

All of these layer 2-5 protections can be classified as infrastructure protection measures. They do have value and the scope analysis indicates what that value is. But they only protect the content – the data – by providing some security to the infrastructure. They do not provide security to the data itself.

The final example is layer 6/7 protections. The best example of layer 6 protection is secure e-mail (S/MIME). Here the data is protected. It is transformed (the definition of layer 6) either by appending a digital signature, encrypting, or both. The scope of the protection can be end-to-end; some secure e-mail implementations can illustrate: outgoing e-mail is secured by encryption and digital signature at origin. This is done before the data ever leaves the end system. It is then communicated to one or more message transfer agents (slang: mail servers) who forward and store data, but are not allowed to change it (if they did, the digital signature would not verify and an encrypted message would not decrypt). Eventually the message is delivered to the receiving end system and is passed through the operating system and into memory (e.g. hard drive) with the protections intact. Only when the message is read are the protections removed, and even then often only for the viewing – they remain intact on the stored copy (some features are implementation-dependent, they're outside the scope of the standard). This greatly limits the exposure of unprotected data: it is never unprotected over the internetwork infrastructure and only under limited conditions in the end systems.

Another implementation example of layer 6 end-to-end security scope is security protections built into SNMP version 3 which allow attachment of digital signatures and (as applicable) encryption to each SNMP message, entirely independent of how it is delivered. The layer 6 protections are vital to security of content, regardless of what other infrastructure protection mechanisms are implemented.

Table 1 organizes the scope observations in tabular form. The important observation of the sort is that layer 6-7 security measures protect the data; layer 2-5 security measures protect the infrastructure.

Table 1. Security scope table

Reference Model Layer	Object Protected	Scope	Example
6-7	Content data	End to end	S/MIME email, XML-sign/-crypt SNMPv3
4-5	Connection (e.g. TCP connection)	TCP socket to TCP socket	SSL, e.g. https connections
3	IP datagram	Network enclave (excluding end systems)	Vendor or company specific VPN
1-2	Frame (ethernet)	Single network segment	WPA

- **Uses and Requirements:** The management requirement discussed above in the third principle of high availability is a perfect example of the need for end-to-end, application layer, security. Consider for a moment the consequences of someone injecting bogus SNMP 'get' message results into the management console. Or, worse, someone injecting bogus SNMP 'set' messages into critical equipment. In this use case, confidentiality is not particularly important, but authenticity is vital.

But this is only a start. Consider the casualty data (e.g. vital signs) in the instrumented ambulance use case: that data must be both authentic and confidential. And the scope requirement is end-to-end. And consider the data from the ambulance's radio-navigation receiver – the consequences of the wrong position showing up on the dispatcher's common operational picture are not good. The ambulance may grow into a case of 'virtual siren' where it is broadcasting it's position to geographical neighbors – here confidentiality is useless and counterproductive but authenticity is again vital. This kind of security agility is easily attainable with layer 6/7 solutions but not by use of lower layer tools.

Another requirements example is an incident commander dealing with a fire. He clearly needs authenticity in his communications with the firefighting team and he needs confidentiality in some of the data (e.g. previously mentioned medical data). But the incident commander needs communications with the general public, for example, to disseminate evacuation orders. This is an example where authenticity is very important but confidentiality is of no value – the evacuation orders must be en claire. In all these variants the security requirements are end-to-end in scope.

- **Security Requirement Generalization:** All applications require authenticity in some form or another, explicit or tacitly assumed. There are no exceptions. And the required scope of this authenticity is always end to end. These two facts enormously simplify the planning problem. Digital signatures are all dependent on Public Key Infrastructures so the obvious requirement is that all end systems need a key pair. But once you have the key pair in hand, addition of encryption to the authenticity capability costs nothing.

- **Applications:** While most of the availability discussion applies to internetwork infrastructure, the requirement for fault monitoring includes end systems and their applications as well. A fireman engaged in fighting a fire cannot stop to diagnose a fault in his handset and voice application, for example.

End-to-end security features are all built into applications that run over the internetwork; they are not part of the infrastructure (terrestrial WANs, radio-WANs, routers,...).

- **State of the Industry:** Most operating system distributions include an SNMP agent in the distribution (but it's either turned off or not installed). But many applications (like a voice app in your cell phone) do not. If the application is to be considered mission critical, an SNMP agent should be part of it's structure along with end-to-end signatures and encryption option.

There are a variety of e-mail user agents (UA), many of which implement signing and encryption. Most, but not all, implement the S/MIME in a satisfactory way limiting the range of unprotected data within an operating system (hint: check the Sent mail directory for unprotected body parts). Some of these UAs are automated user agents that allow automated insertion of data into e-mail envelopes – it's still e-mail but not necessarily human-to-human (webcams often have such). Once the reader understands all this one can think of lots of applications that can use e-mail for their communications envelope!

Extensible Markup Language (XML) provides -sign and -crypt primitives as part of the language that, if used, have end-to-end scope. An XML statement that has been signed will have authenticity attributes and those attributes remain until the statement is interpreted at destination. The test is easy: is the protection applied before the data leaves origin? And does it remain intact until it reaches destination?

Secure shell (ssh) also provides a layer 6 security means; the scope is end-to-end. Ssh can be programmed into shell scripts and is therefore common in file transfer implementations and file synchronization applications, particularly in the open source world. Some of the history of ssh is germane: the protocol was engineered in the early 1990s, a quarter century after the internet was first invented (about the same time that we started seeing serviceable implementations of S/MIME). The effect is secure communications over an untrusted internetwork, which is a corollary of the original internet ethos: reliable communications over unreliable infrastructure.

- **Security Planning Observations:** Since the internet is made up of one infrastructure and 1001 applications (with new ones appearing regularly), we can observe that end-to-end security can be built into those applications. For mission critical applications, end-to-end scope of security should be a central requirement with authenticity as a ubiquitous, universal requirement. This does not require changes to a pre-existing internetwork infrastructure (other than addition of support services like PKI white pages servers). Infrastructure planning and application development can be on largely separate tracks. This observation should not be used as an excuse to ignore the security problems though.

QUALITY OF SERVICE

Warning to reader: this topic contains more misinformation and mythology than any other. Worse, in requirements discussions, it seems to be the first topic to be thrashed when it should be the last. Never discuss quality of service issues before disposing of the availability issue.

- **Nomenclature:** The quality of service actually experienced by users of an internetwork is normally noted in lower case: qos. Upper case QoS denotes Quality of Service Control or those configuration tweaks that change the defaults in some way. This distinction is crucial, especially for those who enter this discussion from the experience and viewpoint of circuit-switched voice. An example is the behavior of routers: the default behavior is for a router to have a single queue for each outgoing port and datagrams are fed into the queue in FIFO order – first in, first out. The qos experience is what is called 'best effort'. But if the router enables Differential Services, multiple (usually four) queues are set up for each output port. Datagrams are sorted into these queues by examining the Differential Services Code Point in each datagram header. These queues are then drained to the output starting with the highest priority first. The behavior within each queue remains FIFO but the highest marked traffic queue is sent first.
- **Experienced qos:** In circuit-switched telephone systems, qos is simply whether one gets a dial tone or not. In internetworks there are more parameters. For the infrastructure operator, qos generally means bandwidth efficiency – providing the best service to the most users. To an end user, qos can be measured in interactivity, latency and jitter.

Be careful what you ask for. First, in the terrestrial WAN and LAN portions of your internet, over-provisioning is not only possible but usually happens as a side effect of meeting the availability requirements. If there is no congestion, there is no point in QoS controls – they can't possibly improve things and it's quite likely that some measures will degrade qos. For example, in the above example the router is using CPU cycles to sort. This over-provisioning phenomenon is true for servers too – the end systems that are also susceptible to overload. By the time you've met the system replication needs to satisfy availability requirements, the load-sharing will ameliorate congestion problems. The remaining part of our internetwork that needs attention is the radio-WAN.

- **QoS in the Radio-WAN:** As noted above extending the internet to mobile platforms can be assumed to result in some mission-critical applications being implemented on such an internetwork. Which, in qos terms, means that some packets are more urgent than others. In the radio-WAN it is important to be able to distinguish those packets and give them 'head of line' privileges. There are solutions both at layer 2 and layer 3 that need to be considered together.
- **Layer 3, Differential Services:** In the internet, standards exist (RFC 2474) (RFC Base, 1998). The protocol allows an end system to specify an urgency value known as the Differential Services Code Point in IP datagrams. This allows routers to sort these packets to the head of the queues in the router. The effect is that these privileged packets are dispatched first from the router once capacity is available. In a radio-WAN, this means when it is that station's turn to transmit. In protocols like IEEE 802.16 (IEEE 802.16) and TIA LTE (WiMAX) every active station in the radio-WAN gets a turn to transmit every frame, so the urgent traffic will be sent in that time slice.

- **Layer 2, QoS Control in Radio-WAN:** Within the radio-WAN segment, there are QoS Controls that allow a subscriber station to request more capacity (at the expense of other stations) and several other 'knobs'. But before going here, ask whether 1) we have a decent means for controlling and 2) given differential services and the near-deterministic behavior of these radio-WANs whether we can gain any real improvement.

You can't violate the laws of physics. If, for example, one of your radio-WANs is a satellite system using geosynchronous satellites, you have a 300 msec propagation delay that no protocol can improve.

- **State of the Technology:** It should be evident that most of the parts for necessary QoS Control exist (along with a truckload of unnecessary parts). Some thoughts on system and application design:
  - Differential services consists of a set of settled standards and hardly any implementation. Routers generally can recognize the DSCP and act accordingly (but have this feature routinely turned off). Some end system operating systems have the latent capability to set the DSCP. But hardly any applications call on these features. Not every application needs to be differential-services capable, but those mission-critical ones in the hands of our emergency services folks do. And not every router needs to have differential services turned on – only those at the border to the radio-WAN do.
  - View layer 2 QoS Controls with jaundiced eye. It's not clear that they'll help any, particularly in a near-deterministic MAC environment.

○ Some applications are very 'chatty' in that they depend on high interactivity (ironically low round trip latency times) between client and server. These applications are the first to suffer in poor qos environments. Such applications usually do not fail outright, but their performance is likely to be viewed as poor by an end user (a lot of poor-interactivity problems tend to be misdiagnosed as low-capacity problems). In an all-wired internetwork, this is usually not a problem but with the advent of radio-WANs in the topology the issue does become important and it must be solved by adjusting application design and selecting those mission-critical applications that minimize the issue.

CONCLUSION

Investigation of extending the internet to mobile platforms parallels the investigation of 'plowshares into swords': that is, upgrading the office automation internet to meet emergency services' (or military) needs (I particularly like the instructions from Joel, Chapter 3, verse 10). Emergency services require reach to mobile platforms; similarly it's a safe bet that extension of the internet to mobile platforms will require ability to handle mission-critical applications. This chapter illustrates several design characteristics that tend not to need particular emphasis in an all-wired internetwork or an internetwork with wireless LANs at its fringe. But they become critical in an internet that reaches to mobile platforms. The good news is that the sword version retains all the usefulness of the plowshares version of the internet. These observations can be distilled into a few concluding recommendations:

- Build a routed internetwork – extend the internet. Don't be lulled into shortcuts like bridged (layer 2) networks or layer 7 gateways that represent both poor modularization and Ao-defeating single points of failure.
- Pay attention to the availability (Ao) requirement. It is the easiest to quantify and defend in a budget and it will be the capitalization driver. And do it early in the requirements analysis. You need not have every conceivable application in hand, only the one that needs the availability the most (what's commonly referred to as the tall pole in the tent). If the sponsor has not stated an Ao requirement, then the sponsor requirements document is badly flawed. Get that fixed pronto.
- Focus on the radio-WAN often tends to divert attention from the supporting terrestrial WAN. That terrestrial WAN is the foundation, not an afterthought backhaul. The terrestrial WAN design and provisioning is vital to support the availability and reach for the radio-WAN. Further, the trend is to lower power radios meaning that a given level of coverage requires more base stations. This takes advantage of things that the terrestrial internet does best. Out of sight should not man out of mind.
- End systems and applications therein for mission critical jobs should do three things, regardless of the function of a particular application:
  ○ Secure their content end-to-end (that is, with layer 7 scope). Assume that anyone can both eavesdrop and insert data onto an internetwork – a practical fact given radio-WANs – and protect accordingly. Authenticity is a universal, ubiquitous requirement – get it right first.

- ○ Multicast. The effectiveness need only be tested in one place: the radio-WAN. The radio-WAN is the place where the bandwidth conservation payoff has value. The rest of the internetwork can be over-provisioned.
- ○ Implement an SNMP agent that allows remote fault monitoring. As with any other application, authenticity of the SNMP data is vital.
- Implement differential services in applications that require it (non-implementation in an application simply means that it gets routine best-effort service that all other applications do).

Yours to Lose. The internet is a naturally modular technology. It is entirely in accordance with internet ethos to segment the network into terrestrial-WANs, radio-WANs, and LANs. And it is entirely natural to attach end systems only to the LANs. But this natural, by-design, modularity does not pertain to other communications systems, so it is an easy mistake to slip into the mode of implementing internet technology, but using the inherited (non)modularity.

There are two cardinal reasons for good modularity:

- Interoperability
- Life cycle maintainability

Interoperability has to do with interoperation with other infrastructure outside the scope of your own program. Can your corner of the internetwork be routed into the rest of the Internet (constrained only by policy-driven configuration)? Interoperability also has to do with ability to implement applications that are not of your own program or built later. Can your corner of the internetwork implement next year's hot new app (again, constrained by policy not engineering)?

The test of good modularity is a simple life cycle maintenance one: can one component (such as the radio-WAN technology) be changed (or replicated) without requiring cascading changes? In this case, changes on the other side of the routers? If changes are required, the modularity model is inadequate.

If your reach to mobile can be characterized as 'extend the internet to mobile platforms', then the modularity problem is a solved one that requires action on your part to derail.

REFERENCES

Base, R. F. C. (1998). Retrieved from http://www.rfc-base.org/rfc-2474.html

Configuring Voice over IP. (n.d.). Retrieved from http://www.cisco.com/c/en/us/td/docs/ios/12_2/voice/configuration/guide/fvvfax_c/vvfvoip.pdf

IEEE 802.16. (2014). Retrieved from: http://en.wikipedia.org/wiki/IEEE_802.16

Nichols, K., Blake, S., Baker, F., & Black, D. (n.d.). *RFC 2474, Definition of the Differentiated Services Field (DS Field) in the IPv4 and IPv6 Headers.* Academic Press.

Operational Availability. (n.d.). *Operational Availability.* Retrieved from http://en.wikipedia.org/wiki/Operational_availability

POTS, Plain Old Telephone Service. (2014). Retrieved from http://en.wikipedia.org/wiki/Plain_old_telephone_service

Wi-Fi. (n.d.). In *Encyclopedia Brittanica.* Retrieved from http://www.britannica.com/EBchecked/topic/1473553/Wi-Fi

WiMAX. (2014). *WiMAX.* Retrieved from http://en.wikipedia.org/wiki/WiMAX

KEY TERMS AND DEFINITIONS

3G: Third generation cellular telephone. 3G and earlier cellphone technologies are all circuit-switched. 4G cellphone is packet switched.

Availability (Ao): Defined as up-time/total-time. Availability is an instantaneous probability that the system it applies to is functional at any moment in time.

Bridging, Routing, Layer 7 Gatewaying: Bridging means interconnecting multiple network segments by use of layer 2 bridges. Homogeneity (common frame addressing and format) is generally required. Routing means internetworking multiple network segments at layer 3. Frame structure is irrelevant because it's not present at layer 3 so considerable heterogeneity is tolerable, provided each of the network segments is routable. Layer 7 gateways are means of translating non-IP traffic into internet traffic and injecting it into the internetwork infrastructure (and vice versa). Layer 7 gateways are commonly used to interconnect legacy communications systems and applications (such as POTS phone).

LAN: Last network in an internet – reaches from last router to end systems. May be wired (ethernet) or wireless (WiFi, sometimes abbreviated WLAN for wireless LAN). The radio portion of 3G cellphone, despite its circuit-switch nature, is of same topological character – reaches from the pylon to end system.

Multicast: Delivery of data to more than one destination for the price of a single transit over the media.

Network: An overloaded term that means lots of things to different people. Author tends to not use it, preferring 'network segment' for a single segment and 'internetwork' for the larger multiple hop infrastructure.

QoS: Quality of Service Control – those measures applied to the default behavior of the internet to change the quality of service defaults.

qos: Quality of service that is experienced. Components include bandwidth efficiency, latency, jitter, interactivity.

Radio-WAN: Topologically identical to generic WAN but uses radio.

SNMP Get, Set, Trap: Simple Network Management Protocol contains three kinds of messages. Get messages are requests for information by the management console to an agent who replies with a get-response. Set messages set configuration parameters. Trap messages are generated by a management agent in response to some stimulus. For purposes of this paper, traps would be fault indicators.

Terrestrial-WAN: WAN that is made up of wired connectivity.

WAN: Network infrastructure in interior of internetwork. In a pure case, there are no end systems – the WAN is solely performing router-router interconnect.

This work was previously published in Enabling Real-Time Mobile Cloud Computing through Emerging Technologies edited by Tolga Soyata, pages 342-357 copyright year 2015 by Information Science Reference (an imprint of IGI Global).

Chapter 10
Telemedically Augmented Palliative Care:
Empowerment for Patients with Advanced Cancer and their Family Caregivers

Romina Nemecek
Medical University of Vienna, Austria

Stefanie Porkert
Medical University of Vienna, Austria

Patrick Huber
Medical University of Vienna, Austria

Barbara Hofer
Medical University of Vienna, Austria

Sophie Schur
Medical University of Vienna, Austria

Herbert Watzke
Medical University of Vienna, Austria

Eva Masel
Medical University of Vienna, Austria

Christoph Zielinski
Medical University of Vienna, Austria

Michael Binder
Medical University of Vienna, Austria

ABSTRACT

Patients with advanced cancer have a substantial symptom burden, which deteriorates their quality of life. Palliative care improves well-being of patients and their family caregivers. Within the scope of a controlled pilot study, a user-friendly telepresence system is developed, which enables patients and family caregivers to send a direct request to a palliative care team. Additionally, a specially tailored database is developed, which contains up to date patient information. Twenty patients with advanced non-small cell lung cancer are consecutively assigned in a control and an intervention group. The intervention group receives the telemedically augmented care, whereas the control group receives standard care. The primary goal of this chapter is to determine the usability and feasibility; the secondary goal is the assessment of the intervention's impact on quality of life and the number of unscheduled hospital admissions. To sum up, telemedically supported ambulatory palliative care may synergistically help to improve safety and quality of life.

DOI: 10.4018/978-1-4666-8756-1.ch010

INTRODUCTION

In the context of this telemedical project, the quality of life (QoL) of patients with end-stage lung cancer and their family caregivers will be improved through the possibility of obtaining medical advice 24 hours a day by means of a telemedical system. The system will link them to a palliative care team with the click of a button. During daytime, this team usually consists of several nurses and physicians, as well as of one dietician, one psychologist, one pastor, one social worker and volunteers. Furthermore, a specially tailored database including up-to date important patient information, which can be fed by both the palliative care team and the patients themselves, will be developed. Thus, we hope to improve not solely the QoL of these patients, but also the QoL of their family caregivers.

Although the overall cancer mortality is decreasing, 20,000 people still died of cancer in Austria in 2010[1]. Utilizing palliative care is a only feasible alternative to respond to urgent needs of chronically sick people by improve their wellbeing and quality of life[2].

Most patients with chronically deteriorating incurable disease prefer to spend their last days of life at home[3]. Mobile hospice teams are a well-accepted alternative to provide medical support outside hospitals. A mobile hospice team supports the family caregivers, who are entrusted with the highest amount of the patient's daily care. The term family caregiver is used for all non-professional caregivers, such as family, friends and neighbors. The mobile hospice team consists, depending on individual requirements, of physicians, nurses, social workers, pastors and volunteers. It works together closely with general practitioners, hospitals and home nursing services and offers support in legal issues and organizational problems. The aim is to sustain QoL of patients and their family caregivers.

Generally, mobile hospice care is well accepted by patients and family caregivers. Nevertheless, the major problem is the general scarcity of mobile hospice teams available. Resources are usually not sufficient to manage acute medical problems, especially after hours. If a patient encounters medical problems during the night, usually the emergency service is called and patients are frequently admitted to a hospital. This happens mostly because of lacking information on history and current development of the patient's medical problems.

The primary aim of this project is to improve the QoL of patients and family caregivers by reducing stress and increasing safety. The secondary aim of this study is to reduce the heavy costs due to unnecessary hospital admissions.

Our system proposed comprises an integrated telemedical system, including a telepresence system and a database. Patients and family caregivers will have the possibility of obtaining medical advice 24 hours a day by telemedical support. Due to the organizational structures in the General Hospital of Vienna, they have the possibility to talk to a pastor/ social worker/ psychologist/ dietician only during daytime and if available. The telemedical system will enable patients and their family caregivers to videoconference with the Unit of Palliative Care (Department of Internal Medicine, General Hospital of Vienna), providing professional medical care and psychosocial support. Additionally, a database will be made available to document the patient's condition. This database will not only be fed by medical professionals, but also by patients and family caregivers themselves to document the patient's individual needs. Thus, QoL of these patients and their family caregivers will be improved through the possibility to send a medical request at any time, to receive medical advice quickly and by the reduction of hospital admissions.

BACKGROUND

Past and Current Status
of Palliative Care

According to the World Health Organization (WHO), palliative care is the active total care of patients whose disease is not responsive to curative treatment. The goal is the achievement of the best possible QoL for patients and their families [4]. Control of pain, other symptoms, and psychological, social and spiritual problems is paramount [4]. Palliative care in hospitals and hospices requires a multi-disciplinary team, consisting of nurses and physicians with according training, and, if required, physiotherapists, social workers and psychologists.

The terms "palliative care" and "hospice" describe the same idea, namely the symptom-orientated care for patients with incurable diseases. Hospice is rather associated with the idea itself, palliative care with the professional act. A palliative care unit is integrated into a hospital, whereas a hospice is independent, has advanced standard care and often engages volunteers [5]. The terms "palliative care" and "hospice" therefore characterize the administrative model, but do not state anything about the quality or extent of care [5].

In England, palliative care and hospice have developed rapidly since the late 1960s thanks to Cicely Saunders, who drew attention to the end-of-life care needs of patients with advanced malignant diseases [6]. More than 10 years elapsed before the first services began to appear in Austria. The first mobile hospice care in Austria arose in 1989, funded by the Caritas (Erzdioezese Wien), consisting of 2 physicians, 4 nurses, 1 coordinator and 1 assistant. This team worked in honorary capacity, it did not receive funding from the local authority of Vienna until 1990 [7]. The first Austrian palliative care unit was opened in 1992 in Vienna at the hospital Goettlicher Heiland. The number of hospices, palliative care units and mobile hospice care units substantially increased over the past few decades.

Lung Cancer

This project will focus on patients with advanced non-small-cell lung cancer. The reason why is because end-stage lung cancer is a disease with a very foreseeable course: Initially, the patients are mobile and feel good, but within few weeks or months symptoms such as shortness of breath and pain accumulate. Most patients die within one year. Therefore it seemed appropriate to add a small background section about lung cancer.

Lung cancer is one of the most common malignant diseases worldwide and it is the most common cause of cancer-related mortality. In 2010 more than 4200 Austrians have been diagnosed with this disease and about 3650 people die of lung cancer in Austria every year [8]. It occurs more commonly in men, usually between 50-70 years. It is most predominantly associated with long-term cigarette smoking, but can also occur in non-smokers.

The two main categories of lung cancer are as follows: small-cell lung cancer (SCLC) and non small-cell lung cancer (NSCLC). NSCLC accounts for approximately 85% of lung cancer. It is further divided into histologic subtypes, namely: squamous cell carcinoma, large cell carcinoma and adenocarcinoma of the lung [9].

Diagnostic examinations include chest X-Ray, CT scan and bronchoscopy with biopsy and histological assessment. There are, however, no established screening modalities for lung cancer, and the disease tends to get symptomatic at an advanced stage. Therefore, more than 50% of lung carcinomas are diagnosed after metastasis has occurred, leading to poor prognosis [9].

Most commonly, clinical symptoms associated with lung cancer are shortness of breath, cough, hemoptysis, chest pain, decreased appetite, fatigue, and weight loss. Furthermore, a high number of patients suffer from psychological problems such as depression, emotional distress and anxiety [10]. Especially patients with newly diagnosed, advanced NSCLC (stage IIIB and IV) strongly suffer from disease-related physical and psychological symptoms and have a short life expectancy. In addition to treating the cancer, an important focus is to manage the psychological distress and manage occurring symptoms of these patients.

Staging of NSCLC is performed according to the TNM-classification. The extent of disease influences the therapeutic management. Treatment options comprise surgery, chemotherapy and radiation therapy. Patients with advanced disease (stage IIIB and IV) rarely qualify for surgery and are usually offered palliative chemotherapy, and/or radiation therapy [9]. However, these treatment modalities usually prolong the patients' life for only a few months. In total, the median survival for those patients is less than a year [11]. These treatment options are associated with medical complications and are cost intensive. Therefore, appropriate palliative care is crucial for the management of patients with NSCLC [12].

Lung cancer patients endure the greatest level of distress from their disease relative to other cancer populations. Therefore, it is essential to maximize their QoL from the time of diagnosis. Multiple studies demonstrate that symptoms such as pain, fatigue, and dyspnea are prevalent at diagnosis and worsen over time. As a result, suffering increases throughout the course of the illness. To be most effective, palliative care with intensive symptom management and psychosocial support should begin at the time of diagnosis, not once life-prolonging therapies have failed.

To sum up, in light of their especially high burden of disease together with a poor prognosis and a very foreseeable course of disease, patients with metastatic NSCLC present an appropriate population that could most benefit from a mobile telehomecare service.

After having proved the usefulness of telemedical support, future studies should include other oncological diseases or chronic illnesses such as end-stage leukemia or pancreatic cancer, and patients with severe heart diseases.

MAIN FOCUS OF THE CHAPTER

Issues, Controversies, Problems

In 2005, 180 hospice and palliative care services existed in Austria, thereof 131 were mobile units. In the year 2010, the number of services has doubled to 252, whereas 179 thereof were mobile, respectively. This data is within the European average. The United Kingdom, being pioneer of palliative care, is still the European country with the most palliative care services, closely followed by Sweden; whereas Estonia, Slovakia and Portugal bring up the rear. Since the inpatient and mobile care merges, it is difficult to obtain an exact number of patients who are taken care of.

The mean age of patients receiving palliative care is between 66 and 74 years, and more than 75% suffer from cancer. The increasing service numbers, particularly of mobile hospice teams, reflect the population's need for help. Therefore, to upgrade and extend this particular sector is an important mission.

Main Outcome Parameter: Quality of Life of Patients and their Family Caregivers

End-of-life care for many patients with advanced disease is provided by a family member who undertakes and/or coordinates the majority of care. Unfortunately, the duty of providing care often results in experiencing elevated levels of emotional distress, resulting in a deteriorated QoL [13-16]. One of the main stress factors is the amount of given care, which severely affects the lifestyle of the family caregivers [17].

Tamayo et al. [18] explored the QoL, well-being and learning needs in 194 family caregivers by self-developed questionnaires. He found that they need more information on drug administration and the management of side effects. Communication, positive attitudes, support, and education were important in promoting QoL of family caregivers.

Fleming et al. [19] assessed the association between perceptions of health care quality and quality of life, for both patients and family caregivers. They showed that the presence of depression in family caregivers correlate with family caregivers being less satisfied with the quality of health care being given to their patients, whereas family caregiver satisfaction was associated with a more positive mood. Interestingly, they demonstrated that patient's mental health and depression scores correlate with those of their family caregivers. These data suggest that terminally ill patients and their family caregivers share similar perceptions and evolve as a "unit of care".

This finding is also supported by Northouse et al. [20]. When patients and family caregivers were treated simultaneously with psychoeducational interventions, skills training and therapeutic counseling, important synergies were achieved contributing to the well-being of each person. Programs of care that are directed to patients alone are seldom sufficient to meet patients' needs, because a lot of the patient's care depends on family caregivers. A meta-analysis was performed to analyze data obtained from 29 randomized clinical trials, published from 1983 to March 2009. The analysis showed that interventions (e.g. providing information regarding symptom management, skills training, therapeutic counseling) that are delivered to family caregivers of cancer patients had a significantly positive effect on multiple outcomes, such as better QoL. Interestingly, interventional effects for some outcomes were evident soon after the intervention.

In 2005, Kurtz et al [21] demonstrated that clinical nursing interventions that focused on teaching family caregivers to improve management of patients' symptoms failed to reduce the family caregivers' depressive symptomatology. Apart from the fact that the intervention period in this study lasted only 20 weeks, this finding additionally confirms that the patient-caregiver-situation is very complex.

A recent study by Temel et al. [12], published in the New England Journal of Medicine in 2010, focused on advantages and patient-related outcomes of introducing early palliative care for patients with advanced NSCLC as compared with patients that received standard palliative care. They reported an increase in QoL and decrease of depressive symptoms. Notably, they found an increase in median survival of about 2 months for those patients receiving early palliative care (11.6 months vs. 8.9 months, P = 0.02). As a conclusion, palliative care with intensive symptom management and psychosocial support should begin as early as possible in patients with NSCLC who have a high burden of disease together with high mortality.

Regarding this valuable information, it became clear that we would include family caregivers in our study. Accordingly, the aim of our research will be achieving an improved QoL of both patients and their family caregivers. For details on how QoL will be assessed, please see the "evaluation of quality of life" section below.

Telemedicine in Mobile Hospice Care

Teunissen et al. [22] evaluated the most frequent causes why patients or family caregivers seek medical consultation by analyzing the results of a telephone helpdesk for palliative care. More than thousand telephone consultations were made in the observational period of 5 years. Most questions referred to pain (49%), delirium (20%), nausea and vomiting (16%) and dyspnea (12%). Of the questions, 54% were related to pharmacological problems, 19% to psychological problems and 21% to the organization of care. Supported by other studies, most requests included reassurance concerning medication usage, symptom management and anxiety [22-24]. These requests do not necessarily require the presence of a physician and thus could be easily solved by telemedicine.

Audio-visual technologies may be useful in home-based palliative care. Morgan et al. [25] observed that videoconferencing for patients with severe congenital heart disease decreased anxiety levels compared with telephone calls, as it was associated with improved clinical information. In a study by Miyazaki et al. [26], the use of ISDN video-phones in palliative and antenatal home care was examined. The palliative care patients and their families commented that visual features of their mobile phones enhanced the received care. Video-phones might allow more personalized communication between family caregivers and members of the palliative care team and they can improve the effectiveness and efficiency of communication. Visualization of patients also allows a (limited) physical assessment to be undertaken, which can assist with patient management and care [27].

Various models of telemonitoring have been proven useful in different situations. Maiolo et al. [28] showed that homemonitoring of arterial oxygen saturation and heart rate was reliable and decreased the number of hospital admissions and acute home exacerbations during the telemonitoring phase. In this study, measurements were obtained twice a week and data were automatically transmitted to the hospital's processing centre via a standard telephone line. On the same morning, a respiratory physician analyzed the transmitted data to create monitoring plans and telephoned the patient for comments on symptoms and changes in prescriptions. About 96% of the patients were satisfied with the quality of the personal home-monitoring process. The frequency of hospital admissions and acute home exacerbations during the telemonitoring phase of the study decreased by 50% and 55%. [28]

Scalvini et al. [29] showed that telecardiology in patients with chest pain, using a 12-lead electro-cardiogram transmitted by telephone line, showed a sensitivity of 97.4%, a specificity of 89.5%, and a diagnostic accuracy of 86.9% for chest pain. About 74% of these cases could be solved by the telemedical service.

To sum up, telemedicine can be useful in supporting patients with a variety of chronic diseases. Due to the high psychological strain it is evident that telemedicine and telecare are particularly sensible when it comes to oncological diseases. This is why this project deals solely with patients with advanced lung-cancer.

Solutions and Recommendations

Telemedical support for patients with advanced cancer and their family caregivers may improve their quality of life substantially. Within the scope of this project, a specially tailored database will be developed at the Medical University of Vienna in cooperation with the Technical University of Vienna (Institute of Software Technology and Interactive Systems). Furthermore, a convenient videoconferencing system will be used to link oncological patients and their family caregivers with the Palliative Care Unit, Department of Internal Medicine.

Technical requirements include immediate availability, convenient handling, connectivity to an already existing internet connection, and data security. To access the database, a web interface will be used. The database acts as the server component and the web interface as the client component. The web interface should be user friendly. Ideally, the telepresence system will consist of a monitor with touch-screen function, having one particularly striking button, which is for emergency requests. An installation should not be necessary. Every request to the palliative care unit should be documented in an audit repository.

Development of a Database

The database will include the necessary information concerning participating patients and should be collaborative, meaning that physicians/nurses as well as patients and/or family caregivers will be able to add important information to continually update the database. The process of updating should be as easy as possible. Therefore, it should be possible to use the web interface via mobile devices (e.g. smartphone, tablets). If the study participants desire to speak to a psychologist, pastor or social worker, the main points of the consultation will be documented in the "Comments" section (see below).

Weight, pulse, blood pressure, pain, body temperature and diet should be documented. Important nursing information (e.g.: patient's ideal rest position) should be documented too. Automatic data transmission (e.g. SpO2 as a triage tool for medical emergencies) is desirable and will be one major aim in subsequent studies. Essential requirements are data security (encrypted data transmission, password protected login) and usability. From the medical point of view, the challenge is to support the physician in charge by providing a quick overview of the patient's history and characteristics, thus facilitating decision-making.

Ergonomic aspects for patients with special needs (e.g. mobility problems) will be considered. In order to assess the patients' needs and expectations of such a telemedical support system, structured interviews with 10 oncological patients and 10 family caregivers will be performed.

In a first step, the telemedical database will be implemented at the palliative care unit (Division of Internal Medicine) at the Medical University of Vienna / General Hospital of Vienna. The advantages are found in the multidisciplinarity of the palliative care team, which usually consists of: physicians, nurses, a pastor, a social worker (specialized on organizing mobile hospice care, nursing home places and applications for oncological rehabilitation), a dietician (specialized on diets for oncological patients and parenteral nutrition) and trained volunteers (help with organizational requests, are available if patients want to bare their souls in a conversation with somebody uninvolved). Usually, all members of the team are available during daytime, whereas during nighttime two nurses and one physician are available. In future projects, further departments

or hospices can be affiliated to the telemedical service. Additionally, mobile hospice teams can be involved.

One of the first software development tasks will be the design of Graphical User Interface (GUI) mockups. These mockups are useful tools for the requirements engineering part of the project. Instead of single textual descriptions, mockups can help to get a glimpse what the final product, in our case the GUI of our database will look like. Therefore we already created some example mockups that can be used for further development, especially for the programming of the database frontend.

Regarding to the use case, two different clients for the database are necessary. In detail, it could be one client, but depending on what user role is currently logged in, the view and functions would be different. As mentioned before, the clients have to be implemented as web applications. The following Figures are mockups of the patient's view on a tablet-PC. The first version of the database frontend will only be a responsive web application, and not a native app. That means the web application responsively adjust their design to the specific screen resolution. The main advantage of a responsive web application is the independence of the operating system (e.g. Windows, Mac OS X and also mobile operating systems like iOS or Android). The downside is usually the slower performance against a native app.

Keeping the usability in mind, the home screen of the database frontend should be self-explanatory as possible. This requirement can be reached with big symbol-like icons that can easily be clicked on (or touched on a tablet-PC).

Generally, the patient's/ family caregiver's view of the client is for entering the daily parameter values. Clicking on the icons will open the screen for the specific parameter. Figure 2 shows a mockup for the parameter "Body Temperature".

The physician's view of the web application will open with the ability to find patients, in form of a patients list. Selecting one patient shows im-

Figure 1. Database: Home screen for patients/family caregivers

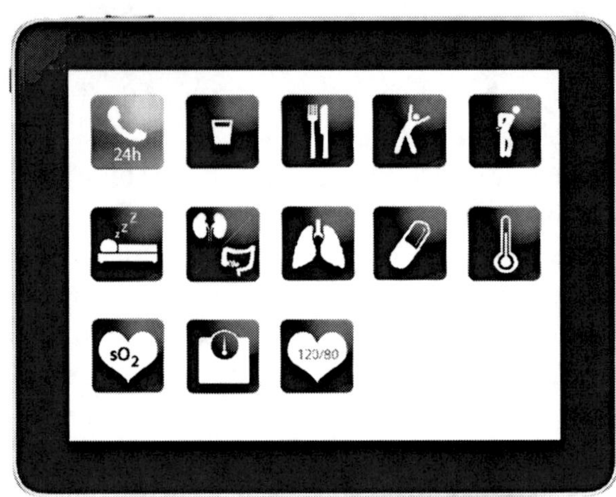

Figure 2. Documenting body temperature: Patient's/ family caregivers' view

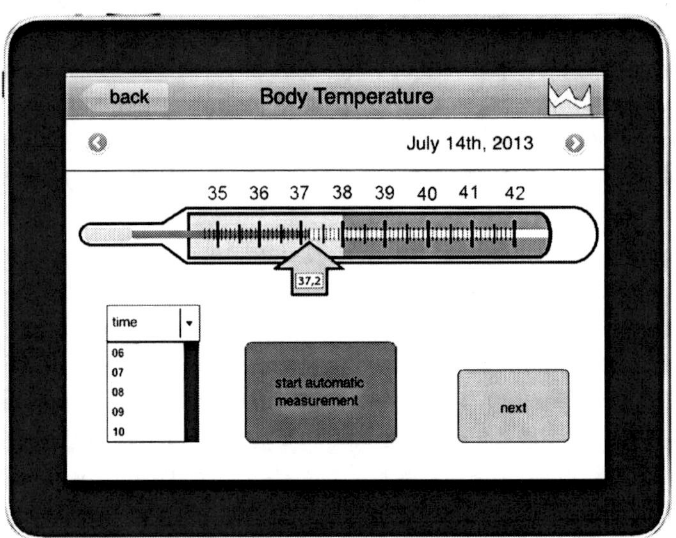

mediately the most-recent values. On this screen a medication list and the recent overall status of the patient will be displayed. The medication data in conjunction with the proposed parameters will help the physician to adapt the therapy.

Furthermore, a time-dependent visualization of the parameters will be provided like in Figure 3. One possible solution would be a full-screen chart of a single parameter. Another approach could be the combination of multiple parameters into multivariate data visualization.

Finally, some words to the database backend. Due to the small number of parameters and the existing relation to a patient, a relational database design is appropriate. Instead of showing an Entity-Relationship model, Figure 4 shows a domain analysis model in UML notation. The reason for this representation is primarily the fact, that the web client will be implemented in an object-oriented programming language like Java or Ruby. The rapid application development of the database-driven application will be supported by

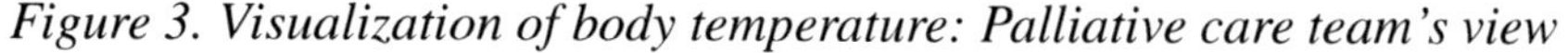

Figure 3. Visualization of body temperature: Palliative care team's view

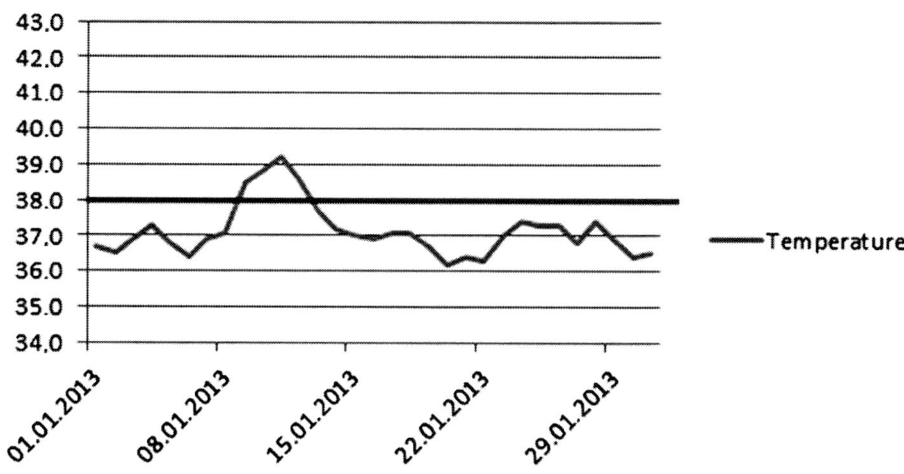

Figure 4. Domain analysis model (draft)

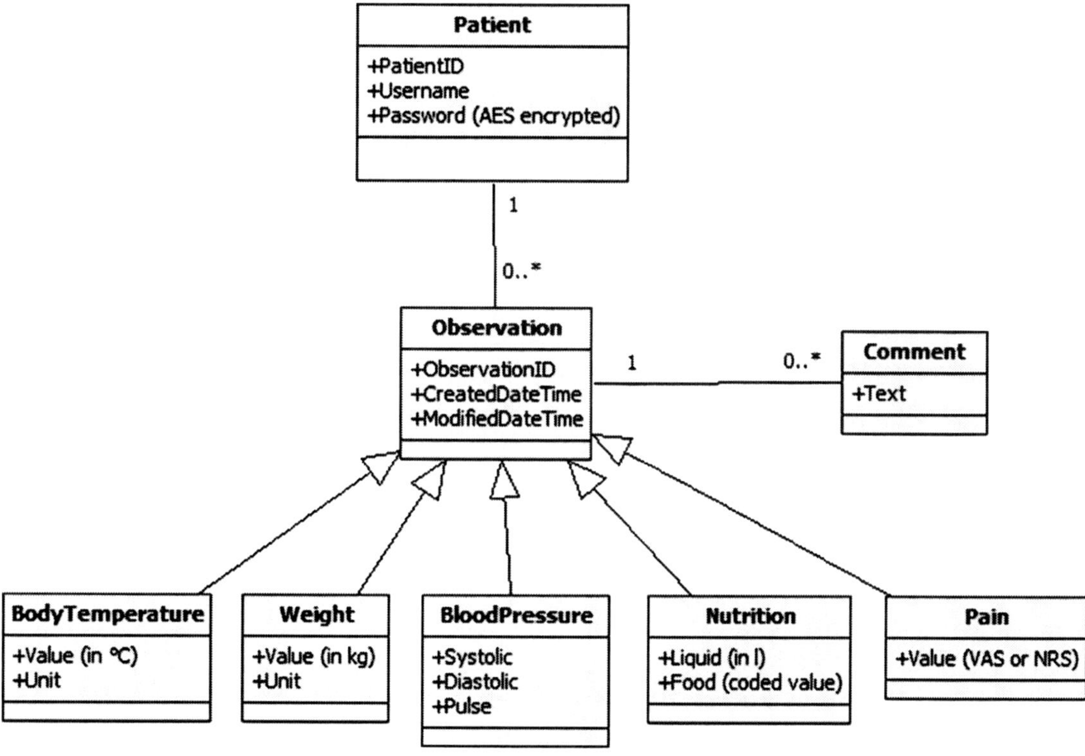

either the "Play Framework" for Java or the "Rails Framework" for Ruby. Both are web application frameworks that promise high velocity web development. With regard to these frameworks a modern web application with all expected features is more comfortable to implement.

The first draft of the domain analysis model in Figure 4 consists of eight classes. During active development of the web application with a concrete web application framework, the domain analysis model could be adapted to the needs of the project. This opportunity also applies after the first release of the web application. The three main classes are *Patient, Observation* and *Comment*. The *Observation* class is a generalization of the stored parameter classes. The classes for the parameters are *BodyTemperature, Weight, BloodPressure, Nutrition* and *Pain*. The units of the parameters are degree Celsius, kilograms, liters, mmHg and bpm. The parameter *Food* will be stored as a coded value (e.g. 0 to 4 for each dish). The parameter for *Pain* will be captured either with the Visual Analog Scale (VAS) or the Numerical Rating Scale (NRS). Both scales will be stored as discrete values between 0 and 10 in the database. The *Comment* class will be a free text field where the patient can write some additional information of experienced symptoms. This free text field will also be used to document consultations with the psychologists, social worker, pastor and dietician.

Another informative parameter could be the overall being of the patient. It is considered to add this parameter to our Domain Analysis Model. The reason why it isn't already included is that possible overlaps with other parameters are present. A parameter for anxiety is maybe a more valuable parameter.

Data Transmission and Security

All participants will receive a unique ID-number. Two databases will be used: the first one will store the personal data (first name, last name, date of birth, address) related to the ID-number, and the second one will store the patient's medical data according to her/his ID-number (e.g. medical history, medical background, current therapy). These databases will be stored independently from each other. This separation guarantees that only physicians have access to the personal data. The collected medical data will be stored according to the ID-number, thus ensuring anonymity.

The telemedical database will be protected by a firewall. The collected data will be used exclusively by the study group at our University. Physicians already registered as medical users at the Medical University of Vienna, will have to identify themselves with a username and password to access the database. The connection to the Medical University of Vienna will be protected via SSL (secure socket layer). Additionally, the physicians will get a detailed training for data security to ensure maximal safety precautions.

Maintaining these specifications, the database will be in accordance with the Austrian Data Protection Act.

Project Workflow

Altogether 40 study participants (20 patients each with one family caregiver) are going to be recruited consecutively. The recruitment will take place at the Day Ward at the Medical University of Vienna, Department for Internal Medicine I.

Inclusion criteria are:

- Patients with end stage lung cancer (stage 4, non-small cell lung cancer).
- Diagnosis within the past 8 weeks.
- Inclusion before any therapy was started.
- <75 years old.
- GOOD general condition of the patient.
- One of their family caregivers agrees to participate too.

The study participants will be divided in two groups – one intervention and one control group.

The intervention group will receive the telemedical support (including an extensive instruction for the use of the personal care devices and the database by an expert). In case of an emerging problem, patients and their family caregivers will have the possibility to start a videoconference with the palliative care team at the Department of Internal Medicine I, Medical University of Vienna. The medical team will be available around the clock, whereas the other services can only be engaged during daytime. Furthermore, the palliative team will be equipped with the previously described database which provides all-important information about the patient in need of help and which will serve the responsible physician as decision support. We assume that most cases will be solved by telemedicine. If the medical request cannot be solved by telemedicine, the patient must be admitted to hospital. Although the focus of this project lies in usability-testing, the main objective is to achieve an improve QoL for patients and their family caregivery by supporting them in stressful situations. To evaluate the effect of the telemedical intervention, QoL will be assessed using validated questionnaires (see chapter below).

To illustrate the workflow, we will describe a realistic case example that could be solved by telemedicine: A patient suffering from end stage lung cancer was recently discharged from a palliative care unit. At home, he is updating his database every day by filling in information about his diet and pain level as well as by using his personal care devices (pulse oximeter, blood pressure gauge). All of a sudden, he is short of breath and quickly starts to feel troubled. His wife is very concerned and decides to establish a teleconsultation. After briefly describing the symptoms to the nurse on duty, the physician in charge is fetched. The physician in charge now has the possibility to consult with the patient and his wife. The visualization of the patient allows him to undertake a limited physical assessment. He notices the patients' respiratory distress in terms of shallow breathing and an increased breathing frequency. The patient's complexion appears to be healthy; the color of his lips is inconspicuous as well. By accessing the patient's database on his computer, the physician in charge gets a quick overview about the patient's condition: About an hour ago, he showed normal blood pressure levels as well as an oxygen saturation rate of over 95%. Two weeks ago, the patient started taking hydromorphone for pain. Since the patient's oxygen saturation rates as well as his complexion are unremarkable, the physician in charge advises the patient to add an additional dose of his hydromorphone aiming to relieve shortness of breath. The patient complies and soon feels remarkably better. One hour the event a brief communication with the patient's wife demonstrates significant improvement of the patient's condition

Figure 5. Project workflow

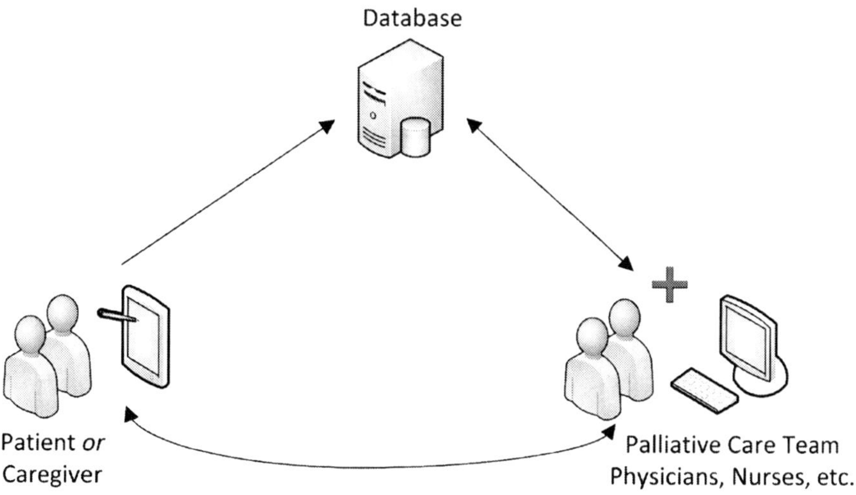

Patient's Parameters as Triage Tool for Hospital Admission

Palliative care patients often suffer from pain, nausea or breathlessness. These symptoms do not necessarily require the presence of a physician or even a hospital admission. Certain vital parameters can be used as triage tools to differentiate between real emergencies requiring immediate admission and potentially solvable situations. Here is a small excerpt (without any claim of completeness) how vital parameters can be used as triage tools.

Pain

Patients with advanced cancer almost always suffer from pain (e.g. abdominal pain because of peritoneal carcinosis or back pain because of osseous metastasis). Usually, cancer pain is treated with short acting opioids like hydromorphone or morphine. Once the patients become accustomed to these substances, their dosage can easily be adapted following medical guidelines (e.g. Clinical practice guideline for management of opioid therapy for chronic pain, US Department of Health and Human Services).

Blood Pressure and Pulse

Low blood pressure levels in combination with tachycardia (high pulse) can indicate a septic, hypovolemic (e.g. due to vascular hemorrhage) or cardiogenic shock.

Breathlessness

Oxygen saturation the bloodstream can easily be measured by pulse oximetry. High oxygen saturation indicates a subjective feeling of breathlessness, whereas low oxygen saturation can be a sign of a pulmonary disorder, severe circulatory disorder (shock), chronic kidney failure or result of a metabolic misbalance due to diarrhea or emesis.

Body Temperature: Fever or Hypothermia

Body temperature can provide vital information about the patient's condition. Certain chemotherapies result in a pronounced weakness of immune response, thus promoting infections that can be potentially life threatening. A body temperature over 37.5 degree Celsius in these vulnerable patients is a clear indication for admission and intravenous antibiotics administration. In elderly patients, the body temperature often fails to rise in case of infection, but in combination with other symptoms like disorientation and/or agitation, even a slightly increased body temperature can be a sign of infection.

Study Results

Every consultation, its participants and purpose will be documented in a case report form, as well as its outcome (hospital, admission, treatment recommendation, reassurance, etc.) Additionally, technical aspects will be assessed too (image and sound quality, technical breakdowns, etc.).

Patients and family caregivers of the intervention group, who will be supported by telemedicine, will fill in a questionnaire regarding their experiences with the telemedical service. This structured questionnaire will include the following exemplary topics:

Patients' Subjective Opinion of the Doctor-Patient Relationship by using Electronic Media

The end of life is one of the most demanding times during a doctor-patient relationship. Communication between the doctor, patient, caregiver and family plays a significant part when taking care of patients with diseases that are not responsive to curative treatment. A well functioning communication line might ease physical symptoms and provide social, emotional and spiritual support to the patient and his/her caregiver as well. By means of approximately 5 parameters, we will assess patients' subjective view of the effects electronic media have on doctor-patient relationship.

Patients' and Family Caregivers' Subjective Opinion of the Quality of Care Received through the Telepresence Systems

Even though face-to-face visits play a crucial role when establishing and maintaining a good doctor-patient relationship, studies have shown that a well maintained telepresence system has the potential to effectively substitute face-to-face meeting while maintaining the same quality of medical care [30].

By means of approximately 5 parameters (e.g. quality of medical care received, trust into the telepresence system), an additional assessment if the telepresence system is eligible to fully replace face-to-face visits will be performed.

Investigation of Participants' Acceptance of and Satisfaction with the Telepresence System and Potential for Improvement

The future implementation into clinical practice of the telepresence system will highly depend on its acceptance by all participants. Therefore, it is crucial to assess perceived usefulness, ease of use and joy of use of patients, family caregivers and also of the palliative care team with this method and evaluate their suggestions for improvements before implementing it on a larger scale.

We will assess satisfaction by means of approximately 7 parameters and include room for free text feedback including suggestions for improvement.

To assess QoL and mood, the validated questionnaires EORTC QLQ-C15-PAL, Hospital Anxiety and Depression Scale (HADS) and FAM-CARE (Caregiver Satisfaction with Advanced Cancer Care) will be used. These questionnaires will be filled in at 3 different points of time. All patients (both study groups) will fill in HADS and QLQ-C15-PAL, whereas the family caregivers

(also both study groups) will fill in HADS and FAMCARE. The first survey will be performed at the beginning of this project (baseline), the second survey will be conducted 10 weeks after baseline and the last survey will be conducted 20 weeks after baseline.

After the study is completed, all questionnaires and case report forms will be analyzed. Although we will not be able to draw definite conclusions with this sample size, the results will help to identify in which direction further research has to go.

Objectives

The main objective of this project is to assess the feasibility, benefit and limitations of telemedical support for palliative care patients and their family caregivers. We expect that by providing a telepresence system to palliative care patients, most problems can be solved by telecommunication, thus sparing the patient and family caregivers additional distress. Furthermore, the possibility to get medical advice at any time may improve symptom management, decrease emergency room visits and enhance support for families and friends who are taking care of patients at home. Thus, QoL of oncological patients and family caregivers will be improved.

The secondary endpoints are the evaluation of quality of life of oncological patients with lung cancer and their family caregivers within the telemedical support. The results will be compared with a control group who received standard care. Frequency of hospital admissions between both groups as well as acceptance of the telemedical system, adherence to the telemedical service (number of teleconsultations), the number of occurrences where the teleconsultation was not possible (data transmission errors, etc.).

We are aware of the fact that we may not get statistically valid results with such a small sample size, but due to the high manpower requirements for such a study (telemedical/ IT-experts, the palliative care team's willingness and feasibility to participate at any time) it is not possible to include more patients right now. Nevertheless, this study will shed light on the patients' needs, their perception of this special form of care and their motivation to actually use the telemedical intervention. Moreover, the study results on quality of life will give direction to further research.

Some potential pitfalls:

- Hardware breakdowns.
- Internet connection failure.
- Patients'/family caregivers' reluctance to use the telemedical support.
- Drop-out due to death.
- Unavailability of the palliative care team.

In order to avoid a high drop-out rate due to technical problems, study participants will get a special instruction from an IT-expert, who will be available also during the study period. To achieve an optimal usability, all occupational groups as well as patients and caregivers will be included in the development of the database. Nevertheless, it is not possible to debunk all possible pitfalls. One big issue will be the availability of the medical team, especially during nighttime. Although there's always (24/7) one physician on duty, there's the possibility that he's engaged with medical problems at the ward and may not be available for the teleconsultation. This could lead to waiting times and hence to resentment of the study participants. Unfortunately, there is no way to avoid these unfavorable situations.

To sum up, future studies should focus on optimizing organizational parameters and motivation of all study participants.

FUTURE RESEARCH DIRECTIONS

Since compliance is the determining factor for success in telemedicine, future research will focus on optimizing usability. Tablets and smartphones are now commonly used and should be integrated

in telemedical solutions. They are usually easy to handle and require a lot less time to get acquainted with. One of the main problem will be legal aspects. The present situation in Austria is very unsatisfying. Telemedicine can be practiced in the context of scientific studies, but when it comes to actual implementation, multiple problems arise:

- Are all devices certified for medical use?
- How reliable is the internet connection?
- How can telemedical services be accounted in the health care system?
- Who is going to be responsible for the technical support?

To obtain statistically significant results, a randomized controlled study with a higher sample size has to be conducted. This also implicates considerations about engaging more staff in order to preserve a high quality of care for each study participant. To motivate patients and their family caregivers to participate, it seems obvious that more publicity for this new kind of care should be done. If study results are promising, the telemedical care should be considered for other diseases as well. It is also desirable to include other medical care providers and mobile services (e.g. mobile hospices).

CONCLUSION

Patients with advanced cancer and their family caregivers suffer from considerable distress and are often overstrained when medical problems occur. Telemedicine may be very well suited to alleviate this potentially agonizing situations. We hypothesize that telemedically augmented palliative care will improve patients' and caregivers' quality of life, provide reassurance when needed and may reduce the frequency of hospital admissions without increasing risk.

Since compliance is the crucial factor for a well accepted system, our study focuses on usability and maximizing the perceived usefulness. Further research projects will aim for automatic data transmission in order to keep the patients' effort hardly noticeable and to ensure a consistent monitoring of all-important patient parameters. Randomized-controlled trails have to be conducted in order to get valid data on quality of life and number of hospital admissions. Besides, the potential use of telemedical care should be tested for a spectrum of suitable diseases.

REFERENCES

Bensink, M., Armfield, N., Russell, T. G., Irving, H., & Wootton, R. (2004). Paediatric palliative home care with Internet-based video-phones: Lessons learnt. *Journal of Telemedicine and Telecare*, *10*(1), 10–13. doi:10.1258/1357633042614465 PMID:15603596

Cameron, J. I., Franche, R. L., Cheung, A. M., & Stewart, D. E. (2002). Lifestyle interference and emotional distress in family caregivers of advanced cancer patients. *Cancer*, *94*, 521–527. doi:10.1002/cncr.10212 PMID:11900237

Clark, D. (2007). From margins to centre: A review of the history of palliative care in cancer. *The Lancet Oncology*, *8*, 430–438. doi:10.1016/S1470-2045(07)70138-9 PMID:17466900

Fleming, D. A., Sheppard, V. B., & Mangan, P. A. et al. (2006). Caregiving at the end of life: Perceptions of health care quality and quality of life among patients and caregivers. *Journal of Pain and Symptom Management*, *31*, 407–420. doi:10.1016/j.jpainsymman.2005.09.002 PMID:16716871

Goldstraw, P., Ball, D., & Jett, J. R. et al. (2011). Non-small-cell lung cancer. *Lancet*, *378*, 1727–1740. doi:10.1016/S0140-6736(10)62101-0 PMID:21565398

Grivaux, M., Zureik, M., & Marsal, L. et al. (2011). Five-year survival for lung cancer patients managed in general hospitals. *Revue des Maladies Respiratoires*, *28*, e31–e38. doi:10.1016/j.rmr.2008.07.001 PMID:21943545

Höfler, A.E. (2001). *Die Geschichte der Hospizbewegung in Österreich*. Zukunft braucht Vergangenheit.

Hopwood, P., & Stephens, R. J. (1995). Symptoms at presentation for treatment in patients with lung cancer: Implications for the evaluation of palliative treatment: The Medical Research Council (MRC) Lung Cancer Working Party. *British Journal of Cancer*, *71*, 633–636. doi:10.1038/bjc.1995.124 PMID:7533520

Hospiz - Palliativ Ein Beitrag zur Begriffsbestimmung. (n.d.). Retrieved April 14 2014, from http://www.hospiz.at/pdf_dl/broschuere_hospizgeschichte.pdf

Kidd, L., Cayless, S., Johnston, B., & Wengstrom, Y. (2010). Telehealth in palliative care in the UK: A review of the evidence. *Journal of Telemedicine and Telecare*, *16*, 394–402. doi:10.1258/jtt.2010.091108 PMID:20813893

Krebserkrankugnen - Luftröhre, Lunge, Bronchien. (n.d.). Retrieved April 14 2014, from http://www.statistik.at/web_de/statistiken/gesundheit/krebserkrankungen/luftroehre_bronchien_lunge/index.html

Kuenzler, A., Hodgkinson, K., Zindel, A., Bargetzi, M., & Znoj, H. J. (2011). Who cares, who bears, who benefits? Female spouses vicariously carry the burden after cancer diagnosis. *Psychology & Health*, *26*, 337–352. doi:10.1080/08870440903418877 PMID:20309780

Kurtz, M. E., Kurtz, J. C., Given, C. W., & Given, B. (2005). A randomized, controlled trial of a patient/caregiver symptom control intervention: Effects on depressive symptomatology of caregivers of cancer patients. *Journal of Pain and Symptom Management, 30,* 112–122. doi:10.1016/j.jpainsymman.2005.02.008 PMID:16125026

Maiolo, C., Mohamed, E. I., Fiorani, C. M., & De Lorenzo, A. (2003). Home telemonitoring for patients with severe respiratory illness: The Italian experience. *Journal of Telemedicine and Telecare, 9,* 67–71. doi:10.1258/135763303321327902 PMID:12699574

McBride, T., Morton, A., Nichols, A., & van Stolk, C. (2011). Comparing the costs of alternative models of end-of-life care. *Journal of Palliative Care, 27,* 126–133. PMID:21805947

Miyazaki, M., Stuart, M., Liu, L., Tell, S., & Stewart, M. (2003). Use of ISDN video-phones for clients receiving palliative and antenatal care. *Journal of Telemedicine and Telecare, 9,* 72–77. doi:10.1258/135763303321327911 PMID:12699575

Morgan, G. J., Craig, B., Grant, B., Sands, A., Doherty, N., & Casey, F. (2008). Home videoconferencing for patients with severe congenital heart disease following discharge. *Congenital Heart Disease, 3,* 317–324. doi:10.1111/j.1747-0803.2008.00205.x PMID:18837809

Northouse, L. L., Katapodi, M. C., Song, L., Zhang, L., & Mood, D. W. (2010). Interventions with family caregivers of cancer patients: Meta-analysis of randomized trials. *CA: a Cancer Journal for Clinicians, 60,* 317–339. PMID:20709946

Payne, F., Shipman, C., & Dale, J. (2001). Patients' experiences of receiving telephone advice from a GP co-operative. *Family Practice, 18,* 156–160. doi:10.1093/fampra/18.2.156 PMID:11264265

Phillips, J. L., Davidson, P. M., Newton, P. J., & Digiacomo, M. (2008). Supporting patients and their caregivers after-hours at the end of life: The role of telephone support. *Journal of Pain and Symptom Management, 36,* 11–21. doi:10.1016/j.jpainsymman.2007.08.017 PMID:18411012

Rhee, Y. S., Yun, Y. H., & Park, S. et al. (2008). Depression in family caregivers of cancer patients: The feeling of burden as a predictor of depression. *Journal of Clinical Oncology, 26,* 5890–5895. doi:10.1200/JCO.2007.15.3957 PMID:19029423

Scalvini, S., Zanelli, E., & Conti, C. et al. (2002). Assessment of prehospital chest pain using telecardiology. *Journal of Telemedicine and Telecare, 8,* 231–236. doi:10.1258/135763302320272211 PMID:12217107

Schulz, R., Visintainer, P., & Williamson, G. M. (1990). Psychiatric and physical morbidity effects of caregiving. *Journal of Gerontology, 45,* 181–191. doi:10.1093/geronj/45.5.P181 PMID:2144310

Sepulveda, C., Marlin, A., Yoshida, T., & Ullrich, A. (2001). Palliative Care: The World Health Organization's global perspective. *Journal of Pain and Symptom Management, 24,* 91–96. doi:10.1016/S0885-3924(02)00440-2 PMID:12231124

Song, J. I., Shin, D. W., & Choi, J. Y. et al. (2011). Quality of life and mental health in family caregivers of patients with terminal cancer. *Supportive Care in Cancer, 19,* 1519–1526. doi:10.1007/s00520-010-0977-8 PMID:21479527

Statistik Austria - Todesursachen 2010. (n.d.). Retrieved April 14 2014, from http://www.statistik.at/web_de/statistiken/gesundheit/todesursachen/index.html

Tamayo, G. J., Broxson, A., Munsell, M., & Cohen, M. Z. (2010). Caring for the caregiver. *Oncology Nursing Forum, 37,* E50–E57. doi:10.1188/10.ONF.E50-E57 PMID:20044332

Temel, J. S., Greer, J. A., & Muzikansky, A. et al. (2010). Early palliative care for patients with metastatic non-small-cell lung cancer. *The New England Journal of Medicine*, *363*, 733–742. doi:10.1056/NEJMoa1000678 PMID:20818875

Teunissen, S. C., Verhagen, E. H., Brink, M., van der Linden, B. A., Voest, E. E., & de Graeff, A. (2007). Telephone consultation in palliative care for cancer patients: 5 years of experience in The Netherlands. *Supportive Care in Cancer*, *15*, 577–582. doi:10.1007/s00520-006-0202-y PMID:17165090

World Health Organization. (1990). Cancer pain relief and palliative care: Report of a WHO Expert Committee. *World Health Organization Technical Report Series*, *804*, 1–75. PMID:1702248

ADDITIONAL READING

Foley, K. M., & Gelband, H. (2001). *Improving palliative care for cancer*. Washington: National Academy Press.

Gothelf, J. (2013). *Lean UX: Applying Lean Principles to Improve User Experience*. Sebastopol: O'Reilly Media Inc.

Hanks, G., Cherny, N. I., Nicholas, A. C., Fallon, M., Kaasa, S., & Porteno, R. K. (2009). *Oxford Textbook of Palliative Care*. Oxford: Oxford University Press. doi:10.1093/med/9780198570295.001.0001

Hoyt, R. E., Bailey, N., & Yoshihashi, A. (2012). Health Informatics: Practical Guide For Healthcare And Information Technology Professionals.

Mazza, R. (2009). *Introduction to Information Visualization*. London: Springer-Verlag.

Murray, S. (2013). *Interactive Data Visualization for the Web*. Sebastopol: O'Reilly Media Inc.

Trotter, F., & Uhlmann, D. (2011). *Hacking Healthcare: A Guide to Standards, Workflows, and Meaningful Use*. Sebastopol: O'Reilly Media Inc.

Wootton, R., Craig, J., & Patterson, V. (2006). *Introduction to Telemedicine*. London: Royal Society of Medicine Press Ltd.

KEY TERMS AND DEFINITIONS

Empowerment: Empowerment strategies aim at increasing the degree of autonomy and self-determination of people by enabling them to express their interests arbitrary.

EMR: Electronic medical record, collection and storage of medical parameters.

Family Caregivers: Family caregivers are relatives, friends or neighbors who provide assistance but are not paid for their services.

Palliative Care: Palliative care focuses on symptom management and aims improvement of quality of life when a disease is not responsive to curative treatment.

Quality of Life: Quality of life is a subjective parameter and indicates the overall well being of an individual, including social, spiritual and mental well being.

Telemedicine: Telemedicine bridges the regional distance between physician and patient using information and telecommunication technology.

Telepresence System: A telepresence system is a device, which can be used for videoconferencing. The videoconference creates the illusion that the conference partners are actually present.

Chapter 11
Evaluating Integrated eCare:
Discussions and Guidance of a Diverse Field

Anne-Kirstine Dyrvig
Center for Innovative Medical Technologies, Denmark

ABSTRACT

Evaluation of projects on integrated eCare is key to implementation and widespread use. The evaluation must, though, be thorough and include research methods from multiple different research traditions simultaneously. This implies a necessity of knowledge from all research paradigms and understanding of proper reporting. In this chapter, guidance for evaluation of integrated eCare is provided, along with discussions of advantages and disadvantages related to certain decisions that must be made during the research process. As an aid for understanding, real-life examples of evaluation are provided to illustrate challenges and possible solutions throughout the chapter.

INTRODUCTION

Resource scarcity combined with the interest in always doing what serves the community best, are the primary drivers of both implementation of and research within integrated eCare. Integrated eCare is aiming to solve problems for those of us who use both health and social care, i.e. most of us during the period of a lifetime. It is well known, that across health and social care systems in different countries, the simultaneous use of both kinds of services imply problems and barriers for the end users (Kodner & Spreeuwenberg, 2002).

Current demographic developments with decreasing workforce and increasing number of frail elderly people further challenges the health care delivery as of today, so part of the solution is sought within better integration of systems combined with eCare. The aim of enhanced integration supplemented by eCare is to improve effectiveness while increasing quality and decreasing costs (Kodner & Spreeuwenberg, 2002).

Meanwhile, it is important to make sure that the attempts at increasing effectiveness and quality and lowering costs, does not imply decreased level of care for the individual or impose a huge

DOI: 10.4018/978-1-4666-8756-1.ch011

risk for adverse events. Thus, scientific methods are used to follow up the changes made along with the outcomes of the changes.

The trend in health care has, since primo the 1970ies developed in direction of so called evidence-based health care. The idea is that if treatment A in scientific studies has proved more efficient than treatment B, doctors should prescribe treatment A, unless good causes are presented against that choice (Mar, Glasziou, & Mayer, 2004). Good causes could be patient values or ethical objections or unclarity in the scientific studies, such as the impact of co-morbidity. In these cases, the clinical judgment, which is still informed by the evidence and patient values, will be the guide.

In recent years, this trend towards evidence in decision making has spread to decision makers outside of health care. Evidence is becoming a prerequisite for political decisions to change or implement new technologies, routines and interventions. And for a good cause: all citizens are interested in ensuring that health and social care services are indeed helpful and not inducing unnecessary risks. Also, integration of services can be quite resource demanding, and it is in the best interest of our populations that resources are spent wisely on interventions with known consequences.

In this chapter, challenges and requirements for producing reliable evidence for the consequences of integrated eCare is discussed. The discussion is illustrated with current examples of the challenges and solutions from real life scientific work within the field of integrated eCare. The objective of the chapter is to provide guidance on evaluating integrated eCare in the process of developing evidence for decision makers.

BACKGROUND

Due to differences in organization and reimbursement of health and social care in different countries, definitions are necessary to ensure a common understanding. In this section central terms are defined for use throughout the chapter.

Integrated Care

Integrated eCare is usually designed in order to solve different types of problems in overall health and social care provision simultaneously.

Examples of problems that are thought solved through implementation of eCare include duplication of work (e.g. GP and hospital making the same blood tests), or communication across sectors (e.g. ensuring that home care service providers are informed on a patient being discharged from hospital). In line of this thinking, Leichsenring et. al. (2013) defined integration of care as:

"Integration is usually conceptualized as a process through which new methods of working together bring actors and/or things closer to one another and allow them to become more tightly bound to each other. In this perspective a care system is integrated when dysfunctional barriers are overcome and smoother system function is attained".

The aim of providing ICT supported integrated care thus comprises the aspects of collaboration that causes problems in health service provision.

Complex Intervention

Integrated eCare as a solution to problems on collaboration or duplication of efforts consists of several components, i.e. a database of tests performed, diagnosis, medication etc. along with a communication system. The scientific community regards such interventions consisting of *"multiple interconnected parts"* (Collins, 1979) as complex interventions.

Craig et al. (2013) define an intervention as complex, if it includes:

- [A] number of interacting components within the experimental and control interventions.
- [A] number and difficulty of behaviors required by those delivering or receiving the intervention.

- [A] Number of groups or organizational levels targeted by the intervention.
- [A] Number and variability of outcomes.
- [A] degree of flexibility or tailoring of the intervention permitted.

Integrated eCare include all these aspects, and can thus be regarded a complex intervention. Therefore, the evaluation of integrated eCare needs to take into consideration that these characteristics are present. In practice, this implies using a complex set of evaluation methods to comprise the total contents of evaluation (Kodner & Spreeuwenberg, 2002).

EVALUATION OF COMPLEX INTERVENTIONS/ INTEGRATED CARE

Evaluation is the use of the scientific method, and the rigorous and systematic collection of research data, to assess the effectiveness of organizations, services and programs (e.g. health service interventions) in achieving predefined objectives ((Bowling, 2009) referring to Shaw 1980)

Since integrated eCare is complex, there are a number of different stakeholders involved and a number of different possible outcomes. This means, that a full evaluation of effectiveness requires careful consideration beforehand and careful monitoring of all aspects during follow-up. Thus, a number of authors recommend an initial assessment of study phase and evaluation ambition before taking on the outcome evaluation (Campbell et al., 2000; Kidholm et al., 2012; Parry, Carson-Stevens, Luff, McPherson, & Goldmann, 2013).

Campbell et al. (2000) suggests four phases of complex interventions. First, the definition phase, where aims are clarified and the technology is developed to accomplish the aims. Second, acceptability and feasibility of the technology is tested. This is best done through qualitative study designs, where all involved stakeholders are interviewed or observed regarding their use of the technology and attitudes towards it. The third phase is called the main trial, or in this chapter, the outcome evaluation, where multiple scientific methods are combined in order to obtain knowledge on all wanted and unwanted consequences of implementing the technology. Finally, the fourth phase is the implementation of the technology. The four phases depend on each other in that it does not make sense to move from one phase to the next, if negative results are obtained. It is possible, though, to accommodate the unwanted results and carry out a re-test in the same phase.

Once initial assessments and evaluations have indicated that the technology is complying with the wishes of all users and decision making stakeholders, it is time to plan the outcome evaluation, which is the main focus of this chapter.

The most challenging aspect of evaluating outcomes of complex interventions is to find the balance between measuring the right and enough aspects, while not spending too many resources measuring. It is given by the commonly used statistical approach with significance given at a 5% level, that for each 20 measurements, one will turn out statistically significant simply by the accepted level of chance. Therefore, consideration needs to be given to why each outcome is important and how it is best measured.

In order to aid the phase of identifying all possible wanted and unwanted outcomes and decide on method of measurement, a number of models exist (Kidholm et al., 2012; Kodner & Spreeuwenberg, 2002; Schünemann et al., 2013). The common aspects are that they provide a certain structure for outcome identification, and recommend using any suitable qualitative or quantitative scientific method to measure the effect. Thus, the differences are related to the given structure rather than the content or preferred methodology, which means that one might be just as useful as the other. For this chapter, the MAST model was chosen as point of departure due to the one particular aspect that MAST was developed to structure evaluations of telemedicine specifically. While there are a few differences between telemedicine and eCare, the model has been amended to include the wider range of stakeholders and service providers.

Originally, MAST introduces seven domains that have to be considered when evaluating a telemedicine application;

1. Health problem and characteristics of the application.
2. Safety.
3. Clinical effectiveness.
4. Patients' perspectives.
5. Economic aspects.
6. Organizational aspects.
7. Socio-cultural, ethical and legal aspects.

These domains comprise a selection of possible important outcomes of implementing eCare. The selection of domains was based on a thorough systematic literature review and roundtable discussions with stakeholders in health care (Kidholm et al., 2012). Thus, the domains will be used as point of departure for the more thorough model for evaluation of integrated eCare suggested in this chapter.

Evaluating Integrated eCare Cookbook

Both qualitative and quantitative research methods include multiple choices that need to be made and documented during the evaluation process. This starts before launching the project and stops after reporting.

In this section of the chapter, each step in a typical research process will be worked through explaining choices and recommendations along the way. This includes choice of study design, inclusion of patients/citizens and other stakeholders, measures of outcomes, statistics and reporting.

PROJECT PLANNING: STATE OF THE ART SOLUTION

The single most important phase of planning evaluation of integrated eCare, is determining priority or emphasis given to each aspect. Since integrated eCare is a complex intervention, the possibilities for evaluations consequently is unlimited. Complex interventions might have an impact on a number of different aspects, and while MAST serves as a guide to structuring the comprehensiveness of the evaluation, it does not suggest any priority among the domains.

So, if enough resources are available, the optimal solution is to collect evidence for all the aspects through the appropriate research methods. Thus, this chapter proceeds with descriptions of how to assess all relevant outcomes of integrated eCare. While reading through, it should be noted though, that in reality an important task is to priorities among the aspects and possibilities in accordance with local circumstances.

In order to illustrate the complexity and derived evaluation consequences, this section is supported by an illustration taken from the Region of Southern Denmark. The Region is implementing a project for integrating health and social care supported by ICT for heart failure patients admitted to hospital.

Usually, heart failure patients are admitted to hospital due to chest pain and/or collapse. After diagnosis, they undergo surgery or have medication prescribed. When being discharged from hospital, they are told that they will be contacted by the municipality (responsible for social care in Denmark) and that they should visit their GP for follow-up on their condition. They go home. Usually frightened and without fully understanding what happened and why, but knowing that death was close by. The follow-up from municipalities differs, and depends on the referral, which is often unclear, e.g. states 'heart failure follow-up'. The workers in the municipality contact the citizen, and when they meet, nobody knows what happened and in terms of follow up intervention, the choice is an educated guess rather based on what the patient remembers being told by hospital staff. There is no official sharing of information between sectors. GP visits are the sole responsibility of the citizen. And any meetings with the GP are similar to those with social care workers – no official sharing of information – putting the patient at the centre of communication across sectors.

As a possible solution to the lack of sharing of information, an ICT system has been developed. It collects data from records across sectors, and is available to all carers and the patient.

Imagine that this is the starting point of an evaluation. It is clear, that a problem is present. It involves communication across sectors and the ability of patients to handle the responsibility of providing information to different care professionals. Also, the example suggests integrated eCare as a possible solution.

Defining Aim and Objectives

The first question stated by any professional evaluator would always be: What is the aim of this intervention? Establishing the aim is a very important input in that it is used for clarification for a number of derived aspects, i.e. population of interest, study design, choice of outcomes, necessary sample size (sample is number of patients necessary for the evaluation).

So, in this case, the aim of implementing the intervention could be 1) Improved communication between professionals in different sectors, 2) Improved quality of care in terms of relapse, 3) Improved quality of care as determined by patients, 4) Improved feeling of coherence in the patient pathway, 5) Decrease in replication of work done by different sectors etc.

Each of these questions could stand alone as research questions in different projects. But separating the questions would not reflect the real world very well. In the real world, implementation of the intervention would most likely influence all aspects including communication, quality, coherence and economy. Therefore, setting up a research project to answer only one of the questions would not make much sense.

The MAST approach to evaluation acknowledges all these different possible aims in that data can be collected for all aspects, and provides a structure to decrease the complexity without violating comprehensiveness. So, using the original MAST structure, the possible aims can be described as questions to answer for each domain as presented in table 1.

Table 1. Original MAST structure including questions to answer in a full evaluation

MAST Domain	Questions
Health problem and characteristics of the application	Is the health problem relevant? Can the application serve as a solution to the problems related to the treatment of patients?
Safety	Is it safe for the patients to use the system?
Clinical effectiveness	Does the treatment of patients work at least as well as the current treatment?
Patients' perspectives	Do patients have any concerns related to using the application? What are their preferences and experiences?
Economic aspects	Do the costs from of the current treatment differ from the suggested solution? If so, how and how much and for which stakeholders?
Organizational aspects	Does implementation of the application change organizational aspects? In terms of tasks, staff satisfaction, replication of work and communication? Does implementation of the application affect the communication across sectors of health and social care?
Socio-cultural, ethical and legal aspects	What socio-cultural, ethical or legal aspects might influence the ability to obtain the estimated effects of the application?

Table 2. MAST framework applied to integrated eCare

MAST Domain	Health Care	Social Care	Volunteers/Relatives
1. Health problem and characteristics of application	1. Health problem and characteristics of application	1. Social problem and characteristics of application	1. Health and social problem and characteristics of application
2. Safety	2. Safety	2. Safety	2. Safety
3. Clinical effectiveness	3. Clinical effectiveness	3. Care effectiveness	3. Clinical and care effectiveness
4. Patient perspectives	4. Patient perspectives	4. End-user perspectives	4. End-user perspectives
5. Economic aspects	5. Economic aspects	5. Economic aspects	5. Economic aspects
6. Organizational aspects	6. Organizational aspects	6. Organizational aspects	6. Organizational aspects
7. Socio-cultural, ethical and legal aspects	7. Socio-cultural, ethical and legal aspects	7. Socio-cultural, ethical and legal aspects	7. Socio-cultural, ethical and legal aspects

The table is derived from using the original MAST framework, which needs to be elaborated in order to include all the possible stakeholders and outcomes of implementing integrated eCare. Therefore, it has been elaborated in table 2 below to include all stakeholders in integrated eCare.

Table 2 presents the aspects of MAST that needs to be included in a full outcome evaluation of integrated eCare. Also, it includes the perspectives of different stakeholders involved in providing or receiving integrated eCare.

Table 3. Example of MAST applied to integrated eCare

MAST Domain	Health Care	Social Care	Volunteers/Relatives
1. Health problem and characteristics of application	Heart failure acute treatment and an electronic portal that collects pre-defined, relevant data from existing system	Heart failure rehabilitative treatment including needs assessment and an electronic portal that collects pre-defined, relevant data from existing system	Heart failure and derived consequences related to work- and social life
2. Safety	Patient safety/adverse events, data safety, privacy	Patient safety/adverse events, data safety, privacy	Patient safety/adverse events, data safety, privacy
3. Clinical effectiveness	Clinical effectiveness	Care effectiveness and quality	Clinical and care effectiveness including possible other aspects
4. Patient perspectives	Access to data, usefulness of portal, feasibility and acceptance	Access to data, usefulness of portal, feasibility and acceptance	Access to data, usefulness of portal, feasibility and acceptance
5. Economic aspects	Economic aspects from hospital perspective, including costs and reimbursement	Economic aspects from municipality perspective, including costs and income (tax based)	Economic aspects from organizational/private perspective, including income, costs and payers
6. Organizational aspects	Changes in tasks or task distribution among personnel or organizations, including impacts on culture, work flow and process	Changes in tasks or task distribution among personnel or organizations, including impacts on culture, work flow and process	Changes in tasks or task distribution among personnel or organizations, including impacts on culture, work flow and process
7. Socio-cultural, ethical and legal aspects	Socio-cultural: changes related to the new treatment plan for heart failure Ethical: provision of the best possible treatment Legal: data safety, privacy protection	Socio-cultural: changes related to the new treatment plan for heart failure Ethical: provision of the best possible treatment Legal: data safety, privacy protection	Socio-cultural: changes related to the new treatment plan for heart failure Ethical: provision of the best possible treatment Legal: data safety, privacy protection

In order to enhance understanding of the practical application of MAST, table 3 below has been developed. Table 3 returns to the example from Region of Southern Denmark with patients suffering from heart failure.

In Table 3, the different changes that might occur have been listed, although still on a rather superficial level. The different changes and outcomes reflecting these changes will be more detailed later in this chapter. The main purpose at this level is to go through the table and assess whether all relevant aspects have been considered, or if any additional changes should be added to ensure comprehensiveness in the evaluation.

Study Design and Sample Selection

With the aim clearly defined the navigation through the proceeding steps of evaluation are easier to manage, due to reduced complexity. So, still relying on the MAST outline, the study design for each of the domains is specified in table 4 below:

In Table 4, a number of different methods for data collection are mentioned, combining quantitative and qualitative data. This reflects that complex interventions require data collections using a broad range of scientific methods. The advantage is that it is possible to combine data collections for different domains and the disadvantage is

Table 4. MAST domains including descriptions of information collection methods and advice on measurements

MAST Domain	Type of Information	Measurement Advice
Health problem and characteristics of the application	Qualitative descriptions	Narratives explaining the impact of the disease
Safety	Quantitative intervention studies	Recording of any event happening in either intervention group or control group throughout the study period. Including problems with equipment, and health related outcomes i.e. falls, deaths
Clinical effectiveness	Quantitative intervention studies	Randomized trial, case-control, before/after study etc. The most important aspect is to find a proper control group to increase the likelihood that the intervention was in fact causing any change during the research phase. To control for "dosage" of the intervention log-information from ICT systems can be valuable
Patients' perspectives	Qualitative interviews and quantitative intervention studies	Questionnaires can be distributed during the study phase. Interviews, observations and/or diaries can supplement questionnaires
Economic aspects	Quantitative intervention studies and qualitative observations	Information on costs and revenue can often be obtained through records. For more detail, observations, interviews and/or diaries can supplement or replace record information. Effects in economic analyses are measured similarly as in clinical trials regardless of study design, so those outcomes are covered in other domains
Organizational aspects	Qualitative interviews and observations	Understanding of culture, process, communication and workflow can be sought through interviews with relevant staff, observations and/or diaries from key personnel
Socio-cultural, ethical and legal aspects	Qualitative descriptions	Descriptions of certain local circumstances that affect either the intervention or the implementation requires in-depth knowledge from the setting. If researchers do not have this knowledge, it can be obtained through interviews with key stakeholders. Also, there might be relevant information in any material on subcontracting or invitations to tender

that this type of comprehensiveness is resource demanding. Locally, it is possible to priorities between domains or data collection methods or sample sizes in order to accommodate the budget.

It is widely debated in research communities which study design is most appropriate for complex intervention, particularly within the quantitative paradigm. Since it is beyond the scope of this chapter to identify which is best, it is recommended to consider the weighting of practicality and trustworthiness of results. In order to determine an effect, you wish to compare like with like (Evans, Thornton, Chalmers, & Glasziou, 2011). So, preferably, the only difference between people receiving the intervention and those not receiving it is the intervention itself. The study design most suitable for this setup is randomized controlled trials. This type of study includes a number of people as similar as possible and randomly divides them into groups. The easiest way to make sure that other factors do not have an impact on results is to apply strict inclusion criteria, so the population is highly selected. This provides results that are highly trustworthy in terms of the effects of the intervention. On the other hand, in reality people differ – e.g. in terms of co-morbidities or use (dosage) of the intervention. The number of people necessary in a randomized controlled trial for determining an effect increases exponentially with the types of variability allowed among the people. So, if people with co-morbidities are excluded from the sample, fewer patients are necessary to show an effect of the intervention. No co-morbidity is, however, not a proper reflection of real life patients. Therefore, other study designs allowing more flexible inclusion criteria are sometimes preferred in order to provide a more solid reflection of real life. This is done with the knowledge that it means increasing the likelihood of bias in the estimated effectiveness of the intervention. The decision on one study design, is always based on local circumstances, which is acceptable as long as it is clearly state which study design is chosen and why.

Data Collection

Quantitative Data

Thorough planning of data collection means less trouble during the study phase. For quantitative data, it is helpful to set up a database with the variable that should be measured and a codebook explaining how to type data from each patient into the database.

If quantitative data can be accessed through existing databases, it needs to be possible to link the specific data to the specific patient for later analyses to make sense. If such databases exist, it can make the data collection less resource demanding.

Data that needs to be obtained from users can be collected through questionnaires. If questionnaires are completed while waiting for an appointment in hospital or elsewhere, the likelihood of high response rate is greater than by postal mail. Again, local circumstances play a large role in terms of what is possible for gathering all necessary data. Also, it is possible to have questionnaires developed in software that enables electronic reading of responses rather than people having to type the answers into a database.

A database can be created directly in the statistical software that will be used for calculations or in any type of database software as long as no laws on data safety are violated. E.g. Googledocs has some privacy problems. But Microsoft Excel or Access or Epidata, which is available online can be used. The only requirement is that if the information is stored on a level which provides personally attributable data may not be sent via email.

The figure below shows part of a database created in Excel with the top row explaining each variable and a number of additional rows representing one participant, and finally summaries for each period.

Figure 1. Part of a database for quantitative data collection

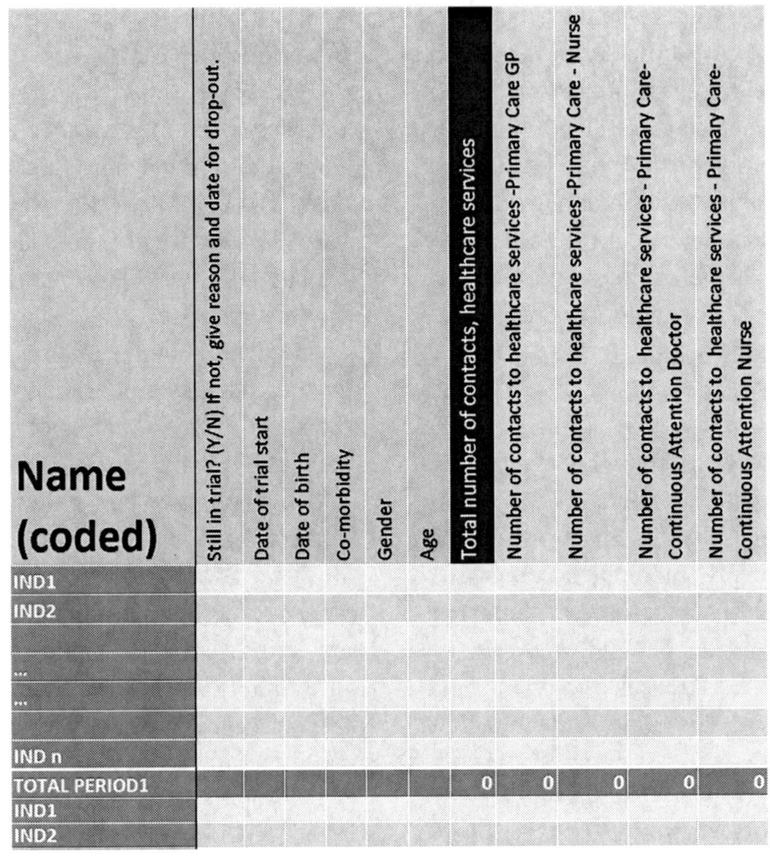

Qualitative Data

Data from interviews can consist of notes and/or recordings of the session. Observations are easiest to handle, if they are provided in a predefined form which can include room for notes toward the end. Likewise, if patients or staff are asked to use diaries during the study phase, it is possible to structure parts of the diaries to make sure that certain information are repeatedly provided. Personal notes should be allowed as well, to enable participants to give any – even unexpected information – related to the study.

For example, a diary entry might include a few headlines, e.g. date, time, place, overall well-being, chest pain, other symptoms, activities and room for personal notes.

Outcome Measures

An infinite number of outcomes can be measured. So when it comes to establishing which outcomes to measure in an evaluation of integrated eCare. The domains in the MAST model can be helpful in ensuring that all important outcomes are included.

Returning to the heart failure example from the Region of Southern Denmark, the table below has been elaborated. For each domain of MAST, a number of measurements have been chosen that reflects the domain. Also, it is explained who the respondent is, the necessary level of data and level of detail along with possible collection methods and the reason given for including the specific outcome measure.

Another important aspect for outcome measures is to keep the number of outcomes reasonable. On the one hand, the collected data should be comprehensive so that analyses are possible. On the other, study participants being overwhelmed by the number of questionnaires or interviews can be reluctant to participate, or report lower satisfaction levels. Finding the balance can be aided by carrying out pilot tests of involved questionnaires and interview guides.

One example from the above table is that two different measures of frailty are included. It might make sense to use only one. In addition, sometimes hospital records include a frailty measure. If that is the case, no additional measures should be necessary.

Analyses

The specific statistical and qualitative analyses should follow guidelines for the chosen study design. It is important to consider which analyses will answer the aims and objectives of the study from the planning phase. If this is not kept in mind from the beginning, there is a risk to finish the study without being able to answer the study questions due to lack of data. Also, an early focus on analyses ensures that the scale used, reflecting the level of detail for each variable, is sufficient – i.e. is age can estimated as levels (0-9, 10-19…) or as a numeric variable. Therefore the research group needs to include statisticians from the outset. Table 5 above includes this information under the 'level of detail' heading.

The preliminary strategy for analyses should be documented as a specific plan for analysis, which then serves as a useful guideline when carrying out the analyses after data collection. Also, if there is a wish to publish in scientific journals, the knowledge on which analyses were planned and which were carried out post hoc, is necessary.

Keep in mind, that data can sometimes be recycled. In an organizational analysis, for instance, it is common to calculate the use of time for different types of staff or organizations. This information is also used in economic evaluations and can thus serve as input for this. The study group only needs to collect the data once, but can use it in analyses for several MAST domains. Also data on clinical effectiveness is used in economic analyses.

In practice, a strategy for analyses would usually include the following items:

1. Prepare a log of any changes that are made in the dataset. All changes should be noted along with the reasons for changing. This will come in handy later on.
2. Check distribution of variables (normally distributed variables is an assumption in all parametric tests later on. If normally does not exist, non-parametric tests should be used).
3. Check for outliers or odd values (including a strategy for handling, i.e. dele the observation, the entire set for the patient or go back in records to see if a mistake was made during typing data into the database).
4. If necessary, change variables to log-scales.
5. Combine any variables that are included in a total scale.
6. Check for correlations between variables.
7. Carry out the combined analyses, most often logistic or multiple regressions.

Reporting and Communication

The type of reporting to follow an evaluation is highly dependent on the channels that should be used after the project has finished. Also, a communication strategy will help ensuring that the necessary stakeholders are informed throughout the project. Communication should not solely be considered after finishing data collections.

If any scientific publications are planned, it is important to keep in mind the timing of publications. Most scientific journals do not accept articles that have had results published elsewhere. Thus, timing of providing information to media, on conferences or to politicians can impact the possibility of having results published in scientific journals.

Table 5. Outcomes for chronic heart failure project (I)

Measurement	Respondent/ Target Group	Level of Data	Level of Detail	Collection Method	Reason
1. Overall service effectiveness and specific outcome measures.					
Number of contacts, healthcare services	Citizen / client / carer	Individual level	Number	Registries	Total number of contacts is 1) easy to establish (was there a contact or not), and 2) it is available in all relevant care providing sites
Unplanned contacts, healthcare services	Citizen / client / carer	Individual level	Number	Registries	Unplanned contacts is chosen because it is 1) easy to establish (was there an unplanned contact or not), and 2) it reflects both the aim of the interventions in clinical terms but also safety issues, organizational and economic aspects.
Number of contacts, social care services	Citizen / client / carer	Individual level	Number	Registries	Total number of contacts is 1) easy to establish (was there a contact or not), and 2) it is available in all relevant care sites
Unplanned contacts, social care services	Citizen / client / carer	Individual level	Number	Registries	Unplanned contacts is chosen because it is 1) easy to establish (was there an unplanned contact or not), and 2) it reflects both the aim of the interventions in clinical terms but also safety issues, organizational and economic aspects.
Number of contacts, volunteer sector services	Citizen / client / carer	Individual level	Number	Registries	Total number of contacts is 1) easy to establish (was there a contact or not), and 2) it is available in all relevant care sites
Unplanned contacts, volunteer sector services	Citizen / client / carer	Individual level	Number	Registries	Unplanned contacts is chosen because it is 1) easy to establish (was there an unplanned contact or not), and 2) it reflects both the aim of the interventions in clinical terms but also safety issues, organizational and economic aspects.
1.a Disease specific health status measures.					
Blood pressure	Citizen / client	Individual level	Number	Registries	Indicator for health status
Cholesterol	Citizen / client	Individual level	Number	Registries	Indicator for health status
Status/severity of primary condition	Citizen / client	Individual level	Scale or number	Registries	Predictor of health outcome
1.b Generic health related / functional quality of life.					
Health related quality of life (instrument: SF 36 v2)	Citizen / client	Individual level	Scale	Questionnaire or interview	Might be affected by the intervention
Frailty measure (instrument: Barthel index)	Citizen / client	Individual level	Scale	Clinical measurement	Indicator for health status
Frailty measure (instrument: Timed up & go)	Citizen / client	Individual level	Number	Clinical measurement	Indicator for health status

continued on following page

Table 5. Continued

Measurement	Respondent/ Target Group	Level of Data	Level of Detail	Collection Method	Reason
CASP-19 family carer QoL	Carers	Individual level	Scale	Questionnaire or interview	The CASP-19 is used to specifically measure QoL of family carers. The measure has four domains: control, autonomy, pleasure and self-realization. The scale contains 19 items. The domains have Cronbach's αs between 0.60 and 0.80. Correlations between the four domains range from 0.40 to 0.70. Concurrent validity has been assessed using the Life Satisfaction Index – Wellbeing. A strong and positive association was found between the two scales.
1.c Psychological measures.					
Anxiety and depression (instrument: HADS)	Citizen / client	Individual level	Number	Questionnaire or interview	The HADS is used to determine the levels of anxiety and depression in end users. It is a 14-item scale. Seven of the items relate to anxiety and seven related to depression.
Depression according to GDS	Citizen / client	Individual level	Number	Questionnaire or interview	The Geriatric Depression Scale-15 (GDS-15) is a short, 15-item instrument specifically designed to assess depression in geriatric populations. Its items require a yes/no response. The Geriatric Depression Scale was first introduced by Yesavage et al. in 1983, and the short form (GDS-15) was developed by Sheikh and Yesavage in 1986.
Isolation according to Perceived Isolation Questionnaire	Citizen / client	Individual level	Number	Questionnaire or interview	Previous research has identified a wide range of indicators of social isolation that pose health risks, including living alone, having a small social network, infrequent participation in social activities, and feelings of loneliness. However, multiple forms of isolation are rarely studied together, making it difficult to determine which aspects of isolation are most harmful to health. Cornwell and Waite (2009) used population-based data from the National Social Life, Health, and Aging Project to generate questions combining multiple indicators of social isolation into scales assessing social disconnectedness (e.g., small social network, infrequent participation in social activities) and perceived isolation (e.g., loneliness, perceived lack of social support). These questions can be ascribed numerical values so that, when repeated, they provide a way for people to self-rate whether they are more or less socially disconnected and isolated from others than at the previous time of measurement

continued on following page

Table 5. Continued

Measurement	Respondent/ Target Group	Level of Data	Level of Detail	Collection Method	Reason
Carer burden according to ZBI (short version)	Carers	Individual level	Number	Questionnaire or interview	The Zarit Burden Interview was developed to measure subjective burden among family carers of adults with dementia. Items were generated based on clinical experience with family carers and previous research, resulting in a 22-item self-report inventory that examines burden associated with functional or behavioral impairments and the home care situation. Most researchers use the 22-item version of the ZBI. However, the length of the instrument may be a deterrent to its use in clinical and research environments. Bédard et al produced a short version consisting of 12 items, with results comparable to the full version. Cronbach's α for the 12-item version is 0.88.
Carer burden according to CADI-CASI-CAMI suite	Carers	Individual level	Number	Questionnaire or interview	Carers are also assessed for difficulties, satisfaction and management in caring using the CADI-CASI-CAMI suite. The CADI-CASI-CAMI suite is a collection of three instruments used to assess family carers' perceptions of difficulty, satisfaction and management (coping strategies). The Carer Assessment of Difficulty Index (CADI) is a 30-item index and contains a series of statements which carers have made about the difficulties they face. Carers are asked to tick the box next to each statement that applies to them the most from the following options: 'this does not apply to me', 'not stressful', 'stressful', and 'very stressful'. The Carer Assessment of Satisfaction Index (CASI) is also a 30-item index and contains a series of statements about the satisfaction carers experience. The Carer Assessment of Management Index (CAMI) is a 38-item questionnaire and contains a series of statements about the coping strategies used by family carers.

Table 6. Outcomes for chronic heart failure project (II)

Measurement	Respondent/target group	Level of data	Level of detail	Collection method	Reason
2. Safety.					
Technological functioning	Citizen / client	Individual level	Continuous count of not-functioning	Log files	Easy to establish, common as adverse event
Deaths	Citizen / client	Individual level	Yes/no (dichotomous)	Registries	Easy to establish, common as adverse outcome
Measurement	Respondent/target group	Level of data	Level of detail	Collection method	Reason

Table 7. Outcomes for chronic heart failure project (III)

Measurement	Respondent /Target Group	Level of Data	Level of Detail	Collection Method	Reason
3. End user / client / carer perspectives.					
End user / client / carer empowerment	Citizen / client / carer	Individual level	Scale for each question	Questionnaire	Reflects part of the aim of the intervention - to empower the users
End user / client /carer satisfaction	Citizen / client / carer	Individual level	Scale for each question	Questionnaire, IFIC	This would be based on the eCare Client Impact Survey developed in CommonWell and INDEPENDENT measuring impacts on older end-users and informal carers beyond clinical outcomes and with particular focus on impacts occurring from combined social and health care.
End user perception of integration	End-users	Individual level	One question with visual scale	Questionnaire	Visual scale to reflect the level of integration as perceived by the end-users

Table 8. Outcomes for chronic heart failure project (IV)

Measurement		Level Of Data	Level of Detail	Collection Method	Reason
4. Economic measures.					
Efforts related to service development & implementation	Citizen / client / carer	Individual or organizational level	Number	Various	To support the design and implementation of viable and sustainable services. To produce supportive economic for internal decision making processes. To allow for an overall, post-hoc assessment of socio-economic impacts.
	Service providers				
Efforts related to service operation or use	Citizen / client / carer	Individual or organizational level	Number	Various	As above.
	Service providers				
Equipment cost	Service providers	Organizational level	Number	Various	As above.
Service effectiveness benefits	Service providers	Organizational level	Number	Various	As above.
Service efficiency benefits	Service providers	Organizational level	Number	Various	As above.
Revenue streams	Service providers	Organizational level	Number	Various	As above.
Willingness to pay	Citizen / client / carer	Individual level	Scale	Questionnaire	Relevant if a service fee payable by end user / client /carer is considered to become part of the revenue model.

Table 9. Outcomes for chronic heart failure project (V)

Measurement	Respondent / Target Group	Level of Data	Level of Detail	Collection Method	Reason
5. Organizational impact measures.					
Impacts on staff	Service providers: staff members and key informants / decision makers	Organizational level	Scales, qualitative	Questionnaire or interview	Key measures to understand the organizational changes caused by the new service, as well as to get a better understanding of what was actually achieved through the integration of different service silos. Can also capture where staff members and organizational decision makers are (still) not satisfied with the result.
Impacts on organizations	Service providers: staff members and key informants / decision makers	Organizational level	Scales, qualitative	Questionnaire or interview	As above.
Service integration aspects	Service providers: staff members and key informants / decision makers	Organizational level	Scales, qualitative	Questionnaire or interview	As above.
Mainstreaming potential and sustainability	Service providers: key informants / decision makers	Organizational level	Scales, qualitative	Questionnaire or interview	As above.

Having mentioned this possible problem, an advantage of having a strategy enables publication of results to have similar contents. Therefore written material can relatively easy be reused as long as timing does not conflict.

A thorough plan for communication through e.g. newsletters, political summaries, scientific publications, conference abstracts and contact to media enhances the likelihood that knowledge of results becomes widespread. Regardless of having found the expected results, it is important to ensure that all, external as well as internal, stakeholders learn about results in order to enhance the overall benefit of the work carried out in the project.

Scientific reporting follows more or less strict rules on contents and length. A number of pub-lications deal with explanations on the outline and requirements, which is beyond the scope of this chapter. Also, most scientific journals have requirements explained on their webpage.

Ethics

Before starting to include any patients in any project, local authorities need to be informed of the project to know if any permission is required. Usually, ethical approval is required for experimental studies testing new treatments, or studies that collect data that can be back-transferred to identify individuals. Nevertheless, it is recommended to always make sure that a written accept of the study is given to either not require a formal approval, or

Table 10. Outcomes for chronic heart failure project (VI)

Measurement	Respondent / Target Group	Level of Data	Level of Detail	Collection Method	Reason
6. Possible confounders / control variables.					
Date of birth	Citizen / client / carer	Individual level	YYYY-MM-DD	Registries or interview	Age is a strong predictor of any health outcome
Gender	Citizen / client / carer	Individual level	Male/female	Registries or interview	Gender is very often related to health outcomes
Level of education	Citizen / client / carer	Individual level	Categories	Registries or interview	Level of education is a strong predictor of any health outcome.
Marital status	Citizen / client / carer	Individual level	Categories	Registries or interview	Marital status is a strong predictor of health outcomes.
Ethnicity	Citizen / client / carer	Individual level	Categories	Questionnaire or interview	Ethnicity is strongly related to health outcomes
Main work status (last 12 months)	Citizen / client / carer	Individual level	Categories	Questionnaire or interview	Work status is being recognized as a strong indicator of health outcome. It turns out that people belong to the social group in which they work rather than the one in which they are educated.
People older than 18 living in household	Citizen / client / carer	Individual level	Number	Questionnaire or interview	Indicator for the level of informal care received
Household income	Citizen / client / carer	Individual level	Number	Questionnaire or interview	Necessary if willingness-to-pay is analyzed.
Daily tobacco use	Citizen / client	Individual level	Dichotomous	Questionnaire or interview	Indicator for health status
Frequency of alcohol (12 months)	Citizen / client	Individual level	Categories	Questionnaire or interview	Indicator for health status
Height (CM)	Citizen / client	Individual level	Number	Questionnaire or interview	Indicator for health status
Weight (Kg)	Citizen / client	Individual level	Number	Questionnaire or interview	Indicator for health status
Co-morbidity	Citizen / client	Individual level	ICD-10 codes	Registry, questionnaire or interview	Indicator for health status, highly relevant for the usability of results after finishing the trial

the approval itself. In scientific reporting of the evaluation, it is usually a requirement to mention whether approval was necessary and/or given.

People included in evaluations are in most cases obliged to sign an informed consent regardless of being included as receiving or not receiving the intervention. Local ethical boards have standard consent forms that can be adapted to the project.

Follow-Up

If it is decided to implement the integrated eCare solution after the project period ends, continuing data collection – perhaps on a minor number of variables, is of great value. As discussed earlier, scientific studies usually excludes a number of patients from the intervention due to certain characteristics that violates the attempt to compare like with like. When the intervention is implemented in real life, however, these restrictions are usually not required. That means that a larger number of individuals receive the intervention. And in reality, it is unknown whether they benefit the same, more or less from the intervention than those originally included in the evaluation study. Therefore, collecting additional data on the real world patients, contribute greatly to the knowledge of strategic aiming of the intervention towards subgroups benefitting the most, while also contributing to scientific knowledge on the differences between the measured effectiveness (efficacy) and the real life effectiveness.

Follow-up data can be collected more or less automatically and are thus far from as resource demanding as the evaluation itself. It should be noted though, that data should be collected only, if they are used.

In the MAST model, it is advised that a transferability assessment is carried out. Such an assessment is independent of supplementary data and does to a certain degree provide information on what happens if the intervention is extrapolated beyond inclusion criteria or regional/national borders. The recommendations given in MAST include an assessment of how the outcomes or results of the integrated eCare will change if the intervention is extrapolated. Mostly, these assessments should be based on judgment, but when possible, data could support the estimations.

Three different types of transferability are presented in the MAST model. In the table below, the types of transferability are presented along with the questions to answer when assessing and how to handle the assessment in practice.

Table 11. Operationalisation of transferability

Type of Transferability	Assessment Question	Practical Guidance
Cross-border	Validity of results in other countries	Describe the setting in sufficient detail to allow copy-cats Assess changes in results, if setting differs
Scalability	Validity of results if scaled to country-level	Assess changes in results if inclusion of more similar patients Asses within-country similarity of relevant settings
Generalisability	Validity of results if criteria for inclusion are widened	Assess impact of relevant aspects, e.g. disease severity Determine whether inclusion criteria could be extended – asses how results would change accordingly

Protocol and Project Plan

The information that has been reviewed in this chapter can with advantage be summarized in a formal document. In the scientific community this will be known as the protocol – in other communities known as a project plan.

If scientific publication is planned, publication of the protocol is recommended. There are a few guidelines for contents (Chan et al., 2013) and some dedicated databases depending on the chosen study design (clinical.trials.gov, Cochrane trials). This chapter has included information additional to what is required in scientific journals, since a responsible evaluation includes more aspects than merely scientific publication. Currently it is debated to which degree scientists should be held responsible for maximization of the output made from information collected for research purposes. Key stakeholders within the scientific community find it ethically correct to emphasize on communicating research results (alltrials.net).

In summary, the outline of a project plan as presented in this chapter, includes:

- Aim and objectives.
- Study design.
- Data collection.
- Outcome measures.
- Analyses.
- Reporting and communication.
- Ethics.
- Follow-up.

SOLUTIONS AND RECOMMENDATIONS

Set the Team

The one single aspect, that will have the largest possible influence over trouble during the phases of any project, is the team responsible for carrying out any aspect of the project. With complex interventions and integrated eCare, the requirements in terms of competences are great. Thus, the best team reflects the following competences. The number of people representing the competences is less relevant, as long as everybody involved are ready to discuss constructively and make compromise.

- Clinical competences within the relevant field.
- Knowledge on day-to-day routines within the relevant fields of health and social care.
- Understanding of political context.
- Qualitative research methods.
- Quantitative research methods.
- Health economy.
- Project co-ordination.

Furthermore, as within any type of project, the process has highest chances of success, if communication is respectful and deadlines are kept. With a number of people representing each one field of competences, achieving compromise can be challenging. On the one hand, these final considerations are not rocket science, on the other hand, they cannot be taken for granted. If the team is internally unfamiliar with each other, or if previous experiences have ended in conflict, written agreements and documentation of process and decisions can serve as conflict solution tools later in the process.

Prioritizing Domains/Study Designs

MAST allows for several aims to be comprehended within the same evaluation. Nevertheless, in a world of scarce resources, the usual case is that priority has to be given to only a sub-set of the possible studies to answer each aim of the seven MAST domains. It is possible to plan a quantitative study design, pragmatic randomized trial or similar, and supplement with information collected qualitatively. If restriction on resources requires disregard of some domains, it should be considered to select the most important domain based on the aim, or the most comprehensive domain. Economic aspects, for instance are rarely presented without some attention to clinical effectiveness and organizational aspects.

It is not possible to provide much general guidance on the prioritization of domains. That should be decided on a case basis and always clearly describe what has been prioritized and why.

Evidence and Hierarchy

Within the scientific community it is widely debated which study design is most suitable for complex interventions. The discussion centers on the issue of the trade-off between scientific rigor versus reflecting real life. Until now, there has not been any convincing scientific documentation showing that either of the perspectives in this debate is right. Therefore, the currently best possible advice is to explain what reasons justify the decision of one over the other on a case basis. As long as this issue is based on values, people will disagree regardless of the choice, so it should not stop evaluations from being carried out that it is unclear if it is best to go for the best possible evidence or the best possible reflection of real life.

Evidence and Complex Interventions

Integrated eCare usually consists of several aspects such as changing routines while implementing ICT support, and as such it is a complex intervention. One disadvantage of evaluating complex interventions is the inability to attribute parts of the total effectiveness to specific parts of the intervention and to know the interaction of effects caused by the specific combination of interventions.

So, if both routines and ICT are changed simultaneously, as is most times the case in integrated eCare, it is not possible to know the details of causes and effects. Therefore, when reporting evaluation of integrated eCare, it is important to be quite detailed as to what was changed and how. If these details are not provided, the stakeholders reading a report or scientific article will be unable to learn from the reported experiences and therefore the evaluation loses its value to outsiders. This is neither the interests of the people participating in the intervention, project or the evaluation.

Evidence and Policy

When a project has been carried out and thoroughly evaluated, most participants wish for it to be continued and implemented as the usual practice. This is not always the case. Evaluators are not decision makers, and a MAST evaluation is not a decision. Decisions are based often on evidence, but also on other aspects, e.g. values, religion, political pressure etc. Therefore, evaluators need to keep in mind that a project can be well done even if the intervention is not implemented (or implemented when it showed unwanted results). So even though evidence is certainly an important input in decision making, it needs to be acknowledge as no more than that: an input.

FUTURE RESEARCH DIRECTIONS

Due to the rapid speed of technology development, future research needs to focus on transferability and external validity of results. Thorough research takes time, and to make the most of research results, it is worthwhile to focus on how we can extrapolate from studies carried out in other settings. Especially regarding complex interventions, the knowledge on external validity is limited. With the difficulties in attributing parts of the measured effect to specific parts of the intervention, it is even more critical to learn what happens when going from project to implementation.

CONCLUSION

This chapter presents a thorough guide on what to consider when evaluating integrated eCare. Regardless of doing the research while implementing an intervention or as a research project, the recommendations and cook-book approach can be used as a reference for aspects to include a structure that can be applied.

First of all, proper planning will pay out during all project phases. Planning includes definition of aims and objectives, selection of study design along with prioritizing important domains of the evaluation, plan for data collection, outcome measures and analyses. Also, during the planning phase it is recommended to remember reporting and communication strategy, ethical aspects, follow-up plans and the writing of a proper protocol and project plan.

Additionally, it is recommended to include people with knowledge on research and statistics at the beginning of a project to make sure that aims and objectives can be fulfilled by the planned data collection.

Although research sometimes seems straightforward, it should be kept in mind that subjective choices are made throughout the process. Any such decisions along with justifications should be clearly stated in any reporting of results so that readers follow the line of the argument and understand what has happened. Doing this enhances the usability of the study for readers throughout the world.

In conclusion, thorough planning and clear reporting is key to successful communication of evaluation results.

REFERENCES

Bowling, A. (2009). *Research methods in health: Investigating health and health services* (3rd ed.). Open University Press and McGraw Hill.

Campbell, M., Fitzpatrick, R., Haines, A., Kinmonth, A. L., Sandercock, P., Spiegelhalter, D., & Tyrer, P. (2000). Framework for design and evaluation of complex interventions to improve health. *BMJ (Clinical Research Ed.)*, *321*(7262), 694–696. doi:10.1136/bmj.321.7262.694 PMID:10987780

Chan, A. W., Tetzlaff, J. M., Altman, D. G., Laupacis, A., Gotzsche, P. C., Krleza-Jeric, K., & Moher, D. (2013). SPIRIT 2013 statement: Defining standard protocol items for clinical trials. *Annals of Internal Medicine*, *158*(3), 200–207. doi:10.7326/0003-4819-158-3-201302050-00583 PMID:23295957

Collins. (Ed.). (1979). *Collins' English Dictionary*. Retrieved from http://www.collinsdictionary.com/dictionary/english

Craig, P., Dieppe, P., Macintyre, S., Michie, S., Nazareth, I., & Petticrew, M. (2013). Developing and evaluating complex interventions: The new Medical Research Council guidance. *International Journal of Nursing Studies*, *50*(5), 587–592. doi:10.1016/j.ijnurstu.2012.09.010 PMID:23159157

Evans, I., Thornton, H., Chalmers, I., & Glasziou, P. (2011). *Testing Treatments: Better Research for Better Healthcare*. London: Academic Press.

Kidholm, K., Ekeland, A. G., Jensen, L. K., Rasmussen, J., Pedersen, C. D., Bowes, A., & Bech, M. (2012). A model for assessment of telemedicine applications: Mast. *International Journal of Technology Assessment in Health Care*, *28*(1), 44–51. doi:10.1017/S0266462311000638 PMID:22617736

Kodner, D. L., & Spreeuwenberg, C. (2002). Integrated care: Meaning, logic, applications, and implications--A discussion paper. *International Journal of Integrated Care*, *2*, e12. PMID:16896389

Mar, C. D., Glasziou, P., & Mayer, D. (2004). Teaching evidence based medicine. *BMJ (Clinical Research Ed.)*, *329*(7473), 989–990. doi:10.1136/bmj.329.7473.989 PMID:15514319

Parry, G. J., Carson-Stevens, A., Luff, D. F., McPherson, M. E., & Goldmann, D. A. (2013). Recommendations for evaluation of health care improvement initiatives. *Acad Pediatr, 13*(6Suppl), S23–S30. doi:10.1016/j.acap.2013.04.007 PMID:24268081

Schünemann, H. J., Tugwell, P., Reeves, B. C., Akl, E. A., Santesso, N., Spencer, F. A., & Helfand, M. (2013). Non-randomized studies as a source of complementary, sequential or replacement evidence for randomized controlled trials in systematic reviews on the effects of interventions. *Research Synthesis Methods, 4*(1), 49–62. doi:10.1002/jrsm.1078

Chapter 12

The Mobile is Part of a Whole:
Implementing and Evaluating mHealth from an Information Infrastructure Perspective

Tiwonge Davis Manda
University of Oslo, Norway & University of Malawi, Malawi

Terje Aksel Sanner
University of Oslo, Norway

ABSTRACT

A challenge with mHealth in developing countries is that implementations are frequently treated as standalone solutions. Implementations fail because they are not sufficiently aligned with existing health information infrastructures (II). An interesting tool for evaluating implementation efforts in the context of the overall health II strategy, and thus potentially useful for identifying and mitigating risks, is the Bootstrap strategy. Bootstrapping is concerned with addressing take-off challenges facing novel solution implementations through incremental progression, resource maximization, mutual learning, and complexity mitigation. Although the strategy has been previously employed in retrospect to explain how implementation take-off challenges can be alleviated, less is known about its effectiveness as a tool for real time implementation risk assessment. Drawing on an action research mHealth project in Malawi, the study confirms bootstrapping as an effective tool for risk assessment, although the case also reveals that it may not always be easy to mitigate risks identified.

1. INTRODUCTION

Application of theory as a sensitizing device informing conceptualization, design, implementation, evaluation of interventions, and application of evaluations has gained recognition and influence over the past two decades. However, despite apparent recognition and influence of the approach, there is a dearth of case examples which clearly document and recount enactment approaches, procedures and analytic frameworks, and application of evaluation results (Coryn, Noakes, Westine, & Schröter, 2011). This paper reflects on application of conceptualizations on information

DOI: 10.4018/978-1-4666-8756-1.ch012

infrastructure (II) (Bowker, Baker, Millerand, & Ribes, 2010; Hanseth & Lyytinen, 2010; Ribes & Finholt, 2009; Star & Ruhleder, 1996) in the planning, implementation, and evaluation of mHealth pilots for routine health data reporting in Malawi. II can be defined II as shared, open, heterogeneous and evolving socio-technical systems consisting of IT capabilities and their users, operations and design communities (Hanseth & Lyytinen, 2010).

Goals for our mHealth pilots were threefold. First, we set out to investigate the possibility of replacing existing paper-based data reporting between health facilities and district health offices with mobile phone supported reporting. Second, we were interested in studying the interplay between mobile phone supported data reporting and existing reporting practices which centred on the movement of paper-based report forms. The third goal encompassed the first two in that we were ultimately interested in observing how existing socio-technical arrangements in the broader health information system setup would interplay with our efforts. The healthcare industry is characterised by diversity: patients, professional disciplines, treatment options, healthcare delivery processes, and interests of various stakeholder groups (AbouZah & Boerma, 2005). Consequently, building on such a socio-technical setup (installed base) (Hanseth & Lyytinen, 2010) in the implementation and use of mHealth solutions demands the convergence of people, healthcare processes, devices, healthcare information systems, systems development, and wireless communication technologies (Yu, Wu, Yu, & Xiao, 2006). To exemplify the significance of this, some studies posit that IT initiatives in developing countries often fall apart due to inadequate local human and technical capacity (AbouZah & Boerma, 2005; Heeks, 2002); over reliance on external financial and technical support (AbouZah & Boerma, 2005; Heeks, 2002); weak enabling infrastructure, resource constraints, and top-down design and implementation of initiatives (Lippeveld, 2001).

Adopting an information infrastructure perspective can therefore be informative towards design, implementation and evaluation of mHealth interventions due to emphasis placed on heterogeneity and multiplicity of competing, cooperating, converging and diverging composite socio-technical subsystems (Constantinides & Barrett, 2005; Garcı́a-Marco, 2011; Hanseth & Lyytinen, 2010). We adopted an information infrastructure perspective not because the pilots we are running are large scale, but because of the considerable multiplicity and importance of socio-technical arrangements that interplay with our pilots. In addition, previous studies demonstrate that the growing tendency by stakeholders to treat mHealth implementations as standalone solutions despite the obvious existence of multiple solutions and interacting components, hampers mHealth interventions from realising their potential (Braa & Nielsen, 2013; Mechael et al., 2010).

Negotiating complexity that results from heterogeneity of parts and logics at work in information infrastructure innovations is characterised by ambiguity and nonlinearity of outcomes (Baker & Bowker, 2007; Edwards, Jackson, Bowker, & Knobel, 2007; Hughes, 1987). The implication of these observations is that as researchers we could not only focus on possible outcomes of our pilots. Design, implementation, and maintenance of the pilots to address shortcomings in the installed base upon which we were building, as well as making arrangements to enhance prospects for long-term sustainability, were just as important. Design, implementation, and maintenance work has a bearing on the attainment of our first goal. With this realisation we drew upon *bootstrapping* (Hanseth & Aanestad, 2001, 2003; Hanseth & Lyytinen, 2010), a strategy targeted at addressing take-off problems facing IT innovations, as a sensitizing lens in the design, implementation, and evaluation of our pilots. The strategy addresses challenges of reaching a momentum of user adoptions and stability of novel information technology solutions. Momentum is considered a stage of implementation where the initiative is self-sustaining, with little or no assistance (i.e. technical expertise, funding) from external stakeholders.

The rest of this paper is organised as follows: the next section reviews related literature and adopted theoretical framework. This is followed by a presentation of the research methodology used to gather empirical data. After that we present our empirical case, which is then followed by discussion of the case using an information infrastructure perspective and bootstrapping as a guiding lenses. Finally we present concluding remarks.

2. LITERATURE REVIEW

Considering the multiplicity of factors that interplay with information systems efforts, organizations must inevitably respond to risk factors that are both within and outside their immediate control. Some risk factors common to information technology implementations include: diverging logics and interests between a multiplicity of stakeholders and user communities; management and alignment of stakeholder relationships; lack of locally trained skilled personnel resulting to over reliance on external consultants; and failures in external dependencies (Schmidt, Lyytinen, Keil, & Cule, 2001). Mitigation of such challenges for successful implementation of novel solutions requires effective management of technology, human arrangements, and institutional resources (Ribes & Finholt, 2009). It is also important, among other things, to understand how risk factors relate to each other and the trade-offs or contingencies among risk factors (Scott & Vessey, 2002).

Various studies have proposed implementation strategies to try and manage the aforementioned risks (Hanseth & Aanestad, 2003; Ribes & Finholt, 2009; Schmidt, et al., 2001; Scott & Vessey, 2002). Ribes and Finholt (2009) argue that development of information technology solutions must focus on both immediate and long-term goals, align stakeholder interests, and stimulate continued user contribution. Hanseth and Aanestad (2001; 2003) propose *bootstrapping* as an implementation strategy and analytical lens to guide negotiation of take-off challenges facing infrastructure innovations.

2.1. Bootstrapping Technological Innovations

Bootstrapping provides for identification and management of trade-offs between multiple competing path-ways for managing implementation challenges. The strategy advocates an incremental approach to implementing technological innovations (Hanseth & Aanestad, 2001). Hanseth and Aanestad (2001) argue that implementation of novel solutions should aim for immediate usefulness to an initial small base of early adopters, promote learning from on-going implementation efforts, start with supporting less critical and less complex routines, and then actively expand the user base and the scope of the solution to handle more complex and critical tasks. This is bound to lessen contradictions with existing organisational socio-technical arrangements, which can adversely affect on-going solution implementation efforts (Aanestad & Jensen, 2011; Hanseth & Aanestad, 2003). To minimize contradictions with the existing socio-technical setup, identification of the right point of entry is essential. Below is a presentation of the strategy, as an algorithm, by Hanseth and Aanestad (2001):

1. "Start by designing the first, simplest, cheapest solution we can imagine and which satisfy the needs of the most motivated users in their least critical and simplest practices and which may be beneficial by supporting communication and collaboration between just a few users.
2. use the technology and repeat as long as possible: enrol more users

3. If possible: explore, identify and adopt more innovative (and beneficial) ways of using the solution, go to 2

4. Use the solution in more critical tasks, go to 2

5. Use the solution in more complex tasks, go to 2

6. Improve the solution so new tasks can be supported, go to 2" (p. 14).

Application of bootstrapping as an analytical lens has evolved over the last decade. Hanseth and Aanestad (2001) use bootstrapping with a focus on resource maximisation to raise the growth momentum of novel solutions. Hanseth and Lyytinen (2004; 2010) emphasise mutual learning, from an on-going implementation. Skorve and Aanestad (2010) use the concept to analyse the need for complexity mitigation in the introduction of a technological solution aimed at supporting diverse groups of medical practices and practitioners. We contribute towards theoretical application of bootstrapping through our application of the concept to reflect on risks inherent in multi-stakeholder IT innovations, which might be a source of failure should external dependencies collapse.

In addition, previous theoretical development and application of the bootstrapping concept has largely focused on the influence of internal organisational arrangements on implementation efforts. Where interplay between cross-organisational entities has been reflected upon (Aanestad & Jensen, 2011; Hanseth & Aanestad, 2003), it has been in a context where stakeholders have more or less similar goals, albeit with different tactics for managing implementation complexities (Skorve & Aanestad, 2010). This leaves a gap in existing literature when it comes to exploring the potential of applying bootstrapping as an analytical lens to study infrastructure efforts that rely on commitment from multiple stakeholders, across service sectors, geographical boundaries, who although controlling key parts of the socio-technical installed base to be leveraged are not intended solution adopters.

3. METHODOLOGY

This paper reports findings from an on-going action research study on the use of mobile phones for routine health data reporting and access, between Lilongwe district health office and 17 subordinate health facilities, in Malawi. Lilongwe district health office is sub-divided into six administrative health areas and we are running the aforementioned pilots in two of these. One health area has nine health facilities and the other has eight. The health area with nine facilities is rural based, whilst the other health area has a rural-urban blend in the distribution of health facilities. Routine data reporting is often a challenge for these health facilities as members of staff have to fund own travel to the district health office in order to submit reports. In addition, a round trip to the district health office takes an entire day for staff travelling from health facilities in rural areas. Consequently, officers are unavailable to deliver healthcare at their duty stations which are mostly understaffed. During the rainy season travel can also be challenging as the majority of roads in rural areas become impassable, which negatively impacts people's mobility. Against this background, it was considered that the aforementioned challenges could be addressed by enabling health facilities to submit reports remotely, through the use of mobile phones, to an online server accessible to the district health office. An action research approach was, therefore, adopted as the approach provides for the pairing of interventions to solve existing problems with careful study of the interventions, to build knowledge (Davison, Martinsons, & Kock, 2004). In addition, such an involved approach to research also allows in-depth access to people, issues, and data (Walsham, 2006). We were also cognisant of research suggesting that immediate relevance of technological solutions is critical to their wide adoption (Hanseth & Lyytinen, 2004).

The pilots running in Malawi are part of a larger international action research mHealth project, MobiHealth, based at the University of

Oslo in Norway. MobiHealth, itself, is part of a larger action research network called the Health Information Systems Programme (HISP). HISP is an International South-South-North action research network focusing on health information systems strengthening and research. As part of its efforts, HISP is actively developing the District Health Information Software (DHIS 2), a generic server-based solution for collection, validation, analysis, and presentation of aggregate statistical data. Traditionally, DHIS 2 has supported data entry and access using desktop and laptop computers. However, over the past three years MobiHealth has spearheaded development of a module (DHIS Mobile) to enable mobile data communication with DHIS 2. The pilots running in Malawi are based on DHIS Mobile. Software development for DHIS Mobile is mainly done in Norway and Vietnam.

3.1. Research Design

3.1.1. Diagnosis Phase

The first part of our intervention involved consultations with the Ministry of Health's Central Monitoring and Evaluation Division (CMED), Lilongwe district health office, and a selected number of health facilities, on goals and scope of the intended pilots. Through the discussions, it was agreed that we pilot DHIS Mobile solutions in all health facilities under Lilongwe district health office. This was followed by visits to health facilities, to gather baseline data on existing paper-centric data gathering and reporting practices, existing feedback mechanisms on submitted reports, and data utilization at health facility level. This was mainly done between September and December 2011.

3.1.2. Action Planning and Taking

At the beginning of November, our plans for the pilots were revised from a somewhat big bang approach (rolling-out to all health facilities at once) to a phased approach (rolling-out the solutions to one health area, at a time). Informed by the bootstrapping concept (Hanseth & Aanestad, 2001, 2003) we decided to progress with our efforts in small incremental steps. This was done to minimize the possible impact of any unintended consequences, arising from our efforts. Finally, mobile phones, for the pilots, were purchased and the two pilots were rolled out between February and March 2012.

The DHIS Mobile pilots running in Malawi were commissioned to contribute towards ongoing health information system strengthening efforts being undertaken by the Ministry of Health. In 2009 the ministry began efforts to migrate its principal health management information system software solution from DHIS 1.3, a desktop software solution, to DHIS 2, a server-side solution. A national DHIS 2 server was setup in 2009, but national scale-up efforts only picked up in 2012, with the support of various development partners. Figure 1 shows a timeline depicting key milestones in DHIS 2 and DHIS Mobile implementation efforts.

3.1.3. Evaluation and Specifying Learning

After going live with the pilots, we conducted two review meetings in May 2012. In January 2013, we conducted two more review meetings. Between the review meetings in May 2012 and those in January 2013 we also made several ad-hoc visits to health facilities taking part in the pilots. Analysis of empirical findings from the review meetings and visits to health facilities were used to inform the on-going pilots, as well as research publications.

3.1.4. Data Collection and Analysis

Principal data collection methods employed include: semi-structured interviews, focus group

Figure 1. Timeline for key milestones in DHIS 2 and DHIS Mobile implementation efforts

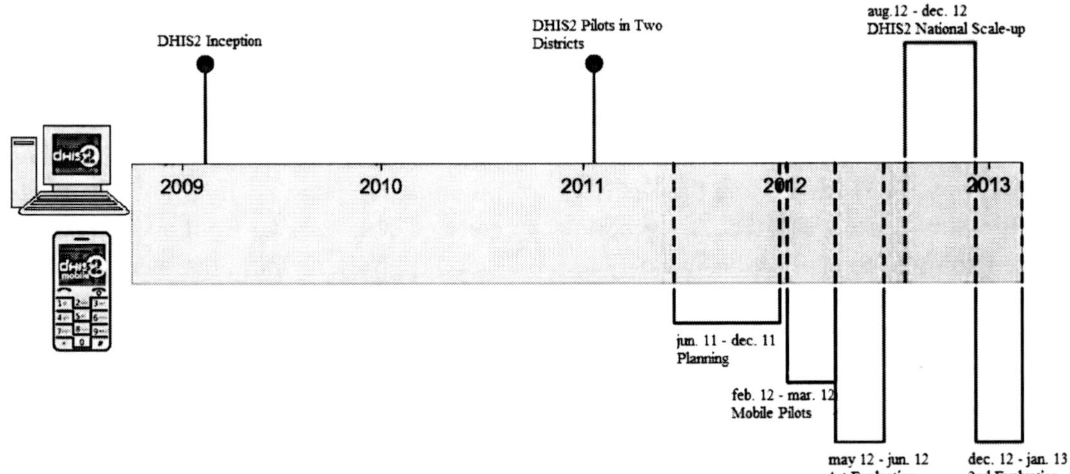

discussions, and three training sessions on the mobile phone solutions being piloted. Key informants for the study include medical officers, health surveillance assistants (salaried community health workers), and statistical clerks. Statisticians, for the national health management information system at district health office and ministry of health levels, were also interviewed. Interactions with the MobiHealth research team in Oslo as well as software developers in Norway and Vietnam have also provided valuable insights. These interactions have been facilitated by face-to-face meetings, exchange of emails, and conference calls. The mobile service operator providing the telecom services required for the two pilots has also played a central role in the implementations. Several planned and ad-hoc meetings between the researchers and various representatives of the operator have taken place. Other data like national health management information system (HMIS) policy documents, status reports, registers, and photographs of existing technologies physically present at health facilities (e.g. radio communication equipment, solar panels, personal mobile phones, ground phones etc.) have served as secondary sources of information to the study. Finally, personal reflections on roles assumed by

the researchers, (one being a Malawian national and the other a Norwegian), in the on-going pilots and empirical data gathering inform this paper. The Malawian researcher is the lead investigator in the on-going pilots and finds himself very much at the centre of coordinating the pilots and interacting with key stakeholders.

Training sessions for would-be users on the solutions under pilot were mainly conducted in December 2011, February 2012, and March 2012. The trainings had three stages. First, we conducted focus group discussions covering topics such as existing paper-centric routine health data collection and reporting practices, and data use at health facility level. Second, we had hands-on training on the DHIS Mobile solutions under pilot. The third part of the training was a feedback session, on issues covered during the training. This was done through another round of discussions and completion of pre-designed feedback forms. Through the feedback forms participants were able to evaluate the training, reflect on the strengths and weaknesses of mobile reporting vis-à-vis paper based reporting, and suggest possible functional enhancements for DHIS Mobile solutions. All interviews and focus group sessions were audio recorded. Selected parts of the extensive audio material were transcribed and coded by each of the researchers separately to allow for subsequent negotiation of shared interpretations. For the most part, our analysis of empirical material was guided by the notion of bootstrapping. Data were analysed to highlight conformance to, and deviation from, the bootstrapping strategy.

4. EMPIRICAL CASE

The pilots involve multiple stakeholders with varying interests and priorities. Key players include health personnel at health facility level, managers at district health office level, the Ministry of Health headquarters, the University of Oslo's MobiHealth project, and mobile service providers in Malawi, a DHIS implementation team based at the Malawi College of Medicine, and a team of postgraduate students who are leading DHIS Mobile pilot implementations. All activities concerning the DHIS Mobile pilots in Malawi are supported financially by MobiHealth. The DHIS implementation team is responsible for all DHIS2 implementation and maintenance related tasks, which among others include system customisation, management of the national DHIS2 server, and end-user training. The Ministry of Health did not have sufficient IT expertise to manage the national DHIS server and other mundane IT tasks. For example, the ministry relied on a different government agency for IT support. Until the end of 2012, the ministry only had one resident IT officer, in the professional grade.

4.1. Planning and Running of the DHIS Mobile Pilots

After consultations with key stakeholders at Ministry of Health, district health office, and health facility levels it was decided that DHIS Mobile solutions be rolled-out in December 2011. The pilots were to start with supporting monthly reporting for only two datasets, HMIS-15 and Integrated Disease Surveillance and Response (IDSR). IDSR monitors epidemic prone diseases, such as Cholera,

and diseases targeted for eradication. HMIS-15 on the other hand contains summary data from all health services delivered at health facilities.

When planning was done, we bought twenty Nokia C2-00 phones from India. This phone model was chosen because it supports two SIM cards. That way, participants in our pilots could use own SIM cards together with those provided as part of the pilots. We decided to buy phones for health facilities participating in our pilots because not all would-be end-users had phones with support for GPRS, which was a necessity for the DHIS Mobile pilots. Figure 2 depicts some of the phones owned by participants in our pilots.

After buying the Nokia C2-00 phones, we planned end-user training and roll-out of the pilots for December 2011. However, we suffered a setback because we could not get the phones configured for internet connectivity in Malawi. Even technical personnel from the mobile service operator we had subscribed to, were unable to resolve the connectivity problems. The phones did not support manual packet data configuration and neither could they get automated configuration settings from the operator's side. Our roll-out efforts were consequently postponed for two months, during which we bought twenty five Nokia C1-01 phones, nine from Malawi and sixteen from Norway. Reasons behind the purchase of phones from Norway and India were cost related. The cost of buying phones was significantly higher in Malawi than in India and Norway. Making cost savings prompted our mother project, MobiHealth, to buy some phones from India and Norway.

In February and March 2013, our team conducted end-user trainings and went live with the pilots. Participants in the pilots were given mobile phones and support for Internet connectivity and voice calls. Support for voice calls was pegged at an equivalent of $9 at the time of implementation, but had reduced to $4 at the time of writing, due to weakening of the local currency. We decided not to revise the amounts upwards in line with our intentions to gradually transfer the responsibility for payment for voice calls to participating health

Figure 2. Participants' mobile devices at a training session in Malawi

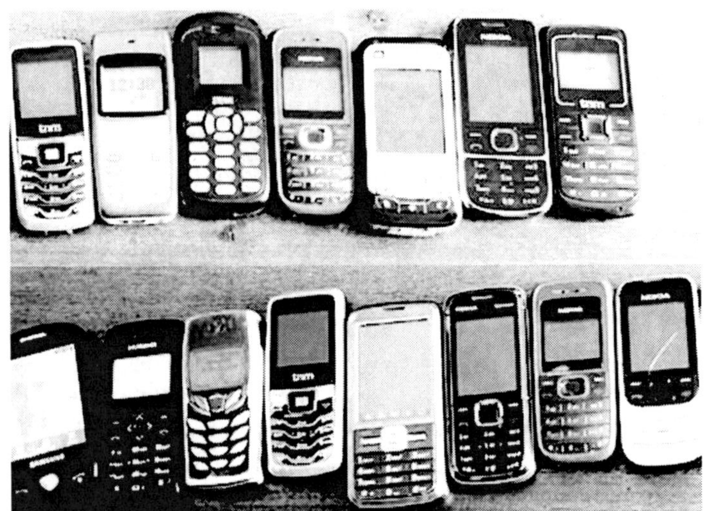

facilities. It was thought that through this we could reduce reliance on external support.

For the pilots we adopted a post-paid mobile service subscription arrangement. The main driving factor behind such an arrangement was that we would only have to deal with the mobile service operator with regard to maintaining monthly subscriptions. With a pre-paid subscription we would have had to manage phone credit transfer to the participants ourselves. A second factor was that Internet connectivity was going to be more expensive had we opted for a pre-paid subscription arrangement. Internet data bundles that fit with the low data demands of our pilots had short validity periods, lasting between one and five days. A third reason for us choosing a post-paid subscription arrangement was our intention to get summaries on Internet data usage, as part of our research. This could not have been possible with a pre-paid arrangement.

4.2. Challenges Faced and Persistent Risks

Progress on DHIS 2 national scale-up remained slow from the start of our pilots until mid-way through 2012. During this period the Ministry of Health lacked funding to support the scale-up process, which required enhancement of poor network infrastructure and provision of stable Internet connectivity at district level. There was also need for training of assistant statisticians at district level and members of district health management teams across the country's twenty eight districts. Unlike with DHIS 1.3, a desktop software solution, reliable Internet connectivity was necessary for districts to ably access the online national DHIS 2 server.

Stalling of the migration efforts from DHIS 1.3 to DHIS 2 negatively impacted DHIS Mobile pilots in at least two ways. First, without DHIS 2 becoming the mainstream health management information system (HMIS) solution, DHIS Mobile solutions had limited significance in the larger HMIS setup. Second, the Central Monitoring and Evaluation Division (CMED) of the Ministry of Health which was responsible for the HMIS function was also still on DHIS 1.3, which meant that districts submitting reports to CMED had to do so in DHIS 1.3 compliant format. In addition to these factors, being PhD students, our time was split between Malawi and Norway, meaning that we were, at times, unavailable on the ground to attend to certain problems arising within the pilots.

Furthermore, our studies demanded that we split our time between fieldwork and working towards producing scientific publications, putting us under constant time pressure.

Mobile service delivery, especially with regard to the management of our post-paid subscription on the mobile operator side, also negatively impacted our pilots. At the beginning of each month the operator was supposed to credit participants' phone accounts with call credit, but this process was far from smooth. With the post-paid arrangement users could not top-up their call credit, as is the case with pre-paid subscriptions. Users could also not get queries resolved by the mobile service operator without our involvement, as we were the account managers. When these problems persisted some users just took out the SIM cards we had provided and used their own SIM cards, some from a different service provider. In the end, we decided to switch to a pre-paid subscription arrangement. This would allow participants in the pilots to top-up own call credit, and resolve issues with the mobile service provider without our constant involvement. However, before doing this we had to negotiate with the mobile service operator for a deal allowing the validity period of Internet data bundles we would purchase to last a month, instead of between three and five days. We also had an option to directly pay the mobile service provider for the usual monthly call credit we sent to participants in the pilots and have the service provider manage credit transfers to their phone accounts, together with Internet bundles. The switch to the pre-paid arrangement was made at the start of February 2013.

4.3. Looking Ahead

Towards the end of the year 2012, the Ministry of Health recruited a Technical Assistant (TA), with support from International Training and Education Centre for Health (I-TECH). The TA's task was to oversee IT implementations and policy formulation. We also engaged another TA, in collaboration with the ministry, with the support of MobiHealth. The TA was made responsible for supporting our pilots and other electronic health projects within the ministry. We engaged the second TA to contribute towards development of local capacity as well as ensure constant availability of end-user support for participants in the pilots.

At the time of writing, we were working towards expanding coverage of our pilots to the whole of Lilongwe district. Efforts were also underway to increase the number of supported datasets, based on feedback gathered during review meetings:

The future looks promising, but if possible it would be good to add other datasets, such as those for antenatal care and maternal health. Since this [only supporting two datasets] was like an introduction, we should be moving forward; we cannot stay at the same place. (Statistical Clerk, 2013)

We should also consider some other parts [datasets] …when one is involved in other programmes [whose datasets are not part of the implemented solutions] he/she still has to travel to the district [health office]. (Health Surveillance Assistant - IDSR, 2013)

Some participants in the pilots were responsible for other datasets that were not yet supported, meaning travel to district health offices, for report submission, was inevitable. However, extending coverage to more datasets is dependent upon integration of the national DHIS 2 installation with existing parallel health programme specific reporting solutions. The encouraging news is that despite challenges faced earlier, DHIS 2 scale-up efforts have progressed. Trainings have been conducted in all districts and efforts to strengthen Internet connectivity at district level are close to finalisation.

Beyond our mHealth pilots, we are actively participating in the "mHealth Malawi" forum, which brings together different stakeholders doing mHealth in Malawi. Among other reasons, the grouping was established to deal with the problem of multiple small scales mHealth pilots, which although having similarities did not collaborate. Chaired by the Ministry of Health, the grouping seeks to foster collaboration between members, develop guidelines to regulate future mHealth activities, as well as build on economies of scale in dealing with mobile service providers. Just like us, most members have reported facing challenges when negotiating service arrangements with mobile service providers, individually.

5. DISCUSSION

The empirical case presented in this paper suggests that bootstrapping technological innovations requires coordination of efforts across organisational and geographical boundaries. Envisaging the level of complexity and risk inherent in such a setup we decided early on in our implementation efforts to use bootstrapping as a sensitising lens to minimise implementation related risks. Despite making such a choice early on, the case portrays aspects that both comply with, and deviate from, the bootstrapping strategy.

5.1. Following the Bootstrapping Strategy

In compliance with the strategy, our DHIS Mobile pilots were preceded by efforts to understand existing data collection and communication work practices, as well as gain buy-in from key stakeholders, such as the Ministry of Health, Lilongwe District Health Office, and personnel from health facilities. We also sought to understand existing communications infrastructure and its influence on paper-based data reporting and potential influence on our pilots. This helped us to place our solutions for increased relevance and minimize contradiction of the installed base. For example, our solutions addressed important user concerns such as the need to circumvent transportation by enabling remote

submission of reports. Our understanding of the implementation context also made it possible for us to provide participants in our pilots with mobile phones capable of supporting Internet data. Usage of a single phone model (Nokia C1-01) for the pilots also avoided the complexity of supporting different phone models. These steps correspond with the bootstrapping strategy's recommendation to, as much as possible, build on the installed base, rather than contradict it (Aanestad & Jensen, 2011; Hanseth & Aanestad, 2003; Skorve & Aanestad, 2010). Furthermore, the logic followed here echoes observations from related research that mHealth involves the convergence of heterogeneous socio-technical arrangements, which include information systems, people and healthcare processes, and available technology options, among others (Yu, et al., 2006).

Our pilot strategy also aligns with the bootstrapping strategy in that we started by supporting the critical but less complex task of routine health data reporting. Introducing the use of mobile phones mainly as a data transportation mechanism does not require radical changes in the way people work, in order to accommodate the solutions under pilot. The current use of mobile phones for data reporting mostly compliments, rather than contradicts, existing socio-technical arrangements for data communication. In addition, routine health data reporting is vital to health service delivery, which makes our solutions immediately relevant to stakeholders at various levels of administration.

The decision not to go ahead with a big bang approach, where we would have rolled out DHIS Mobile solutions to all health facilities, also proved beneficial. Starting small facilitated our learning process from implementation decisions taken and challenges faced. Learning from on-going experiences is vital towards improvement of information technology innovations (Hanseth & Lyytinen, 2004, 2010). Table 1 depicts how we made use of the bootstrapping strategy, by showing actions taken, and related compliance to the bootstrapping strategy.

Table 1. Applying the bootstrapping strategy

Action Taken	Way of Compliance with the bootstrapping strategy	Stage in Pilots
Change from big bang approach to starting with implementation in two health areas	Incremental progress, minimizing impact of unintended breakdowns	Action planning
Minimizing mobile phone heterogeneity among participants by buying phones for the pilots	• Minimizing complexity by limiting device heterogeneity • Strengthening the weak installed base of phones, where some participants had no phones with GPRS support	Action planning

Starting with supporting monthly routine data reporting	• Looking for Immediate relevance:
	  o supporting an important task in the HMIS setup – reporting
	  o Trying to minimize transportation challenges
	  o Minimizing need for travel during report submissions – could allow healthcare practitioners more time at health facilities
	• Supporting a critical but less complex task first
		Action planning and implementation

Starting with supporting only two datasets	Avoiding complexity that would have resulted from supporting multiple datasets that are often handled by different departments/ individuals	Action planning and implementation
Subsidizing Internet connectivity and voice calls	• Subsidizing costs of first adopters • Providing an incentive by supporting voice calls	Action planning and implementation
Making arrangements for post-paid mobile service subscription – only one point for settling phone bills	Minimizing the need for our team to manage credit transfers to participants in the pilots	Action planning and implementation
Shifting from a poorly working post-paid subscription arrangement to a pre-paid arrangement	• Minimizing breakdowns from the mobile service operator's inability to timely top-up participants' phone credit • Providing participants with an opportunity to top-up own phone credit • Flexibility in service subscription strategy – applying lessons learned	• Evaluation • Improvement of pilots
Negotiating for Internet bundles with short validity periods to last a month under the pre-paid arrangement	Maintaining control on Internet subscription	• Evaluation • Improvement of pilots

From the table it can also be noted that we tried to minimize complexity and risk of failure by: starting with supporting only two datasets; providing additional incentives to the participants in the DHIS Mobile pilots through subsidizing Internet connectivity and voice calls; making arrangements for post-paid mobile service subscription, so we could have the mobile service operator manage call credit transfers to participants in the pilots. However, the shift to a pre-paid arrangement, later on, demonstrates flexibility in our implementation strategy, as well as an application of lessons learned. This fits with arguments from earlier application of the bootstrapping strategy advancing incremental build upon the installed base, whilst minimizing complexity, and learning from emergent developments in the implementation of technological innovations (Hanseth & Aanestad, 2001, 2003; Hanseth & Lyytinen, 2010; Skorve & Aanestad, 2010). Despite these achievements, it should be noted that not all implementation factors at play can be reconciled nor can all competing stakeholder interests be aligned.

5.2. Challenges to Walking the Bootstrapping Path

The case demonstrates lack of sufficient technical expertise within the Ministry of Health in Malawi to fully support existing technological solutions.

For example, the Ministry is reliant on the DHIS implementation team, based at the Malawi College of Medicine, which is external to the ministry, to lead DHIS2 rollout in the country. The ministry also relies on a different government agency for IT support. This, coupled with dependence on external sources of funding to drive information technology initiatives, requires extensive coordination between stakeholders. Such a setup also introduces multiple points of possible failure, making it harder to bootstrap novel solutions. This situation supports arguments by Lucas (2008) that information technology implementations in developing countries are heavily dependent on external support (Lucas, 2008). Consequently, failure in such external dependencies can be costly to implementations (Schmidt, et al., 2001).

The relevance of cross-organisational arrangements in the bootstrapping of technological innovations is also highlighted by inconsistencies in the quality of mobile service delivery, especially with regard to the post-paid subscription arrangement we had. This is a factor over which the research team managing the pilots in Malawi has little control. Challenges we have encountered with regard to mobile service delivery place the mobile service operator more in the foreground of our routine operations, than is necessary. At the same time only having two major mobile service operators limits our choices, making it harder for us to correct present inefficiencies. These challenges demonstrate inherent complexity in infrastructure initiatives, resulting from heterogeneity of socio-technical arrangements and divergent stakeholder interests (Hanseth & Lyytinen, 2010; Ribes & Finholt, 2009). An integral part of such a setup is multiplicity of competing, cooperating, converging and diverging composite socio-technical subsystems (Constantinides & Barrett, 2005; Garci´a-Marco, 2011; Hanseth & Lyytinen, 2010). Such complexity entails that outcomes from infrastructure initiatives cannot be deterministic but nonlinear, requiring constant negotiation across time scales to push towards desired outcomes (Baker & Bowker, 2007). Table 2 depicts a summary of challenges that made adherence to the bootstrapping strategy challenging, alongside contributing factors.

Table 2. Challenges in adhering to the bootstrapping strategy

Challenge	Tactics deviating from the bootstrapping strategy	contributing factors
Buying Nokia C2-00 phones from outside the implementation context, before ascertaining availability of support	• Building on technology that had not been tested locally • We could not readily access the supplier when challenges emerged	Better utilization of MobiHealth project funds when buying phones – striking a balance between local and cross-context needs

Lack of local IT capacity	• Reliance on teams external to the Ministry of Health for IT support, resulting in:
	  o increased coordination complexity
	  o The ministry being in less control of on-going implementations
		• Historically weak IT capacity
		• Reliance on different government agency for IT support

Reliance on external financial support from multiple development partners	• Increased complexity, resulting from:
	  o heterogeneity of stakeholder interests
	  o increased coordination complexity
		Historically weak local financial base

Quality of mobile service delivery	Having a key enabling component in the pilots outside our control	• Enabling socio-technical arrangements span across organisations and industrial sectors • Mobile service delivery is an industry on its own, so we have to rely on what is already there • Limited choices available with regard to mobile service delivery

The table suggests that factors significantly influencing the implementation of technological innovations can either be within or outside the immediate control of solution implementers (Schmidt, et al., 2001). Having an increased number of factors outside the control of implementers and managers of technological innovations is bound to significantly increase the take-off challenges for novel technologies which the bootstrapping strategy seeks to minimize.

5.3. Multi-Stakeholder Involvement and Associated Risks

In multi-stakeholder initiatives, such as the DHIS Mobile pilots, it is critical that we map key stakeholders; key roles they play; risks inherent in their involvement, over the long-term; and possible steps that can be taken to correct identified risks. Table 3 presents a summary of such dynamics.

Stakeholder roles, associated risks, and possible corrections of identified risks need to be continuously reviewed over the course of interventions. Where possible, it is vital to minimize external dependencies, as failures in such arrangement negatively influence technological innovations (Schmidt, et al., 2001). Minimizing risks inherent in having multiple external dependencies can help address take-off challenges of innovations such as the DHIS Mobile pilots, as well as enhance their institutionalisation (Silva & Backhouse, 1997).

6. CONCLUSION

In this paper we have discussed how we applied bootstrapping as a sensitizing lens in the planning, implementation, and evaluation of mHealth solutions for routine health data reporting in Malawi. Informed by conceptualisations on information infrastructure we applied the bootstrapping strategy to highlight risks inherent in multi-stakeholder interventions that span not only organisational boundaries, but also industrial and geographical ones. The pilots in Malawi are funded by the MobiHealth project at the University of Oslo, have the Ministry of Health, in Malawi, as a host organisation, and rely on mobile service delivery by a commercial provider. The Ministry of Health, in Malawi, also relies on external consultants for technical support. Our application of the bootstrapping strategy suggests that adherence to the bootstrapping strategy can enhance mitigation of unintended consequences that emerge in the implementation of technological innovations. Beyond this, our empirical material suggests that in interventions that involve heterogeneous socio-technical arrangements it may be quite challenging to adhere to the bootstrapping strategy. Some arrangements that significantly influence implementations may be outside the immediate control of solution implementers. Our dependence on problematic mobile service delivery arrangements are a good example of this.

In highlighting the significance of risk in our pilots we demonstrate that weaknesses of the Ministry of Health to adequately support new information technology solutions, both financially and technically, mean that significant alliances with multiple implementation partners cannot be done away with easily. It has been argued in this paper that the nature of such alliances functions in ways that enable or constrain bootstrapping of novel solutions. For example, divergent stakeholder interests require negotiation and there is an increased need for coordination in multi-stakeholder initiatives. All this increases the potential for failure in the event that stakeholder relationships and dependences fail. Successful bootstrapping of novel information technology solutions, therefore, requires effective management of stakeholder linkages. There is need to negotiate access and control to key parts of the existing socio-technical arrangements that must be leveraged, with stakeholders who although in control of

Table 3. Stakeholders roles, enabling role and risk for long-term sustainability

Stakeholder	Key Role	Risk	Correction
Ministry of Health	Parent hosting organisation for the DHIS Mobile pilots	• Weak IT capacity • Weak financial capacity to scale and support DHIS Mobile pilots, when MobiHealth withdraws support	Recent recruitment of Technical Assistants with support from ITEC and MobiHealth – this is however externally supported
District Health offices	Hosts for the DHIS Mobile pilots	• Weak IT capacity • Concerns for Internet connectivity to provide stable access to DHIS 2, which is an enabler for DHIS Mobile • Weak financial capacity to scale and support DHIS Mobile pilots, when MobiHealth withdraw support	Strengthening of local networks and Internet connectivity as part of DHIS 2 scale-up
Health facilities	• Principal users of DHIS Mobile solutions • This is where daily use of the solutions takes place – demonstrating relevance and securing buy in at this level is critical	Weak IT and financial capacity to support own scale up efforts	• Using server based solutions with limited or no application installation on the client side • Subsidizing costs for first set of adopters • Using GPRS solutions, as internet data is affordable • Demonstrating relevance with regard to enhancing reporting, so users would be willing to fund own mobile phone usage
DHIS Implementation team	Champions of on-going DHIS 2 efforts- DHIS2 customization, national server hosting, DHIS 2 capacity development, leading local area network and Internet connectivity strengthening at district level	External entity, loosely attached to the Ministry of Health and externally funded to support the ministry	Need for long-term funding and work arrangements
DHIS Mobile team	• Leading DHIS Mobile pilots • Providing technical advice on DHIS 2 efforts	• Project based arrangement • Externally funded • Mostly PhD students who also have to attend to own academic requirements	Recruitment of a Technical assistant resident, to work under the Ministry of Health
MobiHealth	• Funding DHIS Mobile pilots • Developing and supporting DHIS Mobile software	• A project based arrangement • International project with need to balance cross-context interests – some decisions taken might negatively impact pilots in Malawi, e.g buying phones from India	• Recruitment of Technical assistant residents in Malawi – one year arrangement • Need for identification of long-term funding arrangements • Developing arrangements that focus on the long-term, e.g involvement of Malawian PhD students in DHIS Mobile pilots and other related efforts
Mobile service operator	Providing platform for utilization of mobile technology – providing network connectivity, mobile services, managing subscriptions	• Erratic quality of service delivery • Hard to control – beyond our jurisdiction • Hard to control – large mobile service operator with large customer base, so our small pilots seem not to matter much	Better customer support, **but this is beyond our control**
Structuring of mobile service industry	Promoting better and competitive service delivery	Only two major mobile service operators, so choices for the customer are significantly reduced	Having more service providers, **but this is beyond our control**
Other mHealth implementations	• Sharing expertise and equipment • Economies of scale when dealing with operators	Varied interests, funding arrangements, and implementation strategies	• Creation of the mHealth Malawi forum – co-chaired by the Ministry of Health • Development of guidelines to guide future mHealth activities

such parts are not part of the target user community. This suggests that if mHealth solutions are to become an integral part of wider health information system setups they should not be developed and promoted as standalone solutions. Unfortunately, such is often the case.

Our application of bootstrapping to reflect on risks of potential failure in IT implementations, resulting from failures in external dependences, contributes to its theoretical applications. Previous application of the strategy focused on resource maximisation (Hanseth & Aanestad, 2001), mutual learning (Hanseth & Lyytinen, 2010), complexity mitigation in negotiating heterogeneous work arrangements (Skorve & Aanestad, 2010), and modular implementation and stakeholder mobilization (Aanestad & Jensen, 2011), to raise growth momentum of novel solutions.

ACKNOWLEDGMENT

We are very grateful to all members of MobiHealth, the Ministry of Health in Malawi, all pilot study participants, Kristin Braa, Margunn Aanestad, and our working group at the 35th IRIS seminar, for their valuable contributions.

REFERENCES

Aanestad, M., & Jensen, T. B. (2011). Building nation-wide information infrastructures in healthcare through modular implementation strategies. *The Journal of Strategic Information Systems*, *20*(2), 161–176. doi:10.1016/j.jsis.2011.03.006

AbouZah, C., & Boerma, T. (2005). Health information systems: The foundations of public health. *Bulletin of the World Health Organization*, *83*(8), 578–583. PMID:16184276

Baker, K., & Bowker, G. (2007). Information ecology: open system environment for data, memories, and knowing. *Journal of Intelligent Information Systems*, *29*(1), 127–144. doi:10.1007/s10844-006-0035-7

Bowker, G., Baker, K., Millerand, F., & Ribes, D. (2010). Toward information infrastructure studies: Ways of knowing in a networked environment. In J. Hunsinger, L. Klastrup, & M. Allen (Eds.), *International handbook of internet research* (pp. 97–117). Springer Netherlands. doi:10.1007/978-1-4020-9789-8_5

Braa, K., & Nielsen, P. (2013, May 19-22). Leveraging the potential of mobiles in developing country health initiatives: From ICT4D to information infrastructures 4D. In *Proceedings of the IFIP Working Group 9.4, 12th International Conference on Social Implications of Computers in Developing Countries*, Sunset Jamaica Grande, Ocho Rios, Jamaica.

Constantinides, P., & Barrett, M. (2005). Approaching information infrastructure as an ecology of ubiquitous sociotechnical relations. In C. Sørensen, Y. Yoo, K. Lyytinen, & J. DeGross (Eds.), *Designing ubiquitous information environments: Socio-technical issues and challenges* (Vol. 185, pp. 249–260). Springer, US. doi:10.1007/0-387-28918-6_19

Coryn, C. L. S., Noakes, L. A., Westine, C. D., & Schröter, D. C. (2011). A systematic review of theory-driven evaluation practice from 1990 to 2009. *The American Journal of Evaluation*, *32*(2), 199–226. doi:10.1177/1098214010389321

Davison, R. M., Martinsons, M. G., & Kock, N. (2004). Principals of canonical action research. *Information Systems Journal*, *14*, 65–86. doi:10.1111/j.1365-2575.2004.00162.x

Edwards, P. N., Jackson, S. J., Bowker, G. C., & Knobel, C. (2007). Understanding infrastructure: Dynamics, tensions, and design. *NSF Report of a Workshop: History and theory of infrastructure: Lessons for new scientific cyberinfrastructures.* Retrieved from http://deepblue.lib.umich.edu/handle/2027.42/49353

Garcı'a-Marco, F.-J. (2011). Libraries in the digital ecology: Reflections and trends. *The Electronic Library, 29*(1), 105–120. doi:10.1108/02640471111111460

Hanseth, O., & Aanestad, M. (2001). Bootstrapping networks, communities and infrastructures. On the evolution of ICT solutions in health care. In *Proceedings of the ITHC*, Erasmus University, Rotterdam, The Netherlands. Retrieved from http://heim.ifi.uio.no/~oleha/Publications/On%20the%20evolution%20of%20telemedicine%20networks4.pdf

Hanseth, O., & Aanestad, M. (2003). Design as bootstrapping: On the evolution of ICT networks in health care. *Methods of Information in Medicine, 42*(4), 385–391. PMID:14534638

Hanseth, O., & Lyytinen, K. (2004). Theorizing about the design of Information Infrastructures: Design kernel theories and principles. *Sprouts: Working Papers on Information Systems, 4*(12). Retrieved from http://sprouts.aisnet.org/4-12

Hanseth, O., & Lyytinen, K. (2010). Design theory for dynamic complexity in information infrastructures: The case of building internet. *Journal of Information Technology, 25*(1), 1–19. doi:10.1057/jit.2009.19

Heeks, R. (2002). Information systems and developing countries: Failure, success, and local improvisations. *The Information Society, 18*(2), 101–112. doi:10.1080/01972240290075039

Hughes, T. P. (1987). The evolution of large technological systems. In W. E. Bijker, T. P. Hughes, & T. Pinch (Eds.), *The social construction of technological systems* (Vol. 2, pp. 52–81). MIT Press.

Lippeveld, T. (2001, March 14-16). Routine health information systems: The glue of a unified health system. In *Proceedings of the The RHINO Workshop on Issues and Innovation in Routine Health Information in Developing Countries*, The Bolger Center, Potomac, MD.

Lucas, H. (2008). Information and communications technology for future health systems in developing countries. *Social Science & Medicine, 66*(10), 2122–2132. doi:10.1016/j.socscimed.2008.01.033 PMID:18343005

Mechael, P., Batavia, H., Kaonga, N., Searle, S., Kwan, A., Goldberger, A., et al. (2010). *Barriers and gaps affecting mhealth in low and middle income countries: Policy white paper.* Center for global health and economic development earth institute, Columbia University.

Ribes, D., & Finholt, T. A. (2009). The long now of technology infrastructure: Articulating tensions in development. *Journal of the Association for Information Systems, 10*(5), 375–398.

Schmidt, R., Lyytinen, K., Keil, M., & Cule, P. (2001). Identifying software project risks: An international Delphi study. *Journal of Management Information Systems, 17*(4), 5–36.

Scott, J. E., & Vessey, I. (2002). Managing risks in enterprise systems implementations. *Communications of the ACM, 45*(4), 74–81. doi:10.1145/505248.505249

Silva, L., & Backhouse, J. (1997). Becoming part of the furniture: The institutionalization of information systems. In *Proceedings of the IFIP TC8 WG 8.2 International Conference on Information Systems and Qualitative Research*, Philadelphia, PA.

Skorve, E., & Aanestad, M. (2010). Bootstrapping revisited: Opening the black box of organizational implementation. In K. Kautz & P. Nielsen (Eds.), *Scandinavian information systems research* (Vol. 60, pp. 111–126). Springer Berlin Heidelberg. doi:10.1007/978-3-642-14874-3_8

Star, S. L., & Ruhleder, K. (1996). Steps toward and ecology of infrastructure: Design and access for large information spaces. *Information Systems Research, 7*(1), 111–134. doi:10.1287/isre.7.1.111

Walsham, G. (2006). Doing interpretive research. *European Journal of Information Systems, 15*, 320–330. doi:10.1057/palgrave.ejis.3000589

Yu, P., Wu, M. X., Yu, H., & Xiao, G. C. (2006, June 21-23). The challenges for the adoption of m-health. In *Proceedings of the IEEE International Conference on Service Operations and Logistics and Informatics (SOLI 2006)*, Shanghai, China.

Chapter 13
Giving Up Smoking Using SMS Messages on your Mobile Phone

Silvia Cacho-Elizondo
IPADE Business Schoolm, France

Niousha Shahidi
EDC Paris Business School, France

Vesselina Tossan
CNAM, France & EDC Paris Business School, France

ABSTRACT

The current tendency to use cell phones or other mobile devices for healthcare purposes offers a huge opportunity to improve public health worldwide. In that direction, mobile devices make it easier to offer coaching services through text/video messages, to support individuals trying to break addictions such as smoking. Given that use of such services is still low in France and other countries, it is important to have greater understanding of what leads users to adopt them. Therefore, we propose and validate an explanatory model for the intention to adopt a mobile coaching service to help people to stop smoking. This chapter uses the concepts of vicarious innovativeness, social influence, perceived monetary value, perceived enjoyment, and perceived irritation.

INTRODUCTION

Addictions to tobacco, alcohol, drugs, over-eating, caffeine and pathological gambling are a serious problem for society. Breaking the habit takes enormous willpower, and in many cases the help of therapists or support groups. The rising popularity of smartphones, has led to a dramatic increase in mobile services through apps. The current tendency to use cell phones or other mobile devices for health offers a very interesting opportunity to improve public health worldwide (Stanford Social Innovation Review, 2011). One such service could provide support for giving up smoking. According to the report of PwC (2013), by 2017, mHealth has the potential to save 2.6 billion EUR by helping people quit smoking. This type of service is relatively new in France, hence the relevance of studying the profile of potential adopters.

DOI: 10.4018/978-1-4666-8756-1.ch013

In France, almost 66,000 deaths each year are directly attributable to smoking (5 million in the World), which is the primary cause of avoidable premature death, and the problem of nicotine addiction continues to grow despite efforts to curb it (INPES, 2007). Across the whole French population aged 15-75, the proportion of daily smokers rose from 26.9% to 28.7% between 2005 and 2010, and cigarette sales saw a slight upturn between 2008 and 2009 (from 53.6 billion to 55 billion packets) after dropping significantly between 2001 and 2004 (from 82.5 billion to 54.9 billion, due to substantial increases in the price of tobacco products). However the proportion of smokers that smoke more than ten cigarettes a day is diminishing. The French smokers are usually very young and represent 50% of the smoker people (about 94% of the smokers in EU start smoking before they turn 25). Considering 15 million of French smokers (more than 100 million in the world), more than half would like to stop smoking. Only 750 000 (5% of the smoker people) people stop smoking each year. More than 2 million of smokers used skin patches, nicotine substitute or pharmacological processing in 2010.

Tobacco companies are investing in a new generation of smokeless alternatives to cigarettes as the industry faces growing regulatory threats across the globe. The world's four biggest tobacco companies outside China –Philip Morris International, British American Tobacco, Japan Tobacco International and Imperial Tobacco – are positioning themselves for an increasingly smoke-free future as they seek to entice smokers to non-combustible substitutes such as electronic cigarettes, tobacco vaporizers and nicotine inhalers over the next decade (Wembridge & Thompson, 2012). Nevertheless, the benefits of electronic cigarettes are still controversial. Coaching people to avoid taking a cigarette or an e-cigarette seems to be a better option. According to PcW estimates, out of the 102 million smokers, 48.8 million can potentially use mHealth solutions regularly and 3.9 million smokers could quit smoking successfully.

Since January 2010, Health & Human Services (HHS) has invested $5 million dollars to develop its eHealth/mHealth smoking cessation resources aimed at increasing quitting attempts among teens, young adults and adults (Merill, 2011a).

This chapter concerns a mobile coaching service providing support for people trying to stop smoking. The service takes the form of short text messages (SMS or MMS) sent to cell phones to help individuals in a range of situations or anti-smoking activities. The principal objective of this study is to identify drivers fostering the intention to adopt such a service in the young smokers segment in France. The chapter is structured as follows. Firstly, the conceptual framework is presented and after that the model of the intention to adopt the mobile coaching service is introduced. The methodology is then described along with the operationalization of the underlying hypotheses. After reporting the main findings and managerial and social implications, the chapter concludes by considering limitations and avenues for future research.

CONCEPTUAL FRAMEWORK

The effectiveness of a mobile coaching service has already been tested in various countries, including New Zealand where a program to stop smoking was developed and tried out (Whittaker et al., 2008). But such mobile coaching services are relatively little used in France, and this is why they are considered as an innovation for the purposes of this study. Several definitions of an innovation have been proposed. The one used here is by Rogers (1962), who defines an innovation as an idea, practice or object perceived as new by the individual. Diffusion of an innovation is the process by which it is communicated through certain channels over time among the members of a social system (Rogers, 1962). Rogers identifies three factors that explain how an innovation spreads and is adopted: 1) the characteristics of the product or service, 2) the characteristics of consumers and 3) the profiles of different adopter categories through the innovation diffusion process.

Adoption of an innovation can be defined as the initial purchase or repeated purchase of the innovation, depending on the context. For frequent-purchase products, repetition of the purchase is necessary to consider a product adopted, and the threshold of three purchases appears to be an acceptable threshold for judging whether a product has been adopted by the consumer (Cestre, 1996), whereas for durable goods and services, adoption is generally considered to take place from the very first purchase, regardless of regular use or replacement purchases (Le Nagard-Assayag & Manceau, 2011). Gatignon and Robertson (1985) propose a general model of innovation diffusion, taking the conceptual bases proposed by Rogers (1983) (which include the concept of innovation, diffusion over time, influence of interpersonal communication and opinion leaders, the adoption process, the role of innovators and other adopter categories, and the social system in which the diffusion takes place) and adding the influence of marketing campaigns and competitors' actions.

D'Hauteville (1994) develops an attitudinal model of factors that enhance the acceptability of an innovation for consumers that he seeks to explain not only by consumer characteristics but also by product attributes. His empirical studies confirm the results of other studies on innovation, particularly the finding of Ostlund (1974) that perceived attributes play a decisive, more important role in the acceptability of a new product than individual variables, including the specific variable of innovativeness. He also confirms the predominant role of consumer habits in forming attitudes.

Consumer Innovativeness

The concept of consumer innovativeness is not unanimously accepted among researchers (Cestre, 1996; Masson, 2010). Some (Hurt, Joseph & Cook, 1977; Foxall & Haskins, 1986; Venkatraman & Price, 1990) see it as a core personality trait, possessed to varying degrees by all individuals. Midgley and Dowling (1993), Roehrich (1994) and Le Louarn (1997) consider it at the level of all consumer products as a consumer's *generalized unobservable predisposition to purchase new products and brands* rather than sticking to habitual choices and models (Midgley & Dowling, 1993). Others (Goldsmith & Hofacker, 1991; Goldsmith, d'Hauteville & Flynn, 1998) see innovativeness at the level of a product category as a combination of personality traits and attitudes.

For Subin, Mason and Houston(2007), empirical studies paint an inconsistent picture of the relationship between the consumer's innovative predisposition and an innovative behavior (adoption of a new product). They demonstrate that innate innovativeness does not influence adoption behavior *directly*, but *indirectly* through two of the three components of indirect or vicarious innovativeness (defined later), namely modeling and involvement in word of mouth, but not exposure to advertising.

Hirschman (1980) identifies three types of innovativeness: *adoptive innovativeness*, *indirect innovativeness* or *vicarious innovativeness* and *use innovativeness*. Adoptive innovativeness concerns the actual adoption of a new product. Vicarious innovativeness can be defined as *openness to information on new products of any kind*. This vicarious innovativeness is followed by adoptive innovativeness when consumers actually adopt the product. Finally, use innovativeness involves solving consumer problems with products already available to the consumer. In other words, the consumer invents new uses for an existing product. For the purposes of this study the focus is on the vicarious innovativeness specific to a given field, i.e. the consumer's attitude to new services, namely *mobile coaching services via cell phone*.

Intention to Adopt the Mobile Coaching Service

It is established that intention is a good predictor of actual behavior (Davis, Bagozzi & Warshaw 1989; Ajzen, 1991; Venkatesh & Brown, 2001). Intention is determined by the attitudes to that behavior, and by subjective norms (Ajzen & Fishbein, 1980). Subjective norms relate to the way the subject perceives the opinion of people important to him/her about his/her decision to engage or not engage in a certain behavior. When an information technology-based service is in the early stages of diffusion, as is the case for mobile coaching services to help people stop smoking, the intention to adopt appears a more appropriate object of study than adoptive behavior (Hong & Tam, 2006). This is why we seek to explain the intention to adopt rather than adoptive behavior.

The Technology Acceptance Model (TAM) constructed by Davis (1989) is an adaptation of the theory of Reasoned Action (Fishbein & Ajzen, 1975) designed to model the intention to adopt information systems. Perceived usefulness is defined as the degree to which a person believes that using a particular technology would enhance his or her job performance (Davis, 1989). It determines both the attitude and the intention to use. The perceived ease-of-use is defined as the degree to which a person believes that understanding and using a particular technology would be free from effort (Davis, 1989). This leads the individual towards a perceived usefulness but also to an attitude that directly affects the intention to use (Davis, Bagozzi & Warshaw, 1989, p. 985).

Later, Hong & Tam (2006) showed that the perceived usefulness exercises a direct positive influence on the intention to adopt multi-purpose information services. Information services are devices or instruments that are used to supply users with various types of information: data, video, images (Bergman, 2000). Hong and Tam (2006) define multi-purpose information services as information technology (IT) artifacts that: 1) improve the personal, individual link with the user, 2) offer mobile services and 3) supply a suite of functions for both work and leisure needs. These authors also demonstrate that the perceived monetary value exerts a positive influence on the intention to adopt these services, and that the perceived enjoyment has a positive influence on the intention to adopt. Their study also confirms that the perceived enjoyment has a positive influence on perceived usefulness and perceived ease-of-use, and that social influence has a positive influence on the intention to adopt.

Explanatory Factors for the Intention to Adopt a Mobile Coaching Service and Hypotheses

- **Vicarious Innovativeness:** Vicarious innovativeness towards cell phone coaching services should influence the intention to adopt a specialist service such as help with stopping smoking. Therefore, we propose the following hypothesis:

H1: Vicarious innovativeness towards coaching services exerts a direct, positive influence on the intention to adopt a text-message based mobile coaching service to stop smoking.

Apart from the innovativeness related to the above field, other variables may influence the adoption process. In this study, we consider social influence, perceived monetary value, perceived enjoyment, perceived irritation and demographic profile. Future research could examine the influence of other variables.

- **Social Influence:** This is defined as the measure of a subject's belief of whether significant referents will approve or disapprove of the subject adopting a certain behavior (Ajzen, 1991).This social influence is exerted through messages and signals that help to form perceptions concerning the value of a product or activity (Venkatesh & Brown, 2001). Various studies confirm that peers, superiors and family members all influence consumer behavior and the decisions associated with adoption of products or services (Venkatesh & Brown, 2001; Hong & Tam, 2006).

In the theory of planned behavior, intention, as a determinant of behavior, is conditioned by attitude, subjective norms (or social influence) and perceived behavioral control, which is a kind of perceived ease of adoption (Ajzen, 1991). Mathieson (1991) developed a scale to measure this social influence that was used by Hong & Tam (2006) to demonstrate that social influence has a direct, positive effect on the intention to adopt mobile data services. They define such services as a set of digital data services accessed by a mobile device across a vast geographical zone that can be used to exchange messages, pictures and emails, check flight times, book concert tickets and play games, making no distinction between the services and the devices used to access them. Mobile coaching services, such as support with stopping smoking, are services in which messages of encouragement are sent at random intervals to users, and are therefore a specific category of mobile services. Based on past studies, we propose the following hypothesis:

H2: Social influence (SOCIAL) has a direct, positive effect on the intention to adopt a text-message based mobile coaching service to stop smoking.

- **Perceived Monetary Value:** Most consumers encode prices along a scale and classify products as "expensive" or "cheap" even when they are not familiar with the products concerned. This happens because individuals call on references associated with similar experiences. In general, consumers mentally consider the perceived quality and perceived sacrifice associated with a price. This consideration brings about a perceived monetary value in the consumer's mind, which has an effect on the consumer's intention to adopt a product (Dodds, Monroe, & Grewal, 1991).

When the consumer attaches high importance to the use value, he is willing to make a greater monetary sacrifice. If the consumer perceives the mobile coaching services as having a higher use value than other methods of stopping smoking then he will have the intention to adopt them. Based on these premises, we propose the following hypothesis:

H3: The perceived monetary value (MONEY) exerts a positive influence on the intention to adopt a text-message based mobile coaching service to stop smoking.

- **Perceived Enjoyment:** Seeking pleasurable, fun experiences is a typical personal desire (Rokeach, 1973). The value of enjoyment as regards use of an innovation is conceptualized as the extent to which use of an innovation is agreeable in itself, independently of the expected consequences of its performance. The variables of enjoyment and irritation are rooted in study of the affect and its influence on behavior in general and innovative behavior in particular. Several studies show that the perceived enjoyment value explains adoption of information technologies (Hong & Tam, 2006).

Venkatesh and Morris (2000) and Venkatesh and Brown (2001) argue in their research that perceived enjoyment can have an indirect impact on intention through the perceived ease-of-use. Hong and Tam (2006), meanwhile, suggest that services such as downloadable games, horoscopes or videos can help to pass the time agreeably while a person is waiting for a train. They show that the perceived enjoyment has a positive influence on the intention to adopt mobile data services. In this view, the "fun" aspect of the mobile service will facilitate its adoption and have a positive effect on attitudes. But other researchers such as Chowdhury et al. (2006) find that the influence exerted by perceived enjoyment on the attitude towards mobile advertising is negative and non-significant. To verify this, we propose the following hypothesis:

H4: The perceived enjoyment (ENJOY) exerts a positive influence on the intention to adopt a text-message based mobile coaching service to stop smoking.

- **Perceived Irritation:** Based on the fact that mobile advertising may be perceived by the consumer as invasive, irritating or boring, Chowdhury et al. (2006) propose a scale of perceived irritation, which is not the same thing as the absence of perceived enjoyment. They set out to demonstrate that this construct is negatively associated with the consumer's attitude to mobile advertising.

However, their research leads to the opposite finding, namely that the *influence of irritation on the attitude to mobile adverting is positive but non-significant*. As regards the intention to adopt a mobile coaching service for support while stopping smoking, this leads us to propose the following hypothesis:

H5: Perceived irritation (IRRITA) exerts a negative influence on the intention to adopt a text-message based mobile coaching service to stop smoking.

Considering the conceptual framework developed above, we propose the following model in Figure 1.

The following hypotheses compare different groups of individuals:

H6a: The intention to adopt the Mobile Coaching Service differs between individuals who have never tried to stop smoking before and the others.

H6b: The effect of perceived enjoyment is greater in individuals who have never tried to stop smoking before than in others because others know how difficult it may be to stop and not to start again

As this is a model of intention to adopt a technological service, it would appear interesting to compare the model by gender (Venkatesh & Morris, 2000). Gender differences are often addressed in health reports about smokers (Griffith et al, 2012;Briones-Vozmediano et al, 2012).

H7: The impact of vicarious innovativeness on the intention to adopt the mobile coaching service differs according to gender.

Figure 1. Model of adoption of a text-message based mobile coaching service

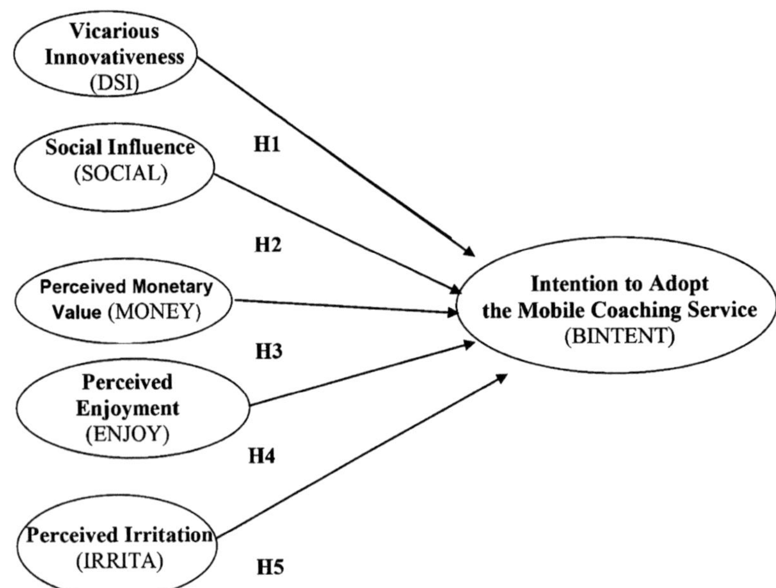

METHODOLOGY

This research originated in a joint project with a French start-up company called

e-Medicis, which was considering introducing a new service to provide support for people who wanted to stop smoking. The study took the form of a face-to-face survey with a convenience sample of 113 people in several Paris locations. The objectives were to measure vicarious innovativeness as regards mobile services, to measure the intention to adopt the mobile coaching service for stopping smoking, and to validate the hypotheses. The analysis also covered the demographic profile of participants, their smoking behavior (heavy smokers/medium smokers/light smokers/non-smokers).

Below is the analysis of the data collected through the face-to-face survey with smokers. The description of the mobile coaching service tested in the survey is provided in Exhibit 1. The analysis done used the structural equations method. Six 5-point Likert scales from "totally disagree" to "totally agree" were used to measure the variables in the model. The scales are described, together with the authors that inspired them, in Table 1.

- **Intention to Adopt the Mobile Coaching Service** (BINTENT). To measure this construct, we used a French adaptation of the scale proposed by Davis et al (1989), itself adapted from Ajzen and Fishbein (1980). This scale consists of three items: (1) I intend to use this mobile coaching service to stop smoking in the future. (2) I would be prepared to use this mobile coaching service to stop smoking in the future. (3) To stop smoking, I will use this service.

- **Vicarious Innovativeness** (DSI). Goldsmith and Hofacker (1991) distinguish global innovativeness from domain-specific innovativeness that can be applied to a specific category of products or services. They propose a scale to measure consumers' tendency to be among the first to try out new products in a specific field. This 5-point scale consists of six items that capture the following constructs: *involvement,*

Table 1. Measurement scales

Concept	Label	Items	Adapted From
Intention to Adopt the Mobile Coaching Service	BINTENT	1. I intend to use this mobile coaching service to stop smoking in the future. 2. I would be prepared to use this mobile coaching service to stop smoking in the future. 3. To stop smoking, I will use this service	Davis (1989)
Vicarious Innovativeness	DSI	1. **Involvement:** If I heard a new mobile coaching service was available, I would be interested in using it. 2. **Intention to adopt:** I would consider adopting a new mobile coaching service even if I had not yet heard about it. 3. **Perceived knowledge:** I know more about new mobile coaching services than other people do. 4. **Ease of use:** If I heard that a new mobile coaching service was available and easy to use, I would be interested enough to adopt it. 5. **Need for change:** I adopt a new mobile coaching service because of the advantages it offers me. 6. **Need for cognition:** Before adopting a new mobile coaching service I consider the benefits provided by innovation and its relationship to the status quo. 7. **Price:** I would adopt the mobile coaching service if the price was right (intention to adopt if you have to pay and at what price level, or if the service is free, sponsored by a private or public organization).	Pagani (2007)
Social Influence	SOCIAL	1. People who are important to me would want me to use this mobile coaching service. 2. People who influence my behavior would think I should use this mobile coaching service. 3. People whose opinions I value would prefer me to use this mobile coaching service.	Mathieson (1991)
Perceived Monetary Value	MONEY	1. I expect that this mobile service would have a reasonable price. 2. This mobile service would offer good value for money. 3. I believe that at the right price, this mobile service would be good value.	Dodds, Monroe & Grewal (1991)
Perceived Enjoyment	ENJOY	1. I expect that using this mobile service would be enjoyable. 2. I expect that using this mobile service would be pleasing. 3. I expect that using this mobile service would be entertaining.	Chowdhury, Parvin, Weitenberner & Becker (2006)
Perceived Irritation	IRRITA	1. I feel that this mobile service is irritating. 2. I feel that mobile coaching services are everywhere and, there is no need for another. 3. This mobile service looks annoying.	Chowdhury, Parvin, Weitenberner & Becker (2006)

usage, intention to adopt, opinion seeking, perceived knowledge and *need for change.* The scale has been validated for durables and other goods as well as for services.

In 2007, Pagani added two further indicators to this scale. The first, *ease of use*, is an indicator that emerges from the theory of reasoned action and the Technology Acceptance Model (TAM) constructed by Davis (1989). The second, the *need for cognition*, is an indicator drawn from psychological studies. Pagani (2007) uses this scale to measure the vicarious innovativeness regarding third generation (3G) mobile music services, which use technology to generate voice, images and video in any place, network or terminal. Pagani showed in her research that the scale gained reliability when the *opinion seeking* and *usage* items were eliminated. Her final modified scale consists of 6 items measuring involvement, intention to adopt, perceived knowledge, ease of use, need for change and need for cognition. In addition to these items, we include a *price* item (I will adopt a mobile coaching service if the price is right, an item used by Pagani (2007) to test the nomological validity of her scale).

- **Social Influence** (SOCIAL). Following Mathieson (1991), three items were used: (1) People who are important to me would want me to use this mobile coaching service. (2) People who influence my behavior would think I should use this mobile coaching service. (3) People whose opinions I value would prefer me to use this mobile coaching service.
- **Perceived Monetary Value** (MONEY). Following Dodds et al. (1991), three items were used: (1) I expect this mobile service would have a reasonable price. (2) This mobile service would offer good value for money. (3) I believe that at the right price, this mobile service would be good value.
- **Perceived Enjoyment** (ENJOY). We adopt the scale devised by Chowdhury et al. (2006). Four items were used: (1) I expect that using this mobile service would be enjoyable. (2) I expect that using this mobile service would be pleasing. (3) I expect that using this mobile service would be entertaining.
- **Perceived Irritation** (IRRITA). As previously, we use the scale devised by Chowdhury et al. (2006). Three items were used: (1) I feel that this mobile service is irritating. (2) I feel that mobile coaching services are everywhere and, there is no need for another. (3) This mobile service looks annoying.

The Table 1 sums up our measurement scales.

STATISTICAL ANALYSES AND RESULTS

Descriptive Analysis

The sample shows a homogeneous distribution between men (52%) and women (48%). Among the participants, 76% of them are aged between 14 and 21 (N=86). More than 80% of participants (N=92) state that they smoke every day or nearly every day. Smokers can be grouped into three categories according to the number of cigarettes smoked per day: *light smokers* (N=32, 28%), *medium smokers* (N=40, 36%) and *heavy smokers* (N=41, 36%) (see Tables 2 and 3). Of the 113 participants in the study, only 37 stated that they intended to stop smoking in the next 12 months; 76 did not share that intention. However, the average intention to adopt the service does not differ significantly between the two groups, i.e. between people who say they want to stop smoking and the rest (F=2.62 (0)).

Among the people who intend to stop smoking in the next 12 months (N=37), most are Heavy Smokers (more than 10 cigarettes a day) and Light Smokers (fewer than 5 cigarettes a day). Medium

Table 2. Classification of smokers by age

Age	Group Size	%
14-17	48	42.5
18-21	38	33.6
22-25	21	18.6
Over 25	6	5.3

Table 3. Classification of smokers by number of cigarettes smoked by day

	Cigarettes per Day	Number	%
Light	< 5 cigarettes	32	28
Medium	5-9 cigarettes	40	36
Heavy	>10 cigarettes	41	36

N = 113 participants.

Smokers (5 to 9 cigarettes a day) have proportionally less intention of giving up smoking; probably because, according to the arguments collected in the exploratory study they are less worried about their budget and their health, or are under less pressure from their entourage.

One of the barriers to adopting the service that emerges from the study is the lack of human contact in the coaching service. This is observed more with individuals over 18 than individuals under 18. The reason may be that the latter who are digital natives and so more used to digital services without human contact. Analysis of the variance shows a significant difference between the averages for the two groups of individuals (F=2.969 and p-value=0.088). Of the 43 individuals who would not use this service because of the lack of human contact, 22 think it could help someone else to stop smoking. This is consistent with extant literature that shows that consumer acceptance of the mobile Internet is linked with a low desire for social contact (Koenigstorfer & Groeppel-Klein, 2012), the mobile Internet being a replacement of social contact (Syed & Nurullah, 2011).

Hypotheses H1 to H7 (except H6a) were tested using the structural equations technique. The maximum likelihood fit function was applied. A two-stage approach was used as recommended by Anderson and Gerbing (1988). First, the measurement instruments for the constructs were assessed by examining the reliability and validity of scales. Then, the relationships were tested.

Scale Reliability and Validity

The reliability of all instruments was tested by the Cronbach's alpha reliability coefficient (see Table 4). All coefficients are acceptable, except those associated with the perceived irritation construct ($\alpha=0.56$). Consequently, the IRRITA construct was eliminated from the model and hypothesis H5 was not tested. As Table 4 shows, the Jöreskog ρ values are high (except for the IRRITA construct). Each item is better explained by the construct it relates to than by chance. Concerning convergent validity, the influence of relationships (between the measures and their construct) is statistically different from 0. The average extracted variance

Table 4. Scale reliability and validity

	DSI	Social	Money	Enjoy	Irrita	Bintent
Cronbach's alpha	0.86	0.76	0.76	0.83	0.56	0.84
Standardized item loading (> 0.5)						
Item 1	0.64	0.80	0.84	0.76	0.56	0.86
Item 2	0.84	0.84	0.87	0.79	0.72	0.89
Item 3	0.87	0.83	0.74	0.90	0.48	0.85
Item 4	0.72					
Item 5	0.50					
Item 6	0.50					
Item 7	0.76					
Average extracted variance ($\rho vc>0.5$)	0.50	0.53	0.55	0.67	0.35	0.64
Jöreskog ρ (>0.70)	0.86	0.77	0.78	0.86	0.62	0.84

between a construct and its measures is always above 0.5 (except for the IRRITA construct).

To test discriminant validity, we conducted a Chi squared difference test (by reference to the difference in degrees of freedom). To test the discriminant validity, the analysis recommended by Bagozzi and Yi (1991) relies on a comparison between the χ^2 values of a model that leaves the correlations between the different constructs free, and a model in which the correlations between constructs are fixed at 1. If the difference is significant in view of the difference in degree of freedom, it can be concluded that the model tested is better than the constrained model and that the constructs are different. The results for the indicators used in our study are satisfactory *(difference of Chi squared= 22 and difference of ddl =6).*

Estimation of the Model

Having established that the goodness of fit is satisfactory, interpretation of the estimations of linear relationships can begin. Our model has two sub-models one to measure independent variables, one to measure dependent variables and a structural model connecting the latent dependent variables to the latent independent variables. There are several observed independent variables that depend on 4 latent variables. These latent variables are correlated. There are also 3 observed dependent variables (3 items concerning intention) that depend on a latent variable. The indicators are fairly satisfactory (see Table 5). The data thus show a satisfactory goodness of fit for the theoretical model.

This model explains 69% of the variance in intention (R^2). As shown in Table 6, the "perceived enjoyment", "vicarious innovation" and "social influence" variables make a significant contribution to the intention to adopt the mobile coaching service (critical ratio>1.96 or very similar).

Consequently, hypotheses H1, H2 and H4 are validated. However, the direct influence of the "perceived monetary value" variable on inten-

tion to adopt the mobile coaching service is not significant, and consequently hypothesis H3 is not validated.

The validated model is illustrated in Figure 2.

COMPARISON OF RELATIONSHIPS BETWEEN VARIABLES IN THE SUBSAMPLES

For the first analysis two subsamples are considered:

Sample 1 consists of individuals have already tried to stop smoking (N=56).
Sample 2 consists of individuals who have never tried to stop smoking (N=57).

According to the Table 7, Perceived Monetary Value and Intention to adopt differ between individuals who have never tried to stop smoking before and the others (H6a is validated).

The data are a good fit for the model in each sample (samples 1 and 2:RMSEA=0.068, NFI,

Table 5. Goodness of fit

RMSEA (< 0.08)	0.07
NFI	0.77
CFI (> 0.90)	0.90
TLI (> 0.90)	0.82

Table 6. Effects of variables on the intention to adopt the mobile coaching service

Relationships to Test		Estimation	Critical Ratio
Vicarious Innovativeness	Intention	0.26	2.32
Social Influence	Intention	0.22	1.90
Perceived Monetary Value	Intention	-0.17	-1.43
Perceived Enjoyment	Intention	0.75	4.73

Figure 2. Result of the model tested

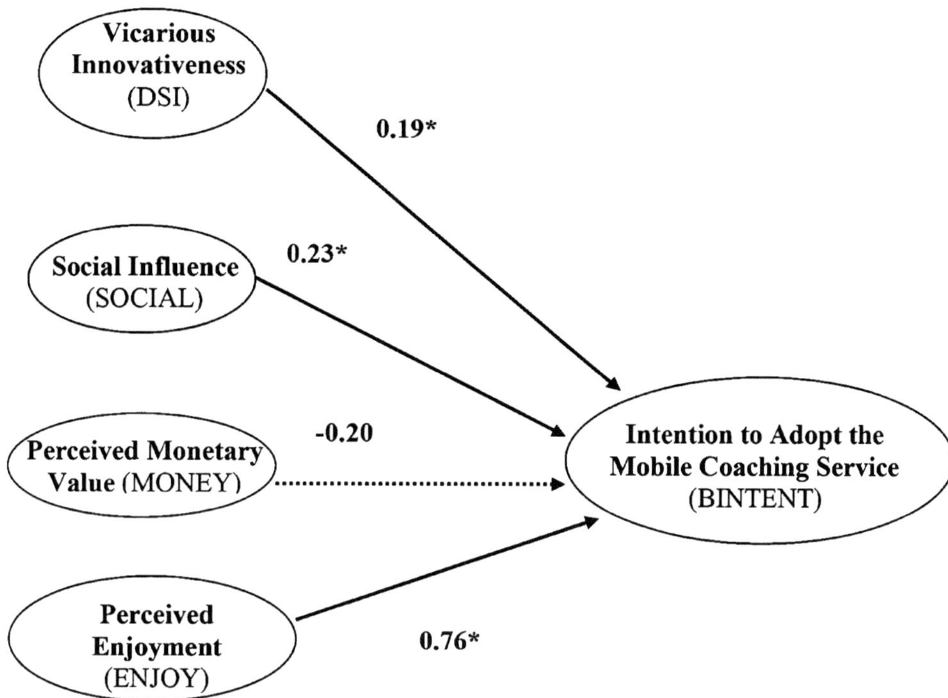

(*): Significant Coefficient (standardized effect), No asterisk: Non-significant

CFI and TLI close to 0.90). The percentage of variance in the intention to adopt the mobile service explained by the model is higher for individuals who have never tried to stop smoking (78.6%) than for the others (60.1%).

Table 8 reports the standardized effects of the model's variables on the intention to adopt the mobile coaching service in each of the two subsamples.

For reasons of clarity, only estimations significant at the 0.05 level are shown. Some variables are significant in one sample but not the other. The "perceived monetary value" variable, which was not significant in the full sample, becomes significant in sample 2. Perceived monetary value exerts a negative effect on the intention to adopt the mobile coaching service in individuals who have never tried to stop smoking. The greater the perceived enjoyment, the more consumers who have never tried to stop smoking will have the intention to adopt the mobile coaching service (double the coefficient of the other group). Hypothesis H6b is thus confirmed.

Vicarious innovativeness has a significant effect on the intention to adopt the mobile service in individuals who have already tried to stop smoking. In individuals who have never tried to stop smoking, the intention to adopt the mobile service will depend more on the perceived enjoyment than on other variables.

Otherwise, if we compare individuals who would like to stop smoking (stopped smoking in the past or not) and the others, there is no difference.

The model tested is now estimated for the same population, this time split by gender. In both subsamples, the data show fairly satisfactory goodness of fit for the model. The portion of variance explained is approximately 65%. Table 9 reports the standardized effects of the model's variables on the intention to adopt the

Table 7. Comparison between variables

Variables	Sample 1 Individuals Who Have Already Tried to Stop Smoking (N=56)	Sample 2 Individuals Who Have Never Tried to Stop Smoking (N=57)	F (df=1)	p	Eta^2	Full Sample
Vicarious Innovativeness	2.89 *(1)* .95 *(2)*	2.68 .57	1.23	.269	.01	2.79 .99
Social Influence	2.55 1.31	2.19 1.03	2.73	.101	.02	2.37 1.18
Perceived Monetary Value	3.57 1.23	3.01 1.34	5.23	.024	.05	3.29 1.31
Perceived Enjoyment	2.58 1.16	2.35 1.17	1.07	.303	.01	2.46 1.16
Intention to adopt	2.46 1.30	2.00 1.12	4.17	.043	.04	2.23 1.22

(1) The mean (2) The standard deviation

Table 8. Standardized effects on the intention to adopt the mobile coaching service

Variables	Sample 1 Individuals Who Have Already Tried to Stop Smoking (N=56)	Sample 2 Individuals Who Have Never Tried to Stop Smoking (N=57)
Vicarious Innovativeness	0.35	-
Social Influence	-	-
Perceived Monetary Value	-	-0.51
Perceived Enjoyment	0.52	1.01

NB: Only significant coefficients (5%) are reported

mobile coaching service in each of the two gender subsamples.

For reasons of clarity, only estimations significant at the 0.05 level are shown. Vicarious innovativeness has a significant effect on the intention to adopt the mobile service in women but not in men. Validation of our conceptual model is higher in the female sample than the male sample. Hypothesis H7 is validated.

Table 9. Standardized effects on the intention to adopt the mobile coaching service

Variables	Females (N=54)	Males (N=59)
Vicarious Innovativeness	0.29	-
Social Influence	-	-
Perceived Monetary Value	-	-
Perceived Enjoyment	0.75	0.82

NB: Only significant coefficients (5%) are reported

CONTRIBUTIONS, MANAGERIAL IMPLICATIONS, LIMITATIONS, AND AVENUES FOR FUTURE RESEARCH

This study has broad social and managerial implications. The field of mobile health services is providing opportunities to make improvements and reduce costs in the French and wordwide health sector. Worldwide, the mobile health market has an estimated value of $50 billion (Ascari, Bakshi, & Grijpink, 2010). However, attention should not be focused solely on the business opportunities offered by the market, but rather on its social impact. Because these mobile health services can offer continuous "24/7" monitoring and have no geographical barriers, thus, mobile coaching services are open to a larger range of benefits (see Exhibit 2 and 3). With their positioning as accessible services that are complementary to other medical and psychological methods, they also offer a less formal approach to support in the fight to break addictions.

The intention to adopt the text message-based mobile coaching service to help stop smoking was tested with a mostly young target. This is precisely the group with the greatest risk of developing tobacco-related illnesses in the long term, since the lower the age at which people start smoking, the higher their risks of serious tobacco-related illnesses. Yet the study observed that these young smokers do not always intend to stop smoking in the short term. It is important to find innovative ways to motivate them to try and start the process of giving up smoking. With this in mind, mobile services can play an important role because young people are generally heavy users of cell phones and generally find new technologies attractive (Syed & Nurullah, 2011).

Two factors of influence should be taken into consideration: peer influence and the enjoyment generated by this type of remote coaching service, habitually perceived as a game. The more enjoyment consumers get out of using these services, the more they will be prepared to use them in the future. The designers of this type of service need to develop amusing messages to convince early adopters to talk about the effectiveness of the service and how much fun it was to use. Furthermore, if the service is perceived to be at a reasonable price or free because sponsored by a government health organization, the potential user will get more enjoyment out of trying it. The influence exercised by smokers' families and

general entourage can also play a decisive role in diffusion of these services by their word of mouth.

The above findings also underline the fact that stimulating curiosity and the smokers' intrinsic interest are more important factors than the perceived monetary value. It would be judicious to ensure that the most favorable techniques and functions are selected, to give the consumer a higher level of perceived enjoyment and intrinsic inter-user motivation.

The negative impact of perceived monetary value for individuals who have never tried to stop smoking before could be explained by the existence of free applications. The smoker may prefer his coaching service for stopping smoking to be free, or provided free by a company or health sector body. However, it is conceivable that when a person really wants to stop smoking, the price to pay will not be a barrier to adoption.

The limitations of this study relate to its small sample size and the overrepresentation of young people, which limits its external validity. Larger-scale studies with samples of different population types (multi-country, different age brackets, different types of smoker) will still be required for closer examination of each segment's needs and preferences. Another possible bias is the low number of participants who had stated a clear intention of stopping smoking in the next 12 months. A much greater effort should have been made to recruit people intending to stop smoking in the near future.

We recommend that an online study should be undertaken with a broader sample comprising subjects of all ages, to determine how the desire (or lack of desire) to stop smoking influences the smoker's perception of the mobile coaching service. Some experience of the service would also be advisable in more advanced stages of the research, once the beta version is available, because the measure of attitude to these new services used in this study is based on respondents' own statements and does not involve them much. A measure that allows closer observation of a behavior could be more effective. It would also be useful to test the perceived enjoyment of this type of service, in order to increase numbers giving up other addictions and/or pay greater attention to other illnesses.

Another interesting avenue to explore is the impact of mobile coaching service in conjunction with e-cigarettes which could grow as greater regulation looms, for example, plain packaging proposals that would remove brands from cigarette packs (Wembridge & Thompson, 2012).

In their research Andrews, Cacho-Elizondo, Drennan and Tossan (2013) showed that perceived usefulness continually proves to be the most important predictor of intentions to use an SMS-assisted smoking intervention. Based on this, health practitioners offering an m-health service must consider its design and delivery to ensure its usefulness to the target group. For Andrew and her colleagues, this could include whether it is used as an additional component to a web-based intervention or a standalone mobile phone-based intervention.

CONCLUSION

This chapter has explored the factors that determine the intention to adopt a text message-based mobile coaching service designed to help people stop smoking. We obtained a fairly robust model in which vicarious innovativeness, social influence and the perceived enjoyment exert a positive influence on the intention to adopt the mobile coaching service. The perceived enjoyment has more influence on the intention to adopt the mobile coaching service in smokers who have never tried to stop smoking before than in smokers who have already tried to stop smoking.

At the methodological level, this research contributes with an improved approach to test the acceptance and potential adoption of new services, not yet available, through the use of a scenario script where the mobile coaching service to quit smoking is described (Exhibit 1).

Kihyun, Gyenung-Min, and Eun Sook (2009) concluded in their research that adoption of an amusing mobile service is a direct reflection of users' way of life insofar as that adoption is in line with socio-economic conditions. In future research, it would be interesting to explore further both the enjoyment aspect of the service and the socio-economic conditions of potential adopters. On this point, male-female differences also require more attention, as our model turned out to be more suited to women. One possible explanation for this could be the level of curiosity associated with this segment, and its usage of mobile applications.

Steenkamp and Gielens (2003) found in their study that the probability of trying an innovation is higher in individuals with a high degree of innovativeness than those with a low degree of innovativeness. These authors compared consumer innovativeness as measured by the attitude scale with innovativeness as measured by affective purchasing behavior for new products, and observe that the results by either measure are equivalent.

Another factor for consideration is the level of involvement. Bloch (1982) and Valette-Florence (1989) noted that a high-involvement individual will have a greater propensity to adopt an innovative behavior than a low-involvement individual.

An additional lesson to be drawn from this study is the discovery of smokers' preference for multimedia communications including images and videos. This trend would certainly help to compensate for the lack of human contact that has often been considered as one of the weaknesses of this type of remote coaching service. A further online study of people from different countries could measure how intending (or not intending) to give up smoking in the short term influences the perception of a mobile coaching service to help people stop smoking. It could also measure the impact of cultural and socio-economic factors, including isolation.

According to Varshney (2014), "Mobile technologies allow information to be made available quickly, but cannot improve the quality of information it is presenting to the patients or healthcare professionals". It remains still true for a mobile phone smoking cessation programme. Therefore, an important challenge is to have a medical approach while coaching people what is not actually verified in the free mobile coaching services.

In addition, it would be interesting to replicate this study with people who want to break other addictive habits such as excessive consumption of medicines, drugs or food or alcohol, or people suffering from health problems such as depression. Support could be provided through prerecorded messages sent by cell phone alone, or in conjunction with other media, for instance as a complement to an internet application, personalized coaching, or treatments such as nicotine patches to stop smoking. In a more advanced stage of research, the service itself could be tried out, to determine the value of using theoretical approaches to examine factors influencing the perceptions and attitudes of participants who use the service.

The future of mobile health or m-health services is promising, it is necessary to continue encouraging further interdisciplinary research to improve them and spread their adoption and wide application in the health sector worldwide. Special focus should be given to developing countries where m-health services or apps could have a significant impact on low-income sensible groups.

ACKNOWLEDGMENT

The authors acknowledge the helpful comments and suggestions of Professor Jean-Pierre Helfer, Dean and Professor at IAE, Paris Panthéon Sorbonne University, President of the Scientific Council at EDC Paris Business School. We would additionally like to thank anonymous referees for their comments, which strengthened this chapter and the support received from our institutions.

REFERENCES

Ajzen, I. (1991). The Theory of Planned Behavior. *Organizational Behavior and Human Decision Processes*, *50*(2), 179–212. doi:10.1016/0749-5978(91)90020-T

Ajzen, I., & Fishbein, M. (1980). *Understanding Attitudes and Predicting Social*. Englewood Cliffs, NJ: Prentice-Hall.

Anderson, J. C., & Gerbing, D. W. (1988). Structural Equation Modeling in Practice: A Review and Recommended Two-step Approach. *Psychological Bulletin*, *103*(3), 411–423. doi:10.1037/0033-2909.103.3.411

Andrews, L., Cacho-Elizondo, S., Drenna, J., & Tossan, V. (2013). Consumer Acceptance of an SMS-assisted Smoking Cessation Intervention: A Multi Country Study. *Journal of Health Marketing Quarterly*, *30*(1), 47–62. doi:10.1080/07359683.2013.758015 PMID:23458481

Ascari, A., Bakshi, A. & Grijpink, F. (2010). mHealth: A New Vision for Healthcare: McKinsey & Company, Inc., and GSMA.

Bagozzi, R. P., & Yi, Y. (1991). Multitrait-Multimethod Matrices in Consumer Research. *JMR, Journal of Marketing Research*, *17*, 426–439.

Bloch, P. H. (1982). Involvement beyond the Purchase Process: Conceptual Issues and Empirical Investigation. *Advances in Consumer Research. Association for Consumer Research (U. S.)*, *9*(1), 413–417.

Briones-Vozmediano, E., Vives-Cases, C., & Peiró-Pérez, R. (2012). Gender Sensitivity in National Health Plans in Latin America and the European Union. *Health Policy (Amsterdam)*, *106*(1), 88–96. doi:10.1016/j.healthpol.2012.03.001 PMID:22465154

Cestre, G. (1996). Diffusion et Innovativité: Définition, Modélisation et Mesure. *Recherche et Applications en Marketing*, *11*(1), 69–88. doi:10.1177/076737019601100105

Chowdhury, H. K., Parvin, N., Weitenberner, C., & Becker, M. (2006). Consumer Attitude toward Mobile Advertising in an Emerging Market: An Empirical Study. *International Journal of Mobile Marketing*, *1*(2).

d'Hauteville, F. (1994). *Un Modèle d'Acceptation du Nouveau Produit par le Consommateur: Cas du Vin allégé en Alcool*. Unpublished Doctoral Dissertation, Université Montpellier II, France.

Davis, F. D. (1989). Perceived Usefulness, Perceived Ease of Use, and User Acceptance of Information Technology. *Management Information Systems Quarterly*, *13*(3), 319–340. doi:10.2307/249008

Davis, F. D., Bagozzi, R. P., & Warshaw, P. R. (1989). User Acceptance of Computer Technology: A Comparison of Two Theoretical Models. *Management Science*, *35*(8), 982–1003. doi:10.1287/mnsc.35.8.982

Dodds, W. B., Monroe, K. B., & Grewal, D. (1991). Effects of Price, Brand, and Store Information on Buyers' Product Evaluations. *JMR, Journal of Marketing Research*, *28*(3), 307–319. doi:10.2307/3172866

Foxall, G., & Haskins, C. G. (1986). Cognitive Style and Consumer Innovativeness: An Empirical Test of Kirton's Adaptation-Innovation Theory in the Context of Food Purchasing. *European Journal of Marketing*, *20*(3/4), 63–80. doi:10.1108/EUM0000000004755

Gatignon, H., & Robertson, T. S. (1985). A propositional Inventory for New Diffusion Research. *The Journal of Consumer Research*, *11*(4), 849–867. doi:10.1086/209021

Goldsmith, R. E., d'Hauteville, F., & Flynn, L. R. (1998). Theory and Measurement of Consumer Innovativeness. *European Journal of Marketing*, *32*(3/4), 340–353. doi:10.1108/03090569810204634

Goldsmith, R. E., & Hofacker, C. H. (1991). Measuring Consumer Innovativeness. *Journal of the Academy of Marketing Science*, *19*(3), 209–221. doi:10.1007/BF02726497

Griffith, D.M., Gunter, K., Watkins D.C. (2012). Measuring Masculinity in Research on Men of Color: Findings and Future Directions. *American Journal of Public Health*, *102*(S2), S187-S194.

Hirshman, E. (1980). Innovativeness, Novelty Seeking and Consumer Creativity. *The Journal of Consumer Research*, *7*(3), 283–295. doi:10.1086/208816

Hong, S., & Tam, K. Y. (2006). Understanding the Adoption of Multipurpose Information Appliances: The Case of Mobile Data Services. *Information Systems Research*, *17*(2), 162–179. doi:10.1287/isre.1060.0088

Hurt, H. T., Joseph, K., & Cook, C. D. (1977). Scales for the Measurement of Innovativeness. *Human Communication Research*, *4*(1), 58–65. doi:10.1111/j.1468-2958.1977.tb00597.x

INPES (French National Health Prevention and Education Institute). (2007), "Le tabac tue un fumeur sur deux. L'industrie du tabac compte sur vous pour les remplacer", *Espace Presse*, retrieved April 4, 2015 from www.inpes.sante.fr/70000/cp/07/cp070820.asp

Kihyun, K., Gyenung-Min, K., & Eun Sook, K. (2009). Measuring the Compatibility Factors in Mobile Entertainment Service Adoption. *Journal of Computer Information Systems*, (Fall): 141–148.

Koenigstorfer, J., & Groeppel-Klein, A. (2012). Consumer Acceptance of the Mobile Internet. *Marketing Letters*, *23*(4), 917–928. doi:10.1007/s11002-012-9206-1

Kotler, P., & Armstrong, G. (2006). *Principles of Marketing* (11th ed.). Pearson Prentice-hall.

Le Louarn, P. (1997). La Tendance à Innover des Consommateurs: Analyse Conceptuelle et Proposition d'une Échelle de Mesure. *Recherche et Applications en Marketing*, *12*(1), 3–19. doi:10.1177/076737019701200101

Le Nagard-Assayag, E., & Manceau, D. (2011). *Le Marketing de l'Innovation, de la Création au Lancement de Nouveaux Produits* (2nd ed.). Paris: Dunod.

Masson, J. (2010). Effets de la Modification d'un Attribut Constitutif d'un Produit Alimentaire sur son Adoption par les Consommateurs: Le cas du Vin à teneur réduite en Alcool. Unpublished Doctoral Dissertation, Montpellier Supagro, Centre International d'Etudes Supérieures en Sciences Agronomiques, France.

Mathieson, K. (1991). Predicting User Intentions: Comparing the Technology Acceptance Model with the Theory of Planned Behavior. *Information Systems Research*, *2*(3), 173–191. doi:10.1287/isre.2.3.173

McArdle, M. (2014). Thank You For E-Smoking, Bloomberg Businessweek, 00077135, October 2, Edition 4366.

Merrill, M. (2011a). HHS mHealth initiatives target smoking cessation, *Healthcare IT News*, retrieved April 4, 2015 from www.healthcareitnews.com/news/hhs-mhealth-initiatives-target-smoking-cessation

Merrill, M. (2011b). Study finds potential in social media tools for smoking cessation, *Healthcare IT News*, retrieved April 4, 2015 from www.healthcareitnews.com/news/study-find-potential-social-media-health-tools-smoking-cessation

Midgley, D. F., & Dowling, G. R. (1993). A Longitudinal Study of Product Form Innovation: The Interaction between Predispositions and Social Messages. *The Journal of Consumer Research*, *19*(4), 611–625. doi:10.1086/209326

Ostlund, L. E. (1974). Perceived innovation attributes as predictors of innovativeness. *The Journal of Consumer Research*, *1*(2), 23–29. doi:10.1086/208587

Pagani, M. (2007). A Vicarious Innovativeness Scale for 3G Mobile Services: Integrating the Domain Specific Innovativeness Scale with Psychological and Rational Indicators. *Technology Analysis and Strategic Management*, *19*(6), 709–728. doi:10.1080/09537320701711207

Poe, M. (2014). 'The issues are complicated' with e-cigarettes, *The Times West Virginian*, March 9.

PwC (PricewaterhouseCoopers) report June 2013, Socio-economic impact of m-health, An assessment report for the European Union, Retrieved November 2014, from http://www.pwc.fr/socio-economic-impact-of-mhealth-an-assessment-report-for-the-european-union.html

Rodgers, A., Corbett, T., Bramley, D., Riddell, T., Wills, M., Lin, R.-B., & Jones, M. (2005). Do u Smoke after txt? Results of a Randomised Trial of Smoking Cessation Using Mobile Phone Text Messaging. *Tobacco Control*, *14*(4), 255–261. doi:10.1136/tc.2005.011577 PMID:16046689

Roehrich, G. (1994). Innovativités Hédoniste et Sociale: Proposition d'une Échelle de Mesure. *Recherche et Applications en Marketing*, *9*(2), 19–42. doi:10.1177/076737019400900202

Rogers, E. M. (Ed.). (1962). *Diffusion of Innovations*. New York: The Free Press.

Rogers, E. M. (Ed.). (1983). *Diffusion of Innovations* (3rd ed.). New York: The Free Press.

Rokeach, M. (1973). *The Nature of Human Values*. New York: The Free Press.

Steenkamp, J.-B. E. M., & Gielens, K. (2003). Consumer and Market Drivers of the Trial Probability of New Consumer Packaged Goods. *The Journal of Consumer Research*, *29*(December), 368–384. doi:10.1086/378615

Subin, I., Mason, C. H., & Houston, M. B. (2007). Does Innate Consumer Innovativeness relate to New Product/ Service Adoption Behavior? The Intervening Role of Social Learning via Vicarious Innovativeness? *Journal of the Academy of Marketing Science*, *35*(1), 63–75. doi:10.1007/s11747-006-0007-z

Syed, S. F., & Nurullah, A. S. (2011). Use of Mobile Phones and the Social Lives of Urban Adolescents: A Review of Literature. *Trends in Information Management*, *7*(1), 1–18.

Thompson, C., & Wembridge, M. (2012). Big Tobacco Push for Cigarette Alternatives. *Financial Times, August* 12.

Valette-Florence, P. (1989). Conceptualisation et Mesure de l'Implication. *Recherche et Applications en Marketing*, *4*(1), 57–78. doi:10.1177/076737018900400104

Varshney, U. (2014). A model for improving quality of decisions in mobile health. *Decision Support Systems*, *62*, 66–77. doi:10.1016/j.dss.2014.03.005

Venkatesh, V., & Brown, S. (2001). A Longitudinal Investigation of Personal Computers in Homes: Adoption Determinants and Emerging Challenges. *Management Information Systems Quarterly*, *25*(1), 71–102. doi:10.2307/3250959

Venkatesh, V., & Morris, M. (2000). Why don't Men ever Stop to Ask for Directions? Gender, Social Influence and their Role in Technology Acceptance and Usage Behavior. *Management Information Systems Quarterly*, *24*(1), 115–139. doi:10.2307/3250981

Venkatraman, M. P., & Price, L. (1990). Differentiating between Cognitive and Sensory Innovativeness: Concepts, Measurement, and Implications. *Journal of Business Research*, *20*(4), 293–315. doi:10.1016/0148-2963(90)90008-2

Wembridge, M., & Thompson, C. (2012), Big Tobacco bets on e-cigarette future, Financial Times, August 12. Retrieved November, 2014, from http://www.ft.com/cms/s/0/cb76997e-e0a5-11e1-b465-00144feab49a.html#ixzz23RJXFAJZ

Whittaker, R., Maddison, R., McRobbie, H., Bullen, C., Denny, S., Dorey, E., & Rodgers, A. et al. (2008). A Multimedia Mobile Phone-Based Youth Smoking Cessation Intervention: Findings from Content Development and Piloting Studies. *Journal of Medical Internet Research*, *10*(5), e49. doi:10.2196/jmir.1007 PMID:19033148

KEY TERMS AND DEFINITIONS

Breaking Addictions: Reduce addictive behaviors like cigarettes, drugs, alcohol adoption of an innovation: use an innovation at least 3 times for consumer goods, buy an industrial item.

Health & Human Services (HHS): "It is the United States government's principal agency for protecting the health of all Americans and providing basic human services".

Mobile Health or mHealth: It considers all the declinations of health care using mobile portable or wireless devices.

Perceived Enjoyment: The fun you may have while playing with an application.

Perceived Irritation: Based on the fact that mobile advertising may be perceived by you as invasive, irritating, or boring.

Perceived Monetary Value: The value you obtain according to the price quality ratio.

Social Influence: Influence of the people who matter for you towards your behavior.

Technology Acceptance Model (TAM): It was constructed by Davis (1989). It is an adaptation of the theory of Reasoned Action (Fishbein & Ajzen, 1975) designed to model the intention to adopt information systems.

Vicarious Innovativeness: It is defined as *openness to information on new products of any kind*. This kind of innovativeness is followed by adoptive innovativeness when consumers actually adopt the product.

This work was previously published in Human Behavior, Psychology, and Social Interaction in the Digital Era edited by Anabela Mesquita and Chia-Wen Tsai, pages 72-94 copyright year 2015 by Information Science Reference (an imprint of IGI Global).

APPENDIX

Exhibit 1: Description of the Mobile Coaching Service provided in the Interviews

We are now going to describe the main characteristics of a SMS assisted smoking cessation service which allows you to receive SMS or MMS message on your mobile phone to help you quit smoking:

Every morning you would receive an SMS or MMS message on your mobile phone to encourage you to not smoke all day.

If during the day, you feel that you will break your effort to not smoke, you can send an SMS message to a special mobile phone number to ask for help.

You will receive a supportive SMS message back immediately that would be specifically adapted to your needs.

In the middle or at the end of the day, if you haven't sent any alert messages, you'll receive an SMS or MMS message of congratulations and encouragement.

You would be able to modify the timing of receiving the messages to suit the times of day that are most convenience for you.

Exhibit 2: Smokeless Trends and the Tobacco Industry

According to Thompson and Wembridge (2012):

Tobacco companies are changing their strategic focus. The change in direction comes as the industry faces increased regulatory pressure both in mature markets and emerging economies. For instance, Australia has passed the world's most strident anti-tobacco regulation, dubbed "plain packaging", whereby tobacco products are sold in drab, standardised packs with graphic health warnings replacing brands. Plain packaging has also being considered in the UK and the European Union.

In 2011, Euromonitor estimated that the smokeless tobacco market, which also includes chewing tobacco and snuff, was already worth $14bn of the $664bn world, with cigarettes still accounting for over 90 per cent of the total. The smokeless tobacco category has continued its upward trajectory in the last years. According to Information Resources Inc.(IRI), in the 52 ended Jan 20, 2014,the category rang up $5.16 billion at U.S. c-stores.-

In order to affront all these pressures and new consumption trends, tobacco companies are seeking alternative solutions, Philips Morris plans to launch a cigarette under the Marlboro brand in 2016 where the tobacco is heated rather than burnt creating less smoke and tar. This product innovation is done to attract more health-conscious smokers. In 2011, British American Tobacco set up a new business unit, Nicoventures, which focuses on smoking alternatives. Nicoventures is working towards launching an inhalable pure nicotine product within the next two years or so. The expected goal is that his product will offer a safer alternative to smoking while still meeting smokers' cravings.

Electronic cigarettes (e-cigarettes), still unregulated, are the biggest component of the current market for cigarette substitutes, however in the past, companies have invested in smokeless alternatives with mixed results. As an illustration we can mention the case of the US conglomerate RJR Nabisco who pioneered one of the first smokeless cigarettes in the 80s, called Premier, at an estimated cost of more than $300m, but it sold poorly due to consumer concerns over the taste and smell.

Another issue affecting e-cigarettes is that they have nicotine inside and the effects on health of inhaling nicotine vapor are not completely known. Experts consider that it is better than inhaling nicotine and byproducts from tobacco on fire.

Matt Myers, president of *Campaign for Tobacco-Free Kids* says: *"The concern with e-cigarettes is that it will re-glamorize smoking, the gesture. Therefore, people who used to smoke may be lured back"* *(Poe, 2014).*

Neutral Packs: Another Recent Trend on Tobacco

The neutral cigarette packs were rapidly accepted by smokers in Australia after their introduction in December 2012 according to a research published by Tobacco Control on November 11th 2014. 28% of them approved this new regulation before it was implemented and they became 49% afterwards.

The same measure is planned to be introduced in France in 2016 to dissuade consumers from cigarettes: all packagings of cigarettes are going to have the same shape, the same size and the same typography without any logo. The brand name will continue to appear in small letters.

This measure combined with a price rise allowed to decrease the number of Australian daily smokers above 14 from 15,1% in 2010 to 12.8% in 2013 according to a research reported by *French journal Libération* on November 11th.

Exhibit 3: Some Examples of Smoking Cessation Mobile Apps

Coaching people to avoid taking a cigarette seems to remain a better option than smokeless alternatives such as the e-cigarette. In that contest, mobile apps emerge as a promising medium to deliver different treatments to promote health, which include smoking cessation. The first research study about a mobile phone smoking cessation program was published by (Rodgers et al., 2005). Nowadays, there are an increasing number of Mobile apps to coach smokers during their smoking cessation efforts offering them different features.

One of these apps is Livestrong *MyQuit Coach*. A related study of social media tools for smoking cessation that surveyed 266 users, released by the University of Southern California's Institute for Communication Technology Management (CTM) and the USC Center for Body Computing (CBC) found that the ability to immediately and continually track cigarette consumption along with encouragement and social support can lead to smoking cessation (Merryl, 2011b).

Another app, *QuitNow*, indicates for how long you haven't smoked, the number of cigarettes you have avoided and the money saved. Based on indicators of the World Health Organization, this app analyses your progresses and you can exchange on the chat with other concerned people.

Other apps available are: *iCoach*, an online digital health coaching platform that helps individuals quit smoking. *SmokefreeTXT* is a mobile text messaging in the United States that propose smokers to send them messages. *Texquit* asks details about the smoker's habits (frequentation, quantity, spending, reasons for quitting, difficulties to resist smoking…). The messages are personalized and sent 4 weeks before and 4 weeks after the quit date (1-5 messages per week).

Chapter 14
Wireless Connected Health:
Anytime, Anyone, Anywhere

Florie Brizel
Brizel Media, USA

ABSTRACT

Wireless connected health is the most current, inclusive phrase to describe healthcare that incorporates wireless technologies and/or mobile devices. It represents one of the fastest growing sectors in the global mobile and wireless ecosystem, with extraordinary change occurring daily. According to the World Health Organization, 80 percent of people in greatest medical need live in low- to middle-income countries. Not enough has been written about how they will afford wireless connected health, or how it can bring positive benefits to patients everywhere with non-lethal chronic illnesses. It also remains to be seen whether people outside the healthcare industry, without any special interest in science, technology, medicine, or illness prevention, will adopt new and future behavior-changing connected health technologies. This chapter provides a current overview of the global health crises created by noncommunicable diseases, explains the evolution of the global wireless connected health sector, includes information about BRICS nations, and offers observations, insights, and recommendations from a socio-economic and political standpoint for responsible and effective future industry growth.

INTRODUCTION

Wireless connected health is the most current and inclusive phrase to describe personal healthcare that incorporates mobile devices and/or wireless technologies. It represents one of the fastest growing sectors in the mobile and wireless ecosystem, with extraordinary change occurring daily.

Today, simply by using their smartphones, people around the world can watch their diets, track their exercise, log their sleep, access motivational fitness coaches and/or programs, and do myriad other things to support lifelong wellness.

Rapid advances in technology now make possible a global initiative to ultimately eradicate disease by empowering individuals to make informed, positive lifestyle choices that are disease-preventive. This bodes well not only for increased human longevity, but also, and perhaps even more importantly, for improved quality of life (WHO, 2013a).

DOI: 10.4018/978-1-4666-8756-1.ch014

The early literature and focus concerning the advent of wireless connected health addressed the successful linkage of systems and networks so machines could communicate with machines, and data – specifically, a patient's electronic health record (EHR) – could be accessed ubiquitously (Chronaki et al., 2007).

Current literature (Sejdić et al., 2013) focuses on the engineering and software behind new and innovative wireless medical devices and mobile medical applications (MMAs).

Furthermore, now that a variety of wireless medical devices and MMAs have entered into progressive clinical practices and mainstream teaching centers, a growing body of literature has begun to examine the clinical performance of products already on the market. Weight loss, weight management and weight gain all have mobile-inclusive protocols (Turner-McGrievy and Tate, 2011; Patrick et al., 2013; Carter et al., 2013; and Cardi, Clarke & Treasure, 2013).

Behavioral sciences and mental health have noteworthy studies and pilot programs that address everything from bipolar disorder (do patients prefer using mobile phones for charting moods or traditional pen-&-paper diaries?) (Depp et al., 2012), to psychosis (Palmier-Claus et al., 2013), to depression, anxiety and stress (Proudfoot et al., 2013), to the effectiveness of a suicide prevention app for indigenous Australian youths (Shand et al., 2013).

Two excellent studies (Spyridonis, Ghinea and Frank, 2013; Kristjánsdóttir et al., 2013) address pain as a significant component of many chronic illnesses and how wireless and mobile technologies can help alleviate this aspect of noncommunicable chronic disease (NCD).

Unfortunately, too few papers focus on ways the changing healthcare landscape affects the end-user as a patient, beyond becoming a personal source of biological data points. One that does is "Telecare, Surveillance, and the Welfare State" (Sorrell & Draper, 2012), which examines whether or not bringing a variety of health and wellness monitoring devices into the sanctity of the home strips individuals living there of autonomy, depersonalizes their care and, as an unintended consequence, actually increases their isolation.

Another excellent paper, entitled "How places matter: Telecare technologies and the changing spatial dimensions of healthcare," (Oudshoorn, 2012, p.124) argues that "Places are not only important because assumptions about the contexts of use are inscribed in technologies…. They also matter because places shape how technological devices are used, or not, and (de)stabilize the specific identities of technologies. Equally important, technologies participate in redefining the meaning and practices of the spaces in which they are used and…introduce new spaces in which people and objects interact." The author goes onto say, "The idea that places matter thus provides an important point of departure for an investigation of how reciprocal relationships between people, places and technologies enable or constrain the identities of users, places and technologies (Oudshoorn, 2012, p. 124)."

Clearly, wireless connected health already has begun to help many people with chronic illnesses. Four chronic illnesses typically used to illustrate its benefits – diabetes, hypertension, heart disease and asthma – are such that if a patient ignores unusual, fluctuating symptoms, results can prove catastrophic or fatal. New wireless medical devices and apps make regular surveillance of signs and symptoms remarkably easy, and they empower these patients to enjoy better health as a result of having better tracking systems to prevent undesired health crises.

However, not enough has been written about whether or how wireless connected health can bring significant, positive outcomes to resistant patients and those with lesser known and rarely fatal chronic illnesses…patients who tax the global healthcare system with a never-ending variety of very real, perplexing ailments that defy easy diagnosis or standard remedy.

And it remains to be seen, despite all arguments to the contrary, whether regular people outside the healthcare industry, without any special interest in science, technology, medicine, or illness prevention, will adopt the plethora of new and future behavior-changing technologies.

This paper provides a current overview of the global wireless connected health sector and offers observations and recommendations from a socio-economic standpoint for responsible industry growth going forward.

A PubMed literature review conducted in Q4/2013 at the Louise M. Darling Biomedical Library at UCLA David Geffen School of Medicine, using search terms *mobile, wireless, mobile health, healthcare, patients*, and *patient perceptions*, returned over 150 papers related to wireless connected health. Abstracts were read for all, eliminating those that dealt exclusively with systems design, engineering, software and strict technology issues. Those abstracts selected for further review broke out as 11 papers about mobile and physical activity; eight (8) about mobile and behavior modification; seven (7) about mobile and mental health; six (6) about mobile and older adults; five (5) about chronic disease; four (4) about mobile and pain management; three (3) about mobile and diabetes management; two (2) papers about mobile and asthma; and, numerous papers that contained an amalgam of relevant material. In addition, there were individual papers about wearables (wireless technology built into clothing or wearable accessories); social networks; games; alcoholism; access to care; medical residents' education; privacy; digital communication failure; and, cancer.

The wireless connected health sector has seen unprecedented growth over the last five years, and major news organizations have given it increased coverage accordingly, in print and online. As it changes significantly on an almost daily basis, a wide variety of industry-specific websites, newsletters, and blogs also served as reliable information sources. Finally, two major governing and regulatory bodies – the World Health Organization (WHO) and the United States Food and Drug Administration (USFDA or FDA) – provided invaluable statistical, regulatory and practical information essential to understanding some of the reasons why the wireless connected health industry, and specifically, mobile medical devices and mobile medical applications, have developed in the initial trajectories they have.

TECHNOLOGIES AND HEALTHCARE

The practice of medicine has a long tradition of incorporating new scientific knowledge through responsible applications. Within the last 200 years, many new technologies have been developed and taken their place in the annals of medicine. In 1816, Laennec introduced the stethoscope to better hear the beating heart. In 1884, the autoclave was introduced to sterilize tools used in the operating theatre. Nine years later, in 1895, Roentgen introduced the radiograph x-ray. French surgeon Alexis Carrel and American aviator Charles Lindbergh introduced the external perfusion pump in 1935. By 1957, the first artificial heart was implanted in a dog; the first artificial heart was placed in a human for 64 hours a mere twelve years later, in 1969. Artificial vertebral discs were introduced at the end of the 20th century and their successful implantation record has greatly minimized the need for more restrictive spinal procedures.

Today, thanks to advances in mobile and wireless technologies, smartphones also can function as medical devices, such as stethoscopes, ultrasound machines, cardiac monitors, and more. In the United States, any medical device must receive approval from the Food and Drug Administration (FDA) prior to use by physicians or the general public (U.S. Food and Drug Administration, 2012a). This law includes mobile and wireless devices intended for diagnostic or therapeutic use, or disease management.

The FDA defines a medical device as "an instrument, apparatus, implement, machine, contrivance, implant, in vitro reagent, or other similar or related article, including a component part, or accessory which is recognized in the official National Formulary, or the United States Pharmacopoeia, or any supplement to them; intended for use in the diagnosis of disease or other conditions, or in the cure, mitigation, treatment, or prevention of disease, in man or other animals; or intended to affect the structure or any function of the body of man or other animals, and which does not achieve its primary intended purposes through chemical action within or on the body of man or other animals and which is not dependent upon being metabolized for the achievement of any of its primary intended purposes (FDA, 2013a)."

Many wireless medical devices already have received clearance for use and are on the market. The GE Vscan ultrasound is a smartphone-based professional medical ultrasound with a probe attached by USB. The AliveCor Heart Monitor is a single-channel smartphone-based electrocardiogram for prescribed patients and their physicians. A number of glucose monitors are on the market. The Infrascanner Model 2000 is a new and exciting addition to medical diagnostics. It is a portable screening device that uses Near-Infrared (NIR) technology to screen patients for intracranial bleeding, identifying those who would most benefit from immediate referral to a CT scan and neurosurgical intervention (InfraScan, 2013).[1] The RP-VITA™ Remote Presence Robot – with audio/video capabilities – can rove throughout a hospital and permit remote telepresence between doctors and patients.

Wireless medical devices should not be confused with mobile medical applications (MMAs), some of which are intended solely for health and wellness, while others are intended for managing or treating a condition (or pre-condition). The FDA has draft guidances for MMAs, with fairly clear distinctions between the two.

"Apps that have the following functionalities will not be regulated by FDA:

- Mobile apps that are solely used to log, record, track, evaluate, or make decisions or suggestions related to developing or maintaining general health and wellness, if not intended to cure, treat, diagnose, or mitigate a specific disease, disorder, patient state, or any specific, identifiable health condition.
- Mobile apps that are used as dietary tracking logs and appointment reminders, or provide dietary suggestions based on a calorie counter, posture suggestions, exercise suggestions, or similar decision tools that generally relate to a healthy lifestyle and wellness and are not intended to cure, mitigate, diagnose, or treat a disease or condition.

Examples of software products intended for use by consumers that the draft guidance says may be subject to "device" regulation include:

- Apps that allow users to input their health information and through the application of formulas, data comparisons, or processing algorithms, issue a diagnosis or treatment recommendation that is specific to that person, such as his or her risk for colon cancer or heart disease, or recommend that the patient take a certain medication or seek a particular treatment.
- Software that is intended to be used to physically or wirelessly connect to and download information from a diagnostic device like a glucose meter to allow the user to display, store, analyze, and/or keep track of his or her medical data values (Hyman, Phelps & McNamara, 2013)."[2]

While the FDA historically has stayed away from MMAs whose intent has been restricted to general health and wellness, it always has maintained regulatory power with respect to MMAs that are more integrally involved in disease diagnosis, treatment and management. However, the FDA also has the prerogative to eliminate the regulatory burden on certain MMAs, such as those whose intent is to help patients better manage their own disease(s).

"The following is a list of mobile apps that FDA believes fall within the medical device definition, but that FDA would like not to regulate:

1. Medication reminder apps for therapy adherence.
2. App for tabulating an Apgar score.
3. App for calculating drip rate for IV solution.
4. BMI calculator apps for use by patients and physicians.
5. Apps that help flag drug-drug interactions for physicians as they prescribe.
6. Diabetes management guide apps such as nutritional guides or pre-diabetes risk assessments.
7. Apps that offer behavior guides to help, for example, wean off smoking.
8. Calorie counters that would be specifically marketed to obese people or other people with health conditions trying to manage weight.
9. Cancer management apps manage medication schedules, and allow the patient to diary side effects and symptoms for reporting to their doctor.
10. Asthma management apps to assess symptoms, medication use and breathing data entered by the user to tell the user when their risk is changing.
11. Hypertension apps to help users log and chart their blood pressure, set medication reminders, record medicine taken, and share data with their doctor.
12. Arthritis management apps containing screening tools and questionnaires to help users determine the type of arthritis, provide treatment strategies and medication information, as well as information on diet and nutrition.
13. Chronic pain (fibromyalgia, headaches) management apps to help users track symptoms and triggers; weather conditions (humidity, pressure); photo attachments to document swelling, rash, discoloration; and interactive graphs of symptoms vs. weather to be shared with their doctor.
14. An app to help users who suffer from Chronic Kidney Disease (CKD) or End Stage Renal Disease (ESRD) make better decisions about their diet, by tracking their daily intake of certain nutrients and comparing their consumption to guidelines their nephrologist and nutritionist have set for them.
15. Digestive disease (Crohn's disease) management apps to help users record and track their food and fluid intake along with when symptoms arise and the time they take pain medication, all logged so a report may be generated for the doctor to review and analyze (Thompson, 2013)."[3]

As of August 2013, the FDA had approved just 75 mobile medical apps (MMAs), although many others are in various stages of development or approvals processes (FDA, 2013b).

The current global spend on MMAs is US$1.3 billion (as of 2012). The U.S. is the major contributor with $700 million. Right now, over 100,000 health and wellness apps are available and this number is expected to double by 2020. As more regulations come into play concerning security issues, future focus most likely will be on the quality of the apps. Also, there will be a significant increase in the number of downloads (Goel, 2013).[4]

Figure 1. Health apps by general categories
Graphics courtesy of Amit Goel (Used with permission)

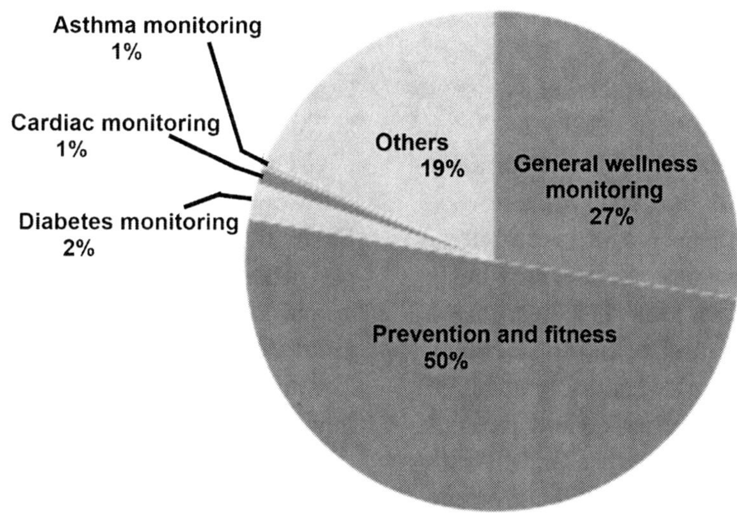

Figure 2. Detailed segmentation of health apps
Graphics courtesy of Amit Goel (Used with permission)

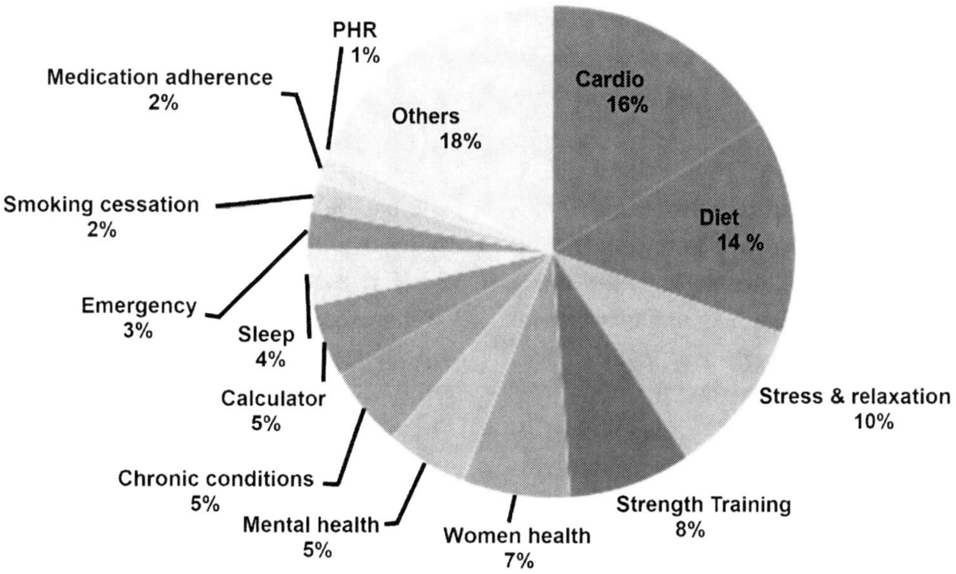

Clearly, opportunities exist for creating apps that support health and wellness for practically every biological function, and innovators around the world are competing in a robust market for the attention of global consumers. New offerings show up almost daily in the various platforms' app stores. These are some of them: Tictrac, Fitocracy, Fitbit, UP by Jawbone, Zombies, Run!, and, Withings.

Physicians and patients both have a vast array of new mobile medical devices and MMAs to help diagnose disease, treat it, and begin, where possible, to promote wellness and even prevent certain illnesses.

One might easily assert that technology, itself, is the driving force behind the practice of medicine and the direction of healthcare in the 21st century. By using an array of digital and wireless technologies, modern healthcare providers can deliver first-world medical care to people who previously would not have had access to any healthcare at all.

They do this through eHealth, or electronic health, defined by the World Health Organization (WHO) as "the use of information and communication technologies (ICT) for health." eHealth is a very broad term – which is good, according to three authors of a compelling editorial in the *Journal of the International Society for Telemedicine and eHealth:* "...how do you define something that is incomplete? Do you know where – or what – eHealth will be in five, 20, 50 years' time? The WHO definition is simple, powerful, clear, descriptive, and flexible enough to accommodate future areas of application (Scott et al., 2013, p.53)."

If ICTs are used (at all) to provide healthcare to patients any time, by physicians almost anywhere, then that is colloquially known as connected health care. If wireless and mobile technologies are used, it's known as wireless connected health or mobile connected health, and sometimes expressed as mHealth. All are subsets of eHealth.

As previously stated, the FDA wields considerable power in the approval of pharmaceuticals, medical devices, and medical software applications. Without FDA approval, no drug, device or software application can be put on the market for sale in the United States, even if it already has gained approval elsewhere by other internationally recognized regulatory organizations.

According to the FDA, connected health "refers to electronic methods of health care delivery that allow users to deliver and receive care outside of traditional health care settings. Examples include mobile medical apps, medical device data systems, software, and wireless technology. The FDA's role in connected health continues to evolve along with medical device technology. The FDA's Center for Devices and Radiological Health (CDRH) plays an important role in enabling a connected health environment while assuring that patients stay safe and the new technologies work as intended. Currently, CDRH is focusing its efforts in several different areas including the convergence of wireless technologies with medical devices (in partnership with the Federal Communications Commission (FCC); medical devices used in a home environment; mobile medical apps; medical device data systems; and, the role of software in medical devices (FDA, 2013c)."

Another subset of eHealth is wireless medical telemetry, which is generally used "to monitor a patient's vital signs (e.g. pulse, and respiration) using radio frequency (RF) communication. These devices have the advantage of allowing patient movement without restricting patients to a bedside monitor with a hard-wired connection (FDA, 2013d)." Wireless medical telemetry deserves credit for reducing the number of hospital re-admissions post-30 days because it allows physicians the ability to better monitor their patients after they originally leave the hospital.

Finally, telemedicine is another type of eHealth. Telemedicine allows patients to have remote access to physicians and medical/healthcare resources via a variety of means, including telephone, video monitoring, video chat, etc. It can bring the world to patients in the most remote locations, and likewise, it can bring some of the most difficult and fascinating patients' cases to world-renowned physicians, wherever they practice.

The single-most important vehicle for facilitating all the above listed forms of eHealth to work optimally is an electronic health record (EHR) – sometimes known as an electronic medical record (EMR). Just as each person has a unique fingerprint by which to be identified, so, too, each person will have a unique EHR that will include information about allergies, pharmaceutical history, lab results, doctors' notes, digital imaging and reports, and (eventually) full genetic blueprints. Authorized healthcare providers anywhere should have digital access to this vital information in order to deliver both *symptom*-appropriate and *patient*-appropriate treatment, irrespective of either the healthcare provider's or the patient's location.

This long-awaited convergence of technology, innovation and delivery makes it possible for eHealth to begin to tackle, on a global basis, the most prevalent noncommunicable diseases (NCDs) and chronic health conditions that account for the bulk of healthcare costs. "Of the 57 million deaths globally, NCDs contribute to an estimated 36 million deaths every year, including 14 million people dying between the ages of 30 and 70. Using mobile telephone technology mHealth practices can help save lives, reduce illness and disability, and reduce healthcare costs significantly (WHO, 2012a)."

The WHO has targeted five of the most pervasive NCDs (and two contributing factors) for global reduction or eradication. They are listed alphabetically below. It is important to understand the direction of the wireless connected health sector's development, including research and development funds for wireless medical devices and mobile medical applications, has taken its cue from this WHO global initiative. Many other diseases and illnesses deserve attention, but they will not garner significant funds for wireless R&D until these first priorities are met.

Cancer

About 30 percent of cancer deaths are due to the five leading behavioral and dietary risks: high body mass index; low fruit and vegetable intake; lack of physical activity; tobacco use; and/or alcohol use.

Tobacco use is the most important risk factor for cancer causing 22 percent of global cancer deaths and 71 percent of global lung cancer deaths. About 70 percent of all cancer deaths in 2008 occurred in low- and middle-income countries. Deaths from cancer worldwide are projected to continue rising, with an estimated 13.1 million deaths in 2030 (Globocan 2008, IARC, 2010). Tobacco use, alcohol use, unhealthy diet and physical inactivity are the main cancer risk factors worldwide. Cervical cancer, which is caused by HPV, is a leading cause of cancer death among women in low-income countries (WHO, 2013b).

Cardiovascular Diseases (CVDs)

CVDs are the number one cause of death globally: more people die annually from CVDs than from any other cause. An estimated 17.3 million people died from CVDs in 2008, representing 30 percent of all global deaths (WHO, 2011a). The number of people who die from CVDs, mainly from heart disease and stroke, will increase to reach 23.3 million by 2030 (WHO, 2011a; Mathers & Loncar, 2006). Most cardiovascular diseases can be prevented by addressing risk factors such as tobacco use, unhealthy diet and obesity, physical inactivity, high blood pressure, diabetes and raised lipids (WHO, 2013c).

Chronic Respiratory Diseases

Some 235 million people currently suffer from asthma. It is the most common chronic disease among children. The strongest risk factors for developing asthma are inhaled substances and particles that may provoke allergic reactions or irritate the airways. These would include indoor and outdoor allergens, tobacco smoke, chemical irritants in the workplace, and/or air pollution. Other triggers can include cold air, extreme emotional arousal, such as fear or anger, and/or physical exercise (WHO, 2011b).

Chronic Obstructive Pulmonary Dysfunction (COPD) is a lung ailment that is characterized by a persistent blockage of airflow to the lungs. It is an under-diagnosed, life-threatening lung disease that interferes with normal breathing and is not fully reversible. Symptoms are breathlessness, abnormal sputum, and a chronic cough. COPD is more than a 'smokers cough. (WHO, 2012b).'

An estimated 64 million people have COPD worldwide in 2004 (WHO, 2008). More than 3 million people died of COPD in 2005, which is equal to 5 percent of all deaths globally that year. The primary cause of COPD is tobacco smoke (through tobacco use or second-hand smoke). The disease now affects men and women almost equally, due in part to increased tobacco use among women in high-income countries. Total deaths from COPD are projected to increase by more than 30 percent in the next 10 years without interventions to cut risks, particularly exposure to tobacco smoke. Because COPD develops slowly, it is frequently diagnosed in people aged 40 or older (WHO, 2012b).

Diabetes

Diabetes is a chronic disease that occurs either when the pancreas does not produce enough insulin or when the body cannot effectively use the insulin it produces. Insulin is a hormone that regulates blood sugar. More than 80 percent of diabetes deaths occur in low- and middle-income countries. (WHO, 2013d) 347 million people worldwide have diabetes (Danaei et al., 2011).

WHO projects that diabetes will be the 7th leading cause of death in 2030 (WHO, 2011). Diabetes increases the risk of heart disease and stroke. 50 percent of people with diabetes die of cardiovascular disease, including primary heart disease and stroke (Morrish et al., 2001). Combined with reduced blood flow, neuropathy (nerve damage) in the feet increases the chance of foot ulcers, infection and eventual need for limb amputation (WHO, 2013d). One percent of global blindness can be attributed to diabetes (WHO, 2012c). The overall risk of dying among people with diabetes is at least double the risk of their peers without diabetes (Roglic et al., 2005).

Obesity

While obesity is categorized as a chronic illness with high priority for improving global health, it has many different components and causes. As such, it commands an arsenal of health and wellness/fitness apps geared toward education as well as behavioral changes to promote healthier living. Some of these include the following: weight charts, caloric intake diaries, caloric output (exercise) monitors, and nutritional values of foods and food groups, etc.

There is a medical distinction between overweight and obesity. The WHO defines a person with a body mass index (BMI) greater than or equal to 25 as overweight. A person with a BMI greater than or equal to 30 is obese (WHO, 2013e). BMI is calculated as weight in kilograms divided by height (in meters) squared.

Worldwide obesity has nearly doubled since 1980. In 2008, more than 1.4 billion adults, 20 and older, were overweight. Of these over 200 million men and nearly 300 million women were obese. More than 40 million children under the age of five were overweight in 2011. Overweight and obesity are the fifth leading risk for global deaths. At least 2.8 million adults die each year as a result of being overweight or obese. In addition, 44 percent of the diabetes burden, 23 percent of the ischaemic heart disease burden, and between seven percent and 41 percent of certain cancer burdens are attributable to overweight and obesity. Obesity is preventable (*emphasis by author*) (WHO, 2013e).

Hypertension (high blood pressure) is one of the key risk factors for cardiovascular disease. Hypertension is a silent, invisible killer that rarely causes symptoms. Many developing countries are seeing growing numbers of people who suffer from heart attacks and strokes due to undiagnosed and uncontrolled risk factors such as hypertension. Researchers have estimated that raised blood pressure currently kills nine million people every year. Preeclampsia is hypertension that occurs in some women during pregnancy. Women who experience preeclampsia are more likely to have hypertension in later life (WHO, 2013f).

Tobacco is an indisputable contributing factor to cancer and to chronic respiratory diseases. It kills up to half of its users. Nearly six million people die annually: over five million deaths result from direct tobacco use; over 600,000 non-smokers perish from second-hand smoke from cigarettes and water pipes. Unless urgent action is taken, the annual death toll could rise to more than eight million by 2030 (WHO, 2013g).

"Tobacco users who die prematurely deprive their families of income, raise the cost of health care and hinder economic development. In some countries, children from poor households are frequently employed in tobacco farming to provide family income. These children are especially vulnerable to 'green tobacco sickness,' caused by nicotine that is absorbed through the skin from the handling of wet tobacco leaves.

Tobacco smoke has over 4000 chemicals in it, with 250 of them known to be harmful and 50 known to cause cancer. Simply put, there is no safe level of exposure to second-hand smoke. In adults, second-hand smoke causes serious cardiovascular and respiratory diseases, including coronary heart disease and lung cancer. In infants, it causes sudden death. Over 40 percent of children have at least one smoking parent. In 2004, children accounted for 28 percent of the deaths attributable to second-hand smoke (WHO, 2013g)."

Today the world has one billion smokers, of which almost 80 percent live in low- and middle-income countries. This fact plays an important role in the disparity between a particular population's health (or lack thereof) and healthcare distribution. Those people with the greatest medical need typically have the least means with which to get it. Wireless connected health can help level the playing field.

Mobile telephony and mobile technologies have jumpstarted the economic growth of five specific populations that merit attention. They are Brazil, Russia, India, China, and South Africa. Colloquially, they are known as BRICS. Their vast geographies and unique cultures play an integral role in, and present enormous challenges to, providing adequate healthcare to their people living in remote locations.

For this reason, BRICS also offer some of the greatest opportunities for improving healthcare and quality of life through existing and emerging eHealth technologies, individually tailored to each place. All these populations face the WHO-identified global health challenges; each one also faces unique health challenges. Wireless connected health can address all of them right now.

In Brazil, the greatest health risk factors for adults come from diabetes, hypertension, obesity and tobacco use, according to the World Health Organization (WHO, 2013h). Brazil currently has five of Latin America's 23 mobile health projects running live, and one of its 10 pilots (Goel, 2013).[5]

According to a 2012 PriceWaterhouseCoopers (PwC) report[6], "U.S. mobile health development will trail developing countries like Brazil and India in the near future (Comstock, 2013)."[7]

In Russia, different sources give differing statistics, all based on data compiled over different periods of time. Essentially, the top health issues, in no particular order, are smoking, cancer, CVDs, chronic respiratory conditions, HIV/AIDS, and alcoholism. Alcoholism takes an enormous toll on Russia and its people, contributing to alcohol poisoning, road traffic injuries, other unintentional injuries, as well as suicides (WHO, 2009; WHO, 2006; Curtis, 1996). Furthermore, "a very high proportion of decedents whose death was attributed to 'other' or 'not classified' cardiovascular diseases had lethal or potentially lethal concentrations of ethanol in blood (Zaridze et al, 2009 p. 149)."

Cancer, CVDs, diabetes, tuberculosis, under-nutrition, malaria, and maternal/infant mortality account for the most serious national healthcare challenges in India (WHO, 2013i). Out of 80 live- and 37 pilot-stage mobile health projects running in the entire Asia Pacific region, India has more (24 live and 10 pilot) than any other single country (Goel, 2013).[8]

As of 2009, the major causes of death from noncommunicable diseases in China were cancer, CVDs, respiratory ailments, and injuries and poisoning (WHO, 2011d). "Studies show that few people understand the specific health risks of tobacco use. For example, a 2009 survey in China revealed that only 38 percent of smokers knew that smoking causes coronary heart disease and only 27 percent knew that it causes stroke (WHO, 2013g)."

Finally, the "S" in BRICS stands for South Africa, geographically smaller than Brazil, Russia, India or China, but economically vibrant and pro-gressive in terms of its adoption of mobile. How-ever, to focus only on South Africa, which must reduce the devastation of HIV/AIDS among its people, and exclude thinking about other African nations would be a grave mistake when consider-ing wireless technologies as means for improving healthcare and quality of life. This paper focuses on sub-Saharan and southern African countries.

Kenya, South Africa, Uganda and Nigeria rep-resent sub-Saharan Africa's healthiest economies, but they, too, have health burdens to overcome. Out of a total of 106 live and 46 pilot mobile health projects in place in sub-Saharan Africa, Kenya has the most: 20 live and eight in pilot stage (Goel, 2013).[9]

CHANGES, CHALLENGES, AND CHANCES IN WIRELESS CONNECTED HEALTH

Daily advances in wireless medical devices and software make it increasingly possible for phy-sicians and patients to benefit from easier and/

or earlier diagnosis of adverse medical condi-tions. As previously described, the GE Vscan ultrasound is a striking example of positive and possible change in wireless connected health. AliveCor Heart Monitor is another, allowing pa-tients to monitor adverse cardiac events and then relay the information through a secure website to their doctor, or store less critical information for later.

In addition to wireless medical devices used only by professionals or in tandem with prescribed patients, numerous new wireless medical devices are currently in the pipeline either for diagnosis by physicians or for prevention through personal monitoring by patients. One, called Eclipse, is a mobile breast imaging tool for home use in between regular mammograms. Still in the early stages of development, its team has chosen to use social media as a tool for generating further public awareness, building interest, and seeking funding for additional development. Another device, currently awaiting final FDA clearance, is QardioCore, a lightweight wearable heart monitor that comfortably can be worn continu-ously and frequently as required or desired, and for years (if needed). It sends clinical-grade, continuous monitoring of ECG, heart rate, heart rate variability, intensity of physical activity and skin temperature up to a secure cloud, where the data can be downloaded to practitioners who can monitor patients remotely in real-time (Qardio, 2013).[10]

For someone with a family history of breast or heart disease, both of these devices (along with myriad others), if approved by the FDA, may provide patients with self-empowering tools to regularly monitor their own health.

Finally, the very well publicized (and very well funded) Qualcomm X-PRIZE Tricorder global competition aims to foster development of a handheld diagnostic device, ultimately intended for consumer use, which will read for a minimum of 15 separate conditions. The expected date of the prize award is sometime in mid-2015, to be followed by the necessary FDA approval process, with consumer rollout as soon as possible after that.[11]

Prevention and wellness require knowledge, which can be gained with ease or effort depending where one lives in the world. While developed nations may have an edge in established health-care and medical protocols, they can be rather entrenched and somewhat resistant to change. Developing nations and regions have the advantage of leapfrogging over such structure (and restriction) and going straight to eHealth through a mashup of means of delivery. Some places use telemedicine. Some places depend on portable kiosks and clinics as first lines of healthcare, with referrals to specialists after an initial evaluation from a certified healthcare professional.

Gamification is a purposely-broad umbrella term used to encompass the process of using 'gaming' elements to motivate and engage people in non-game contexts (Deterding et al., 2011). It is an especially valuable tool since it engages young people – and *very* young people – through two forms of learning and entertainment they already validate: interactive games with a competitive aspect, plus incentives to win prizes or ranking; and, interactive storytelling games with role playing game (RPG) mechanics that keep players coming back to play more. "The 'gamification' of health care is the latest strategy for motivating pediatric patients and their parents to make efforts to adopt a healthier lifestyle. Gamification is driven by data collection and interpretation. Patients use applications and monitoring devices to document compliance with treatment regimens and to visualize progress and goals achieved (Schuman, 2013, p.33)."[12]

Games have been used in a feasibility study in Sweden and the United States to teach high school students how to learn cardiopulmonary resuscitation (CPR) using avatars in massively multiplayer virtual worlds (MMVWs). Conclusion? "A high level of appreciation was reported among these adolescents and their self-efficacy increased sig-

nificantly. The described training is a novel and interesting way to learn CPR teamwork, and in the future could be combined with psychomotor skills training (Creutzfeldt et al., 2013, abstract)."

"Games have also been created for specific health conditions. An example is Bant, a mobile app targeted at adolescents with diabetes that has successfully used incentives to improve the frequency of glucose monitoring (Cafazzo, 2012)." "If we show patients that we feel mobile devices are accurate and reliable enough for office use, we encourage patients and parents to consider using mobile health technology at home when indicated (Schuman, 2013)."

Vaccinations remain one of the most important tools for success in the global fight to eradicate communicable diseases. Unfortunately, many people fear inoculating their children because they mistakenly believe a relationship exists between vaccines and autism, among many other health issues. TiltFactor, a game company/research lab out of Dartmouth, has created a board game with a free app called ZombiePox. (Apparently, anything with zombies seems to motivate kids!) The app is a learning tool for children so they, themselves, will understand the importance of vaccinations. "When people see that the only way to win the game is to focus on vaccinations rather than trying to cure a rapidly spreading disease, the developers believe they will internalize the lesson and hopefully will be motivated to get their shots (Comstock, 2012)."[13]

An enormous number of MMAs on the global market target health, fitness, nutrition, hygiene and disease prevention, among a whole host of other health and wellness topics. Notably, African life and health experiences bear little to no resemblance to life outside of Africa. Thus, in order to deliver region- and experience-appropriate health care and wellness/prevention resources, providers must use different models than elsewhere.

In South Africa, Anne Githuku-Shongwe, the 2013 Schwab Social Entrepreneur of the Year and founder and CEO of Afroes Transformational

Games, has created a company whose *raison d'être* is to "build games, simulations and interactive engagements to inform, inspire and challenge young Africans using the mobile phone as an educational platform…. With over 450,000 users, we have built a series of mobile games designed to shape new choices and conversations. We built MORABA, an award-winning mobile game addressing difficult questions of gender-based violence and challenging the user to contemplate what he or she believes about sexual relations and sexual violence (Githuku-Shongwe, 2013)."[14]

While these games seem, perhaps, to be more socially driven than health-centric, they actually play a vital role in preventive healthcare individually, and societal wellness as a whole. Domestic and gender-based sexual violence and their consequences place incalculable economic burdens on healthcare systems around the world due to physical injuries, emotional trauma, psychosocial disruption, and the fact that many survivors of sexual violence never admit the true nature of their injuries to healthcare providers.

The biggest push for disease prevention and wellness in Africa has just begun, with the announcement that Samsung has created the Smart Health Hub, a pan-African mobile health platform. Initially, it will be featured on all new Samsung smartphones and tablets sold and distributed across the African countries in which Samsung operates.[15] It will be free to anyone who already has a Samsung smartphone or tablet, and available for free through Google Play and the Samsung Store for travelers to the region. Tapping on the Smart Health Hub button will take you into the following sub-platform areas (Simon, 2013):

1. Pre- and post-natal care.
2. Nutrition (providing guidelines for healthy African nutrition, since Africa has its own food groups and fruit groups pertinent to the African experience).
3. HIV-AIDS.[16]
4. Tuberculosis.[3]
5. Malaria.[3]
6. Symptom checker with colloquial relevance for Africa.
7. Aerobics and general exercise (games custom-designed in Ireland with motion sensor capture for interaction with a low-cost touch screen smartphone or a Samsung).
8. SafePoint Single-Use Syringe Safety and Information Campaign.[17] (This sub-platform area shows what happens if one needle is used on a number of patients, and educates how secondary infection can be curbed and HIV-AIDS can be prevented by not using any needle twice. Videos and other tools teach good patient and clinical safety regarding injections.)

Wellness also depends upon motivation. Much of the thought behind mHealth revolves around, and depends upon, the theory that, given the ability and opportunity, most people gladly will wear a variety of body sensors to monitor everything that's quantifiable about their physiology, moment-to-moment. Enough people already have started doing this to earn the moniker "Quantified Self." Trendsetters in the Quantified Self movement have been, predominantly, athletes and dieters, according to Alexandra Sifferlin in a March 14, 2013 article she wrote for *Time.com* (Sifferlin, 2013).[18]

Convincing people to purchase and wear a wireless monitoring device or sensor, as well as to perform different and specific behaviors related to it, may not be as easy as it seems.

Renowned Stanford University behavioral psychologist Dr. B.J. Fogg has written extensively about the three specific conditions necessary for an individual to make a change in behavior: motivation, ability, and a trigger.

His Fogg Behavior Model (www.behaviormodel.org) asserts, "For a target behavior to happen, a person must have sufficient motivation, sufficient ability, and an effective trigger. All three

Figure 3. Graphic illustration of the Fogg behavior model (Fogg, 2011)
BJ Fogg. (2007). [Graphic illustration of the Fogg Behavior Model]. BJ Fogg's Behavior Model. Retrieved from http://behaviormodel.org/. Used with permission.

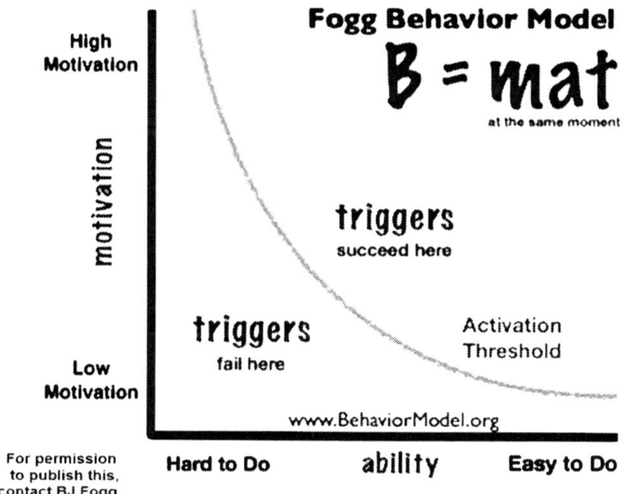

factors must be present at the same instant for the behavior to occur (Fogg, 2009)."[19]

In other words, it will take more than ability and opportunity for most people to adopt radically new behaviors to secure their own wellness and access their health data. According to Dr. Fogg, motivation and ability can trade off, but "the FBM makes clear that motivation alone – no matter how high – may not get people to perform a behavior if they don't have the ability." Without the trigger, a behavior *will not happen* (Fogg, 2009).

The FBM is perhaps most instructive because it provides insight into the user experience. Who is the user of eHealth? The user is a person. A real, live – sometimes quite ill – human being. Paradoxically, this same person will be perceived as a consumer by those selling a product and interested in profit, efficiency and statistics, and seen as a patient by those people on the frontlines (real or remote) providing vital healthcare to him or her.

Advances in wireless connected health make it possible and practical to provide improved healthcare delivery to rural and outlying distances through the portability of technology and digital communications. Telemedicine has proved itself to be especially effective in this realm. The study "1,000,000 Electrocardiograms by Distance: An Outstanding Milestone for Telehealth in Minas Gerais, Brazil," provides an excellent example (Alkmim et al., 2013).

The telehealth model developed to support primary healthcare in Minas Gerais has produced good clinical and economic results. As a consequence, it is now a regular health service in the State, covering 660 of the 853 municipalities, and integrated to the healthcare system. The model and technology characteristics permit the replication in other parts of the world (Alkmim et al., 2013).

The 'connected' in wireless connected health refers to the ability to electronically link multiple departments within the same hospital; multiple hospitals in the same network; and, ideally, different hospital networks and clinics, locally and globally. Interoperability (to be addressed later) will be mandatory for this last linkage to happen.

With the ability to digitally input all of a patient's data – her protected health information

Figure 4. Background for Minas Gerais State, Brazil
Alkmim, M.B. et al. Used with permission.

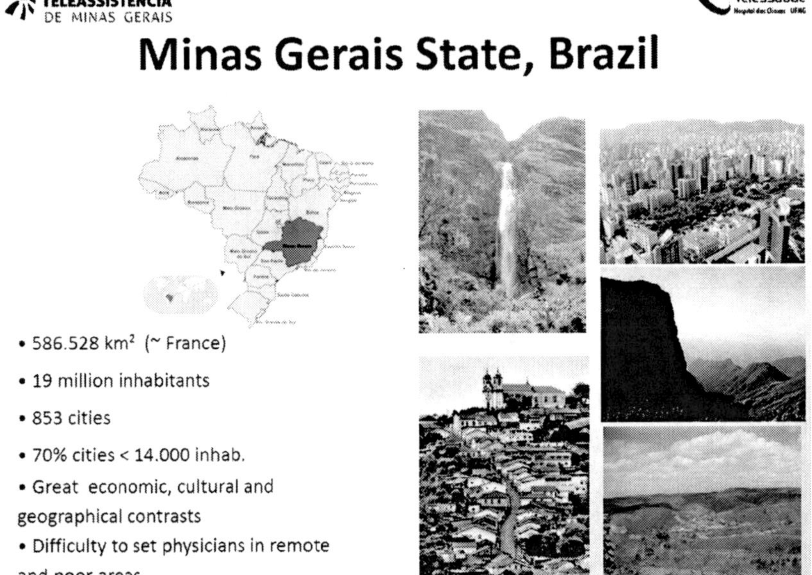

Figure 5. Telecardiology in Minas Gerais, Brazil
Ribeiro, A.L., Alkmim, M.B., et al. Implementation of a telecardiology system in the state of Minas Gerais: the Minas Telecardio Project. Arq Bras Cardiol 2010, 95(1): 70-78. Used with permission.

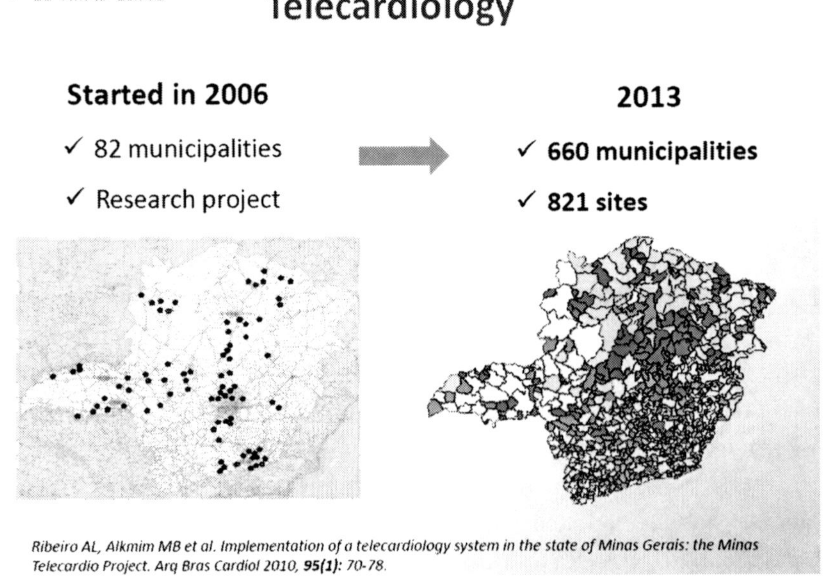

Ribeiro AL, Alkmim MB et al. Implementation of a telecardiology system in the state of Minas Gerais: the Minas Telecardio Project. Arq Bras Cardiol 2010, 95(1): 70-78.

(PHI) – doctors and other healthcare providers can create a unique, comprehensive electronic health record (EHR), or electronic medical record (EMR), that also should include allergies, complete pharmaceutical records, and, eventually, pharmacogenetic information. This then can be accessed directly by the patient, doctors, and other authorized people, irrespective of location or mobile device. This will absolutely have a positive impact on healthcare globally.

In other words, wireless connected health frees doctors to practice medicine from within or outside the confines of a physical healthcare facility. It gives people the security of knowing that wherever they may be – at home or globally – if they fall ill or need medical assistance, their protected health information can be retrieved from their electronic health record for a local doctor to attend to them, or for any specialist in the world to connect via eHealth.

Mobile communication has tilted toward text; medical tests have drifted toward digital; and impatient patients now insist on instant. The effects these changes will have on private practitioners cannot be overstated.

Some practices will upgrade to mobile and wireless ICTs and remain relevant. The up-front costs of doing business will increase, but they can be mitigated by the age of the medical practitioner and the potential number of years he or she likely will continue to practice.

Those people who do not shift to incorporate mobile and wireless ICTs into their practices likely may find themselves with fewer and fewer patients since they will be perceived as having lost relevancy in a digital age. Older physicians who foolishly think they can stick with their ways may find themselves forced into unanticipated early retirement.

Before we can examine how these changes will impact patients, we must address the greatest challenge, by far, to the success or failure of the entire eHealth initiative: interoperability. This refers to the ability for all healthcare IT systems

around the world to be able to 'talk' to each other. It is not enough that all the healthcare facilities in one country run on the same operating system and software. "Health information stored in one IT system must be retrievable by others, including doctors and hospitals that are a part of other health systems. This is particularly important in emergency situations (Kellerman & Jones, 2013a)." If a patient from one country winds up in another needing medical assistance, his or her local doctor(s) must have meaningful access to that patient's complete health record. If there is incompatibility between or among systems that prevents this, then meaningful access to a patient's EHR does *not* exist and the patient is ill-served, indeed.

So far, patients have greater ability than ever before to access information in order to understand their own medical issues. They have improved opportunity to actively participate in their own healthcare decisions. They have better access to physicians, relevant medical information, and advanced technology anywhere around the world. And with myriad MMAs and games to educate, motivate and monitor compliance, as well as encourage wellness and illness prevention, patients have an arsenal of support to help them live longer, healthier and, hopefully, happier lives.

Changing over to connected health presents daunting behavioral challenges – for patients, physicians and other healthcare providers, plus institutions. As previously mentioned, motivation will play a key role in determining whether or not healthy individuals and existing patients successfully integrate wireless technologies as a fundamental part of a new medical paradigm. Older patients, many of whom are either not tech savvy or not tech inclined, may find this especially challenging.

Perhaps the most perplexing obstacle to the gospel of mHealth preached by its zealots comes from age-old human behaviors such as denial, exhaustion, and hedonism, to name but a few. There may, indeed, be excellent wireless medical devices and mobile medical apps available to help corral people into better health…provided they truly want it. People commonly say, "Without good health, nothing else matters." But in reality, people's actions speak louder than their words.

As long as someone with a bad knee is in denial, then he won't acknowledge that playing one more game of soccer could sideline him forever. As long as someone with hypertension regularly skips exercise in favor of a hot bath and a hot toddy, then no amount of body sensors and data tracking can incent that person toward better health. And if a clearly overweight person has a lousy day at work and seeks comfort later with "just a single piece of pie…maybe with a little ice cream on top," then obesity will eventually win. Healthcare industry entrepreneur and angel investor, Esther Dyson, refers to this paradox as one of "the most interesting unsolved problems in health care and human behavior (Regalado, 2013)."[20]

Consumers will make any number of impulse purchases based on an incalculable number of different factors at any given time. Yet, for all the hoopla surrounding the ever-increasing number of MMAs available to help folks "become 'Quantified Self' types who can never have too much data on themselves (Wieners, 2013)"[21] as they track their vital signs, count calories, log their footsteps (and the list goes on), "most of the apps are merely part of the entertainment industry," comments Robert B. McCray, president and CEO of the influential Wireless-Life Sciences Alliance (www.wirelesslifesciences.org).

Unless the apps receive FDA certification as to the science behind their design, and the genuine health and wellness benefits they can confer, they're likely to become one-hit wonders. Still, there's still a benefit in these apps in that they make personal health and quantification fashionable and, in my view, cultural shifts have the potential to produce more health benefits, more efficiently, than the health care system (McCray, 2013).[22]

Health clearly fascinates doctors, medical device makers, and MMA developers. Presumably, that's why they choose the work they do. The mistake they make is in assuming the rest of the world is as focused on health, body sensors, data monitoring, fitness tracking, etc., as they are. Cars take up most of an auto mechanic's attention during the day. A fashion designer concentrates on fabric, texture and color. A chef wants to know who has the freshest ingredients and how to use them in an original recipe, and a political journalist cares most about getting the story first and getting the story right.

Someone who already *is* healthy and is *not* a fitness buff may not necessarily have an interest in taking up the sport of 24/7 health monitoring. And people with non-fatal, yet painful chronic illnesses (e.g., chronic migraine, osteoarthritis, fibromyalgia, Ehlers-Danlos syndrome[23]) typically don't want to think about their health on days when they feel good. They want to live for that day and enjoy it completely without thinking at all about when they're going to feel bad next.

This is actually when people with non-fatal chronic illnesses are at risk for acting outside their own best interests medically. To people living with chronic pain, sometimes having a bit of fun *is* worth the price of pain later, since almost everyone with chronic pain knows the pain will inevitably return, no matter what. "The development and maintenance of chronic widespread pain and fibromyalgia involve a complex dynamic process with biological, cognitive, and psychosocial factors…. Maladaptive thoughts and feelings seem to play an important part in the negative spiral resulting in the maintenance of chronic pain (Kristjánsdóttir et al., 2013; Flor, 2011).

Change never happens without resistance, particularly in medicine, according to Dr. Eric Topol, who wears many distinguished hats. He is director of Scripps Translational Science Institute; chief academic officer for Scripps Health; the Gary & Mary West Chair of Innovative Medicine;

professor of genomics at The Scripps Research Institute; and senior consultant for the division of cardiovascular diseases at Scripps Clinic. "Of all the professions represented on the planet, perhaps none is more resistant to change than physicians. If there were ever a group defined by lacking plasticity, it would first apply to doctors (Topol, 2012, p. 177)."

Not all doctors or healthcare workers like the changes they have begun to see as a direct result of connected healthcare. "The typical 15-minute office visit is rarely enough time to fully address the clinical needs of patients with multiple chronic illnesses, and the onerous documentation demands of electronic medical records ensure that doctors spend most of that visit interacting with the computer rather than with the patient (Ofri, 2013)."[24]

The costs of re-tooling a large health system for eHealth can be staggering. Memorial Healthcare System (MHS) (www.mhs.net) in Hollywood, Florida, is the second-largest public healthcare system in the United States. It has five hospitals (not including Joe DiMaggio Children's Hospital), numerous outpatient facilities throughout South Broward County, and over 1800 in-patient beds. Although MHS provides more than $200 million in direct costs for uncompensated care, it receives only $15 million (one percent) of its $1.5 billion annual budget from local taxes. The System's revenue is generated primarily by fees for healthcare services. A relatively small, but meaningful, amount also comes from donors through the System's two foundations (Janser, 2013).

MHS recently finished installing EPIC software across its entire health system (clinical data, financial data, EHRs, MyChart portal for patients, etc.) to achieve true connected healthcare among its different hospitals and facilities, and to begin empowering every MHS patient with meaningful access to his/her own health record. EPIC also offers secure messaging and scheduling apps that run on smartphones and tablets for those doctors who choose to use them.

The entire transition took three years, at a cost of approximately $130 million. MHS has invested extraordinary capital to keep the healthcare system at the top in its field, not only in terms of technology and innovation, but also in its commitment to patient care by engaging patients earlier and more comprehensively in making medical decisions for themselves. The greatest resistance to change came from…the doctors (Blanton, 2013).

In commentary co-written by Arthur Kellermann and Spencer S. Jones, appearing on *Project-Syndicate.org*, they, too, address physician resistance to change: "…a newly hired neurosurgeon with 27 years of education may have to read a thick user manual, attend tedious classes, and accept periodic tutoring from a 'change champion' to master the various steps required to use his hospital's IT system. Not surprisingly, despite its theoretical benefits, health IT has few fans among health-care providers. In fact, many complain that it slows them down (Kellerman & Jones, 2013b)."[25] In a recent PricewaterhouseCoopers report in which a number of health industry leaders were interviewed, the difference between doctors and patients, according to Steinar Pedersen[26], "is the centre of the battlefield" over mHealth. Misha Chellam[27] adds that such technology "changes the balance of power. It is not surprising that doctors would be concerned (PricewaterhouseCoopers, 2012)."

Educating new doctors and other healthcare providers, as well as re-educating older ones, present additional challenges for realizing the promise of eHealth. Many medical schools (and nursing schools) already have begun to incorporate mobile and wireless tools for teaching, diagnosis and therapeutics. Students can use mobile technology for reference tools, for virtual anatomy practice in place of cadavers, and as stethoscopes and ultrasound devices, for example. While these schools train future caregivers to use and trust data provided by spectacular wireless technologies, they also must teach students to trust their patients, too.

Today's medical schools must educate for a new "connected bedside manner." Students weaned on smartphones and wireless technologies are at risk, themselves, of forgetting to make eye contact with patients. Doctors cannot practice good medicine without this.

Skillful, compassionate and well-aligned care takes time. It goes slowly. It requires face-time, not computer time. We have to listen to the fellow human in our midst, examine her, go over both relative and absolute risks and benefits of treatment options, and then be clear about expectations. You don't really think an EMR is capable of removing fear and ignorance from medical decisions, do you? And the 6-page office note…this helps align care with a patient's goals (Mandrola, 2013)?[28]

Dr. Eric Topol is uniquely poised to envision and describe the future of medicine, not only because he is brilliant and leads an extraordinary team in the field of human genetics research, but also because he literally sees the future become reality each time another genetic mystery unfolds. He refers to the ability to unlock every detail of human DNA as the ability to 'digitize humans.' "Digitizing a human being is determining all of the letters ('life codes') of his or her genome – there are six billion letters in a whole genome sequence. It is about being able to remotely and continuously monitor each heart beat, moment to moment blood pressure readings, the rate and depth of breathing…all the things that make us tick (Topol, 2012, p.vi)."

With all due respect to Dr. Topol, the things that make us tick go well beyond mere genetic data. In Act IV of Shakespeare's *The Tempest*, Prospero says, "…We are such stuff / As dreams are made on, and our little life / Is rounded with a sleep." The phrase "digitizing humans" speaks to a dispassionate, clinical approach to issues that go to the very figurative heart of who we are as people. As a person *and* as a patient, I take offense at it. Dr. Topol concedes, with the various technology convergences that make digitizing humans possible, "there will be legitimate worries about depersonalization, about treating the digital information instead of the individual (Topol, 2012, p.xi)."

There can be little argument left against the benefits wireless connected health can bring. It will facilitate better prevention of illness or disease, thus engendering sustained wellness of most people. People want to feel well and they want to feel good getting there. Mobile games and other mobile means of education allow individuals to learn and process at their own pace and according to their own schedules. Peer pressure advocating for healthy living that promotes wellness will increase, just as peer pressure to stop smoking, reduce drinking and driving, etc., has had a positive effect on human behavior. As good healthcare becomes available ubiquitously, excuses for poor health will no longer be socially acceptable.

Wireless connected health will bring improved diagnostic and treatment opportunities for people living in rural and distant communities. Telemedicine has already proved itself a viable and desirable option for first line healthcare in remote areas. Lab work and other diagnostics performed on site can be interpreted at distant locations by transmitting data/images via mobile and wireless devices. Patients need not wait days and weeks for results, which benefits them if they have conditions meriting immediate treatment. As smaller mobile medical devices become standard tools for both health providers and patients, alike, problems can be detected sooner, therapeutic treatment can begin more expediently, and people with chronic illnesses have greater opportunity for extended periods of wellness through active health maintenance.

Another clear benefit of wireless connected health comes from using mobile and wireless media for faster containment of disease outbreaks. Upon discovery of the presence of any highly communicable disease, such as an influenza outbreak, healthcare providers can utilize many forms of instant communication to prevent epi- and pandemics. Mobile social media can alert local and global populations at highest risk. Mobile apps (such as GPS) can direct these same populations to safety zones. And mobile devices such as Propeller Health (www.propellerhealth.com formerly known as Asthmapolis) can be used to detect poor breathing conditions for at-risk asthmatics or people with COPD, both chronic respiratory conditions among the top global NCDs to address.

Opportunities for innovation will increase as more people become stakeholders in the healthcare process itself. Mobile social media makes it possible for online support groups and communities to connect patients with the same disease or chronic illness living anywhere in the world. People often innovate in those areas where they have a personal interest or need, and by joining forces and funds with mutually motivated people, they potentially can fast-track research, new products, therapeutics, and more.

SOCIAL, POLITICAL AND ECONOMIC IMPLICATIONS OF WIRELESS CONNECTED HEALTH

Health and wellness, illness and disability all contribute to self-image and how others perceive us. Based on our health status, we may gain or lose social standing, political power, and/or economic opportunity. The expectation of connected health is that, individually, people will be empowered to monitor and safeguard their health or improve it by using an ever-increasing number of mobile medical devices and mobile medical apps (and general health and wellness apps) powered by wireless technologies. On a larger scale, entire populations will eventually be enabled to shift from poor health toward wellness.

Psychology, sociology and culture play important and interconnected roles in the social implications of connected health. The extraordinary popularity of social media such as Facebook and Twitter prove (if ever there were doubt) that humans are social creatures.

Chatting online or via mobile social platforms about personal experience validates toward personal empowerment, and experience sharing among groups via social networks and online support groups further helps to validate an individual's own experience.

James Fowler, PhD, is professor of medical genetics and political science at the University of California, San Diego. His work lies at the intersection of the natural and social sciences, with a focus on social networks, behavioral science, evolution, politics, genetics, and big data. A panelist at the 8th Annual Convergence Conference of the Wireless-Life Sciences Alliance in San Diego, California, he asserted, "Friends will be critical over the next ten years." He discussed friends as data ("Data from your friends can predict your political party."); friends as sensors ("Data can predict, academically, by Twitter, about where there are H1N1 virus outbreaks."); and friends as motivators[29], referring to a Brown University paper called "The Social Context of Dietary Behaviors: The Role of Social Relationships and Support on Dietary Fat and Fiber Intake" (Dube, 2010). Not surprisingly, among the authors' conclusions: social support improved results.

Researchers repeatedly have shown the health benefits of belonging to a community (Helliker, 2005). Communities contribute to wellness. When it comes to connected health, the definition of community, itself, expands beyond geographic boundaries (it can exist online or locally), social similarities, or religious or moral values. Community can derive from people who share the same chronic illness, genetic expression, or other health-related similarity, and it also can develop around non-professional people who provide care to others with health issues.

In the United States, the National Multiple Sclerosis Society offers community not only to people with MS, but also to their families and friends. Alzheimer's support groups provide community for an increasing number of people who personally understand the challenges of caring for a loved one with Alzheimer's dementia. Perhaps the best-known example, globally, of healthful benefits from belonging to a community comes from Alcoholics Anonymous.

Dr. Fowler wants to "unlock the 'socio' for bio-pharmaceutical prediction and prevention," describing his own work as "tapping the social side for prediction and prevention. We need to uncover the emotional drivers of crazy decisions regarding our own healthcare (Fowler, 2013)." We need his expertise now.

Distracted driving, by using mobile media for texting, talking, or otherwise not paying complete attention to the road-train tracks-bus lane-bicycle lane-or-boating conditions (or others) invites potential injury or death for the driver-pedestrians-passengers-cyclists- swimmers-oncoming vehicles…or all of them. Still, people continue making a crazy decision regarding their own well being, and the sanctity of others' lives, every time they consciously make the choice to do this.

Cultural will figure enormously in the ultimate success or failure of global eHealth initiatives. "Culture is a term that refers to the inherited set of implicit and explicit rules guiding how a group's members view, feel about, and interact with the world. Cultural expressions and, to a lesser extent, cultural values change over time and are influenced by others (García, 2006)."

We already know wireless medical devices and MMAs work. They can help patients more precisely self-monitor chronic health conditions to enjoy extended periods of wellness, and they can help people learn to adopt new and healthy behaviors. This holds true for children as well as adults. However, the cultural drivers behind Western medicine do not necessarily have relevance for other cultures holding differing values, beliefs, and perspectives on health.

A commonly-held Western assumption that all people everywhere strive for excellent health in order to have the longest life possible is just that…an assumption. Many Eastern cultures give higher importance to living a balanced life, rather than achieving longevity. Some cultures are more present- than future-oriented, so trying to 'sell' the long-term benefits of changing behaviors now for better health in the future may have little impact. Still other cultures are group-oriented. Anything that places sustained focus on individual change – be it diet, exercise, or lifestyle – can seem threatening to the group as a whole (García, 2006).

Poverty is its own culture, or rather, a subculture within nearly every known culture around the world, and a subculture most every member would happily abandon if only he or she knew how. Poverty affects attitude and expectations. If a person grows up with nothing, is told to expect nothing, gets nothing, and finds no visible means of improving her lot in life, then by being told that simply changing certain behaviors will dramatically improve her life, she probably won't believe it.

eHealth can make enormous inroads to improve the quality of life for the world's most disadvantaged or at-risk populations if it first can crack the mindset that says, essentially, "Life is hard and suffering is inevitable."

In many countries other than the United States, healthcare is viewed as a human right and basic costs are covered by a national health plan. For these people, eHealth already has begun to take hold and likely will continue to grow. eHealth also has caught on quickly in developing nations without a pre-existing medical infrastructure. According to a 2013 PricewaterhouseCoopers report, "Patients and doctors in emerging markets are much more likely to use mHealth than those in developed countries – and more payers in emerging markets cover the cost of mHealth than in developed countries. Why? Existing healthcare is scarce – in many cases, mobile technology is the only (rather than alternative) affordable tool to reach people. The lack of existing infrastructure means fewer entrenched interests, so lower barriers. Change is more welcome (PricewaterhouseCoopers, 2013, overview)."[30]

As time passes and technology advances, savvy healthcare providers will lean more and more on eHealth innovations to accurately and efficiently manage chronic diseases, ameliorate or eradicate non-chronic medical conditions, and prevent illness in the first place. Prevention – wellness – will become the focus and new mindset in medicine.

It is good public policy to emphasize population wellness. However, population wellness cannot be achieved if people cannot afford the tools necessary for their health, such as a basic eHealth tool kit (for instance, a thermometer, blood pressure cuff and reader, ECG device, pulse oximeter[31], and glucometer). How will patients pay for additional devices when they already can't adequately cover the costs of their existing health burdens?

In the U.S., it remains to be seen how long it will take for eHealth to become the standard of care (beyond the federal mandate to implement EHRs by 2015). In our current political climate, private insurers dictate the economics of healthcare. Will insurers penalize patients who do not use eHealth tools because they can't afford to? And if so, will this stratify our society into a post-modern "caste system" based on health status, with healthy people being 'Brahmins' and chronically ill and/or low-income patients being 'untouchables?' As much as these may seem like economic questions, they are actually highly political in nature.

In our near future, wireless and mobile medical devices and MMAs will help us to avoid adverse health events (heart attack, brain attack/stroke, asthma attack) in the first place. Soon, using an ever-increasing variety of wireless medical devices and mobile apps, everyone (who can afford them, that is) should be able, theoretically, to prevent anything unmanageable from happening. Theoretically, then, no one would ever get sick.

Preventive medicine using eHealth technologies would make unnecessary, or greatly reduced, the social and medical "safety nets" governments have struggled to sustain in the face of shifting political winds and economic realities. It sounds almost too good to be true, and there's a reason.

Over 80 percent of the world's deaths from CVDs occur in low- and middle-income countries. People in low- and middle-income countries who suffer from CVDs and other noncommunicable diseases have less access to effective and equitable health care services that respond to their needs (including early detection services) (WHO, 2013c).

The promise of wireless connected health is just that – a promise – if it's out of reach for the very people who need preventive healthcare the most. Furthermore, women in low-income countries suffer disproportionately, simply for lack of access to early detection services. A woman who dies young often leaves behind young children, stunting their growth for loss of a provider, especially if the woman was nursing, and crippling their economic opportunities should they survive into adulthood.

Many other obstacles exist (besides the loss of one or both parents) to threaten a person's well being. All it takes is a vehicle crash, or tick bite, or fire, for our health status to permanently change in an instant.

Fortunately, technology is in place and enough data already exists for us to know on a day-to-day basis, and even on an hourly basis, for example, where air quality exceeds safe breathing conditions for people with chronic respiratory diseases; or, where climate conditions have created breeding grounds for mosquitoes. The truth is mosquitoes can actually drive public health policy.

In a 2013 broadcast on National Public Radio in the U.S., Beenish Ahmed reported on a two-year concerted effort by the local government in Lahore, Pakistan, to stop the spread of dengue fever, a deadly tropical disease caused by mosquitoes. Mosquitoes can breed just about anywhere there's standing water. In 2011, one of the world's worst epidemics of dengue fever hit Punjab (Ahmed, 2013).[32]

The government hired Umar Saif, a Cambridge-educated computer scientist who developed a smartphone app called Clean Lahore "to track all efforts to prevent the disease." Local investigators first canvassed the city to identify trouble spots and take a photo using the app. City workers then went about doing their jobs. If their jobs happened to involve prevention activities at known trouble spots, an investigator would follow, taking pictures of the workers in action.

With 'before' and 'after' documentation, workers knew they could not be accused of skipping work or shirking their full responsibility. "If Punjab averted another epidemic in 2012, then it didn't happen by accident," said Saif. "There were 67,000 different prevention activities [that] were performed and photo-logged by the smartphones." Saif went on to develop a Google map that correlates the locations of dengue cases and mosquito larvae for "a clear pattern of disease outbreak that corresponds to reports of positive dengue larvae (Ahmed, 2013)."

Sending patients across national borders for critical care transcends local politics and can sometimes be good for international relations. Almost everyone knows the story of Malala Yousafzai, the young, outspoken Pakistani schoolgirl who advocated for girls' education. The politically powerful and highly feared Taliban targeted her for assassination, but failed. Nevertheless, she suffered life-threatening injuries. Local Pakistani doctors and resources could not treat her severe wounds, so they airlifted her to a hospital in Birmingham, England, for critical care and long-term rehabilitation. What began as a gesture of good will between two nations turned an extraordinary young women into an international symbol of hope and a U.N. advocate for worldwide access to education for children.

When a crisis of almost any nature occurs anywhere, brave men and women show up to help, often traveling great distances and sometimes at their own expense: doctors, medics, engineers, trained rescuers, and others with the expertise needed to solve immediate problems on the ground. Telemedicine can play an increasing role as an international "partner" and "global ambassador" when disaster strikes. As long as a wireless signal can be accessed, ICTs can connect caregivers on the ground with expert doctors and caregivers all around the world. Having access to EHRs will help treat injured people promptly and *appropriately* to reduce serious casualties and possibly avert fatalities.

Politically, there is one very compelling reason to encourage and facilitate the adoption of eHealth to support population wellness locally and nationally, and that is to *sustain* population wellness. Illness and communicable diseases, such as influenza, cross borders without discrimination. Today, the global mobility and migration of people mean disease can spread rapidly. One infected passenger on an international flight can scatter sickness around the world. The best defense against illness is a foundation of good health and good public health policy.

Wireless medical devices and MMAs are quickly becoming "go to" tools for diagnosing, monitoring and/or management of a variety of health conditions that affect people worldwide. Costs and benefits go along with this wireless makeover – for the healthcare industry, for local and global economies, and for individuals. Most all of it is good.

Initially, healthcare providers, especially institutional ones, will face significant upfront costs to transition their facilities into eHealth entities. Not only will a variety of ICTs be involved, but also, new hardware and software may need to be installed or upgraded, and if pre-existing systems aren't replaced, then new systems will need to be compatible with them, at least for some time. Some of the costs were addressed previously in this chapter. The benefits show up as added jobs in the work force: real people sell the systems and must oversee every installation.

There are costs affiliated with training end users, too. These include doctors, nurses and other hospital personnel, who must actively train anywhere from eight to 16 hours per person (anesthesiologists are required to train the maximum time) – time and billing which is taken away from regular patient care (Blanton, 2013). For some providers, the high costs and complexities may force them out of business altogether, or to align with larger medical groups that can absorb them.

Hospitals and large medical groups also will need to spend money on community outreach to market and promote the new, user-friendly EHR systems that allow patients to access their entire medical record. Not all people will recognize or understand EHRs as a benefit, at first. However, most systems have been created to be highly intuitive, so users learn quickly how to navigate them once they try.

People who join the "Quantified Self" movement, whether out of vanity or for medical necessity, will face increased costs for the privilege or necessity of non-stop monitoring. Currently, it is not clear who will pay for these expenditures. As of October 2013, a pulse oximeter can cost approximately \$250, a blood pressure reader and cuff, \$129, and a heart monitor that can generate an ECG runs about \$200. A high-end baby monitor costs \$250, while the same company's baby scale is \$180, and its fitness scale costs \$150.[33] These costs are out of reach for most low- and many middle-income families.

Most MMAs currently range in price from free to a few dollars, while medical devices cost much more. One new market has emerged as a clear economic winner in the race toward connected health: "wearables." Until recently, "wearables" went by another, more clinical name: body sensors. "Wearables" is definitely cooler. Last year, nearly 30 million wearable wireless medical devices were shipped, according to ABI Research (Slabodkin, 2012).[34] Wearables are the *sine qua non* of any bona fide "Quantified Self." Some people sport multiple types of wearables simultaneously. UP by Jawbone, for one example, currently lists at \$130. Clearly, paying for the ability to "know (about) thyself" is not for the faint of heart or wallet.

Wearables allow for 24/7 monitoring, collection, and/or transmission of a garden variety of physiological data, ranging from body tem-

perature, skin temperature, amount and quality of sleep, to number of steps taken in a day, heart rate during exercise and rest, and more. They have become a new fashion statement, taking the form of bracelets, rings, watches, and even 'smart' tattoos. Fabric has been explored for its wearability for several years already, which says everything about its greater potential and absolutely nothing about how it looks or feels.

As people become healthier through the benefits available via connected health, the social cost of poor health should decrease. More households' incomes can be allocated for education and other opportunities previously unavailable due to financial resources being usurped by healthcare.

One unstoppable vehicle for health education is mobile games. Within the mobile games market, educational games are referred to as "game-based learning" or "serious games." Games that are used for such things as corporate training are referred to as "simulation-based learning." If there is any lesson to be learned, it's this: games make serious money.

According to Sam Adkins, chief research officer at Ambient Insight, "Mobile educational games are now outselling PC educational games. And the entrepreneurs are incredibly passionate about what they are doing (Takahashi, 2013)."[35]

In a report from research firm Ambient Insight, forecasters predict the serious games market will grow from \$1.5 billion in 2012 to \$2.3 billion in 2017, with the total market (including simulation-based learning) to grow to \$8.9 billion in 2017 (Takahashi, 2013). The global mobile health market is estimated to generate \$56.6 billion[36] in revenue by 2020, with the number of mobile apps on the market at approximately 200,000. The number of smartphone users by 2020 will grow to over four billion. Approximately half of these users are likely to use health and wellness apps, which indicates there will be numerous downloads and great usage of these apps (Goel, 2013).

While games-based learning offers many choices for youngsters and adults, it doesn't cater well to learners after the 4th grade because teachers seem to prefer using other methods to teach older learners. "There's a lot of debate still about the effectiveness of game-based learning, but it has long since proved its worth," Adkins asserted. "I don't know why we are still having that debate (Takahashi, 2013)."

Wireless connected health augurs economic growth locally and globally. As the field expands, it will create a need for new wireless medical devices, wearables, and apps. Every product will go through research and development, manufacturing and sales, and any aspect of the process can take place anywhere in a connected world. Globally, one source of growth will come through greater dispersion of population centers since adequate, even excellent, healthcare will no longer be restricted to major metropolitan areas. As the cost of healthcare delivery goes down, more people can enter into the system to access it. As the benefits of healthcare delivery go up, and an emphasis on illness prevention becomes the norm, overall population wellness will help maintain economic stability.

CONCLUSION

The high penetration rates of smartphones around the world now make the promise of wireless connected health a reality. Wireless medical devices and mobile medical apps have become the primary means for bringing mainstream medicine and healthcare to previously overlooked or underserved populations, especially in remote locations around the world. People unable to access regular healthcare, most notably in developing nations, now have another option for improving their lives through better health. They adopt eHealth quite readily.

While the road ahead remains uncharted in some ways, it also offers the opportunity for industry leaders to establish a connected health ecosphere that truly responds to the needs of end-users, taking into consideration not only best medical practices, but also the social, cultural, educational, economic, and political issues that contribute to a patient's experience of the world.

In the following paragraphs, I will provide my observations, insights and recommendations regarding people behavior, community, culture, education, entertainment/games, economics, public policy, and international relations in a wireless connected health world.

Behavior

Observations: In a wireless connected health world, a plethora of medical devices and MMAs can monitor conditions and provide massive data about one's health status, moment-to-moment, to the patient, the doctor, and others. From this data, preventive or corrective recommendations can be made and appropriate action taken, accordingly. Wireless connected health technologies allow us to create tailored communication to support patients and encourage compliance. Data alone does not persuade people to change their behavior, and patient non-compliance remains one of the most vexing issues in the fight against illness.

Insights: We need to better understand why patients do crazy things and don't comply with sound medical advice. We have the ability to track people's moods. This could be a part of every tool used in service to patient compliance. An empowered patient is one who will tend to do what is beneficial, not detrimental. If current technologies can predict which patients likely will not comply, then we have the choice of doing nothing and, ultimately, letting that patient fail, or else helping to provide whatever support is needed. If we can prevent or cure almost everything, does this mean we could theoretically live forever? Will it be a question of who can afford it?

Recommendations:

- Societal transformation begins by learning how to treat our bodies with respect and admiration for the extraordinary machines they are.
- Begin teaching children their bodies must last them a very long time and they must take good care of them.
- Organize a well-thought out, international clinical trial of known, non-compliant patients to search for insight that will lead to better medical outcomes with less patient resistance.

Community

Observations: Our notion of what defines a community has radically changed in light of social media and mobile social media. Improving health or sustaining wellness has a better chance of success with the support of one's social networks. Fowler tells us we can gather data from a patient's typical activity on social media and track it to see variances, which can indicate when that patient is reaching out to (or isolating from) friends. Evidence shows a well-supported person will be more inclined to do what is good for him/herself.

Insights: There has been much talk about healthcare solutions, but less about patient support, which takes different forms for different problems in different communities. The understanding of community has expanded to mean almost any group of people held together by at least one common interest. Since we know that community support improves patient compliance and health outcomes, helping people find – or create – the right support as soon as possible would benefit patients and caregivers alike. If illness and disease were colloquially (not medically) reframed as "conditions," and support groups were reframed as "communities," then perhaps the disempowerment associated with 'needing support' could be turned into positive participation in a communal group activity. Everyone has something to offer. This could occur either locally or online/mobile. In addition, the concept of rape hotlines and suicide hotlines is well established: chronic and serious health conditions can precipitate crises for patients and caregivers, too.

Recommendations: The various medical societies/sub-specialties should take the lead to create guided frameworks for support groups – caring communities – for the types of patients they treat.

- Create separate support groups/communities for patients from their families/caregivers and/or other support team members to encourage candor. Have at least one facilitator, to prevent the group from devolving into a 'pity party.'
- Engage another co-facilitator who is a trained healthcare professional to answer psychosocial or medical FAQs.
- Facilitators may need training in cultural sensitivity/cultural relevancies.
- Offer additional, trusted resources for reliable information.
- Every country should create these, so each community is language-appropriate. Translation capabilities still may be a digital necessity.

Culture

Observations: Cultural awareness helps when bringing Western-based medicine into developing nations. Working knowledge of customary and traditional local remedies for medical conditions also can prove instructive in building bridges that will integrate best Western medical practices with complementary healing regimens.

Insights: Culture plays a much larger role than possibly we have accounted for in the prescription for health and wellness. Many people around the world have ancient remedies and healing methods indigenous to their culture. We must find a way to bring in 'best practices' of modern medicine while, at the same time, honoring culturally respected traditions, provided they do no known harm.

Furthermore, when we talk about health, we also are *not* talking about death. Cultural beliefs about health, illness, life and death must be known in order to implement best modern medical practices that also respect cultural views surrounding the end of life. This even may extend to death rites of passage. Anthropologists and ethnologists can offer not only insight, but also directed pathways, to identify leaders of cultural communities, who can convey this information back and forth to build trust among all stakeholders. In this way, entire communities can be enlisted all together in the quest for wellness.

Recommendations:

- Identify colloquial relevancies and cultural absolutes.
- Ensure all recommendations are realistic by paying attention to the economic standing of patients and any other considerations that could impede compliance in spite of best intentions.
- Find something of value in each culture and introduce it to another, especially promoting cross-cultural exchange and conversation.
- Pay attention to religious mandates such as gender role expectations, dietary restrictions, and separation of genders so modesty (among other issues) can be observed/preserved as required.
- Above all else: ask leaders from every culture what is important to them!

Education

Observations: Everything about healthcare is always about education and learning for someone. Healthcare professionals' education and learning never stops. People may have rudimentary knowledge about health in general, but they only start serious learning on an as-needed basis when a particular health condition manifests personally.

Insights: Once people discover they "have" something, they become patients. Fear is often their primary emotion that drives everything else, whether it's fast-track learning of latest information, thorough investigation of complementary medicine, prayer/spirituality, or denial. Knowledge can mitigate fear. As our understanding of science and medicine increases daily, we gain greater choices in how to deliver newer, better, more customized care to patients, especially through advances in wireless connected health. One day, genetic mapping may make it possible to prevent NCDs or other conditions by interventional therapeutics. How might this affect our understanding of not "blaming" the patient for the disease?

Recommendations: This could be an extraordinary opportunity to change the entire conversation about health and wellness.

- Teach age-specific and demographic-specific audiences about a variety of health issues well before they would typically occur, including risk factors and known behaviors that can lead to disease.
- Teach how positive behaviors can help prevent disease onset.
- Teach how to recognize important physiological symptoms not to ignore.
- Empower patients, through early and ongoing education, not to deny pain or symptoms, but rather, to recognize them as important messages that our bodies need prompt care, like fixing a flat tire on a car, or watering a wilting plant.
- Start teaching health and wellness in preschool or grammar school. If we teach good habits in a positive way early on, then kids in the schoolyard (another type of community) can support each other in making good food choices and other health-positive decisions.

Entertainment/Games

Observations: MMAs developed as games are being used successfully to educate people while simultaneously entertaining them. They work especially well with young people and pediatric patients, who already play games and validate their design structure of using incentives or rewards to a) encourage repeat play, or b) drive competition with others. Apps for chronic conditions risk boring the very people who need to master what they teach and then maintain what they've learned, which often involves repeating one or more activities indefinitely.

Insights: Games have proved worthy vehicles for edutainment in many different fields. It's still too early to know definitively how effective game-based learning will be for instruction in health and wellness. Time will tell; initial results seem positive. If developers work in an interdisciplinary, collaborative fashion not only with epidemiologists, psychologists, and sociologists, but also with experts in artificial intelligence (AI), then they can develop agile games with compelling player/avatar interaction that not only can educate, but also continue to entertain and challenge players. Structuring games 'learning' in stages would allow players to complete one level of play and then graduate up the learning ladder.

Recommendations:

- Healthcare providers should seek to connect motivated patients with games designer/developers.
- Gamers with chronic diseases can explain, first-hand, what it's like to live with their particular condition and whether or not (or how) it affects their ability to play games being designed potentially for them (e.g., people with fibromyalgia might experience muscle exhaustion or pain from repetitive movements; people with diabetes might have neuropathy in their hands, plus loss of fine motor skills, both of which make using hand controls an issue; people with extreme hypertension might need to avoid stressful games or competitions with elevated emotional involvement; and, people with anything-plus-a-hearing impairment may need on-screen captions).
- Knowing the particulars of a specific condition, games designers could actually create a massive multi-player game for patients all around the world with similar (or same) conditions. This would create entirely new communities of people initially connected by their condition, but united over time by having fun and feeling better.

Economics

Observations: The complexity of networking different ICT systems to each other takes significant time, expertise, and capital. The costs for healthcare providers to transition their facilities into eHealth operations can be staggering, if not lethal barriers. The necessity for interoperability of networks and systems around the world is an imperative for eHealth to live up to its promise of providing excellent, personalized healthcare to any patient anywhere any time.

Much has been made of the costs to providers. Less has focused on the economics of eHealth implementation, especially for people in low- to middle-income countries. Eighty percent of NCDs occur in such places. Poverty, cultural traditions and reduced expectations for quality of life conspire to keep down those populations with the greatest need and least access to modern tools that can change those dynamics.

Insights: A smartphone or tablet is just the first of many costly devices and apps necessary for monitoring one's own vital signs and managing any number of chronic ailments. Who will pay for all the technologies necessary for poor, or even mid-income people to access the benefits of connected health? Will governments or insurers look to the models of telco operators and subsidize the cost of smartphones, wireless medical devices and MMAs to reduce the social cost of poor health? Would there be a value proposition in subsidizing the cost of a smartphone or medical device, and if so, for whom, and in what ways? If governments, for example, spend less on the cost of patient healthcare because of effective medical ICTs, would they pump such newly 'available' resources back into technology development?

As patients learn to better manage their NCDs, remaining healthier for longer, and as preventive healthcare increasingly keeps more people from developing NCDs in the first place, hospitals should see a downturn in admissions. What will this mean in terms of their own budgets, and more so, their fundamental identity? If people don't get sick in the first place, what new purpose might hospitals serve?

Recommendations:

- Hospitals and other qualified care providers should learn from each other about best practices for transitioning large healthcare systems and smaller, independent hospitals and clinics to eHealth.
- Consider alternative ways, besides full payment up front, for patients to afford devices and apps, such as rent-to-own, or micro lending to a small group of people who can share equipment, where feasible.
- As more and more people avoid illness, they will be able, theoretically, to remain productive members of society and enter, or re-enter, the job marketplace. Now is the time to begin thinking about how to maximize this future asset, including creating new job categories, such as interdisciplinary wellness mentors.

Public Policy

Observations: Data from wireless and mobile ICTs can help track disease, recognize adverse environmental and health conditions, and send alerts to people at risk. Wireless technologies can play a vital, positive role in public health policies and initiatives, which can benefit people whose lives are often at the mercy of elements beyond their control.

Insights: Good health doesn't happen by accident. Public policies promoting health and wellness need to be seen as relevant and beneficial by the constituents affected by them.

Recommendations: Leaders in connected health should seek out municipal (or higher) politicos to learn what kind of data sets already exist about their own populations.

- Examine existing data for new insights that specifically relate to health and wellness as they relate to communicable- and NCD patterns.
- In low- and middle-income nations, help frontline healthcare workers validate the efficacy and benefits of wireless connected health by implementing a massive campaign that educates and entertains, showing wireless and mobile as essential and welcome tools in the arsenal of healthcare, prevention and wellness.
- Communicate that effective public policy for healthcare, such as vaccinating school children against a host of illnesses, has contributed globally to the near elimination of smallpox, polio, and other dreaded diseases.
- Clearly communicate tangible benefits to individuals, as well as the community, of every policy initiated and approved.
- If public policy requires individuals to download apps to comply with the policy, then they should be not only free of charge, but also understandable to the broadest diversity of individuals.

International relations

Observations: An old aphorism says, "Good fences make good neighbors." A newer one might say, "Good connected healthcare keeps connected neighbors healthy."

Wireless connected health already has shown results as a vehicle for positive international relations. Telemedicine, especially, builds bridges between nations, benefits patients who might otherwise not receive adequate treatment, and now can turn these patients into lifelong ambassadors of goodwill for their "adopted" nation that helped them.

Insights: Physicians routinely rotate through the various specialties of medicine to attain broad-based knowledge, plus a sense of what it would be like to pursue a particular career direction. As a direct result of this sampling and exploration, they're highly versatile, broadly speaking. Those doctors who opt to specialize after general training often relocate in order to gain specific expertise.

Carrying out effective international relations requires knowledge about a broad range of subjects, too. So does connected healthcare. In a highly mobilized world that increasingly will rely upon wireless connected health, physicians and other qualified care providers could conceivably be called upon at any time, anywhere, to substitute briefly in the absence of a patient's regular doctor or qualified care provider. In essence, they would be conducting international relations *without* regard to nationality or politics because blood is always red no matter where it drips. Wireless connected health could hold a key to healing the world.

Recommendations: A new form of practicing medicine – via wireless connected health – may require a new twist in medical students' education and post-graduate training.

- Medical schools, nursing schools and training programs for other allied healthcare professionals should consider instituting a mandatory pre-graduation 'study abroad' clinical experience in a low- or middle-income country. This will give students even greater insight and connection to patients from different cultures and vastly different circumstances. While this recommendation would certainly entail complicated global negotiations regarding financial underwriting, legal liability, and other considerations, it would challenge the ingenuity of innovation that is the hallmark of exceptional and productive international relations.

- International physician exchange programs should be encouraged and cultivated through all available means.

- Interoperability of systems almost necessitates some level of interoperability among globally connected physicians and qualified healthcare providers, too, so they not only have a wealth of medical knowledge with the ability to collaborate, but they also carry within themselves a breadth of cultural and geographic awareness if called into service anytime anyone, anywhere needs medical help.

REFERENCES

Ahmed, B. (2013, September 16). How Smartphones Became Vital Tools Against Dengue In Pakistan. *NPR: National Public Radio.* Retrieved from http://www.npr.org/blogs/health/2013/09/16/223051694/how-smartphones-became-vital-tool-against-dengue-in-pakistan

AliveCor. (2013). *AliveCor Heart Monitor.* Retrieved from http://www.alivecor.com/en

Alkmim, M. B., Marcolino, M., Figueira, R., Maia, J., Cardoso, C., & Abreu, M. ... Ribeiro, A. (2013, April 10). 1,000,000 electrocardiograms by distance: An outstanding milestone for telehealth in Minas Gerais, Brazil. In Presentation to 2013 Med@Tel/Luxembourg. International Society for Telemedicine and eHealth.

Cafazzo, J. A., Casselman, M., Hamming, N., Katzman, D. K., & Palmert, M. R. (2012, May 8). Design of an mHealth app. for the self-management of adolescent type 1 diabetes: A pilot study. *Journal of Medical Internet Research, 14*(3), e70. doi:10.2196/jmir.2058 PMID:22564332

Cardi, V., Clarke, A., & Treasure, J. (2013, May 16). The Use of Guided Self-help Incorporating a Mobile Component in People with Eating Disorders: A Pilot Study. *European Eating Disorders Review*, *21*, 315–322. doi:10.1002/erv.2235 PMID:23677740

Carter, M. C., Burley, V. J., Nykjaer, C., & Cade, J. E. (2013, April 15). Adherence to a Smartphone Application for Weight Loss Compared to Website and Paper Diary: Pilot Randomized Controlled Trial. *Journal of Medical Internet Research*, *15*(4), e32. doi:10.2196/jmir.2283 PMID:23587561

Chronaki, C., Kontoyiannis, V., Mytaras, M., Aggoutakis, N., Kostomanolakis, S., & Roumeliotaki, T. … Tsiknakis, M. (2007). Evaluation of shared EHR services in primary healthcare centers and their rural community offices: the twister story. In *Proceedings - IEEE Engineering in Medicine and Biology Society*. Retrieved from http://www.ncbi.nim.nih.gov/pubmed/18003492

Comstock, J. (2012, December 4). Real games for health and the trouble with gamification. *MobiHealthNews*. Retrieved from http://mobihealthnews.com/19323/real-games-for-health-and-the-trouble-with-gamification/

Comstock, J. (2013, May 28). Brazil: An up-and-coming mobile health market. *MobiHealthNews*. Retrieved from http://mobihealthnews.com/22654/brazil-an-up-and-coming-mobile-health-market/

Creutzfeldt, J., Hedman, L., Heinrichs, L., Youngblood, P., & Felländer-Tsai, L. (2013, January 14). Cardiopulmonary Resuscitation Training in High School Using Avatars in Virtual Worlds: An International Feasibility Study. *Journal of Medical Internet Research*. doi:10.2196/jmir.1715 PMID:23318253

Curtis, G. E. (Ed.). (1996). *Russia: A Country Study*. Washington, DC: GPO for the Library of Congress. Retrieved from http://countrystudies.us/russia/53.htm

Danaei, G., Finucane, M. M., Lu, Y., Singh, G. M., Cowan, M. J., & Paciorek, C. J. et al. (2011, July 2). National, regional, and global trends in fasting plasma glucose and diabetes prevalence since 1980: Systematic analysis of health examination surveys and epidemiological studies with 370 country-years and 2.7 million participants. *Lancet*, *378*(9785), 31–40. doi:10.1016/S0140-6736(11)60679-X PMID:21705069

Depp, C. A., Kim, D. H., de Dios, L. V., Wang, L., & Ceglowski, J. (2012, January 1). A Pilot Study of Mood Ratings Captured by Mobile Phone Versus Paper-and-Pencil Mood Charts in Bipolar Disorder. *Journal of Dual Diagnosis*, *8*(4), 326–332. doi:10.1080/15504263.2012.723318 PMID:23646035

Deterding, S., Miguel, S., Nacke, L., O'Hara, K., & Dixon, D. (Eds.). (2011). Gamification: Using game-design elements in non-gaming contexts. In *Proceedings of the 2011 Annual Conference Extended Abstracts on Human Factors in Computing Systems* (pp. 2425–2428). doi:10.1177/0141076813480996

Dube, A. R., & Stanton, C. A. (2010). The Social Context of Dietary Behaviors: The Role of Social Relationships and Support on Dietary Fat and Fiber Intake. *Modern Dietary Fat Intakes in Disease Promotion. Nutrition and Health (Berkhamsted, Hertfordshire)*. doi:10.1007/978-1-60327-571-2_2

Flor, H., & Turk, D. C. (2011). *Chronic Pain: An Integrated Biobehavioral Approach. International Association for the Study of Pain Press*. Retrieved from.

Fogg, B. J. (2009). A Behavior Model for Persuasive Design. In *Proceedings of the 4th International Conference on Persuasive Technology*. Retrieved from http://bjfogg.com/fbm_files/page4_1.pdf

Fogg, B. J. (2011). BJ Fogg's Behavior Model. *BJ Fogg 6d*. Retrieved from http://behaviormodel.org/

García, A. (2006). Is health promotion relevant across cultures and the socioeconomic spectrum? *Family & Community Health, 29*(1), 20S–27S. doi:10.1097/00003727-200601001-00005 PMID:16344633

General Electric Healthcare. (2013). *Vscan Ultrasound*. Retrieved from www.vscanultrasound.gehealthcare.com

Githuku-Shongwe, A. (2013, March 6). The Greatest Return of Investment Is Investing in the Mindsets of the Future Generation of Leaders. *The Huffington Post*. Retrieved from http://www.huffingtonpost.com/anne-githukushongwe/afroes-anne-githuku-shongwe_b_2819045.html?view=print&comm_ref=false

Globocan. (2008). Retrieved from http://globocan.iarc.fr/factsheets/populations/factsheet.asp?uno=900

Helliker, K. (2005, May 3). Body and Spirit: Why Attending Religious Services May Benefit Health. *Wall Street Journal*. Retrieved from http://online.wsj.com/article/0,SB111507405746322613-email,00.html

Hyman, Phelps, & McNamara. (2013, March 12). Are All Health and Wellness Mobile Apps Exempt from FDA Regulatory Requirements? *FDA Law Blog*. Retrieved from http://www.fdalawblog.net/fda_law_blog_hyman_phelps/2013/03/are-all-health-and-wellness-mobile-apps-exempt-from-fda-regulatory-requirements.html

InfraScan, Inc. (2013). *The Infrascanner Model 2000*. Retrieved from www.infrascanner.com

Kellermann, A. L., & Jones, S. S. (2013a, Jan). What It Will Take to Achieve the As-Yet-Unfulfilled Promises of Health Information Technology? *Health Affairs, 32*(1), 63–68. doi:10.1377/hlthaff.2012.0693 PMID:23297272

Kellermann, A. L., & Jones, S. S. (2013b, February 26). The Delayed Promise of Health-Care IT. *Project Syndicate*. Retrieved from http://www.project-syndicate.org/commentary/the-delayed-promise-of-health-care-it-by-art-kellermann-and-spencer-jones

Kristjánsdóttir, O. B., Fors, E. A., Eide, E., Finset, A., Stensrud, T. L., & van Dulmen, S. et al. (2013, January 7). A Smartphone-Based Intervention With Diaries and Therapist-Feedback to Reduce Catastrophizing and Increase Functioning in Women With Chronic Widespread Pain: Randomized Controlled Trial. *Journal of Medical Internet Research, 15*(1), e5. doi:10.2196/jmir.2249 PMID:23291270

Mandrola, J. (2013, August 19). *Compassionate, well-aligned healthcare takes time, a luxury few doctors have*. Retrieved from http://medcitynews.com/2013/08/compassionate-well-aligned-healthcare-takes-time-a-luxury-few-doctors-have/

Mathers, C. D., & Loncar, D. (2006). Projections of global mortality and burden of disease from 2002 to 2030. *PLoS Medicine, 3*(11), e442. doi:10.1371/journal.pmed.0030442 PMID:17132052

Morrish, N. J., Wang, S. L., Stevens, L. K., Fuller, J. H., & Keen, H. (2001). Mortality and Causes of Death in the WHO Multinational Study of Vascular Disease in Diabetes. *Diabetologia, 22*(2), S14–S21. doi:10.1007/PL00002934 PMID:11587045

National Institutes of Health. (2010). *Traditional Chinese Medicine: An Introduction*. Retrieved from http://nccam.nih.gov/health/whatiscam/chinesemed.htm

National Institutes of Health. (2013). *Ayurvedic Medicine: An Introduction*. Retrieved from http://nccam.nih.gov/health/ayurveda/introduction.htm

Ofri, D. (2013, August 14). Why Doctors are Reluctant to Take Responsibility for Rising Medical Costs. *The Atlantic.com*. Retrieved from http://www.theatlantic.com/health/archive/2013/08/why-doctors-are-reluctant-to-take-responsibility-for-rising-medical-costs/278623/

Oudshoorn, N. (2012). How places matter: Telecare technologies and the changing spatial dimensions of healthcare. *Social Studies of Science*, *42*(1), 121–142. doi:10.1177/0306312711431817 PMID:22530385

Paiz, J. M., Angeli, E., Wagner, J., Lawrick, E., Moore, K., & Anderson, M. … Keck, R. (2013, March 1). *General Format*. Retrieved from http://owl.english.purdue.edu/owl/resource/560/01/

Palmier-Claus, J. E., Rogers, A., Ainsworth, J., Machin, M., Barrowclough, C., & Laverty, L. et al. (2013). Integrating mobile-phone based assessment for psychosis into people's everyday lives and clinical care: A qualitative study. *BioMed Central Psychiatry*, *13*, 34. doi:10.1186/1471-244X-13-34 PMID:23343329

Patrick, K., Marshall, S. J., Davila, E. P., Kolodziejczyk, J. K., Fowler, J. H., & Calfas, K. J. et al. (2013, November 9). Design and implementation of a randomized controlled social and mobile weight loss trial for young adults (project SMART). *Contemporary Clinical Trials*, *37*, 10–18. doi:10.1016/j.cct.2013.11.001 PMID:24215774

PricewaterhouseCoopers. (2012, June 7). *Emerging mHealth: Paths for growth*. Retrieved from http://www.pwc.com/us/en/press-releases/2012/consumers-are-ready-to-adopt-mobile-health.jhtml

PricewaterhouseCoopers. (2013). *mHealth implementation in emerging markets: PwC*. Retrieved from http://www.pwc.com/gx/en/healthcare/mhealth/opportunities-emerging-markets.jhtml

Proudfoot, J., Clarke, J., Birch, M. R., Whitton, A. E., Parker, G., & Manicavasagar, V. et al. (2013, November 15). Impact of a mobile phone and web program on symptom and functional outcomes for people with mild-to-moderate depression, anxiety and stress: A randomised controlled trial. *BioMed Central Psychiatry*, *13*, 312. doi:10.1186/1471-244X-13-312 PMID:24237617

Qardio. (2013). *QardioCore*. Retrieved from http://www.getqardio.com

Regalado, A. (2013, August 18). Esther Dyson: We Need to Fix Health Behavior. *MIT Technology Review*. Retrieved from http://www.technology-review.com/news/518901/esther-dyson-we-need-to-fix-health-behavior/

Roglic, G., Unwin, N., Bennett, P. H., Mathers, C., Tuomilehto, J., & Nag, S. et al. (2005). The burden of mortality attributable to diabetes: Realistic estimates for the year 2000. *Diabetes Care*, *28*(9), 2130–2135. doi:10.2337/diacare.28.9.2130 PMID:16123478

Schuman, A. J. (2013). Improving patient care: Smartphones and mobile medical devices. *Contemporary Pediatrics*, *30*(6), 33.

Scott, R. E., Mars, M., & Jordanova, M. (2013). Would a Rose By Any Other Name - Cause Such Confusion?. *Journal of the International Study for Telemedicine and eHealth*, *1*(2).

Sejdić, E., Rothfuss, M. A., Stachel, J. R., Franconi, N. G., Bocan, K., Lovell, M. R., & Mickle, M. H. (2013). Innovation and translation efforts in wireless medical connectivity, telemedicine and eMedicine: A story from the RFID Center of Excellence at the University of Pittsburgh. *Annals of Biomedical Engineering*, *41*(9), 1913–1925. doi:10.1007/s10439-013-0873-8 PMID:23897048

Shand, F. L., Ridani, R., Tighe, J., & Christensen, H. (2013). The effectiveness of a suicide prevention app. for indigenous Australian youths: study protocol for a randomized controlled trial. *Trials*, *14*, 396. doi:10.1186/1745-6215-14-396 PMID:24257410

Sifferlin, A. (2013, March 14). South By Southwest (SXSW), Will Collecting Data on Your Body Make You Healthier? *TIME.com.* Retrieved from http://healthland.time.com/2013/03/14/south-by-southwest-sxsw-will-collecting-data-on-your-body-make-you-healthier/

Slabodkin, G. (2012, December 11). Wearable mHealth device shipments to hit 30 million by year's end. *FierceMobileHealthcare.com.* Retrieved from http://www.fiercemobilehealthcare.com/story/wearable-mhealth-device-shipments-hit-30-million-years-end/2012-12-11

Sorrell, T., & Draper, H. (2012, Aug 10). Telecare, Surveillance, and the Welfare State. *The American Journal of Bioethics*, *12*(9), 36–44. doi:10.1080/15265161.2012.699137 PMID:22881854

Spyridonis, F., Ghinea, G., & Frank, A. O. (2013, April 10). Attitudes of Patients Toward Adoption of 3D Technology in Pain Assessment: Qualitative Perspective. *Journal of Medical Internet Research*, *15*(4), e55. doi:10.2196/jmir.2427 PMID:23575479

Takahashi, D. (2013, August 16). With a mobile boom, learning games are a $1.5B market headed toward $2.3B by 2017 (exclusive). *VentureBeat.* Retrieved from http://venturebeat.com/2013/08/16/with-a-mobile-boom-learning-games-are-a-1-5b-market-headed-toward-2-3b-by-2017-exclusive

Thompson, B. (2013, August 27). Set the FDA mobile medical app. guidance free! *Mobihealth News.* Retrieved from http://mobihealthnews.com/25040/set-the-fda-mobile-medical-app-guidance-free/

Topol, E. (2012). *The Creative Destruction of Medicine: How the Digital Revolution Will Create Better Health Care.* New York: Basic Books.

Turner-McGrievy, G., & Tate, D. (2011, December 20). Tweets, Apps, and Pods: Results of the 6-month Mobile Pounds Off Digitally (Mobile POD) Randomized Weight-Loss Intervention Among Adults. *Journal of Medical Internet Research.* doi:10.2196/jmir.1841 PMID:22186428

U.S. Food and Drug Administration. (2012, January 24). *Medical Devices: Premarket Approval (PMA).* Retrieved from http://www.fda.gov/medicaldevices/deviceregulationandguidance/howtomarketyourdevice/premarketsubmissions/premarketapprovalpma/

U.S. Food and Drug Administration. (2013a, February 8). *Medical Devices: Is the Product a Medical Device?* Retrieved from http://www.fda.gov/medicaldevices/deviceregulationandguidance/overview/classifyyourdevice/ucm051512.htm

U.S. Food and Drug Administration. (2013b, June 6). *Mobile Medical Applications: Examples of MMAs the FDA Has Cleared or Approved.* Retrieved from http://www.fda.gov/MedicalDevices/ProductsandMedicalProcedures/ConnectedHealth/MobileMedicalApplications/ucm368784.htm

U.S. Food and Drug Administration. (2013c, August 13). *Medical Devices: Connected Health.* Retrieved from http://www.fda.gov/MedicalDevices/ProductsandMedicalProcedures/ConnectedHealth/default.htm

U.S. Food and Drug Administration. (2013d, August 13). *Medical Devices: Wireless Medical Telemetry Systems.* Retrieved from http://www.fda.gov/MedicalDevices/ProductsandMedicalProcedures/ConnectedHealth/WirelessMedicalDevices/ucm364308.htm

Wieners, B. (2013, August 8). Dude, My Testosterone's Pushing 1290: How About Yours? *Bloomberg Businessweek*. Retrieved from http://www.businessweek.com/printer/articles/142612-dude-my-testosterone-s-pushing-1290-dot-how-about-yours

World Health Organization. (2006). *World Health Statistics 2006*. Retrieved from http://www.cdc.gov/globalhealth/countries/russia/pdf/russia.pdf

World Health Organization. (2008). *The global burden of disease: 2004 update*. Retrieved from http://www.who.int/healthinfo/global_burden_disease/GBD_report_2004update_full.pdf

World Health Organization. (2009). *Public Health and the Environment, Russian Federation*. Retrieved from http://www.who.int/quantifying_ehimpacts/national/countryprofile/russian-federation.pdf

World Health Organization. (2011a). *Global status report on noncommunicable diseases 2010*. Retrieved from http://www.who.int/mediacentre/factsheets/fs317/en/

World Health Organization. (2011b, May). *Asthma fact sheet No.307*. Retrieved from http://www.who.int/mediacentre/factsheets/fs307/en

World Health Organization. (2011c). *Country Health Information Profiles: China*. Retrieved from http://www.wpro.who.int/countries/chn/5CHNpro2011_finaldraft.pdf

World Health Organization. (2012a, October 17). *ITU and WHO launch mHealth initiative to combat noncommunicable diseases*. Joint ITU/WHO news release. Retrieved from http://www.who.int/mediacentre/news/releases/2012/mHealth_20121017/en/

World Health Organization. (2012b, November). *Chronic obstructive pulmonary disease fact sheet No.315*. Retrieved from http://www.who.int/mediacentre/factsheets/fs315/en/

World Health Organization. (2012c). *Global data on visual impairments 2010*. Retrieved from http://www.who.int/mediacentre/factsheets/fs312/en/index.html

World Health Organization. (2012d). *China Health Service Delivery Profile*. Retrieved from http://www.wpro.who.int/health_services/service_delivery_profile_china.pdf

World Health Organization. (2013a, October). *Millennium Development Goals (MDGs) fact sheet No.290*. Retrieved from http://www.who.int/mediacentre/factsheets/fs290/en/index.html

World Health Organization. (2013b, January). *Cancer fact sheet No.297*. Retrieved from http://www.who.int/mediacentre/factsheets/fs297/en/index.html

World Health Organization. (2013c, March). *Cardiovascular Diseases (CVDs) fact sheet No.317*. Retrieved from http://www.who.int/mediacentre/factsheets/fs317/en/index.html

World Health Organization. (2013d, March). *Diabetes fact sheet No.312*. Retrieved from http://www.who.int/mediacentre/factsheets/fs312/en/index.html

World Health Organization. (2013e, March). *Obesity and overweight fact sheet No.311*. Retrieved from http://www.who.int/mediacentre/factsheets/fs311/en

World Health Organization. (2013f, April). *A Global Brief on Hypertension*. Retrieved from http://www.who.int/cardiovascular_diseases/publications/global_brief_hypertension/en/

World Health Organization. (2013g, July). *Tobacco fact sheet No.339*. Retrieved from http://www.who.int/mediacentre/factsheets/fs339/en/

World Health Organization. (2013h). *Brazil: Health profile*. Retrieved from http://www.who.int/gho/countries/bra.pdf

World Health Organization. (2013i, May). *India: Country Cooperation Strategy*. Retrieved from http://www.who.int/countryfocus/cooperation_strategy/ccsbrief_ind_en.pdf

World Health Organization. (n.d.). *Health topics: eHealth*. Retrieved from http://www.who.int/topics/ehealth/en

X Prize Foundation. (2013). *Life Sciences Prize Group | XPRIZE*. Retrieved from http://www.xprize.org/prize-development/life-sciences

Zaridze, D., Maximovitch, D., Lazarev, A., Igitov, V., Boroda, A., & Boreham, J. et al. (2008). Alcohol poisoning is a main determinant of recent mortality trends in Russia: Evidence from a detailed analysis of mortality statistics and autopsies. *International Journal of Epidemiology*, *38*(1), 143–153. doi:10.1093/ije/dyn160 PMID:18775875

KEY TERMS AND DEFINITIONS

eHealth: Electronic health; a broad, general term referring to health care that uses information communication technologies (ICTs) to transmit medical data and healthcare information among patients, qualified caregivers, doctors and healthcare systems. The term eHealth is frequently interchanged with the terms 'connected health,' 'wireless connected health,' and 'mobile connected health (mHealth).'

Electronic Health Record (EHR): The unique digital health record for each person. Ideally it will contain all medical data across the entire healthcare spectrum, allowing any doctor or qualified caregiver to access all relevant medical information about the person they treat.

Health and Wellness Apps: Applications that can be downloaded (or pre-loaded) onto smartphones for the purpose of maintaining or achieving fitness and wellness and would include apps that help count calories, measure footsteps taken in a day, record amount and quality of nightly sleep, measure pulse, etc. Health and wellness apps are not regulated by the USFDA.

Interoperability: Refers to the ability for all healthcare IT systems around the world to be able to 'talk' to each other. Interoperability includes not only text, such as doctors' notes and lab reports, but also imaging, such as x-rays and sophisticated diagnostic radiological scans.

Mobile Medical Apps (MMAs): Typically, these are applications that can be downloaded (or pre-loaded) onto smartphones for the purpose of helping patients manage an existing medical condition (such as through diet, medication scheduling, awareness of exacerbation triggers, etc.) and/or helping qualified caregivers correctly administer medications, obtain vital statistics, or synch with a wireless medical device for performance. In the US, the Food and Drug Administration regulates MMAs.

Noncommunicable Chronic Diseases (NCDs): Long-lasting illnesses that are not spread via person-to-person contact, such as cancer, cardiovascular diseases (heart disease or stroke), chronic respiratory diseases (asthma or chronic obstructive pulmonary disease), diabetes, and overweight/obesity.

Quantified Self: The name of a movement that began in the late 2000s, whereby people collect, analyze and store (through MMAs) data on an increasing number of their biological functions and daily physical activities. People do this, currently, through the use of 'wearables' (see definition below).

Telemedicine: Refers to the transfer of patient information from one place to another via electronic means (e.g., email, video conferencing, telephones, smartphones) for the purpose of direct patient care. It is not a subspecialty of medicine, but rather, an augmented means of communication allowing medicine to be practiced when a patient and physician (and/or the patient's personal health information) are geographically distant.

Wearables: A broad term referring to a category of wireless data-gathering devices that can be worn on the body – either as clothing made from 'smart fabric,' or as accessories, such as wristbands, headbands, etc. – and then synchronized with other wireless devices where that data can be analyzed.

Wireless Medical Devices: Any wireless device that can diagnose disease or a health condition, or is intended for the monitoring, treatment or cure of such. This would include, but is not limited to, devices that monitor/track biological functions such as blood glucose levels, blood oxygenation, or blood pressure. It also would include smartphones that can function as an ultrasound machine, or record an ECG, or function as a stethoscope, among many other purposes. Wireless medical devices are regulated by the USFDA.

Wireless Medical Telemetry: The ability to connect patients to data measuring/monitoring/recording devices via radio frequency rather than cables. This untethering allows today's hospital patient to be freer to ambulate short distances without physical connection to vital equipment.

ENDNOTES

1   ©2014 InfraScan. Used with permission.

2   © Hyman, Phelps & McNamara, P.C. Used with permission.

3   © 2013 Chester Street Publishing, Inc. All rights reserved. Used with permission.

4   Used with permission.

5   Used with permission.

6   ©2012 PricewaterhouseCoopers LLP, a Delaware limited liability partnership. All rights reserved. Used with permission. PwC refers to the United States member firm, and may sometimes refer to the PwC network. Each member firm is a separate legal entity. Please see www.pwc.com/structure for further details. This content is for general purposes only and should not be used as a substitute for consultation with professional advisors. ©2012 The Economist Intelligence Unit Ltd. All rights reserved. Used with permission. Whilst efforts have been taken to verify the accuracy of this information, neither The Economist Intelligence Unit Ltd. nor its affiliates can accept responsibility or liability for reliance by any person on this information.

7   ©2013 Chester Street Publishing, Inc. All rights reserved. Used with permission.

8   Used with permission.

9   Used with permission.

10   Used with permission.

11   The dire need to improve healthcare and health in the U.S. is a problem whose solution has evaded the brightest minds. The Qualcomm Tricorder XPRIZE is a $10 million competition to stimulate innovation and integration of precision diagnostic technologies, making definitive health assessment available directly to "health consumers." These technologies on a consumer's mobile device will be presented in an appealing, engaging way that brings a desire to be incorporated into daily life. Advances in fields such as artificial intelligence, wireless sensing, imaging diagnostics, lab-on-a-chip, and molecular biology will enable better choices in when, where, and how individuals receive care, thus making healthcare more convenient, affordable, and accessible. The winner will be the team that most accurately diagnoses a set of diseases independent of a healthcare professional or facility and that provides the best consumer user experience. Visit the competition website to learn more. This prize is made possible by a generous grant from the Qualcomm Foundation. TRICORDER is a trademark of CBS Studios, Inc. Used under license. (X Prize Foundation, 2013)"

12   COPYRIGHT NOTICE: Adapted, displayed and reprinted with permission from *Contemporary Pediatrics*, June 2013. *Contemporary*

Pediatrics is a copyrighted publication of Advanstar Communications Inc. All rights reserved.

[13]   ©2012 Chester Street Publishing, Inc. All rights reserved. Used with permission.

[14]   ©2013 Anne Githuku-Shongwe, Afroes Transformational Games. Used with permission.

[15]   As of September 2013, Samsung operates out of all but six African nations.

[16]   The United Nations Global Fund for AIDS, TB and Malaria is an official participant in Smart Health Hub.

[17]   SafePoint is the inventor of the single-use disposable syringe.

[18]   ©2013 Time Inc. All rights reserved.

[19]   ©2009 ACM. Used with permission.

[20]   ©2014 MIT Technology Review. (www.technologyreview.com) All rights reserved. This quote has been reproduced with permission.

[21]   ©2013 Bloomberg L.P. Used with permission.

[22]   Used with permission.

[23]   An exception to this would be Vascular Type EDS. http://ghr.nlm.nih.gov/condition/ehlers-danlos-syndrome

[24]   ©2013 The Atlantic Monthly Group. All rights reserved. Used with permission.

[25]   ©2013 Project Syndicate. All rights reserved. Used with permission.

[26]   Steinar Pedersen, Chief Executive Officer, Tromsø Telemedicine Consult

[27]   Misha Chellam, Chief Operating Officer, Scanadu

[28]   ©2013 John Mandrola, MD. All rights reserved. Used with permission.

[29]   Used with permission.

[30]   ©2013 PricewaterhouseCoopers LLP, a Delaware limited liability partnership. All rights reserved. Used with permission. PwC refers to the United States member firm, and may sometimes refer to the PwC network. Each member firm is a separate legal entity. Please see www.pwc.com/structure for further details. This content is for general purposes only and should not be used as a substitute for consultation with professional advisors.

[31]   "According to Vancouver-based LionsGate Technologies (LGT Medical), the World Health Organization has recognized the importance of making pulse oximetry available to the developing world, where 64 percent of mobile phone users are found."

[32]   ©2013 Beenish Ahmed. All rights reserved. Used with permission.

[33]   All costs in US dollars.

[34]   ©2012 FierceMarkets and FierceMobileHealthcare.com. All rights reserved. Used with permission.

[35]   ©2013 VentureBeat. All rights reserved. Used with permission.

[36]   All costs in US dollars.

This work was previously published in Interdisciplinary Mobile Media and Communications edited by Xiaoge Xu, pages 305-343 copyright year 2014 by Information Science Reference (an imprint of IGI Global).

Chapter 15

Telemedicine Program for Management and Treatment of Stress Urinary Incontinence in Women:
Design and Pilot Test

Anna Abelló Pla
Escoles Universitàries Gimbernat, Spain

Vanessa Bayo Tallón
Escoles Universitàries Gimbernat, Spain

Anna Andreu Povar
Escoles Universitàries Gimbernat, Spain

Dolores Rexachs
Universitat Autònoma de Barcelona, Spain

Jordi Esquirol Caussa
*Escoles Universitàries Gimbernat, Spain &
Hospital Quirón Teknon, Barcelona, Spain*

Emilio Luque
Universitat Autònoma de Barcelona, Spain

ABSTRACT

Stress Urinary Incontinence (SUI), defined as involuntary urine leakage caused by physical activity and/ or efforts, is a frequently found pathology among women that significantly affects their quality of life. SUI treatments are often less effective than expected because they require a conscious effort by the patient to follow them correctly and usually have drawbacks, such as their high cost, time, and/or schedule requirements. ICT-mediated Physical Therapy treatment programs can be useful to improve Stress Urinary Incontinence symptoms and pelvic floor function in women while maintaining total confidentiality, with an at home treatment, accomplishing a higher adherence to the treatment, keeping a low budget for the patients, and saving the health systems' economic resources.

DOI: 10.4018/978-1-4666-8756-1.ch015

INTRODUCTION

The use of Information and Communication Technologies (ICT) and telemedicine can help improve the adherence to the Physical Therapy treatment, and, additionally, it can improve the possibilities of the healthcare providers to monitor if patients follow the treatment correctly (technically and in the recommended schedule), to control the evolution of the patient, and to interact with every patient individually.

Urinary Incontinence (UI) in women is a very important and prevalent health problem that affects quality of life in patients and can be psychologically threatening for them. Its treatment usually consists in Physical Therapy interventions and exercises in groups of affected women (added or not to a medical/pharmacologic management) and to do some individual exercises regularly at home. So, UI women need to go to the Physical Therapist's practice to do the interventions and exercises, generally twice or three times every week during some months, to learn and do their exercises in order to help improving their incontinence; added to the therapy, patients usually must do some home exercises on a daily basis.

This is a quite non affordable program in many cases, due to the geographical distance to the physiotherapist's practice, and for the time and money expenditure that women have to dedicate to the treatment. So, in many cases, treatment adherence is really low and women do not follow correctly the programs; moreover, pathology frequently does not improve as expected.

An ICT mediated domiciliary intervention program for women with UI and need for Physical Therapy is presented. This program has been designed and tested using ICT comodities, as an Internet connected PC with a regular built-in or USB video camera, Skype® and a specific Biofeedback device (Birdi®) to control the vaginal muscular force or the vaginal closing pressure and

monitor the quality of patient's exercises, sending data by Bluetooth to a mobile phone connected to Internet.

With this program, physical therapists can see and interact with every patient confidentially, receive all medical data from the patient to control the quality of the exercise done and monitor and evaluate how every patient's UI is improving day by day. Neither the patient nor the physical therapist must move from their locations, and quality therapy can be provided to patients anywhere in the world, easily and confidentially.

The aim of this chapter is to show how ICT can be applied to conservative Stress Urinary Incontinence treatments (SUI) (Physical Therapy).

This chapter begins with background information about telemedicine and Urinary Incontinence. The main focus of the chapter explains the current model used in Stress Urinary Incontinence treatment followed by our proposal and recommendations: the use of telemedicine and the ICT aided Physical Therapy management and treatment of SUI. After that, we propose future research directions. Then, at the end, there are our conclusions.

BACKGROUND

Telemedicine Generalities

Telemedicine is defined as the use of telecommunication and information technologies in order to provide clinical health care at distance. The American Telemedicine Association (ATA: www. americantelemed.org) defines telemedicine as "the use of medical information exchanged from one site to another via electronic communications to improve a patient's clinical health status".

Sometimes, the terms telemedicine and telehealth may refer to different meanings or definitions but ATA, for example, usually considers them to be interchangeable, providing a wider definition of remote healthcare. Telehealth is often used when interventions do not always mean clinical services such as patient consultations, transmission of still images, e-health portals, etc.

Telemedicine has been reported (by ATA) to have huge benefits as improved access, improved quality and cost-effectiveness. Telemedicine improves access to patients to healthcare and allows health care providers to expand their reach. It has been shown that the quality of telemedicine-delivered services can be as good as those given on-site. In some fields, the resultant product is even superior, showing greater satisfaction and outcomes. It reduces the cost of healthcare and increases efficiency through a better management of diseases.

Additional benefits are found in the use of telemedicine: it usually is an inexpensive user-friendly service that allows patients to have a flexible schedule and the possibility of doing everything from the comfort of their own home (Figure 1). This technology helps improve the management

of diseases by maximizing treatment adherence and comfort, accomplishing a better fulfillment while maintaining, at all times, the patient's privacy, intimacy and while ensuring confidentiality of patients' data (Figure 2).

ATA affirms that patients and costumers want telemedicine: it reduces travel time and related stress. It shows greater satisfaction and they support its use. The most common use of telemedicine is still consultation: patients use this service to consult different healthcare providers about health-related issues.

The first reference about telemedicine in Pubmed is from 1974 (Pubmed - http://www.ncbi.nlm.nih.gov/pubmed - is a free search engine accessing the MEDLINE database of references and abstracts on life sciences and biomedical topics, part of the United States National Library of Medicine at the National Institutes of Health; it is the most used search engine by healthcare providers and medical scientists). The references for the next decade are about its first applications at the

Figure 1. ICT contribution advantages in telemedicine

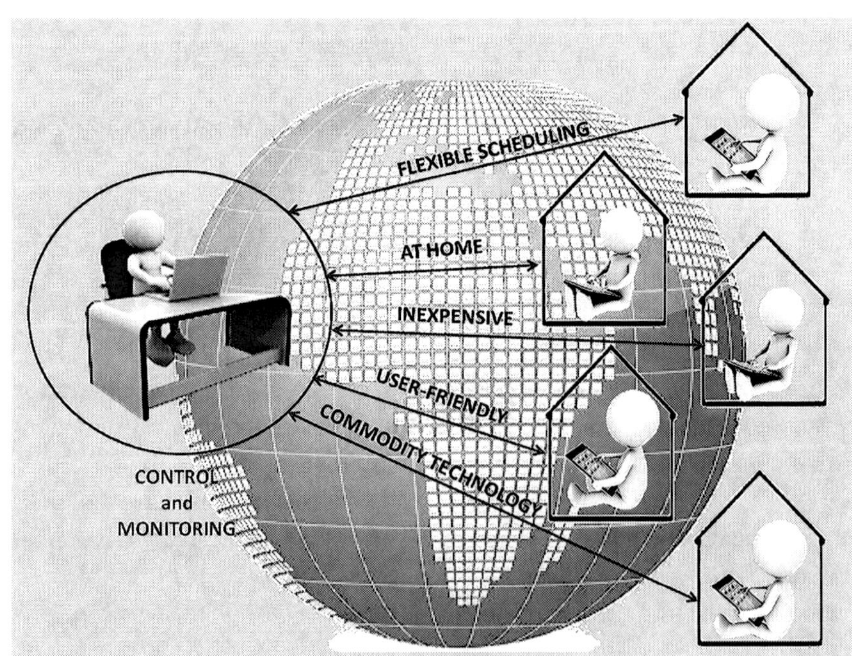

Figure 2. Technology contribution for improving the efficiency of diseases' management

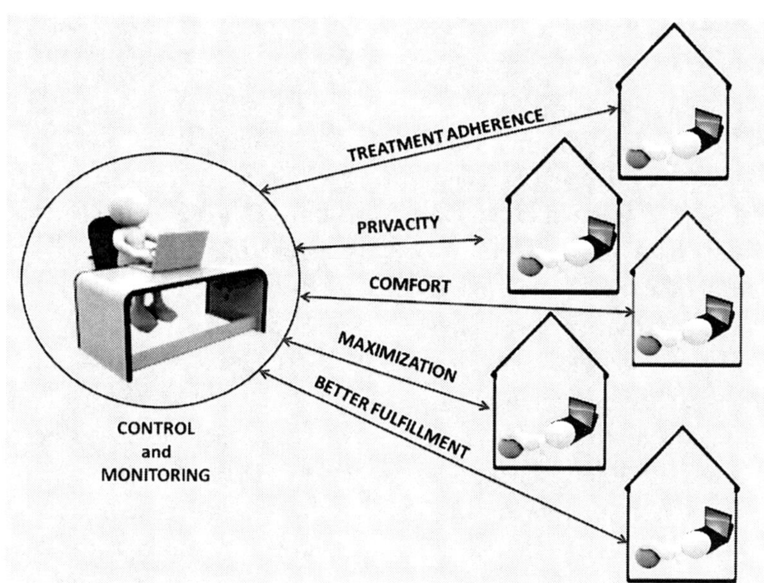

healthcare system and its first outcomes. There are even one or two studies about telemedicine applications in space travel. In the following years, a lot of medical fields adopted telemedicine as a new way of communication and management of their patients' health problems. An unestructured Pubmed search shows that Telemedicine has been used in fields like psychiatry (Lokkerbol, 2014), pneumology (Segrelles Calvo et al., 2014), cardiology (Brunetti et al., 2014), endocrinology (Franc et al., 2014), etc.

In Physical Therapy, telemedicine application began fifteen years ago, more or less. Its first applications in this field were in orthopedic rehabilitation and muscle function improvement. In the following years, other beneficial uses have been tested and showed great results. Nowadays, telemedicine is used to manage acute and chronic diseases, to assess patients' health status, to control their clinical evolution and to treat a lot of different pathologies. In the treatment of Urinary Incontinence, only one study was found that referenced the use of telemedicine (Hui, Lee & Woo, 2006).

Telemedicine has been shown to be a growing and useful tool for all healthcare providers who want to expand their horizons; and for patients, who can have access to this service and can take advantage of its always improving technologies and benefits.

Urinary Incontinence Generalities

In 2009, the International Continence Society (ICS) along with the International Urogynecological Association (IUGA) wrote a joint report where they defined Urinary Incontinence as the "complain of involuntary loss of urine" (Haylen et al., 2010). The US Agency for Health Care Policy and Research (AHCPR) considers that UI is one of the seven medical conditions that have more impact on the health of patients who suffer this condition, comparable to Blood Hypertension or Diabetes Mellitus (Brenes, Dios-Diz & Naval, 2007).

Urinary Incontinence (UI) causes social and family troubles to the patient, being nowadays an important health problem that has a high influence in medical, psychological, social, and economic bearings affecting their quality of life. Urinary Incontinence affects patients' quality of life, restricting their physical activity. The most influential factors for the quality of life decrease in this pathology are age, incontinence severity, symptomatology stage and urinary infections (Córcoles et al., 2008).

Knowing which factors favor, predispose and/or facilitate the appearance of UI and their sequels makes easier to deal with this common pathology that has a huge effect on the emotional sphere. This way, the treatment can be more effective and more efficient, avoiding consequences such as social and emotional exclusion. Nevertheless, one of the biggest problems in treating UI is the adherence to the treatment programs, because it requires all the patients to go to multiple Physical Therapy sessions and, after learning the techniques and exercises, patients must follow their treatments at home. Usually, a lack of adherence entails the therapy's failure (Brenes et al., 2007).

There are three types of Urinary Incontinence, based in symptomatic signs (Espuña Pons, Castro DIaz, Carbonell & Dilla, 2007): Stress Urinary Incontinence (SUI), referred as involuntary urine leakage caused by physical activity, efforts or after simple acts (as sneezing or coughing); Urge Urinary Incontinence (UUI), defined as involuntary urine leakage accompanied or immediately preceded by urgency symptoms; and Mixed Urinary Incontinence (MUI), which includes the simultaneous symptoms of both previously defined types.

The National Health and Nutrition Survey defines the severity of Urinary Incontinence as (Minassian, Stewart & Wood, 2008): Severe, when leakage occurs once or twice a week; Moderate, when there are about two episodes in one month; and Slight, when leakage episodes occur once or twice a year.

Prevalence

The large amount of bibliography about Urinary Incontinence shows the huge importance that the scientific community gives to this pathology in women. Nevertheless, one of the most important

difficulties is establishing its prevalence (Minaire, Sengler, & Jacquetin, 1995; Minassian, Drutz, & Al-Badr, 2003; Minassian et al., 2008).

One of the most important published studies (analyzing all types and severities in middle-aged and elderly women in the general population) estimates that the prevalence of Urinary Incontinence varies between 30% and 60%, also showing that prevalence increases with age (Milsom et al., 2009).

Recognition of suffering UI is an unsolved question, too; among healthy university young women Escoles Universitaries Gimbernat (Barcelona, Catalonia, Spain) published a study about prevalence and recognition of UI in healthy, nulliparous and nuligravid women (n=403), aged between 18 and 25; results estimated prevalence in a 47% (45,5% slight, 47% moderate and 3,5% severe), yet only a 21,8% considered or recognized suffering the disease (Abelló, Esquirol, Salas & Bayo, 2009).

Hunskaar, Lose, Sykes & Voss (2004) gathered information about UI in four European countries (Spain included, too): women older than 18 answered a survey. They estimated a prevalence of 23% with an increase related to age.

Different studies in young, nulliparous and nulligravid women point out the presence of incontinence symptoms: 17% according to Jolleys, 40% to Scout, 57% according to Wolin and 52% to Gemir. In this last one, about 30% of the women had very little but daily leakage.

In a sample of 409 nursing students (mean age 20.4 years), a prevalence of 47.7% was estimated, following a strictly medical diagnosis. 260 women were considered incontinent, 253 of which had minimal occasional leakage. 18 of them were affected psychologically and socially: these socially and psychologically affected women are those that really use to suppose a challenge to the physical therapist (Grosse & Sengler, 1998).

Ueda, Tamaki, Kageyama, Yoshimura & Yoshida (2000) gathered information about women between 40 and 75: Stress Urinary Incontinence

(SUI) was present at all ages but urge incontinence (UUI) was only present in older women, especially in those over 70.

Women who practice high impact sports, as gymnasts and athletes, have higher prevalence rates than those who practice other sports modalities. Eliasson, Larsson and Mattsson (2002), studied Urinary Incontinence prevalence in nulliparous professional trampolinists sports women. 80% of them answered positively to the test about having involuntary urine leakage only during training sessions. Women age and training duration and frequency showed a positively correlation with UI presence. Further investigation should be done in this area to study muscular function and muscular activity in women who practice those kinds of sports professionally (Bø, 2004a).

There are some theories that aim to explain why establishing a global prevalence rate use to be so difficult. It has been suggested that the female population tends to underestimate Urinary Incontinence as a health problem if it's slight: it is often a taboo subject and women have the tendency of not talking about it if the issue is not presented in a way that it is very discreet, confidential and direct (Ricatte, 2004). It seem that a lot of women do not consider UI as a problem: they tend to think that this is the consequence of usual evolution (especially those women who has children). Moreover, UI usually begins as slow beginning irregular symptoms, and patients use to get used to the symptoms.

Added to this, there is also a total lack of homogeneity in epidemiological studies: not every research team use the same definitions, population or mean ages in their samples (Lenoir, 2005).

Diagnosis

In order to diagnose and evaluate UI severity, there are two commonly used questionnaires that help achieve the task: ICIQ-SF and ISI test.

The ICIQ-SF (International Consultation on Incontinence Questionnaire – Short Form)

(Klovning, Avery, Sandvik & Hunskaar, 2009) is a questionnaire designed to detect Urinary Incontinence. It has three items: the first two refer to frequency and quantity, the third asks about how much quality of life is affected. Its final punctuation is obtained after adding up the scores of the first three items. Its graduation varies from zero to twenty-one. There are eight additional questions that do not have a score and their aim is to orientate about the type of the UI among the three types described (SUI, UUI or MUI), helping define in which situations leakage occurs.

The ISI test (Incontinence Severity Index) (Sandvik, Espuna & Hunskaar, 2006), is a questionnaire designed to evaluate the degree of affectation in people who suffer from UI with patients with a positive ICIQ-SF result. It has two questions: the first once refers to leakage frequency and the second asks about leakage quantity. Its final punctuation is obtained after adding up the scores of the two items and it ranges from one to twelve. With these scores, UI can be classified as: slight (1-2), moderate (3-6), severe (8-9), very severe (10-12).

The estimated time for answering both questionnaires is about one minute each.

Conservative Treatment for Stress Urinary Incontinence: Physical Therapy

Physical Therapy is the first therapeutic choice for Stress Urinary Incontinence because it has no secondary effects and is minimally invasive (Berghmans, 2006) (Agennee Nationale d'Ácerédidation et d'Évaluation en Santé., 2000). Although the origin of SUI might not be caused by muscular issues (for example: urethral hypermobility or urethral decreased thickness) (Calais Germain, 1998), the therapeutic basis is centered in restoring or strengthening muscular functions (Grosse & Sengler, 1998); it has been suggested that a deep abdominal co-contraction combined with other interventions that help restoring muscular function might be helpful. Therapeutic approach includes perineum and abdominal muscles exercises, traditionally trained using some kind of special exercises traditionally known as "Kegel exercises" (Bø, 2004b), nowadays known as Pelvic Floor Muscle Exercises.

Pelvic Floor Muscle Training (PFMT) to treat Urinary Incontinence has been described in several ancient texts: "Deer Exercises" were part of an exercise routine in Taoist practices during 16.000 years; ancient Indian texts also reflected similar exercises included in Ashwini Mudra, done by yogis; Hippocrates and Galen also described pelvic floor exercises in ancient Rome and Greece baths and spas (they thought that, by exercising those muscles, they were promoting health, longevity, spiritual development and sexual health) (Haslam & Laycock, 2007).

PFMT in modern medicine began with Margaret Morris in 1936. She described the contraction-relaxation of pelvic floor muscles as a preventive measure and treatment option for fecal incontinence, introducing pelvic floor rehabilitation to British Physical Therapy. Even so, treatment techniques for UI weren't introduced until 1948 by Arthur Kegel, who developed a study with 64 women suffering from SUI and obtaining a functional recovery of pelvic floor muscles (Kegel, 1948).

PFMT is effective to treat SUI in more than 50% of the subjects, in less than three months. Pelvic Floor muscle exercises involve repeated contractions of perineum muscles, improving their strength and tone (Price, Dawood, & Jackson, 2010). In 2010, the European Association of Urology (Schröder et al., 2010) published a clinical practice guideline in with their recommended PFMT as the non-surgical treatment of SUI, UUI and MUI with an A level of evidence.

PFMT (or Kegel exercises) train muscles situated deep inside the body. Sometimes, women do not know how to exercise those muscles or do not have enough strength, which makes training

them extremely difficult (Bø, Sherburn, & Allen, 2003). Unfortunately, this is a common limitation found in daily practice treatments. Even if they repeatedly try, in some occasions, there are women unable of learning these Kegel exercises (PFMT).

Furthermore, we should not rule out that vaginal palpation may deter some women and that might be a problem when trying to correctly perform pelvic floor exercises (Hung, Hsiao, Chih, Lin, & Tsauo, 2010). Biofeedback is used to help solve these problems: it oversees the pressure made by those muscles and shows the results of the contraction in a screen. This technique involves an intracavitary intervention (intravaginal), inevitably. Unfortunately, some women do not feel comfortable with that procedure (Hung et al., 2010).

An alternative has been proposed to treat those women: it is called Hypopresive Abdominal Technique (HAT), created by Marcel Caufriez in the mid 80s. It is defined as a group of postural techniques that lead to a decrease in the intraabdominal pressure and a co-activation of all abdominal and pelvic floor muscles. During the last years, this technique has gained ground in urogynecological Physical Therapy, especially in the post-partum period (Caufriez, Fernandez, Deman & Wary-Thys, 2007; Caufriez, 1993; Esparza, 2007).

The HAT works with both postural and breathing exercises following specific guidelines including, for example, moving forward the body's gravity axis, cervical rectification, spinal column elongation, expiratory apnea and costal aperture (Rial & Villanueva, 2011). HAT provides benefits for the abdominal muscles without producing negative effects on the pelvic floor muscles (Caufriez et al., 2007; Stüpp et al., 2011).

According to Esparza (Esparza, 2007), the HAT includes global and systemic exercises which aim is to regulate muscular and conjunctive tensions at different body levels. During the expiratory apnea, the diaphragm ascends causing a suction effect over the pelvic organs, along with an activation of pelvic floor (Latorre, Seleme, Resende, Stüpp & Berghmans, 2011) and abdominal muscles (Stüpp et al., 2011).

It is used as treatment for a large number of functional pathologies (urinary, digestive, vascular), and it can or cannot be associated to other different therapies (Esparza et al., 2007).

MAIN FOCUS

Current Model: On-Site Physical Therapy

Nowadays, Stress Urinary Incontinence's evaluation, management and treatment, follows an on-site model.

The on-site model begins with the first appointment, when the patient goes to the physical therapist's practice and, for about an hour, answers multiple questions to put together their medical record and undergoes an intracavitary physical exploration. This exploration is done, basically, to measure the patient's intravaginal pressure. Of these sixty minutes, fifty of them are necessary to build a trusty environment between the patient and the physical therapist and, then, ending the appointment with the physical exploration.

During this appointment, the individualized personalized treatment is planned and explained according to the pathology and its severity. Usually, the mean number of on-site sessions is fifteen, including individual sessions and group classes of Hypopresive Abdominal Technique. Sessions frequency is usually once a week even if, ideally, the best thing to do would be doing them daily. Most patients do not have time to go to a daily on-site appointment and that is why they get a recommendation of doing these exercises at home, even if they are not done under a constant supervision.

Individual sessions include doing pelvic floor muscle exercises monitored with a biofeedback; group sessions are done with a group of five patients, where they learn how to do the Hypopresive Abdominal Technique while they are controlled and corrected with all the attention the physical therapist is able to offer.

Solutions and Recommendations: Use of Telemedicine in UI Treatment with Physical Therapy

Telemedicine has become a widely useful tool and its use is growing day by day. With the appropriate tools, telemedicine allows health professionals to monitor their patients without the need of an on-site appointment, avoiding trips or expenditures and optimizing time and health resources.

There is some scientific evidence of telemedicine therapeutic interventions in different Physical Therapy fields but, regarding pelvic floor disorders, the evidence found is very reduced.

An intervention Telemedicine-mediated program would aid patients and health providers to control and improve symptoms of UI, avoiding most of the problems of classical Physical Therapy treatment problems (lack of privacy, higher cost and patient trips to the clinic); in addition, physiotherapists can give the correct treatment to patients located hundreds or thousands of miles away.

New Model: ICT Aided Physical Therapy in Management and Treatment of SUI

A new treatment model has been designed and has been proposed to evaluate, manage and treat SUI, involving the use of ICT to replace on-site appointments, while always trying to maintain and -if possible- improve the efficacy and quality of the treatment, also guaranteeing the patient's privacy and confidentiality.

Once the patient contacts physiotherapist's service (via email, web form or a QR code inserted in different media as business cards, brochures or ads) a brief explanation of the procedure is replied to patient's query via the e-mail. All necessary questionnaires are attached to the same message (Medical Record, ICIQ-SF and ISI) for the patient to fill out before the first appointment. This way, physical therapist can have all patient's relevant information regarding grade and severity beforehand, along with all the clinically relevant data. All information sent by the patient will be revised by the physical therapist and the most important points and issues will be specified during the first appointment with the patient; this first interview will include enough time to clarify whatever questions or doubts the patient could have.

The first appointment is carried out through an individual live on-line videoconference, using Skype® (http://www.skype.com/; Internet connection, PC and a webcam is required). After an initial contact, the physical therapist will talk with the patient about the most relevant items of her clinical record and giving the patient advice on how to use the device and how to do the entire treatment program.

A Birdi® device (http://www.birdisolutions. com, Figure 3) will be shipped to the patient. Birdi® consists in a user-friendly biofeedback device with connection via Bluetooth® with a specific app (named Birdi Kegel Trainer, Birdi Solutions S.L.; available for smartphones, tablets and computers); the shipping pack also includes a friendly user's guide, so the patient can know how to correctly use the device and how to solve most of the problems she could have.

The physical therapist will register every patient on the system and program the first measurement, done with the device; this first measurement will be done before the second on-line appointment with the physical therapist; once the patient has done it, the physical therapist will receive the results of the intravaginal measure instantly and then they will be discussed during the second appointment, also via videoconference.

Afterwards, the physical therapist will propose the individual treatment plan considered to be the most adequate for the patient and will explain all the proposed personalized exercises and actions (Figure 4).

It is recommended that patients do the routines daily. This treatment model includes two different procedures. On one hand, the patients receives group Hypopresive Abdominal Technique classes three times a week, using Skype® Premium, while supervised during all the session by the physical therapist, which explains and corrects all different exercises (Figure 5). Up to nine patients could be simultaneously attended in one session. On the other hand, the patient has individually daily programmed pelvic floor exercises (Kegel exercises) on her Birdi® Kegel Trainer App (Figure 6). All results are transmitted via Bluetooth to the patient's

Figure 3. Birdi Kegel Trainer. Remote biofeedback device.

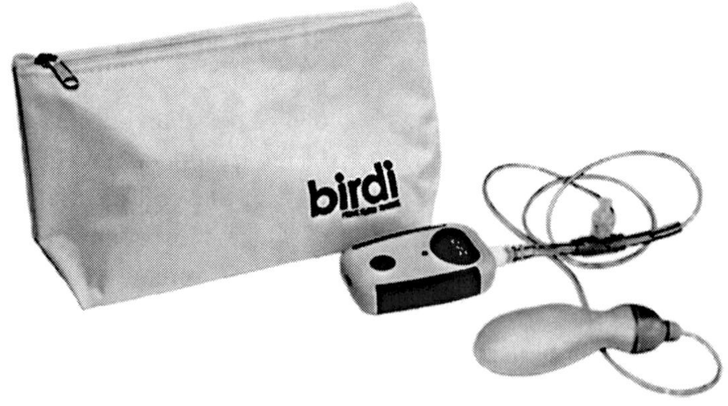

Figure 4. Remote device & treatment plan

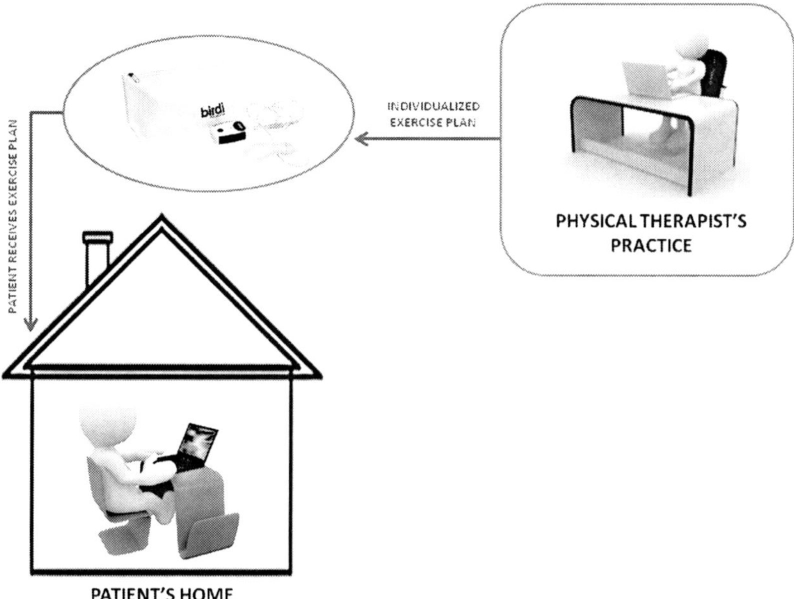

smartphone, tablet or computer and then to the physical therapist's control program; the physical therapist can go over the results of any patient at any time, checking if the patient really does the routines or not. It is also possible to revise the patient's progress and her adherence to the treatment.

Confidentiality can be maintained absolutely in any case if necessary, by not showing one or more of the group participants to the others, while physical therapist can see all of them on the screen. Optimum results can be achieved in groups of five patients.

At any moment, any patient can use different ways of communication with the physical therapist to solve her doubts and/or problems that may develop along the treatment (phone, message apps, videoconference, e-mail, etc.). The Physical Therapist also has specific set appointments for individual consultations using videoconference

Figure 5. Birdi Kegel Trainer APP screenshots

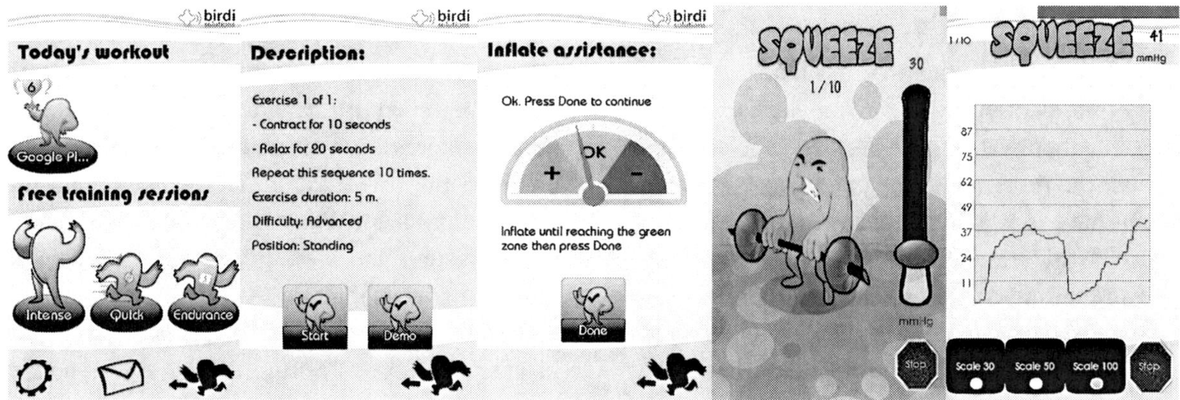

Figure 6. Videoconference and monitoring treatment class

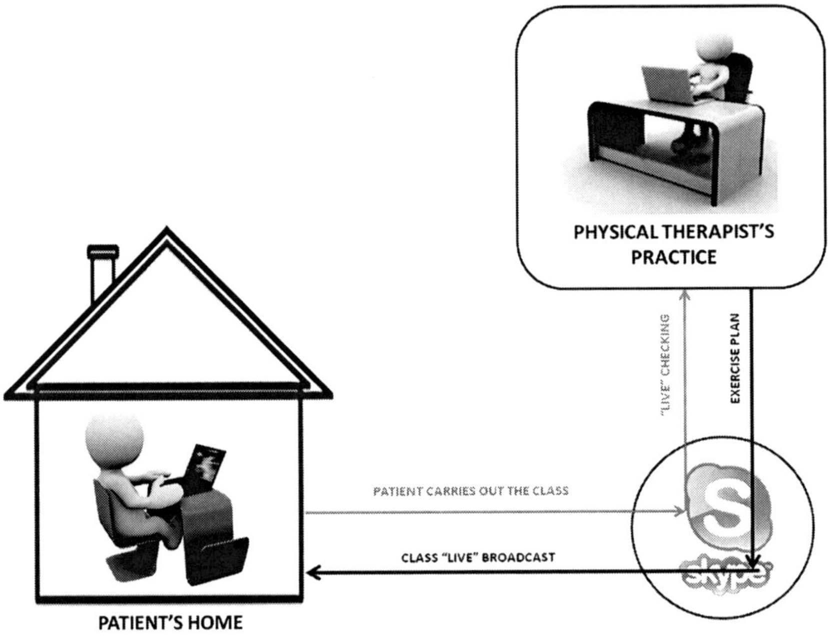

or by phone. They also have a contact email account, revised several times a day by the physical therapist.

All the obtained results are digitally stored in a confidential clinical record.

The progress of patient's intravaginal pressure is easily seen thanks to the Birdi® device, allowing the physical therapist to see and compare the results of all the exercises, day by day (Figure 7). To assess the improvement (or lack thereof) of the symptomatology, patients are asked to monthly answer the questionnaires ICIQ-SF and ISI. Once a month, the patient and the physical therapist will have a short videoconference appointment to go over the results and the progress made.

If treatment's targets are not achieved, the physical therapist will easily detect it and will discuss the results with the patient and whatever means have to be done or changed to accomplish a successful treatment.

Limitations of this model are merely those derived of data line failures, lack of understanding of ICT in some patients or patients that do not have the necessary ICT devices and connections to the Internet at home.

When treatment program ends, Birdi® device can remain with the patient to do follow up exercises by her own, or can be returned to the physiotherapist to be used for another patient by simply changing some expendable parts.

A pilot study has already been started with a first small group of women with SUI. An ad was designed to recruited volunteers for the study. The ad explained what the study was about and clearly indicated its inclusion criteria. A QR-code was included in the poster so the volunteers could download a document with all the relevant information about the study and the inscription form (personal information and ICIQ-SF/ISI questionnaires), which would be, later, sent via email to the investigator. They also signed the informed consent. Participants were introduced in the system and were given a Birdi® device, along with its user guide. After the first measurement, they began three times a week HAT group classes via Skype Premium (Figure 8). Another

Figure 7. Remote evaluation and feedback

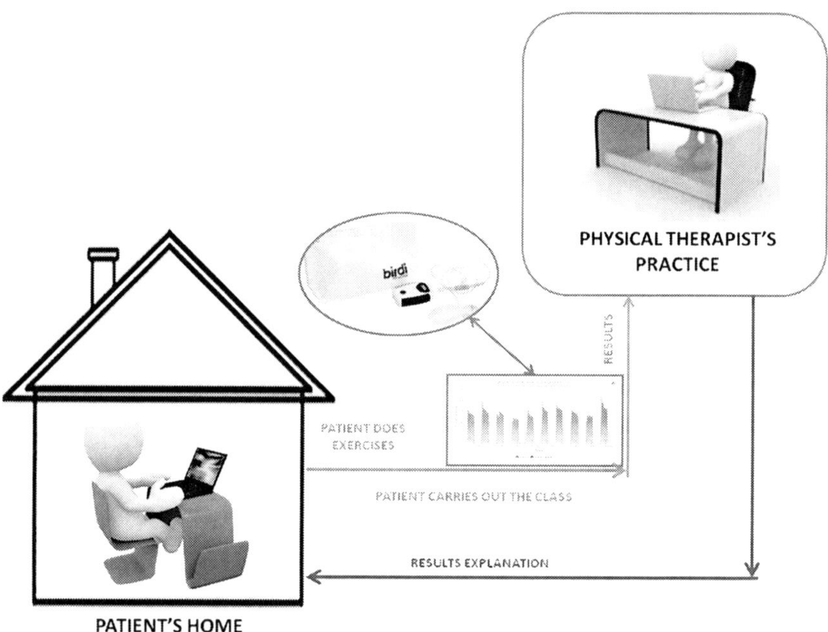

measurement was taken 15 days after the first one: patients showed a great improvement in their vaginal closure pressure (Figure 9).

Evaluation and Discussions

First preliminary results are better than expected while, as expected, adherence to the treatment is really higher than in the classic model of treatment.

The pilot study included 7 patients, all women, with SUI (ICIQ>0). Mean age was 35,86±11,81 years. The severity of UI had a mean value of 7,14±2,11 (moderate-severe). Mean initial pressure was 18,77±6,24 mmHg.

To check if the variables followed a normal distribution, tests of normality were applied to the variables Mean Pressure (Figure 10), ISI (Figure 11) and ICIQ-SF (Figure 12). As the sample size is small, the Kolmogorov-Smirnov Test was performed with a result p>0,05. To confirm that the variables did not follow a normal distribution, a histogram was done.

The non-parametric statistical Wilcoxon Test for related samples was used to assess whether the mean ranks differ. The variable ICIQ-SF showed a non-significant difference between the first and second months of treatment and the initial values (p=0,019 and p=0,104 respectively). The variable ISI showed a non-significant difference between the first month of treatment and the initial values (p=0,059) but, when compared the second month mark with the initial value, the difference showed statistical significance (p=0,042). For the variable mean pressure, neither differences were significant (p=0,173 for the first month, p=0,068 for the second month).

Patients were ask how many days per week (in total) they did the Hypopresive Technique; the mean result was 4,40±2,07 days a week.

To evaluate the patient's acquiescence with the treatment, additional questions were asked once the procedure was completed. When asked about the treatment's usefulness, 100% of them

Figure 8. Global treatment plan

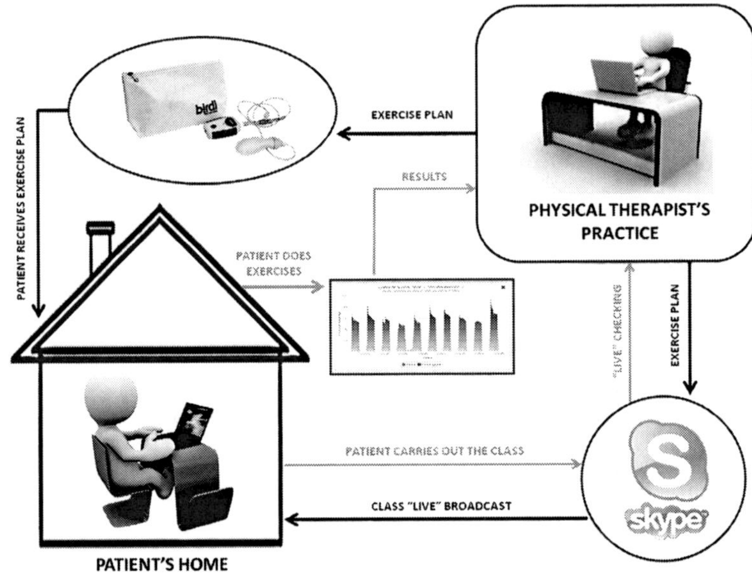

Figure 9. Screenshot of pressure values measured

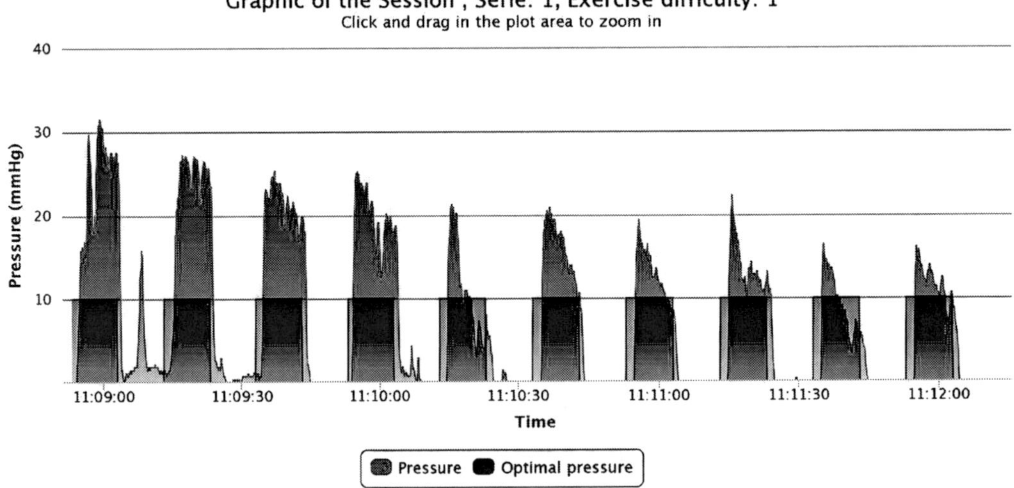

answered affirmatively. To the question: Are you satisfied with this treatment?, 100% replied yes.

Although almost all of the results do not have statistical significance, they are encouraging. The study being a pilot test, the sample size was pretty small; when the sample is increased the results will turn to be, most probably, significant.

These results are quite prosperous and favorable and encourage us to continue working, increasing our sample size and expecting significant outcomes. This pilot test has been useful to validate the methodology and the applied procedure.

Patients feel this program as comfy and friendly; the device is really easy to use. Patients are comfortable with the program and really proud

Figure 10. Mean vaginal closure pressure evolution (mmHg/time)

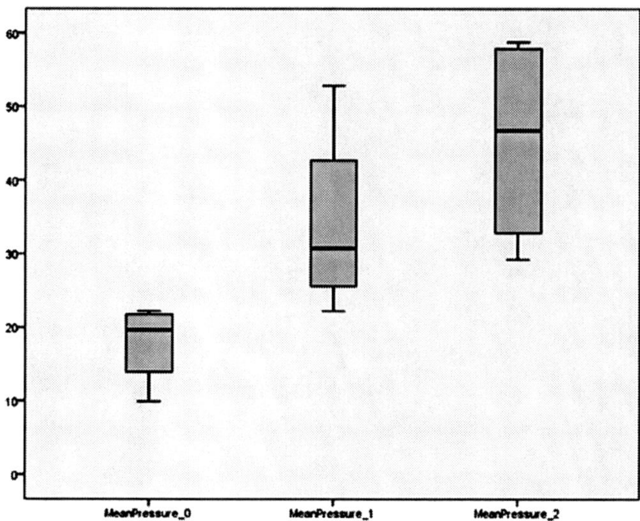

Figure 11. Mean ISI scores evolution (score/time)

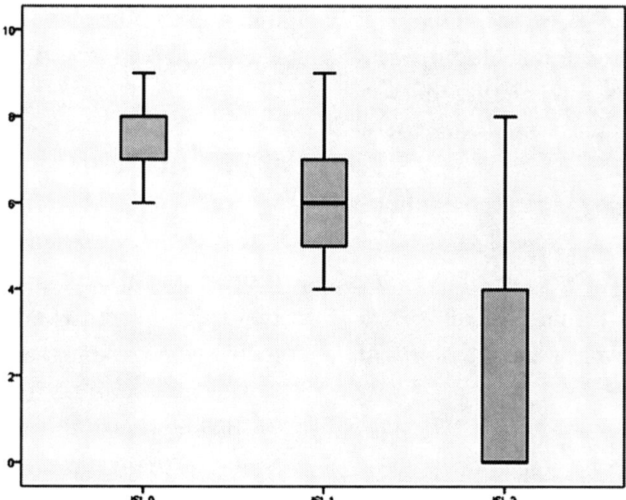

of their progress. They are thankful for not having to go to the physical therapist's practice and they feel that they are saving of time and money (money and time) in their lives. This ICT treatment model is really affordable.

When asked, patients had different things to say about the treatment. Here we reference some of their comments:

- "I think the videoconference-aided treatment is much more effective because you are sure that you are doing the exercises correctly. The physical therapist's supervision and encouragement is always necessary."

- "I think the treatment should always be done with the help of videoconferencing, above all with patients that don't have good body awareness, because the postural cor-

Figure 12. Mean ICIQ-SF scores evolution (score/time)

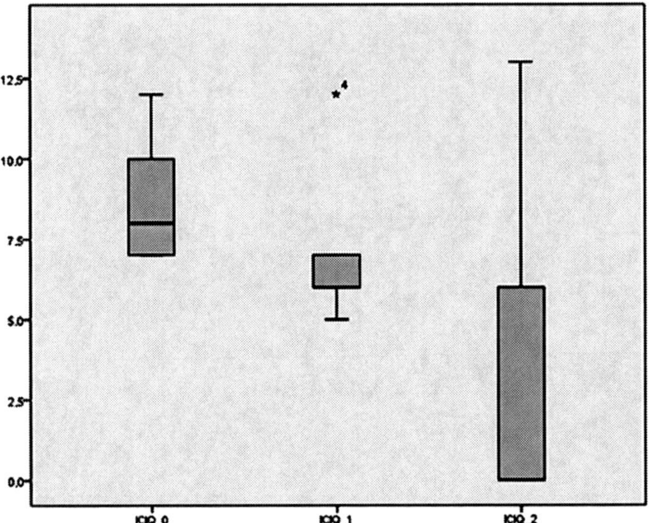

rections are indispensable if you want to do the Hypopresive Technique correctly."

- "I'd like to thank you for teaching me how to do these exercises. I think that the possibility of doing supervised exercises at home is a great idea."
- "I've perceived a great improvement but it hasn't been as good as I expected. It might be related to other pathologies that I have and are related to urinary incontinence. Nevertheless, my level of satisfaction with this treatment is good."

The main possible disadvantage of new treatment model is that physical contact between the patient and the physical therapist is not possible; patients usually feel more confident and at ease with the empathy derived from actual physical contact, even if it is a gentle touch on the shoulder to show support or understanding.

to polish the model. It is also necessary to translate app to other languages (now is available in Catalan, Spanish and English).

CONCLUSION

Stress Urinary Incontinence is a highly prevalent disease that affects quality of life in women. SUI treatment is often less effective than expected due to different circumstances as high costs, time and/ or schedule requirements.

ICT mediated Physical Therapy programs can be useful to improve Stress Urinary Incontinence in women while maintaining total confidentiality, with an at home treatment (anywhere in the world), achieving a higher adherence to the treatment, keeping a low budget for the patients and saving health systems' economic resources, both public or private.

FUTURE RESEARCH DIRECTIONS

From now on, it is necessary to test the new ICT model of treatment in a larger group of patients and solve any problem that it is detected, in order

ACKNOWLEDGMENT

Birdi® is a trademark owned by BIRDI-SOLU-TIONS, S.R.L. with C.I.F.: B18992446, Calle

Collected 24 3° B, registered in the Mercantile Registry of Granada (Spain).

Skype® is is a division of Microsoft Corp., Skype Communications SARL. 23-29 Rives de Clausen, L-2165 Luxembourg. Company No: R.C.S. Luxembourg B100.468 VAT: LU 20981643.

REFERENCES

Abelló, A., Esquirol, J., Salas, D., & Bayo, V. (2009). *Prevalencia y reconocimiento de la incontinencia urinaria en mujeres jóvenes*. Valencia, Spain: Congreso Nacional de Suelo Pélvico. SEGO.

Agence Nationale d'd'Accréditation et d'Évaluation en Santé. (2000). *Bilans et techniques de rééducation périnéo-sphinctérienne pour le traitement de l'incontinence urinaire chez la femme à l'exclusion des affections neurologiques*. Author.

Berghmans, B. (2006). El papel del fisioterapeuta pélvico. *Actas Urologicas Espanolas, 30*(2), 110–122. doi:10.1016/S0210-4806(06)73412-X PMID:16700200

Bø, K. (2004a). Urinary Incontinence, pelvic floor dysfunction, exercise and sport. *Sports Medicine (Auckland, N.Z.), 34*(7), 451–464. doi:10.2165/00007256-200434070-00004 PMID:15233598

Bø, K. (2004b, March-April). Pelvic floor muscle training is effective in treatment of female Stress Urinary Incontinence, but how does it work? *International Urogynecology Journal and Pelvic Floor Dysfunction, 15*(2), 76–84. doi:10.1007/s00192-004-1125-0 PMID:15014933

Bø, K., Sherburn, M., & Allen, T. (2003). Transabdominal ultrasound measurement of pelvic floor muscle activity when activated directly or via a transversus abdominis muscle contraction. *Neurourology and Urodynamics, 22*(6), 582–588. doi:10.1002/nau.10139 PMID:12951667

Brenes, F. J., Dios-Diz, J. M., & Naval, E. N. (2007). *A propósito de un caso en incontinencia urinaria*. Madrid, Spain: Loki & Dimas.

Brunetti, N. D., Dellegrottaglie, G., Lopriore, C., Di Giuseppe, G., De Gennaro, L., Lanzone, S., & Di Biase, M. (2014). Prehospital telemedicine electrocardiogram triage for a regional public emergency medical service: Is it worth it? A preliminary cost analysis. *Clinical Cardiology, 37*(3), 140–145. doi:10.1002/clc.22234 PMID:24452666

Calais Germain, B. (1998). *El periné femenino y el parto: Anatomía para el movimiento: Elementos de anatomía y bases de ejercicios*. Barcelona, Spain: Los libros de la liebre de Marzo.

Caufriez, M. (1993). *Thérapies manuelles et instrumentales en uro-gynécologie (MC Edition.)*. Bruxelles.

Caufriez, M., Fernandez, J., Deman, C., & Wary-Thys, C. (2007). Contribución al estudio sobre el tono del suelo pélvico. *Progresos de Obstetricia Y Ginecología, 50*(5), 282–291.

Córcoles, M. B., Sánchez, S. A., Bachs, G. J., Moreno, D. M., Navarro, P. H., & Rodríguez, V. J. (2008). Quality of life in patients with Urinary Incontinence. *Actas Urologicas Espanolas, 32*(2), 202–210. PMID:18409470

Eliasson, K., Larsson, T., & Mattsson, E. (2002). Prevalence of stress incontinence in nulliparous elite trampolinists. *Scandinavian Journal of Medicine & Science in Sports, 12*(2), 106–110. doi:10.1034/j.1600-0838.2002.120207.x PMID:12121428

Esparza, S. (2007). *Gimnasia abdominal hipopresiva*. San Sebastián: Congreso Franco-Español del Suelo Pélvico y Pelviperineología.

Espuña Pons, M., Castro, D., Iaz, D., Carbonell, C., & Dilla, T. (2007). Comparación entre el cuestionario "ICIQ-UI Short Form" y el "King's Health Questionnaire" como instrumentos de evaluación de la incontinencia urinaria en mujeres. *Actas Urologicas Espanolas, 31*(5), 502–510. doi:10.1016/S0210-4806(07)73674-4 PMID:17711169

Franc, S., Borot, S., Quesada, J. L., Dardari, D., Fagour, C., Renard, E., & Leguerrier, A. M. (2014). Telemedicine and type 1 diabetes: Is technology per se sufficient to improve glycaemic control? *Diabetes & Metabolism, 40*(1), 61–66. PMID:24139705

Grosse, D., & Sengler, J. (1998). *Reeducación del periné: Fisioterapia de las incontinencias urinarias*. Paris: Masson.

Haslam, J., & Laycock, J. (2007). *Therapeutic management of incontinence and pelvic pain: Pelvic organ disorders*. Academic Press.

Haylen, B. T., de Ridder, D., Freeman, R. M., Swift, S. E., Berghmans, B., & Lee, J. et al. (2010). An international urogynecological association (IUGA)/international continence society (ICS) joint report on the terminology for female pelvic floor dysfunction. *International Urogynecology Journal and Pelvic Floor Dysfunction, 21*(1), 5–26. doi:10.1007/s00192-009-0976-9 PMID:19937315

Hui, E., Lee, P. S., & Woo, J. (2006). Management of urinary incontinence in older women using videoconferencing versus conventional management: A randomized controlled trial. *Journal of Telemedicine and Telecare, 12*(7), 343–347. doi:10.1258/135763306778682413 PMID:17059650

Hung, H.-C., Hsiao, S.-M., Chih, S.-Y., Lin, H.-H., & Tsauo, J.-Y. (2010). An alternative intervention for urinary incontinence: Retraining diaphragmatic, deep abdominal and pelvic floor muscle coordinated function. *Manual Therapy, 15*(3), 273–279. doi:10.1016/j.math.2010.01.008 PMID:20185357

Hunskaar, S., Lose, G., Sykes, D., & Voss, S. (2004). The prevalence of urinary incontinence in women in four European countries. *BJU International, 93*(3), 324–330. doi:10.1111/j.1464-410X.2003.04609.x PMID:14764130

Kegel, A. H. (1948). Progressive resistance exercise in the functional restoration of the perineal muscles. *American Journal of Obstetrics and Gynecology, 56*(2), 238–248. PMID:18877152

Klovning, A., Avery, K., Sandvik, H., & Hunskaar, S. (2009). Comparison of two questionnaires for assessing the severity of urinary incontinence: The ICIQ-UI SF versus the incontinence severity index. *Neurourology and Urodynamics, 28*(5), 411–415. doi:10.1002/nau.20674 PMID:19214996

Latorre, G., Seleme, M., Resende, A. P., Stüpp, L., & Berghmans, B. (2011). Hypopresive gymnastics: Evidence for an alternative training for women with local propioceptive deficit of the pelvic floor muscles. *Fisioterapia Brasil, 12*(6), 463–466.

Lenoir, M. (2005). *L'incontinence urinaire de la jeune fille nullipare: etat des lieux dans un collège et rôle du médicin de l'Éducation Nationale*. École Nationale de la Santé Publique.

Lokkerbol, J., Adema, D., Cuijpers, P., Reynolds, C. F. III, Schulz, R., Weehuizen, R., & Smit, F. (2014, March). Improving the cost-effectiveness of a healthcare system for depressive disorders by implementing telemedicine: A health economic modeling study. *The American Journal of Geriatric Psychiatry, 22*(3), 253–262. doi:10.1016/j.jagp.2013.01.058 PMID:23759290

Milsom, I., Altman, D., Lapitan, M. C., Nelson, R., Sillen, U., & Thom, D. (2009). *Epidemiology of urinary (UI) and faecal (FI) incontinence and pelvic organ prolapse (POP)*. Paris: Health Publications Ltd.

Minaire, P., Sengler, J., & Jacquetin, B. (1995). Epidémiologie de l'incontinence urinaire. *Annales de Readaptation et de Medecine Physique, 38*(1), 1–8. doi:10.1016/0168-6054(96)89294-4

Minassian, V. A., Drutz, H. P., & Al-Badr, A. (2003). Urinary incontinence as a worldwide problem. *International Journal of Gynaecology and Obstetrics: The Official Organ of the International Federation of Gynaecology and Obstetrics, 82*(3), 327–338. doi:10.1016/S0020-7292(03)00220-0 PMID:14499979

Minassian, V. A., Stewart, W. F., & Wood, G. C. (2008). Urinary incontinence in women: Variation in prevalence estimates and risk factors. *Obstetrics and Gynecology, 111*(2 Pt 1), 324–331. doi:10.1097/01.AOG.0000267220.48987.17 PMID:18238969

Price, N., Dawood, R., & Jackson, S. R. (2010). Pelvic floor exercise for urinary incontinence: A systematic literature review. *Maturitas, 67*(4), 309–315. doi:10.1016/j.maturitas.2010.08.004 PMID:20828949

Rial, T., & Villanueva, C. (2011). Aproximación conceptual al Método Hipopresivo: Desde el postparto hacia la actividad física saludable. *Móvete,* (5), 14–17.

Ricatte, O. (2004). *Dépistage de l'incontinence urinaire de la femme entre 30 et 50 ans en médecine générale en Franche-Comté en 2003: Étude prospective à propos de 258 cas*. Université de Franche-Comté.

Sandvik, H., Espuna, M., & Hunskaar, S. (2006). Validity of the incontinence severity index: Comparison with pad-weighing tests. *International Urogynecology Journal and Pelvic Floor Dysfunction, 17*(5), 520–524. doi:10.1007/s00192-005-0060-z PMID:16547687

Schröder, A., Abrams, P., Anderson, K.-E., Artibani, W., Chapple, C. R., Drake, M. J., & Thüroff, J. W. (2010). *Guía clínica sobre la incontinencia urinaria*. European Association of Urology.

Segrelles Calvo, G., Gómez-Suárez, C., Soriano, J. B., Zamora, E., Gonzalez-Gamarra, A., & González-Béjar, M. et al. (2014). A home telehealth program for patients with severe COPD: The PROMETE study. *Respiratory Medicine, 108*(3), 453–462. doi:10.1016/j.rmed.2013.12.003 PMID:24433744

Stüpp, L., Resende, A. P., Petricelli, C., Nakamura, M., Alexandre, S., & Zanetti, M. (2011). Pelvic floor muscle and transversus abdominis activation in abdominal hypopresive technique through surface electromyography. *Neurourology and Urodynamics, 30*(8), 1518–1521. doi:10.1002/nau.21151 PMID:21826719

Ueda, T., Tamaki, M., Kageyama, S., Yoshimura, N., & Yoshida, O. (2000). Urinary incontinence among community-dwelling people aged 40 years or older in Japan: Prevalence, risk factors, knowledge and self-perception. *International Journal of Urology : Official Journal of the Japanese Urological Association, 7*(3), 95–103. doi:10.1046/j.1442-2042.2000.00147.x PMID:10750888

ADDITIONAL READING

American Telemedicine Association. (2012). *What is Telemedicine?* Retrieved February 25th, 2014, from http://www.americantelemed.org

Birdi Solutions, S. L. R. (2013). *Birdi Kegel trainer*. Retrieved February 25th, 2014, from http://www.birdisolutions.com

Bø, K. (2012). Pelvic floor muscle training in treatment of female stress urinary incontinence, pelvic organ prolapse and sexual dysfunction. *World Journal of Urology, 30*(4), 437–443. doi:10.1007/s00345-011-0779-8 PMID:21984473

Bø, K., & Hilde, G. (2013). Does it work in the long term? A systematic review on pelvic floor muscle training for female stress urinary incontinence. *Neurourology and Urodynamics, 32*(3), 215–223. doi:10.1002/nau.22292 PMID:22847318

Boyle, R., Hay-Smith, E. J. C., Cody, J. D., & Mørkved, S. (2012). Pelvic floor muscle training for prevention and treatment of urinary and faecal incontinence in antenatal and postnatal women. *Cochrane Database of Systematic Reviews, 10*, CD007471. PMID:23076935

Dumoulin, C., Glazener, C., & Jenkinson, D. (2011). Determining the optimal pelvic floor muscle training regimen for women with stress urinary incontinence. *Neurourology and Urodynamics, 30*(5), 746–753. doi:10.1002/nau.21104 PMID:21661024

Dumoulin, C., & Hay-Smith, J. (2010). Pelvic floor muscle training versus no treatment, or inactive control treatments, for urinary incontinence in women. *Cochrane Database of Systematic Reviews*, (1), CD005654. PMID:20091581

Hay-Smith, J., Herderschee, R., Dumoulin, C., & Herbison, P. (2012). Comparisons of approaches to pelvic floor muscle training for urinary incontinence in women: An abridged Cochrane systematic review. *European Journal of Physical and Rehabilitation Medicine, 48*(4), 689–705. PMID:23183454

Herderschee, R., Hay-Smith, E. J. C., Herbison, G. P., Roovers, J. P., & Heineman, M. J. (2011). Feedback or biofeedback to augment pelvic floor muscle training for urinary incontinence in women. *Cochrane Database of Systematic Reviews*, (7), CD009252. PMID:21735442

Hilde, G., Stær-Jensen, J., Siafarikas, F., Ellström Engh, M., & Bø, K. (2013). Postpartum pelvic floor muscle training and urinary incontinence: A randomized controlled trial. *Obstetrics and Gynecology, 122*(6), 1231–1238. doi:10.1097/AOG.0000000000000012 PMID:24201679

International Continence Society. (2014). Retrieved February 26th, 2014, from http://www.ics.org

International Urogynecological Association. (2013). Retrieved February 26th, 2014, from http://www.iuga.org

Mørkved, S., & Bø, K. (2014). Effect of pelvic floor muscle training during pregnancy and after childbirth on prevention and treatment of urinary incontinence: A systematic review. *British Journal of Sports Medicine, 48*(4), 299–310. doi:10.1136/bjsports-2012-091758 PMID:23365417

Sherburn, M., Bird, M., Carey, M., Bø, K., & Galea, M. P. (2011). Incontinence improves in older women after intensive pelvic floor muscle training: An assessor-blinded randomized controlled trial. *Neurourology and Urodynamics, 30*(3), 317–324. doi:10.1002/nau.20968 PMID:21284022

Sociedad Española de Ginecología y Obstetricia. (2014). *Sección de suelo pélvico*. Retrieved February 23rd, 2014, from http://www.suelopelvico.org/

KEY TERMS AND DEFINITIONS

Biofeedback: Precise instrument that measures physiological activity and provides instant "feed-back" information to the user.

Hypopresive Abdominal Technique: Group of postural techniques that lead to a decrease in the intraabdominal pressure and a co-activation of all abdominal and pelvic floor muscles.

Pelvic Floor Muscle Training: Ensemble of exercises consisting of repeatedly contracting and relaxing the muscles that form part of the pelvic floor.

Physical Therapy: Health profession that promotes, maintains, or restores the physical and physiological well-being of an individual.

Telemedicine: Use of ICT to provide clinical healthcare at a distance.

Urinary Incontinence: All complains of involuntary urine leakage.

This work was previously published in Assistive Technologies for Physical and Cognitive Disabilities edited by Lau Bee Theng, pages 56-77 copyright year 2015 by Medical Information Science Reference (an imprint of IGI Global).

Section 2
Frameworks and Methodologies

This section provides in-depth coverage of conceptual architecture frameworks to provide the reader with a comprehensive understanding of the emerging developments within the field of E-Health and Telemedicine. Research fundamentals imperative to the understanding of developmental processes within E-Health and Telemedicine are offered. From broad examinations to specific discussions on methodology, the research found within this section spans the discipline while offering detailed, specific discussions. From basic designs to abstract development, these chapters serve to expand the reaches of development and design technologies within the E-Health and Telemedicine community. This section includes 11 contributions from researchers throughout the world on the topic of E-Health and Telemedicine.

Chapter 16
Information Architecture for Pervasive Healthcare Information Provision with Technological Implementation

Chekfoung Tan
University of Reading, UK

Shixiong Liu
University of Reading, UK

ABSTRACT

The Pervasive Healthcare Information Provision (PHIP) is a concept that ensures patients are covered with healthcare services with the appropriate information provision together with the technical infrastructure when needed. Clinicians can obtain the real-time information by accessing the electronic patient record that supports decision-making in providing health services. PHIP aims to provide comprehensive healthcare services to its stakeholders covering the social and technical aspect. Information architecture is a high-level map of information requirements of an organisation that possesses business processes and information flows. Organisational semiotics, a fundamental theory for information and communication, helps in understanding the nature of information. It deals with information and information systems in a balanced way, taking account of both the physical space (when physical actions take place) and the information space (which are mainly characterised by information and communication using signs, symbols, and data). Information sharing among multi-stakeholders in decision-making is essential for pervasive healthcare. The information architecture can be reflected in information systems implementation such as Electronic Patient Record (EPR) and other forms. The aim of this chapter is to derive a conceptual model of information architecture for PHIP, including technological implementation via wireless technology. The information architecture serves as requirement engine that covers social and technical needs from both patients and clinicians. The contribution of this research is two fold: 1) establishing the theoretical perspective of information architecture, which serves as backbone to support PHIP, and 2) implementing PHIP via wireless technology and agent-based system.

DOI: 10.4018/978-1-4666-8756-1.ch016

1. INTRODUCTION

Information has played an important role in an organisation. However, information is still not managed well in many organisations (Martin, Dmitriev, & Akeroyd, 2010). This will cost a great deal to an organisation in terms of errors and inefficiencies, and to its client in terms of quality of service. Information architecture would be able to help organisations to deal with the increasing volumes of information to be disseminated, digested and managed effectively. Same applies for a pervasive healthcare environment. Hospitals are always being perceived as a 'data rich, information poor' (Rector, 2001), moreover in pervasive healthcare environment. The concept of pervasive healthcare has emerged in the early twenty first century that aims to provide healthcare to anyone, at any time and everywhere by removing restraints of time and location while increasing both the coverage and the quality of healthcare (Varshney, 2009). Information is vital within a hospital in order to reduce medical errors and increase patient safety (IOM, 2011), hence leading to a better decision making. Hence, information architecture is needed for provisioning information in a pervasive healthcare environment.

Information architecture is defined as a high level map of information requirements of an organisation (Brancheau & Wetherbe, 1986). Same applies for pervasive healthcare. The existing information architecture literature is mostly from the empirical viewpoint. Hence, it opens a new chapter in research to deriving information architecture by adding a theoretical dimension where organisational semiotics is discussed in this paper. Information is a core element in information architecture and yet there are many ways in viewing information. Information can be seen as a sign from a humanistic perspective rather than the bits and bytes from a computer science perspective.

Technology based pervasive healthcare information provision has been proposed for promoting wellness, prevention, disease management, compliance, and reduced incidences of hospitalizations and corresponding expenses (Dishman, 2004; IOM, 2000; Mcgee, 2004). However, the focus so far has been on the development of artefacts with limited attentions given to articulate the process of pervasive patient monitoring and define clear guidelines that can be applied to developing effective, efficient pervasive healthcare solutions. The vision of pervasive healthcare information provision is to improve healthcare delivery by timely and reliable detection of anomalies and enhance the efficiency of the clinicians by assisting them in providing pertinent medical attention as and when needed. In this chapter, a list of requirements, which are the key factors leading to a successful pervasive healthcare solution will be articulated. Wireless network architecture for pervasive healthcare environment, which characterises the processes that can be applied for pervasive patient monitoring will be developed and illustrated with an example. Besides, a detail description and functionality of the various intelligent agents that are tasked with analysing the monitored parameters and the protocols will be given.

This chapter is structured as follow: Section 2 discusses the notion of information provision in the pervasive healthcare environment. Section 3 illustrates information architecture from both empirical and theoretical perspective. As a result, the conceptual design of information architecture is proposed. Section 4 narrates the concept of implementing pervasive healthcare information provision through wireless technology. An example of implementation will be provided. Section 5 draws the conclusion and suggestions for future work.

2. PERVASIVE HEALTHCARE INFORMATION PROVISION

2.1 Pervasive Healthcare

2.1.1 The Concept of Pervasive Healthcare

The concept of pervasive healthcare has emerged in the early twenty first century due to accelerating operational costs, growing numbers of medical errors, insufficient staffing and lack of health services coverage in the rural areas (Varshney, 2003). Pervasive healthcare consists of a wide scale deployment of wireless networks that will improve communications among patients, clinicians, and other healthcare workers and in delivering accurate medical information anytime, anywhere, thereby reducing errors and improving access (Varshney, 2003). Pervasive healthcare delivers services such as mobile telemedicine, patient monitoring, location based medical services, incident detection, emergency response and management, pervasive access to medical data and prevention (Varshney, 2003, 2007).

2.1.2 Benefits of Pervasive Healthcare

Pervasive healthcare has five main benefits (Bardram, 2008), these are 1) continuous care provision where continuous well-being, treatment and care are provided rather than focus on technologies for acute treatment and care, 2) patient self-care where patients treatment and care can be moved from hospitalisation to home-based or outpatient treatment, considering that life expectancy has increased, 3) continuous monitoring where patient can monitor his or her health condition with the assistive decision support system, for example, instead of periodic sampling activities such as blood sampling or x-ray imaging done in the hospital, patients can do it on their own, this will enable pro-active and preventive types of diagnosis, early detection and treatment of various diseases, 4)

patients can play a more proactive role in dealing with their own well-being, health and illness in a larger degree as most pervasive healthcare technologies are more patient-centric rather than designed for clinical professionals, and lastly 5) to improve communication among stakeholders such as clinicians and patients as mass usage of information communication technology (ICT) on information processing, storage, integration, modeling and presentation.

2.1.3 Impact of Pervasive Healthcare on Patient Safety

Pervasive healthcare ensures patients are covered with healthcare services when needed. Clinicians can obtain the real time information by accessing the electronic patient record that supports decision making in providing health services. Pervasive healthcare involves real time systems integration, mobile devices and high-speed wireless network connection. This can improve patient safety and healthcare quality and reduce the elevating operational costs where patients can be monitored remotely without needing to use the facilities in a hospital.

2.1.4 Technology Facet of Pervasive Healthcare

The technology facet of pervasive healthcare is inspired by the notion of pervasive computing. Pervasive computing is defined as to use ubiquitous network capacity within a defined space to integrate devices, usually refers to distributed and embedded sensor networks (Weiser, 1991). A pervasive information system should support nomadic devices that may be carried around by users (Kourouthanassis & Giaglis, 2006). Pervasive healthcare computing, which can be seen as the pervasive information system is defined as ways in which mobile and wireless technologies can be used to implement the vision of pervasive healthcare (Varshney, 2009). In summary, the delivery of pervasive healthcare concept lays on the following technological foundations (Bardram, 2008; Maitland, McGee-Lennon, & Mulvenna, 2011):

- Monitoring technologies such as Body sensor networks in order to reason the functioning of an individual and use this information for early warnings, safety, prevention and assistance.
- Pervasive assistive technologies targeting especially older people such as medication reminder systems and safety systems for detecting falls so they can live independently and well.
- Mobile and context aware applications to support out-patient and home-based treatment patients and persuasive technologies that creates systems that seek to alter people's behaviour, for example making a context aware signs that encourage people to quit smoking
- Wireless technologies for transmitting information between agents such as applications, devices etc.

2.2 Key Requirements of Pervasive Healthcare Information Provision

Pervasive healthcare Information Provision (PHIP) is a concept that roots in pervasive healthcare and information provision. Information provision plays a role in increasing effectiveness of pervasive healthcare providing healthcare service to anyone, anytime and anywhere by integrating seamlessly various healthcare sectors. PHIP ensures patients are covered with healthcare services with appropriate information wirelessly and pervasively when and as needed. The definition of PHIP involves two perspectives, one is the domain of application of technologies using for pervasive communication, and the other is the concept that integrates healthcare service to patient's daily life (Korhonen & Bardram, 2004). PHIP is not just seeking to assist the clinicians in managing

illness of patients by using their expertise, it also allows clinicians to obtain the real time information from EPR in order to support decision making in providing healthcare services. The core responsibilities of the clinicians and professionals will shift from observation of patient's condition and management of diseases to provision of medical expertise. Ubiquitous technology will be used for supporting standards, monitoring vital signs and promoting compliance with medical advice. The enabling technologies such as WSN, RFID, and cellular networks are basically used for ubiquitous communication, monitoring and computing.

2.2.1 Functional Requirements

The key requirements of PHIP are not only diverse supporting information provision for indoor and outdoor, as well as stationary and mobile patients but also involve multiple parameters such as reliability, scalability, and duration of monitoring. Following the research of Varshney (2007), a number of defined requirements can be categorised into two divisions: functional and non-functional requirements. The following overview displays the complexity and diversity of them.

2.2.1.1 Monitoring and Transmission

Monitoring and transmission are the fundamental requirements of pervasive monitoring service. It is continuous, and used for detection of abnormal events at fixed times in a day. In this context, pervasive monitoring indicates the parameters that need to be monitored. For instance: vital signs such as body temperature and ECG need to be monitored periodically and continuously via sensors, thermometer or other physical devices. However, as the pervasive monitoring provides real-time data for analysis and storage, it may lead to an information overload and network traffic. In order to solve the issue, periodic monitoring and transmission sacrifices the real-time advantage in suitable for patients under routing supervision.

2.2.1.2 Patient Accessibility

Patient accessibility defines the mobility of patients in pervasive healthcare environment. In this context, not just stationary patients but also mobile patients are monitored indoor and outdoor by sensors. The variation in mobility pattern relies on a dependable networking solution. Under different circumstance, patient's track is monitored as well in order to improve healthcare quality.

2.2.1.3 Proactivity

Proactivity defines the intelligence of PHIP. The intelligence in the pervasive healthcare environment can sense the intent of the patient by analysing their behaviours and ask built-in agents to take certain actions instead. For instance: if the sensor senses that the patient's body temperature has gone beyond a pre-specified threshold, the agent should be seen as the device to alert the clinicians and schedule an appointment for the patient. However, in order to avoid the false alarm, proactive action should be transparent to the patients so they are able to take prompt action on their own.

2.2.1.4 Intelligent Analysis

Intelligent analysis is the process that analyses the sensed data and proposes solution for diagnoses. As PHIP requires continuous streams of data from monitored patients, analysing the data and making relevant diagnoses would be a complicate task for the clinicians. The network traffic and scalability of the patient monitoring are impacted as well. In order to effectively utilize the computational capabilities of the facilities, intelligent analysis can be adopted for providing a pervasive patient environment. The collected information can be accessed by the intelligent agent for initial analysis and then be passed to the healthcare professionals to make informed decisions and treatments.

2.2.1.5 Context Awareness

Context awareness defines that information in the pervasive healthcare environment can be used to characterize the situation of entities (i.e. whether patient, place or object) that are considered relevant to the interaction between a user and an application, including the user and the application themselves (Dey, Abowd, & Salber, 2001). The concept of context awareness has been described for some time, but technologies (e.g. wireless technologies, mobile tools, and sensors) are now available to support the development of applications and could help healthcare professionals to manage their tasks while increasing the quality of patient care. Nevertheless, new technologies impact the communication between agents. Context awareness plays a decisive role in synch with healthcare intelligence in providing a proactive environment for patients. Decision making process cannot be successful unless the right context information is given. Context awareness can be used for differentiating the abnormities in different situation. For instance: patient's heart rate has gone up which may be caused by excitement, physical exercise or health difficulties. The agent must be aware of the context where and when the heart rate is high and realise the information about who and what.

2.2.2 Non-Functional Requirements

By contrast with functional requirements, which define what the system is supposed to do, the non-functional requirements define how the system is supposed to be. Broadly, it determines the qualities of the system. In this context, the non-functional requirements are reliability, scalability, confidentiality, security, sustainability and privacy.

2.2.2.1 Reliability

As pervasive healthcare relates the potentially life-threatening situation, high reliability of message delivery is critically required for patients and healthcare professionals. Different monitoring messages can be prioritized based on the reliability requirements, which are defined by the tolerance of routine transmission. As part of reliability requirements, any delay in message delivery is hardly allowed as it may cause fatal consequences. The priority of transmitted message determines the routing of messages to reduce delays, which are substantially effected by size of messages, timing of network, broadband speed and the amount of monitored patients.

2.2.2.2 Scalability

The scalability is to measure the quality of monitoring service. It is important in patient monitoring network, which impacts a number of aforementioned patients that can be reliably supported. Factors such as frequency of transmission, bit rate and the amount of information transmitted influence the scalability. However, applying dependable networking solution can eliminate these influences.

2.2.2.3 Confidentiality, Security, and Privacy

PHIP information is transmitted over wireless networks, thus the security of the transmission directly impacts the confidentiality and privacy of patients. Privacy entails the authentication of user to collect and disseminate personal information and security is one of the key requirements toward large-scale adoption (Kara, 2001; Tablado, Illarramendi, Bermudez, & Goñi, 2003).

This section presents the key requirements associated with pervasive healthcare information provision. The requirements are characterize into divisions of functional and non-functional. The benefits of PHIP are implied. However, some of the factors come with their own challenges in

utilisation, information overload and assistance for healthcare clinician. Despite of the technical limitations, the empirical issues associated with the usage and implementation have not been fully explored yet as healthcare sectors are running analysis of the benefits and profits in terms of return on investment, reduction in hospitalizations and financial feasibility. In addition, some of the ethical limitations are also needed to be concerned for future research. For instance: technologies innovations in the practice and healthcare service delivery have been slower adopted by healthcare sectors than industrial sectors because of the acceptance by the healthcare professionals and patients. Furthermore, the value for actual use of innovative technology based PHIP is difficult to be quantified and assessed. Nevertheless, despite of all the issues, there are still massive opportunities associated with pervasive healthcare information provision.

3. INFORMATION ARCHITECTURE TO SUPPORT PERVASIVE HEALTHCARE INFORMATION PROVISION

3.1 Information Architecture in Empirical Contexts

3.1.1 Information Architecture in Information Systems Development

The analogy from building architecture and military aircraft manufacturing is used to define the information system architecture (ISA) with the aim to improve professional communications within the information systems community (Zachman, 1987). The initial Zachman's information system architecture contains six rows and three columns, where the columns cover the what (data), how (process) and where (network) integrates with scope, owner's view, designer's view, builder's view, out-of-context view and functioning system.

It is further extended to include another three columns that covers who (stakeholders), when (time) and why (motivation) (Sowa & Zachman, 1992). Scope corresponds to an executive summary for a planner or investor who wants an estimate of the scope of the system, what it would cost, and how it would happen. Owner's view concerns about the business model that constitutes the design of business and shows the business entities and processes and how they interact. Designer's view adheres to the system model that is designed by system analysts who determine the data elements and functions that represent business entities and processes. Builder's view relates to the technology model that adapts the information system model to the details of the programming languages, I/O devices or other technology. Out of context view refers to the components that contain detailed specifications that are given to programmers who code individual modules without being concerned with the overall context or structure of the system. Functioning system provides a view of programme listings, database specifications, network and so forth that constitutes a particular system.

Zachman's information system architecture is further developed into Information Framework (IF), as shown in which aims to provide a strategy for information management (Evernden, 1996). Information framework is suitable to be applied in a situation where information is used and created. Information framework introduced six dimensions, which are type of information, level of constraints, content, transformation over time and route maps. The content of each cell records knowledge. It is suggested that the framework should be kept in duration, covering a certain periods. Although both information system architecture and information framework are used in technical implementation, the concept in determining the type of information and information flow can be adapted for information architecture development. Comparing to information system architecture, information framework is not easily understood and far away too difficult for implementation.

3.1.2 Information Architecture in Technical Systems Development

As in technical systems development, information architecture is seen as the result of integrated approach to information design that identifies all information elements users need and expect, describing each in terms of content, media and form (Henry, 1998). IA in this context is related to the user centred information design for improving the technical systems usability. There are four tiers in the information architecture. The four tiers are labels, messages, online support elements and printed support elements. Labels and messages are categorised as interaction information, where it is important for completing interaction between technical system and users. Labels are required to identify user objects such as menu options, and messages that provide feedback to users about a user action and a change in system status. Online and printed support elements are support information, which are used to clarify other technical system usability components based on user's request.

3.1.3 Information Architecture in Web Development

Similarly with Henry's (1998) definition for information architecture that is related to technical content design in order to increase usability, Rosenfeld and Morville (2002) associates the definition of information architecture with internet, intranet or any online sharing sites development. Information architecture in this context should contain aspects such as (Rosenfeld & Morville, 2002): 1) the combination of organisation, labelling, and navigation schemes within an information system 2) the structural design of an information space to facilitate task completion and intuitive access to content 3) the art and science of structuring and classifying websites and intranets to help people find and manage information 4) An emerging discipline and community of practice focused on bringing principles of design and architecture to the digital landscape. Therefore, the information architecture needs to be in place in order to effectively study the information within an organisation. This concept is widely applied in web design, e-commerce sites development, information design and needs that relates to improving website usability, and communication or interaction between the website and users.

3.1.4 Information Architecture in Business Process Management

Business process management (BPM) is defined as supporting business processes by using methods, techniques and software to design, enact, control and analyse operational processes involving humans, organisations, applications, documents and other sources of information (Van der Aalst, ter Hofstede, & Weske, 2003). It aims to align the employee of the organisation to the customer, producing customer value through its business processes and associated resources (van Rensburg, 1998). This helps in improving product quality, reducing time-to-market, expanding to new markets, raising customer satisfaction and increasing profit margins (Dyer et al., 2012). The key success factor of BPM is to have the ability to understand change and its effect across all dimensions (people, process, resources and customers) of the organisation.

Van des Aalst et al. (2003) indicates that business process reengineering, business process modeling, business process analysis and business activity monitoring are part of BPM activities. Business process reengineering and information architecture share a common strategic and business process focus (Kettinger, Teng, & Guha, 1996). Information architecture can support or improve existing business processes by managing the deployment of resources and sequencing of deliverables (Dillon & Turnbull, 2005; Kettinger et al., 1996). Business process always involves information, and information always involves

a business process, these two are inseparable (Dyer, 2012). Information architecture serves as a backbone in supplying the relevant information for each activity in the business process. A reusable template can be created when the patterns of information are identified for each activity in a business process.

3.1.5 Information Architecture in Enterprise Architecture

Enterprise Architecture (EA) is defined as the process of translating business vision and strategy into effective enterprise change by creating, communication, and improving the key principles and models that describe the enterprise's future state and enable its evolution (Gartner, 2012). Enterprises are applying EA to ensure that the IT investment is best fit with business purposes. Listed below are a range of EA frameworks that are used in practice where each of them contains an information element or as known as information architecture.

3.1.5.1 Archimate

The Archimate Foundation defines EA as a coherent whole of principles, methods and models that are used in the design and realisation of an enterprise's organisational structure, business processes, information systems and infrastructure (Lankhorst, 2009). This framework identifies a business, application, and technology layer, as well as three elements dealing with passive structure, behaviour and active structure (Op't Land, Proper, Waage, Cloo, & Steghuis, 2009). Lankhorst (2009)derived these three elements are from natural language that corresponds to the subject-verb-object elements that all human languages exhibit. They are the fundamentals to the way in which the world is described. An active structure element is defined as an entity that is capable of performing behaviour, a behaviour element is defined as a unit of activity performed by one or more active structure elements and a passive structure or sometimes referred as information element is defined as an object on which behaviour is performed (TheOpenGroup, 2012).

3.1.5.2 The Open Group Architecture Framework (TOGAF)

TOGAF is an EA framework that provides the methods and tools for assisting in the acceptance, production, use, and maintenance of an EA. It is based on an iterative process supported by best practices and reusable set of existing architecture assets (TheOpenGroup, 2011). TOGAF supports four architecture domains that are widely accepted as subsets of an overall EA. These four architecture domains are: *business architecture* that defines the business strategy, governance, organisation and key business processes, *data architecture* that describes the structure of an organisation's logical and physical data assets and data management resources, *application architecture* that provides a blueprint for the individual applications to be deployed, their interactions and their relationships to the core business processes of the organisation and *technology architecture* that illustrates the logical software and hardware capabilities required to support the deployment of business, data and application services such as IT infrastructure, middleware, networks, communications, processing, standards etc.

3.1.5.3 The Zachman Framework

As illustrated in section 3.1.1, the Zachman framework is applied to information system development. It provides a logical structure to classify and organise the descriptive representations for each columns, associates with various views. This framework has been further transformed into EA (Zachman, 1997). Zachman (1997) illustrates EA as a set of descriptive representations (i.e. models) that are relevant for describing an enterprise such that it can be produced to management's requirements (quality) and maintained over the period of its useful life (change).

3.1.5.4 The Integrated Architecture Framework (IAF)

IAF is Capgemini's enterprise architecture framework developed from best practices. It is a toolbox that contains processes, products, tools and techniques to create all types of architectures which are intended to shape businesses and the technology that supports it (Wout, Waage, Hartman, Stahlecker, & Hofmann, 2010). The framework contains four aspect areas (business, information, information systems, and technology infrastructure), four abstraction levels associated with interrogative pronouns (contextual – why, conceptual – what, logical – how, and physical – with what) and two distinct views in dealing with security and governance issues.

3.1.5.5 Tapscott and Caston's Framework

Tapscott and Caston's framework (Tapscott & Caston, 1993), is represented by five views (business view, information view, work view, application view and technology view) with regards to an enterprise. *Business view* highlights what business is conducted by the organisation. *Information view* provides the information engineering perspective of business solution architecture, focusing on what information will be stored, and to what business rules this should adhere to. *Work view* shows the activities and the resources (i.e. people, information etc) within the organisation. Op't Land et al. (2009) describe *work view* as a way to determine the most effective ways in which the work activities can be supported by IT solutions. *Application view* describes the business realisation activities that will be automated by defining which information resources are needed, and how technology will be used to achieve this. *Application view* is positioned in the centre, that will be impacted directly or indirectly should there are any changes made to other views. *Technology view* provides the required technology to facilitate the other components of the architecture.

3.1.6 Information Architecture in Organisational Change Management

Organisational change management is a process of continually renewing an organisation's direction, structure, and capabilities to serve the ever changing needs of external and internal customer (Moran & Brightman, 2001). Similarly to the purpose of enterprise architecture, information architecture addresses the structure of the information systems at the organisational level for planning and management of information assets and resources (Wang, 1997). In other words, architecting information is to manage both internal and external changes within an organisation. Information is thus helps in decision making.

3.2 Information Architecture in Organisational Semiotics

3.2.1 Information from Semiotics Perspective

Information is defined as processed or interpreted data that has meanings to its users (Evernden & Evernden, 2003; Liu, 2000). There are apparently various views on defining information. Some see information as the conversion of bits and bytes of data from the computing perspective. One of the ways in viewing information is from the semiotics perspective, where information is seen as a sign (Boell & Cecez-Kecmanovic, 2010). Signs are categorised into icon, index and symbol (Peirce, 1935). An icon can either be an object or the effect produced by an object that conveys message or something verbal such as words, an index is a sign that signifies meaning and refers to by a causal process which may be distinguished by repeated observation, and a symbol is a sign that associated with norms or rules which depends upon social conventions to form and sustain them (Peirce, 1935; Stamper, 1985). Information field is contained in a symbol. An information field is a set of shared norms that enables people in community to behave in an organised fashion and determines the information flow in information systems design (Gazendam & Liu, 2003). For example, a blind network spot symbol in a hospital indicates that this particular spot has no network coverage. The hospital has made it as a rule or a common norm as the network connection will interrupt the operation of certain medical devices. Therefore, this norm has to be taken into consideration when designing a pervasive healthcare environment, whether or not the mobile devices are allowed to function in those blind spots. Nake (2002) addresses 'data' in the syntactic level as how does the sign signify, 'information' in a semantic level as does the sign signify, and 'knowledge' in the pragmatic level as why or what for the sign is signifying. This analogy is further mapped to the semiosis process (Nake, 2002).

Figure 1 visualises the notion of turning signs into information by adapting the by taking a field in electronic patient record (EPR) as an example. In the firstness, the sign 'Name' field in the EPR could reflect as the syntactic data in EPR database with certain data structure. This then deduces the secondness of the 'Name' field, which indicates this field should contain a patient's name. When a patient's name is entered in the thirdness, for example John Smith, all the knowledge about John Smith, or John's medical history will be reflected.

3.2.2 Organisational Semiotics

Organisational semiotics (OS) is the study of organisation using concepts and methods of semiotics (Liu, 2000). The study is based on the fundamental observations that all organised behaviour is affected through communications and interpretation of signs by people. There are six key concepts of OS by Ronald Stamper (Gazendam & Liu, 2003). These concepts are the semiotics ladder, social norms, the information field, actualism, the social affordances and ontological dependencies. These concepts are developed based on the social context. Actualism is a philosophical

Figure 1. Semiosis triad (adapted from Liu, 2000;Nake, 2002; Pierce, 1935; Stamper, 2001)

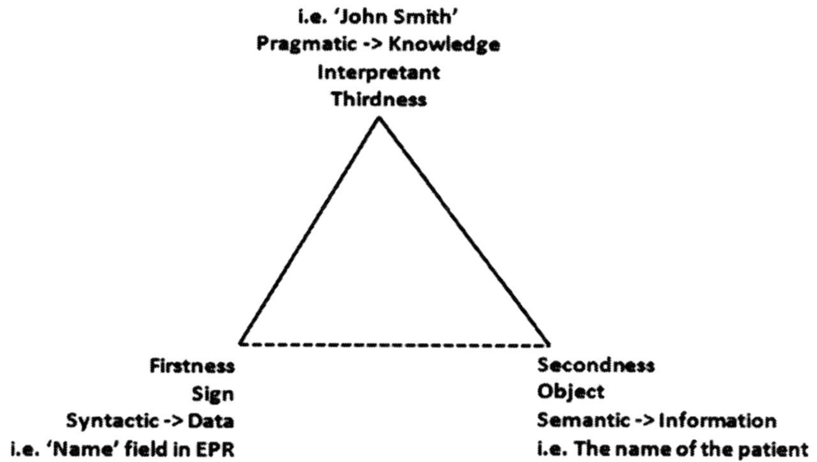

standing of OS transformed from radical subjectivism. The actualism in OS leads to a standce that a responsible agent or human being perceives the world as comprised of affordances. Affordance is actual capability which enables the interaction between human agent and its environment based on behaviour patterns that have evolved over time in the community.

The six key concepts, typically the semiotics ladder and the information field form a theoretical framework in information system development that is to develop an information system by considering the social context. The semiotic ladder (Stamper, 2001) defines the six aspects of signs. Stamper (2001) extended the three semiotics level (Morris, 1946), syntactic, semantic and pragmatic with addition of physics, empiric and social level. The bottom three layers study signs from the technical perspective, such as how signs are produced, transmitted and structured. The top three layers examine the humanistic perspective of signs, such as how signs are interpreted, perceived and used in a particular social setting. The physical or material dimension identifies the basic form of signs, which can be an element usually generated by devices. The empiric level examines the patterns of a set of signs, how they are used or being transmitted. The syntactic level concerns

about the sign structure and how the rules are associated with it. The semantic level deals with the meaning of a sign. It is then being brought up to the pragmatic level, where it is looking into how a sign influences the actions and thoughts of other people. In social level, the interpretation of signs is being examined.

The information field is a set of shared norms that enables people in a community to behave in an organised fashion (Gazendam & Liu, 2003). Norms determine which information is needed in certain occasions. They can be seen as subsets of knowledge. Taking a community as an example, behavioural norms indicate knowledge of what to do, evaluative norms determine how things should be judged, cognitive norms show how things happen, and perceptual norms detail what exists in the world.

MEASUR, the method for eliciting, analysing and specifying user requirements, is a method derived with OS as its theoretical foundation (Stamper, 1994). MEASUR is widely applied in information system design. Same applies to information architecture design. MEASUR consists of five major methods (Liu, 2000), these methods are problem articulation method (PAM), semantic analysis method (SAM), norm analysis method (NAM), communication and control analysis, and meta-system analysis. PAM consists of a set of methods that can be applied in the initial stage of a project where a central task will be identified as a focal system (Kolkman, 1993). The methods are unit system definition which provides a series of actions where stakeholders or agents may be interested on it; valuation framing which reveals the interest of stakeholders towards benefits and drawbacks of the action course; collateral analysis which structures a problem situation into a series of activities with given names; system morphology which clarifies three basic functional areas of social systems such as the organisation onion. Organisation onion contains three level of analysis; informal, formal and technical IS where an organisation is seen as an information system. SAM is a method to assist stakeholders in eliciting and representing their requirement in a formal and precise form based on the input from PAM. NAM specifies the general patterns of behaviour of the agents in the business system. Communication and control analysis analyses the various communications between all responsible agents and unit systems within a focal system. Meta system analysis oversees the whole project of innovation or system development as the object of study.

3.2.3 An Organisational Semiotics Approach for Information Architecture

Organisation is comprehended in terms of the signs and how, through norms to perform certain action, or by other means, organisation is characterised as a structure of social norms from organisation semiotics perspective (Liu, 2000; Stamper, Liu, Hafkamp, & Ades, 2000). Stamper et al. (2000) claimed that information requirements can be deduced once the norms within an organisation are identified. Every norm has the general shape: If CONDITION the CONSEQUENT. The condition part determines what information the norm-subject (an individual person or a group) requires to be able to obey it, while the consequent leads, sooner or later, to the generation of information

for others either directly through sending messages or indirectly through the influence of the norm upon actions.

The organisational onion, an OS view of an organisation, has three layers to define three taxonomies of norms defined for an organisation: technical, formal and informal (Liu, 2000). The informal layer refers to organisational culture, customs and values that are reflected as beliefs, habits and patterns of members within the organisation. The formal layer denotes the rules and bureaucracy to perform the organisational activities. The technical layer contains technical systems that enable actions to be performed for formal and informal layers.

Information requirements have to be identified prior to the development of an information architecture. Norms identified within an organisation by referring the organisation onion can add the analysis of the information requirements for information architecture. For example, in the informal layer, the informal norm indicates information such as the organisational culture to prefer purchasing IT services from local IT service providers as part of the organisation's initiative in supporting local IT entrepreneurs. Therefore, the formal norm in the formal layer will indicate that local IT service providers are preferred in the procurement process. This is then reflected in the company policy. Hence, in the technical layer where the formal norm will be automated, the procurement system will then have an indicator to prioritise the local IT service providers when the request for proposals (RFP) are submitted to the system. This indicator is designed through the information requirement derived from both informal and formal layers.

3.3 Information Architecture to Support Pervasive Healthcare Information Provision

The purpose of information architecture is to provide the right information at the right time, location and process to the right stakeholders with a right motivation and in this context it is to support the pervasive healthcare information provision. The information system architecture proposed by both Sowa and Zachman (1992), associated with the six basic interrogatives is a good foundation for developing an information architecture. The later development of Zachman's framework is a generic classification scheme for descriptive representations of any object (Zachman, 1997). By other means, this framework can be employed and adjusted for various contexts, and in this context, the information architecture development. The six interrogatives, *axis x*, will be fully employed but not the horizontal views. This is because the information system architecture proposed by Sowa and Zachman (1992) is meant for technical systems development, therefore both technical and business views and representations are taken into consideration whereas in the pervasive healthcare context, the aspects of pervasive healthcare information provision are incorporated,

the *axis y*. In addition, there is an additional axis, *axis z* that is called unit system definition in the information architecture. Unit system definition provides a series of actions where stakeholders or agents may be interested (Liu, 2000). This defines the conditions for retrieving information through information architecture. For example, for a care home diabetes patient monitoring process, for the 'how' and 'monitoring and transmission' column, the information returned would be the devices used for this process should the user wants to know what devices are allocated to a particular care home patient. Showing in Figure 2 is the conceptual design for information architecture to support pervasive healthcare information provision

The pervasive healthcare environment is actively involving stakeholders, especially the clinicians in decision making or providing the best consultation to patients, either inpatients, outpatients or care home patient with an adequate level of information provision. Therefore, the social context can't be ruled out for information architecture development

Figure 2. Conceptual design of information architecture to support pervasive healthcare information provision

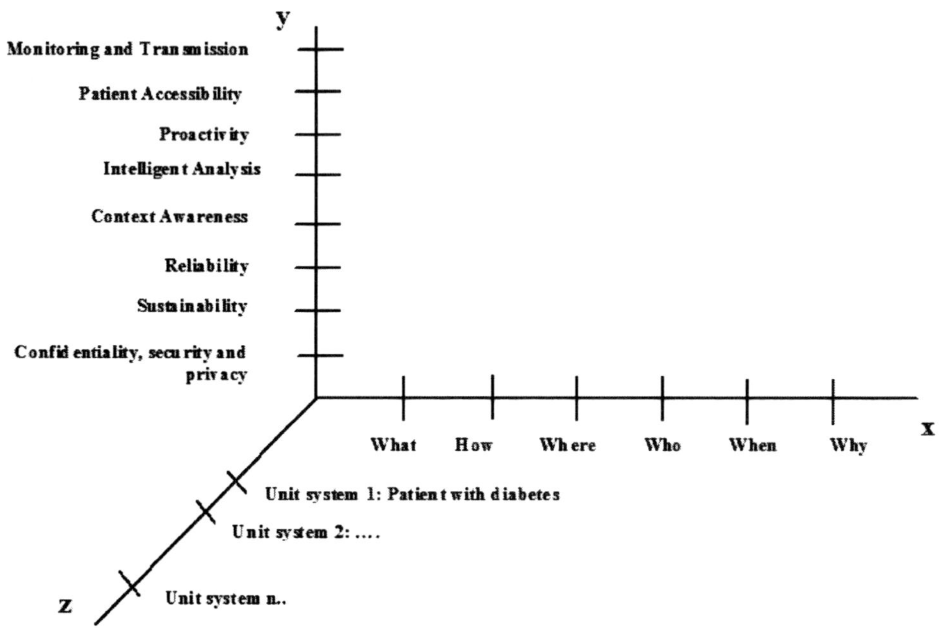

as there is a high involvement of human involvement. The study of norms hence is assimilated in the conceptual design of information architecture. As illustrated in previous section, organisational semiotics is to study the organised behaviours affected through communications and interpretation of signs by people. Information is seen as signs. Information requirements hence can be derived once norms within the pervasive healthcare context are identified. Showing in Table 1 is the interpretation for each interrogative by adopting the six aspects of semiotics ladders with examples. Semiotics ladder is one of the key concepts of organisational semiotics.

4. PERVASIVE HEALTHCARE INFORMATION PROVISION IMPLEMENTATION VIA WIRELESS TECHNOLOGY

To have a complete view of implementation adopting the concept of pervasive informatics in healthcare environment, the main features of the wireless technology used to communicate with Health Information System (HIS) are described in this chapter. Meanwhile, a probable design of an agent-based, seamless healthcare monitoring system is proposed for pervasive healthcare information provision. This system is designed according to the previous research of Multi-Agent System for Building cOntrol (MASBO) which provides automated assessment of the pervasive environment in real-time using readily deployable wireless sensors to personalize occupants' micro-environment and thus achieve optimal wellbeing and productivity (Qiao, Liu, & Guy, 2006). The system and functional architectures, and the deploying agents of the proposed system are described afterwards. Finally, an example applying the information architecture in pervasive healthcare environment via wireless sensor technology is illustrated for extensive understanding of PHIP.

4.1 Overview of MASBO and Supporting Wireless Technology

Several projects in pervasive informatics have been conducted in the Informatics Research Centre and other schools in the University of Reading (Liu et al., 2010). One of the projects "Co-ordinated Management of Intelligent Pervasive Spaces (CMIPS)" is conducted with industry and it has several objectives: automated personalization of the workplace, automated assessment of building environments in real-time and readily deployable sensors by use of wireless sensor networking technology (Yong et al., 2007). This research has one key component which is to deliver a Multi-Agent System for Building cOntrol (MASBO) by using the methods of organisational semiotic in order to balance energy use and occupants' preference, and to learn/predict user's behaviour (Qiao et al., 2006). MASBO provides an agent-based framework that utilises sensory information from sensors to determine the needs of users. In MASBO, mainly four agents (central agent, local agent, monitor & control agent, and personal agent) work with the Building Management System (BMS) and other devices in order to enhance the building performance. The central agent communicates with BMS to control the building; the local agent is to control a defined space, subject to the policies set for each space, and to coordinate with the central agent; the monitor and control agent communicates with devices such as sensors and actuators; and the personal agent analyses user's profile and preference to assist the personalized control of each defined space. The building assessment is to conduct a continuous assessment of building performance for adjustment of policies.

4.1.1 RFID Technology and Applications

A Radio Frequency Identification (RFID) system generally consists of tags and readers. The tag is composed of an integrated circuit for processing data, modulation of radio frequency signal and its

Table 1. Interpretation for each interrogative by adopting the six aspects of the semiotics ladder with examples

	Six Aspects of Signs in the Semiotics Ladder					
	Physical	**Empiric**	**Syntactic**	**Semantic**	**Pragmatic**	**Social**
What (data)	Device / IT application that produce data i.e. blackberry that supports mobile EPR, implantable glucose sensor	Network frequency to transmit data i.e. 3G network, wifi network	Data field / Data structure i.e Name, Age, Gender, Address, NHS number, diagnosis, consultant etc	Information contained in the data field i.e. John Smith, 36, Male, Reading, 123456, high blood sugar level, Mary Jane etc	Interpretation of the information towards patient safety i.e. John Smith has diabetes. He may need the implantable device for further treatment	Social impact derived from the information i.e. the implantable device is widely use in the EU and US. So it is considered safe
How (process)	Data collection i.e. blackberry that supports mobile EPR, implantable glucose sensor	Data transmission i.e. 3G or wifi network installation	Data structure i.e. B-trees, hash table	Information interpretation reflected in business process / clinical pathway i.e diabetes treatment clinical pathway	Intended actions based on business process / clinical pathway i.e. one way for treatment is to get an implantable device to monitor the blood sugar level for long term treatment	Social impact towards the action performed i.e. not every patient can afford an implantable device according to patient feedback. Therefore, they can apply the continuing care from NHS
Where (network)	Physical location where the device / IT application is used i.e mobile clinicians, visiting nurses	'From' and 'To' network points i.e data centres location, server location etc	Databases i.e. data centres location etc	Physical location where the information is used i.e hospital EPR system or mobile EPR system at patient's home	Physical location where this action is performed i.e. hospital or patient home	Social impact towards the location i.e. patient can choose to either to get treatment in hospital or home care from visiting nurses / clinician. Home care treatment usually is less stress
Who (stakeholders)	People who use the devices i.e. Clinicians, patients, patient's family members	People who are impacted by data transmission i.e. Clinicians, patients, patient's family members	People who are able to see the data i.e. Clinicians, patients, patient's family members	People who will interpret the information i.e. Clinicians, patients, patient's family members	People who will perform the action with the interpreted information i.e. a practitioner / clinician	People affected socially through the performed action i.e. patient who gets treatment
When (time)	Time that this device / application is valid for i.e until the hospital decided to retire the application	Response time to get the data transmitted Or Trigger time to transmit data for batch process i.e the response time has to be no longer than 0.01 sec	Time that particular data is used for technical purpose (i.e. data integration) i.e. time for database upgrade	Time when an action is performed that using the information i.e when treating a patient with diabetes	Time when this action is imposed i.e when a patient has diabetes, these are the steps for diabetes treatment	Social impact after the action is imposed i.e. diabetes disease is perceived as no time indication for recovery
Why (motivation)	Justification of the device / IT application usage i.e. software and hardware policy of the hospital	Justification of the network requirement i.e IT infrastructure policy	Justification of the data structure i.e IT infrastructure policy	Justification of the information provision i.e. information protection act	Justification of the action imposed i.e. information protection act	Justification of the observed social impact i.e. information protection act

transmission. The reader is used to retrieve data from tags. The RFID technology plays an important role in pervasive healthcare environment. It provides location-based healthcare services with the main objective of real-time monitoring indoor and outdoor patient's healthcare condition and information collection. For example, healthcare professionals located in the hospital or care home can remotely monitor the real-time health information of the tagged patient. On the other hand, the RFID tag is mounted on patient's wrist bracelet and can communicate with the healthcare sector identifying the patient without requiring additional interrogation to the central repository. In addition, the detailed information of the patient is stored on HIS database to maintain a consistent profile of each patient for further diagnosis. The wireless infrastructure of the medical facility can provide web-based communications among patient, healthcare professionals and caregivers. Furthermore, other applications in addition to monitoring stakeholders and equipment have been proposed for pervasive healthcare based on RFID, like the surgical procedures applications using for reducing medical errors. For example, Bacheldor (2008) develops the Smart Sponge System using RFID tag in surgical operation for recognising if some of the sponges have been inadvertently left in the patient after the operation, and the VeriMed tag which can be implanted on the patient for collecting information such as allergies and medical directives.

4.1.2 WLAN and Mesh Networks

Wireless Local Area Network (WLAN) is an infrastructure-based wireless network that distributes a number of access points (AP) located in fixed positions for supporting control of the network usage in transmission range. The WLAN acts as a router providing Internet connection for transmitted data packet. The reference standard is represented by IEEE 802.11 family (a/b/g) which is based on definition of a service differentiation on transmission in order to set priorities for packets (Ni, 2005). Access categories are defined for several services i.e. real-time services are associating with higher priorities. These parameters during the transmission enhance the network adaptability and improve the quality of services. The traffic prioritisation can significantly support pervasive healthcare while it is applied inside a single service. For example, it can prioritise the data transmission related to alarm message or urgent responses of clinical analysis.

In addition, another approach to extend WLAN coverage is represented by Mesh networks (Bruno, Conti, & Gregori, 2005), which root from the concept of Mobile Ad hoc Networks (MANETs) (Conti & Giordano, 2007). The MANETs consists of a set of self-organised mobile nodes in a multi-hop network topology where the mobile node does not need pre-existing infrastructure for communication and data exchange. Mesh networks allow the mobile nodes to connect the Internet and access through multi-hop path established in wireless backbone. Each mobile node can act as a mesh router: static node can communicate to each other through multi-hop paths. It also can be configured with gateway to enable Internet access to other networks. In order to allow mobile user obtain multi-hop connectivity to communicate with others and access the internet, several mesh networking protocols have been defined (Bruno et al., 2005). These protocols overcomes the interoperability issue i.e. IEEE 802.11s working group (Hiertz et al., 2008) is constantly working on standardisation of mesh network capabilities in Wi-Fi technology.

4.2 Designing Multi-Agent System for Pervasive Healthcare Information Provision

The design of the multi-agent based system for PHIP consists of a Body Area Network (BAN) gateway, routers and a body sensor equipped with RFID tag. The body sensor constantly measures patient's vital signs such as body temperature, blood sugar, and heart rate and the routers relay the data to the BAN gateway which links to the WLAN. A Java program is developed for transmitting sensory data from BAN gateway to the database server via Internet using method of client-server access (Chang & Huang, 2011). Besides, the RFID tag is used for location tracking, i.e. which room the patient is. In this way, when an emergency situation occurs, the location information helps caregivers and healthcare professionals to indicate where the patient is and result in taking a prompt action. In addition, adding sensors embed in buildings, for example, room for delivering more extensive information such as video images, humidity and room temperature can be used in the living environment can extend this design. Sensors with computing and communication capabilities are deployed at specific locations in patient's home to monitor compliance tasks. The sensors are communicated with intelligent agent who analyses the sensory data and sends to corresponding healthcare professionals. The frequency of reporting the health conditions of the patient is adjusted by a healthcare professional as deemed suitable. For example, if the patient is observed to be sitting on the coach in front of the television of personal PC at medication time, then the system will get informed by agent and send a reminder to the hand devices of patient via either internet or cellular network. The scenario of the system implementation is given in Figure 3.

4.2.1 System Architecture

Technically, an implementation of the multi-agent system is an assisted care facility using sensors technology and database. Facility professionals can be alerted when patients need immediate care. RFID plays a key role for communication among patients and staff members and allows long-term health monitoring and easy retrieval of information. Figure 3 is the system architecture describes that how the designed multi-agent system fits into the existing healthcare information system. The system architecture consists of three key layers: 1) software, 2) communication and 3) devices. The software layer contains three contents:

1. **Operational interface:** To provide operational interactions for healthcare provider
2. **Care management:** To provide intelligent analysis for agents
3. **Network management:** To manage network transmission in communication layer

Figure 3. Scenario of system implementation

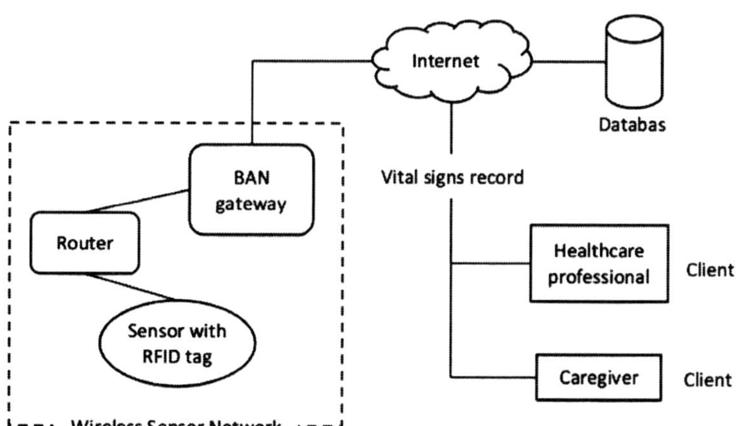

The communication layer has the elements of middleware, backbone network and control network. This layer focuses on providing stable quality of communication. The device layer is where hardware such as sensor resides in and connected the patient.

The architecture is designed by using agent and wireless technology to support healthcare professionals for providing appropriate care. Its capabilities include access to diverse wireless networks and location tracking which supports the system functionalities such as patient position and intelligent emergency response. In addition, the architecture is potentially aiming to reduce long-term cost of healthcare by reducing the burden of healthcare professionals and enhancing the efficiency. Furthermore, a list of commercial applications summarised by Alemdar and Ersoy (2010) are supporting the multi-agent system for monitoring patient. There are five categories of them: 1) location tracing and medication intake reminder – can support monitoring system to provide constant healthcare for patient; 2) daily living activities monitoring – identifies and records patient's routine and anomalies; 3) medical status monitoring – captures healthcare status of patients including heart rate, blood sugar, temperature etc. by using wireless sensor; 4) fall and movement detection – focuses on support for patient who requires special care i.e. patient recovering from an operation.

The mechanism of knowledge representation and reasoning in the agent adopts the EDA (epistemic-deontic-axiological) model which is rooted in organisational semiotics (Filipe & Liu, 2000; Stamper et al., 2000). The EDA model exemplifies the agent informational states, and meanwhile it simultaneously classifies the relationship between them (Booy, Liu, Qiao, & Guy, 2008). As depicted in the Figure 5, the EDA model has four basic component modules: Perceptive Interface (P) which is the initial element perceiving the data that has been sensed by agent or other devices; the epistemic (X) element contains knowledge of the domain (each defined space) and updates tis knowledge and beliefs of the state in the domain through the information received by the perceptive interface; the axiological (Y) element holds the norms, rules related to business process, cultural and personal practice to determine which signs the agent should perceive and what actions are currently available for enabling the evaluation of the current state of the domain using the norms; the deontic (Z) element performs the evaluation and generates commands for actuation through the agent. It determines what actions the agent can perform based on the combination of the perceptual interface, epistemic knowledge and axiological norms. The outcome (S) of the deontic evaluation can result in the health information system for performing recommended actions to the patient.

4.2.2 Functional Architecture

The intelligent agent is developed to perform the task of monitoring and analysing the conditions of patient. The use of the intelligent agent with relevant knowledge has the capability of assisting the healthcare professionals in on-going analysis and diagnosis of sensory data, and it can also support the continuous patient monitoring and alerting in care of anomaly via multi-agent communication (Sneha & Varshney, 2005). The intelligent agent has helped the healthcare professionals to reduce the cognitive overload and promoted timely intervention of healthcare structure as required. The agent carries a large amount of data analysis and communicates with other agent or sends reminder to devices only when required thereby reducing traffic on the wireless networks and enhancing the performance of the healthcare system.

The intelligent analysis is managed by the content of care management at software layer in system architecture. Prior to the first use, professionals based on their expertise and the patient's past condition, thus providing specific personal care, configure the intelligent agent tasked with analysing patient's healthcare condition. The agent

Figure 4. System architecture (adapted from Qiao et al., 2006)

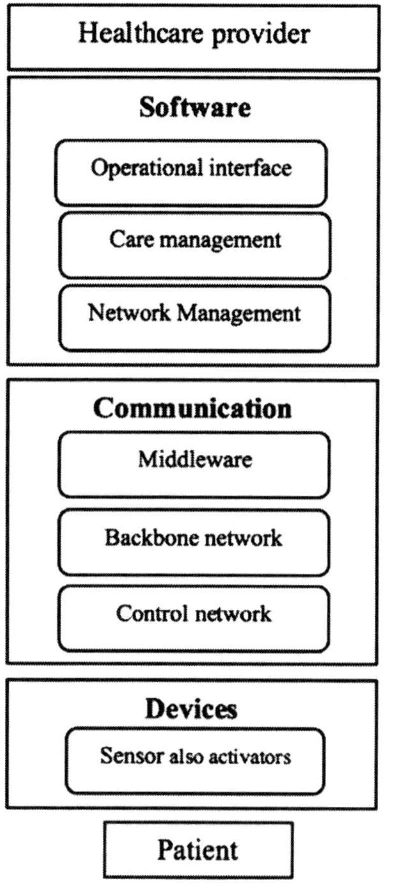

analyses the sensory data derived from sensors equipped on patient, looks for violations of pre-defined thresholds, and alarm patient or healthcare professionals when and as needed. Specialist builds the ontology that categorises different messages. Figure 6 is the functional architecture that elaborates the care management and depicts how agents work on providing continuous care for individual patient.

The intelligent agents are categorised into four agents (Centre Agent, Local Agent, Personal Agent and Manage & Control Agent) for this architecture. With the support of policy management and seamless network connectivity such as WLAN and RFID, the architecture is proposed in order to improve healthcare delivery by timely and reliable detection of anomalies and enhance the efficiency of the clinicians by assisting them in providing medical attention when needed. Figure 4 depicts the agent-based functional architecture for pervasive healthcare environment and the four categories are presented as followed:

- **Personal Agent:** Includes a number of agents such as patient data agent, medical information agent and location which

Figure 5. The EDA agent model (adapted from Duangsuwan & Liu, 2010)

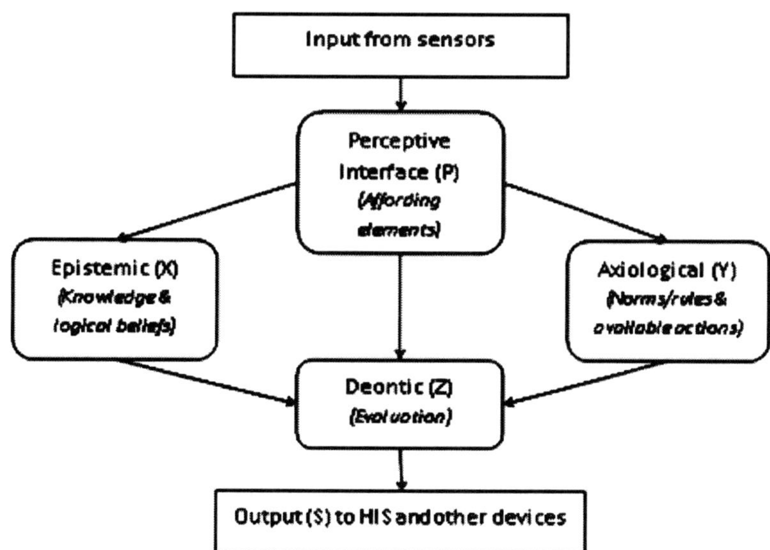

Figure 6. Functional architecture (adapted from Yong et al., 2007)

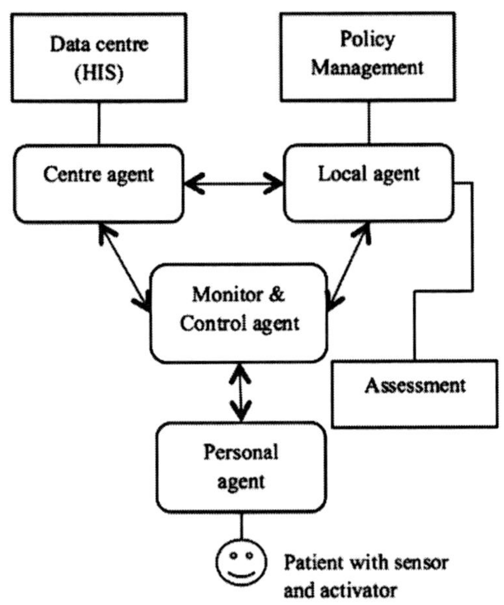

are used for information management and updates.

- **Local Agent:** Plays a central role as a mediator, policy enforcer and information provider. It reconciles patient's behaviour in different contexts, enforces policies and provides structural information for their respective coverage and updates information as needed.
- **Monitor & Control Agent:** Consists of a list of agents such as medication agent, blood sugar agent and weight agent which are used for collecting and monitoring patient's personal information and behaviours. It enforces the operation request given by the patient according to decisions made by the Local Agent.
- **Central Agent:** Has two major functions which are decision aggregation and interface to internal/external services required by other agents. The typical services provided by central agent include agent system configuration and interface to data centre.

In a data centre, a large amount of stored healthcare data which supports the healthcare decision making process is accessed, analysed and updated by the multi agent system. The use of the updated data in the data centre can help related industries such as pharmaceutical authorities, research organisations in analysis of specific health conditions and cost saving. Healthcare professionals, nurses and carers can access patient's information including monitored data. In particular case, they also can be accessed by the third party with authentication. To be aware that following to related data protection acts, the patient's individual healthcare data would not be disclosed to others.

4.3 Illustration: An Implementation of Pervasive Healthcare Information Provision

Based on the literatures (Marzano, 2005; Mitchell, Spiteri, Bates, & Coulouris, 2000), examples adopting the concept of pervasive informatics for designing wireless solution in hospital environment reveal that the experience of hospital stakeholders is improved, and with the assistance of smart home technology, the burden of staff nurses is reduced as well. In this scenario, the designed multi-agent system for pervasive healthcare can be seen as one of approaches for implementing the proposed information architecture in order to provide the right information at right time, location and process to the right stakeholders with right motivation. The section 3.3 has explained that the information architecture contains axis x, y and z and each of them indicates the factors that are taken into consideration for pervasive healthcare information provision. It is worth to note that the axis z in the information architecture is for a number of unit systems which defines the conditions for retrieving information and provide a series of actions where stakeholders or agents may be interested (Liu, 2000). To articulate the process how information architecture can lead a design of multi-agent system to support pervasive healthcare information provision, an example of patient's chronic monitoring and detection is used in following illustration.

As defined in previous section, the unit system is a collection of organised activities based on the Problem Articulation Method (PAM) (Liu, 2000). In this scenario, the unit system depicts that a patient suffering from diabetes living in his/her own house, and this house can be seen as a pervasive healthcare environment monitored by intelligent agents. The pervasive healthcare environment also includes hospital and the social care such as care home. The patient's health conditions are monitored by the embedded sensors, and the sensed data will be immediately transmitted to the healthcare professionals or care givers once anomalies have been detected. In this example, in order to maintain the patient's health condition, a multi-agent system is proposed for applying the concept of PHIP. The system deployed the central agent, local agent, monitor & control agent and personal agent. The personal agent has a list of functions (Blood sugar agent, medication agent, weight agent and sleep agent etc.) to monitor the patient's health condition. The function of blood sugar monitoring is set for frequent detection and alarms once the monitored data exceeds the specified threshold; the function of medication monitoring is to inform the patient to take medicine in every 30 minutes and a weight agent keeps the record of the patient's body weight for intensive diagnoses; the function of sleep monitoring is to detect the anomalies of the patient's sleep which can be reported to clinician in care if they are caused as side effect by mismanagement of diagnoses. As introduced previously the functionalities of the intelligent agents which are responsible for carrying out certain pre-defined tasks and the protocols and functionalities of intelligent agents tasked with the process of analysis. A detail description of each function of the various intelligent agents that are tasked with analysing

the monitored parameters and the protocols is given as followed.

- **Medication monitoring:** The agent set specific time to inform patient to take medicine, and will reminder the patient in every 30 minutes until the patient has confirmed the medication intake. Otherwise, the agent will count the times that patient missed medication intake and send alarm to corresponding healthcare professionals if it exceeded the threshold.

- **Blood sugar monitoring:** The agent set a list of blood sugar levels and defines the thresholds for each level. If the sensed reading of blood sugar has significantly increased or dropped, the agent will request intensive monitoring which reports two consecutive readings, and the agent will send alarm to healthcare professionals if the readings still reveals the anomalies of blood sugar situation.

- **Weight monitoring:** The agent watches patient's body weight and advice the patient on healthy habits if the change in weight is more than 10kg. If the change is more than 15kg, the agent will send alarm to healthcare professionals for further treatment.

- **Sleep monitoring:** The agent observes patient's sleep condition and will send alarm to healthcare professionals if the patient has sleeplessness or too much sleep for more than two consecutive days.

The proposed information architecture from healthcare professional's perspective is implemented in this example for articulating the six interrogatives (What, How, When, Where, Who and Why) and interpreting them by adopting the six aspects of semiotics ladders while retrieving information. Table 2 gives a detailed description of information required for designing the multi-agent system in order to support pervasive healthcare.

Table 2. Information architecture for monitoring patient's health condition (from healthcare professional's perspective)

	Physical	**Empiric**	**Syntactic**	**Semantic**	**Pragmatic**	**Social**
What	Sensor (i.e. medication sensor, blood sugar sensor, weight sensor)	Appropriated radio frequency (i.e. IEEE.11n)	Methods of coding (i.e. ASCII, C++, Java)	Understandable readings (i.e. name, heart rate, monitored data)	Recommended action (i.e. insulin injection, taking tablets)	Social consequence (i.e. diagnosis for diabetes)
How	Sensor installation (i.e. sensor installation manual)	Transmit the sensed data following the protocol and OSI layers (i.e. IPv6)	Data encryption (i.e. SSL, TLS)	Read the information from the clinical pathway (i.e. Clinical pathway for diabetes treatment)	Agree recommended action based on guideline and experience	Social impact towards action performed (i.e patient is embarrassed of having diabetes, so clinician tends to inform patient quietly)
Where	Sensor location (i.e. patient, room, hospital)	Data transmission between the data centre and patient	Database location of data centre (i.e. sequel server)	Health professional reads the sensory information (i.e. blood glucose meter, EPR) at (i.e. patient's home, hospital)	Perform the recommended action at (i.e. patient's home or the hospital)	Social impact where action is perform (i.e. patient feels comfortable to be treated at home)
Who	Clinicians, patients, patient's family members	Clinicians, patients, patient's family members	Clinicians, patients, patient's family members	Clinicians, patients, patient's family members	Clinicians, patients, patient's family members	Clinicians, patients, patient's family members
When	Real-time	Reliable data transmission	Frequent data updates depends on (i.e. computer capacity and amount of users)	Data need to be monitored in every 30 minutes	Time when this action is performed (i.e. when insulin level is high)	Social consequence of when the action is performed (i.e. patient wants to have privacy on his/her own health condition
Why	Hardware implementation policy	Network protocol, IT infrastructure policy	IT infrastructure policy	Health information protection act	Health information protection act	Health information protection act

The example described above articulated the six interrogatives in pervasive healthcare and interpreted them ay using the concept of semiotics ladder. As mentioned in the previous paragraph, the unit system describes a patient suffering from diabetes lives in a pervasive healthcare environment where four types of agents are located for monitoring the patient's health condition. In this context, the interrogative of "what" indicates the contents using for pervasive healthcare information provision. Physically, sensors such as medication sensor, blood sugar sensor are used for detection of signal. Empirically, appropriate radio frequency is the carrier supporting the data transmission. At syntactic level, data and signal are coded by using different methods such as ASCII in order to improve the reliability of transmission. At semantic level, the code can be decrypted into understandable readings which contain meaning such as name, age and condition. Pragmatically, the meaning of health condition reflects the intention of the behaviour, which is the recommended action for the patient. In social, the intention can lead to the social consequences such as rules, diagnoses and treatment. In this case, the social consequence is the specified treatment for dealing with the patient. Based on the proposed information architecture in section 3.3, the rest of interrogatives can be explained by using the same method following to the detail description in Table 2. Noteworthy, the pragmatic level contains the intention of each interrogative. Therefore some of the entities may not directly indicate the interrogative but reflect the effect of them. However, the justification is still in progress and will be discussed in further research.

5. CONCLUSION

5.1 Discussion

This paper outlines the conceptual design of deriving information architecture based upon both theoretical and empirical lens to support pervasive healthcare information provision follows with the technological implementation via wireless technology. The information architecture as illustrated in section 3.3 is derived from the combination of information system architecture and organisational semiotics. The six interrogatives proposed in Sowa and Zachman information system architecture provides a solid background in understanding the information requirement in general. This is further enhanced with organisational semiotics where each interrogative is defined by the six aspects of signs in the semiotics ladder that aims to crystallise the information requirements from technical and social perspective. By other means, the six interrogatives are the main information requirement, followed by the six aspects of signs in the semiotics ladder as the sub information requirement. As shown in Table 2 the interpretation for each interrogative by adopting the six aspects of semiotic ladder serves as an information provision engine. In the context of this paper, it is designed

to support the pervasive healthcare information provision. Therefore, there are two dimensions, the pervasive healthcare information provision requirements dimension and the unit system dimension integrated in the core model. The pervasive healthcare information provision dimension is static as the requirement has been predefined in section 2.2. The concept of unit system is applied so stakeholders can decide under what particular situation the information provisioning is needed. Nevertheless, the three dimensions information architecture is still at the conceptual stage. It is yet to be simulated with more real life situations.

The system architecture to support pervasive healthcare information provision via wireless is proposed. Still, the key challenge is the actual implementation in real life. A critical factor leading to the increasing healthcare expenses is hospitalisation for long term care and monitoring. Hence shifting the site of continuous monitoring and care from the hospital to the patient's home can potentially reduce healthcare cost. The agent-based system for pervasive healthcare environment provides details with respect to the various intelligent agents with their functionalities, and the decision criteria considered by each agent. The contribution of this system architecture is to deliver effective healthcare service, increase compliance with medical advice, and improve quality of life of patients inside and outside of the hospital. Hence, the pervasive healthcare information provision can improve healthcare delivery by timely and reliable detection of anomalies and enhancing the efficiency of the physicians by assisting them in providing pertinent medical attention as and when needed.

5.2 Future Work

This paper proposes the conceptual design for the information architecture for pervasive healthcare information provision with technological implementation. The three-dimensional information architecture is designed as the input for the system architecture of pervasive healthcare information provision via wireless technology and agent based systems. The conceptual design is yet to be further developed for actual implementation with real life situation in hospitals. Feedback from the hospital officials or healthcare professional is needed in order to justify the conceptual design of the whole solution proposed in this paper.

The interpretation for each interrogative by adopting the six aspects of semiotics ladder, as shown in Figure 4, can be further enhanced as an information requirement tool. The six aspects of signs or the sub requirements cover both technical and social aspects in gathering information requirements for each interrogative in developing the information architecture. Questions that are pertinent to the defined unit system can be derived. In addition, the information retrieval mechanism for this three-dimensional information architecture is another aspect to explore in order to ensure stakeholders retrieve relevant information when a meta-data tag from any axis is entered.

The system architecture for pervasive healthcare information provision uses the capabilities of current wireless and mobile networks. As a result, immediate or short-term implementation of the proposed architecture is possible using off-the-shelf components with user devices. Currently, the low to medium bit rate monitoring services can be implemented by the sharing of wireless network capacity among closely located healthcare sectors. Therefore, it can be stated that the architecture is implementable without waiting for future technologies or many resources. As stated throughout this section, the architecture is designed to be available, dependable, and practical. In addition to these characteristics, the proposed architecture can easily be extended for future use as the requirements change or new healthcare sectors emerge. The high-level abstraction and design technique result in a flexible and modifiable architecture.

In the next few years, fourth generation (4G) wireless networks could emerge, allowing users to access multiple wireless networks without manually switching from network to network. This "intelligent" support for network roaming would be even more helpful as the device complexity would be reduced and users could focus more on the healthcare services and less on network access issues. The architecture would benefit from such advances from 4G wireless networks. Besides, there are several factors that have to address before deploying this architecture. These include several known weaknesses in wireless security, and the need for additional training for system operators, healthcare professionals and patients.

REFERENCES

Alemdar, H., & Ersoy, C. (2010). Wireless sensor networks for healthcare: A survey. *Computer Networks*, *54*(15), 2688–2710. doi:10.1016/j.comnet.2010.05.003

Bacheldor, B. (2008). *Surgical sponges get smart.* RFID Journal.

Bardram, J. E. (2008). Pervasive healthcare as a scientific discipline. *Methods of Information in Medicine*, *47*(3), 178–185. PMID:18473081

Boell, S. K., & Cecez-Kecmanovic, D. (2010). *Theorizing information–From signs to socio-material practices.* Paper presented at the 22nd Australasian Conference on Information Systems. Brisbane, Australia.

Booy, D., Liu, K., Qiao, B., & Guy, C. (2008). A semiotic multi-agent system for intelligent building control. In *Proceedings of the 1st International Conference on Ambient Media and Systems*. Academic Press.

Brancheau, J. C., & Wetherbe, J. C. (1986). Information architectures: Methods and practice. *Information Processing & Management*, *22*(6), 453–463. doi:10.1016/0306-4573(86)90096-8

Bruno, R., Conti, M., & Gregori, E. (2005). Mesh networks: Commodity multihop ad hoc networks. *IEEE Communications Magazine*, *43*(3), 123–131. doi:10.1109/MCOM.2005.1404606

Chang, Y.-J., & Huang, W.-T. (2011). A novel design of data-driven architecture for remote monitoring and remote control of sensors over a wireless sensor network and the internet. *Journal of Internet Technology*, *12*(1), 129–137.

Conti, M., & Giordano, S. (2007). Multihop ad hoc networking: The reality. *IEEE Communications Magazine*, *45*(4), 88–95. doi:10.1109/MCOM.2007.343617

Dey, A. K., Abowd, G. D., & Salber, D. (2001). A conceptual framework and a toolkit for supporting the rapid prototyping of context-aware applications. *Human-Computer Interaction*, *16*(2), 97–166. doi:10.1207/S15327051HCI16234_02

Dillon, A., & Turnbull, D. (2005). *Information architecture*. Academic Press.

Dishman, E. (2004). Inventing wellness systems for aging in place. *Computer*, *37*(5), 34–41. doi:10.1109/MC.2004.1297237

Duangsuwan, J., & Liu, K. (2010). *A multi-agent system for intelligent building control-norm approach*. Paper presented at the ICAART. New York, NY.

Dyer, L. (2012). *Information architecture and business process management: A recipe for new business value*. Paper presented at the 2012 Technical Communication Summit. Rosemont, IL.

Dyer, L., Henry, F., Ines Lehmann, G. L., Osmani, F., Parrott, D., Peeters, W., & Zahn, J. (2012). *Scaling BPM adoption: From project to program with IBM business process manager*. International Business Machines Corporation.

Evernden, R. (1996). The information framework. *IBM Systems Journal*, *35*(1), 37–68. doi:10.1147/sj.351.0037

Evernden, R., & Evernden, E. (2003). *Information first: Integrating knowledge and information architecture for business advantage*. London: Butterworth-Heinemann.

Filipe, J., & Liu, K. (2000). *The EDA model: An organizational semiotics perspective to norm-based agent design*. Paper presented at the Agents' 2000 Workshop on Norms and Institutions in Multi-Agent Systems. Barcelona, Spain.

Gartner. (2012). *IT glossary - Enterprise architecture (EA)*. Retrieved 3-September-2012, from http://www.gartner.com/it-glossary/enterprise-architecture-ea/

Gazendam, H., & Liu, K. (2003). *The evolution of organisational semiotics*. Academic Press.

Henry, P. (1998). *User-centered information design for improved software usability*. Artech House, Inc.

Hiertz, G. R., Zang, Y., Max, S., Junge, T., Weiss, E., & Wolz, B. (2008). IEEE 802.11 s: WLAN mesh standardization and high performance extensions. *IEEE Network*, *22*(3), 12–19. doi:10.1109/MNET.2008.4519960

IOM. (2000). *To err is human*. Retrieved 14-August-2012, from http://www.nap.edu/books/0309068371/html/

IOM. (2011). *Health IT and patient safety: Building safer systems for better care*. Institute of Medicine.

Kara, A. (2001). Protecting privacy in remote-patient monitoring. *Computer*, *34*(5), 24–27. doi:10.1109/2.920607

Kettinger, W. J., Teng, J. T. C., & Guha, S. (1996). Information architectural design in business process reengineering. *Journal of Information Technology*, *11*(1), 27–37. doi:10.1080/026839696345405

Kolkman, M. (1993). *Problem articulation methodology.* (PhD thesis). University of Twente, Febo, Enschede, The Netherlands.

Korhonen, I., & Bardram, J. (2004). Guest editorial introduction to the special section on pervasive healthcare. *IEEE Transactions on Information Technology in Biomedicine, 8*(3), 229. doi:10.1109/TITB.2004.835337 PMID:15484426

Kourouthanassis, P. E., & Giaglis, G. (2006). *A design theory for pervasive information systems.* Department of Management Science and Technology.

Lankhorst, M. (2009). *Enterprise architecture at work: Modelling, communication and analysis.* New York: Springer-Verlag. doi:10.1007/978-3-642-01310-2

Liu, K. (2000). *Semiotics in information systems engineering.* Cambridge, UK: Cambridge Univ Pr. doi:10.1017/CBO9780511543364

Maitland, J., McGee-Lennon, M., & Mulvenna, M. (2011). Pervasive healthcare: From orange alerts to mindcare. *SIGHIT Record, 1*(1), 38–40. doi:10.1145/1971706.1971718

Martin, A., Dmitriev, D., & Akeroyd, J. (2010). A resurgence of interest in information architecture. *International Journal of Information Management, 30*(1), 6–12. doi:10.1016/j.ijinfomgt.2009.11.008

Marzano, S. (2005). People as a source of breakthrough innovation. *Design Management Review, 16*(2), 23–29. doi:10.1111/j.1948-7169.2005.tb00189.x

Mcgee, M. K. (2004). E-health on the horizon. *Information Week,* (989).

Mitchell, S., Spiteri, M. D., Bates, J., & Coulouris, G. (2000). *Context-aware multimedia computing in the intelligent hospital.* Paper presented at the 9th Workshop on ACM SIGOPS European Workshop: Beyond the PC: New Challenges for the Operating System. London, UK.

Moran, J. W., & Brightman, B. K. (2001). Leading organizational change. *Career Development International, 6*(2), 111–119. doi:10.1108/13620430110383438

Morris, C. (1946). *Signs, language and behavior.* Academic Press.

Nake, F. (2002). *Data, information, and knowledge.* Academic Press.

Ni, Q. (2005). Performance analysis and enhancements for IEEE 802.11 e wireless networks. *IEEE Network, 19*(4), 21–27. doi:10.1109/MNET.2005.1470679

Op't Land, M., Proper, E., Waage, M., Cloo, J., & Steghuis, C. (2009). *Enterprise architecture: Creating value by informed governance.* Berlin: Springer Verlag. doi:10.1007/978-3-540-85232-2_3

Peirce, C. S. (1935). *Collected papers of Charles Sanders Peirce: Pragmaticisms and pragnoaticism: Scientific metaphysics* (Vol. 5). Belknap Pr.

Qiao, B., Liu, K., & Guy, C. (2006). A multi-agent system for building control. In *Proceedings of the IEEE/WIC/ACM International Conference on Intelligent Agent Technology.* IEEE.

Rector, A. (2001). *From an information poor to an information rich health environment: A research study in health informatics for the UK institute for health informatics.* London: Institute for Health Informatics.

Rosenfeld, L., & Morville, P. (2002). *Information architecture for the world wide web.* Sebastopol, CA: O'Reilly Media, Inc.

Sneha, S., & Varshney, U. (2005). *A wireless ECG monitoring system for healthcare.* Academic Press.

Sowa, J. F., & Zachman, J. A. (1992). Extending and formalizing the framework for information systems architecture. *IBM Systems Journal, 31*(3), 590–616. doi:10.1147/sj.313.0590

Stamper, R. (1985). Towards a theory of information. *The Computer Journal, 28*(3), 195–199. doi:10.1093/comjnl/28.3.195

Stamper, R. (1994). *Social norms in requirements analysis: An outline of MEASUR.* Academic Press.

Stamper, R. (2001). Organisational semiotics: Informatics without the computer. In *Information, organisation and technology: Studies in organisational semiotics* (pp. 115–171). Academic Press. doi:10.1007/978-1-4615-1655-2_5

Stamper, R., Liu, K., Hafkamp, M., & Ades, Y. (2000). Understanding the roles of signs and norms in organizations-A semiotic approach to information systems design. *Behaviour & Information Technology, 19*(1), 15–27. doi:10.1080/014492900118768

Tablado, A., Illarramendi, A., Bermudez, J., & Goñi, A. (2003). *Intelligent monitoring of elderly people.* Paper presented at the Information Technology Applications in Biomedicine, 2003. New York, NY.

Tapscott, D., & Caston, A. (1993). *Paradigm shift: The new promise of information technology.* ERIC.

TheOpenGroup. (2011). *TOGAF version 9.1.* Retrieved 03-September-12, from http://pubs.opengroup.org/architecture/togaf9-doc/arch/

TheOpenGroup. (2012). *Welcome to Archi-Mate® 2.0, an open group standard.* Retrieved 03-September-2012, from http://pubs.opengroup.org/architecture/archimate2-doc/chap02.html#_Toc309639715

Van der Aalst, W., ter Hofstede, A., & Weske, M. (2003). Business process management: A survey. *Business Process Management,* 1019-1019.

van Rensburg, A. (1998). A framework for business process management. *Computers & Industrial Engineering, 35*(1-2), 217–220. doi:10.1016/S0360-8352(98)00068-0

Varshney, U. (2003). Pervasive healthcare. *Computer, 36*(12), 138–140. doi:10.1109/MC.2003.1250897

Varshney, U. (2007). Pervasive healthcare and wireless health monitoring. *Mobile Networks and Applications, 12*(2-3), 113–127. doi:10.1007/s11036-007-0017-1

Varshney, U. (2009). *Pervasive healthcare computing: EMR/EHR, wireless and health monitoring.* New York: Springer-Verlag New York Inc. doi:10.1007/978-1-4419-0215-3

Wang, S. (1997). Modeling information architecture for the organization. *Information & Management, 32*(6), 303–315. doi:10.1016/S0378-7206(97)00025-6

Weiser, M. (1991). The computer for the 21st century. *Scientific American, 265*(3), 94–104. doi:10.1038/scientificamerican0991-94

Wout, J., Waage, M., Hartman, H., Stahlecker, M., & Hofmann, A. (2010). *The integrated architecture framework explained: Why, what, how.* Berlin: Springer Verlag. doi:10.1007/978-3-642-11518-9

Yong, C. Y., Qiao, B., Wilson, D. J., Wu, M., Clements-Croome, D., Liu, K., & Guy, C. G. (2007). *Co-ordinated management of intelligent pervasive spaces.* Paper presented at the Industrial Informatics. New York, NY.

Zachman, J. A. (1987). A framework for information systems architecture. *IBM Systems Journal, 26*(3), 276–292. doi:10.1147/sj.263.0276

Zachman, J. A. (1997). Enterprise architecture: The issue of the century. *Database Programming and Design, 10*(3), 44–53.

KEY TERMS AND DEFINITIONS

Enterprise Architecture: A process of translating business vision and strategy into effective enterprise change by creating, communication, and improving the key principles and models that describe the enterprise's future state and enable its evolution.

Epistemic-Deontic-Axiological (EDA): Model rooted in organisational semiotics, exemplifies agent informational states, and simultaneously classifies the relationship between them.

Information Architecture: A high level map of information requirements of an organisation that aims to provide the right data at the right time, location and process to the right stakeholder with a right motivation.

Multi-Agent System: Computerized system composed of multiple interacting intelligent agents within an environment.

Organisational Semiotics: Study of organisation using concepts and methods of semiotics where it is based on the fundamental observations that all organized behavior is affected through communications and interpretation of signs by people.

Patient Monitoring: Technology to enable monitoring of patients inside and outside of conventional clinical settings, which may increase access to care and decrease healthcare delivery costs.

Patient Safety: A discipline in healthcare professions that applies safety science methods towards the goal of achieving a trustworthy system of healthcare delivery.

Pervasive Healthcare Information Provision (PHIP): Concept rooted in pervasive healthcare and information provision, aims to provide comprehensive healthcare services to its stakeholders covering the social and technical aspect.

Pervasive Healthcare: Consists of a wide scale deployment of wireless networks in order to deliver healthcare services anytime and anywhere, thereby reducing medical errors and improving information access.

Radio-Frequency Identification (RFID): Wireless non-contact use of radio-frequency electromagnetic fields to transfer data, for the purposes of automatically identifying and tracking tags attached to objects.

This work was previously published in the Handbook of Research on Patient Safety and Quality Care through Health Informatics edited by Vaughan Michell, Deborah J. Rosenorn-Lanng, Stephen R. Gulliver, and Wendy Currie, pages 315-343 copyright year 2014 by Medical Information Science Reference (an imprint of IGI Global).

Chapter 17
Monitoring and Assisting Maternity–Infant Care in Rural Areas (MAMICare)

Juan C. Lavariega
Tecnológico de Monterrey, Mexico

Lorena G. Gómez
Tecnológico de Monterrey, Mexico

Gustavo A. Córdova
Tecnológico de Monterrey, Mexico

Alfonso Avila
Tecnológico de Monterrey, Mexico

ABSTRACT

Presented is the project called MAMICare, which is motivated by the alarming number of maternity and infant deaths in rural areas due mainly to a poor monitoring of pregnancy progress and lack of appropriate alerting mechanism in case of abnormal gestation evolution. This work proposes an information technology solution based on mobile devices, and health sensors such as ECG (electrocardiogram), stethoscope, pulse-oximeter, and blood-glucose meter to collect automatically relevant health data for a better monitoring of pregnant women. This article addresses the status of the maternity infant death problem especially in rural areas of Mexico. It reviews some applications of IT in health systems (known also as Electronic Health or simply e-Health) and discusses how these are related to the presented proposal and how they differ. The article presents the proposed solution and discuss the current status of the work.

1. INTRODUCTION

The lack of appropriate maternal and child health in rural areas results in an alarming number of maternity and infant deaths (World Health Organization, UNICEF, UNFPA and The World Bank, 2012). In Mexico, although the infant and maternal mortality has been declining (maternal mortality fell from 89.0 to near 50 per 100 000 live births between 1990 and 2010), the states of

Chiapas, Oaxaca, and Guerrero have high rates, with mortality rates highest among indigenous children. The leading causes of death continue to be associated with hypertension, hemorrhages, and other complications of delivery (World Health Organization, 2006) that could be avoided. It has been demonstrated in other countries that by means of an information technology approach several medical conditions such as maternity care can be intelligently monitored, managed and treated

DOI: 10.4018/978-1-4666-8756-1.ch017

on a long term (Blank et al., 2013, Mougiakakou et al., 2010). Such approaches can be studied and technology can be adapted to the particular conditions of maternity care and information technologies access in the rural areas of Mexico.

Current health conditions in Mexico present a downward trend in overall maternity and infant mortality. However, it is highly remarkable that unequal access to healthcare services prevails as a challenge in the country (World Health Organization, 2006). More specifically rural areas are the ones lacking the high quality services needed to reduce maternal and infant mortality in the whole region. According to a study, health services and human health resources (such as equipped hospitals and well-trained personnel) are more valuable for rural communities (Jennett, Yeo, Scott, Hebert, & Teo, 2005), thus the delivery of these services remotely using accessible technology could help to level up the unequal access to health services. Electronic health records, risk assessment systems, and remote monitoring are just some examples of how technology can be applied in the healthcare field.

The objective of our proposed work is to reduce maternity and child mortality rates in rural areas using information and communication technology (ICT) to strengthen the current health delivery practices for both the mother and child during pregnancy. The goal of this effort is to develop an integrated IT solution similar to our Emergency Remote Pre-Hospital Assistance (ERPHA) project (Muñoz, Avila, Lavariega, González, & Grote 2012). A solution that is suitable for rural areas, focused on the maternity care conditions and considering the technology limitations that prevail in the area are key elements to be considered.

The remainder of the paper is organized as follows: Section 2 presents and discusses current e-Health approaches on which we based our work, including our previous project called ERPHA. In Section 3 we introduce our project to alleviate the maternity infant death situation in rural Mexico.

Finally, in Section 4 we establish our current status and discuss future work in the short and middle term.

2. RELATED WORK

In the past 10 years Information technology (IT) has been used to improve the accuracy of patient records, and health monitoring. Benefits and challenging unsolved problems continue to be the outcomes of such attempts (Bates, 2003), such as electronic health records, remote monitoring, tele-health, health data collection and processing, and clinical decision support systems, to name a few. Groups interested in the IT-Healthcare efforts have gathered and exchanged opinions to identify technological areas with the highest benefits. These groups integrated by members of the public, health care provider and private sectors selected tele-health and electronic health records, in this order, as the most valuable IT approaches. The groups of interest also identified as a disadvantage the changes in the current practices and processes in the delivery of health services (Jennet et al., 2005).

The use of electronic health records (EHR) is one of the most successful examples of the application of IT to support health care services. Research efforts state that EHR is a solution with great potential as EHR strengthens the collaboration between public and primary care (Calman et al 2012). Electronic health records offer additional benefits such as improving public health surveillance by documenting patient data, real-time guiding of the physician interventions using statistical data to generate clinical alerts, improving surveillance and management of a communicable disease, etc. (Calman et al., 2012).

Other research effort focuses in supporting the treatment of patients with type 1 diabetes mellitus. This decision support system (Mougiakakou et al., 2010) provides risk assessment for long-term complications. Data exchange between a unit for the patient and a unit for the management of the patient occurs, and data is also stored in a web server. By combining database technologies, simulation algorithms and data mining, the system provides an advanced processing of the stored data to support the decision making for the physician. Although a study to evaluate the user requirements satisfaction, the cost and the effectiveness of the solution is needed, this work has allowed a proper risk assessment for long-term diabetes mellitus complications. Other risk-assessment technologies have been developed allowing the physician to do a smart diagnosis of the patient.

In Ghana, a software solution was designed in response to the rapid expansion of community health workers in Africa and Asia. This was made taking as an advantage the proliferation of mobile devices. The Mobile Technology for Community Health (MoTeCH) offers features such as calculating the schedule for each patient; and notifying both patient and community workers when care is due. The system automates the delivery of information for routine reports and integrates with existing software applications for mobile data collection. The presented project is the initial part of an iterative process and still requires advanced software development skills, attention to standards and configurable design to make it more readily available to groups of interest within the research (Macleod, Phillips, Stone, Walji & Awoonor-Williams, 2012).

From Brazil and Peru, a Windows-based application called "TeleConsult" proposes to reduce the high mortality on rural areas in Latin America. TeleConsults proposes the establishment of a medical network that communicates using satellite. The system acquires images from ultrasound examinations, electrocardiogram and blood imaging and pretends to cover disciplines such as cardiology, gynecology pediatrics and infections from the region (Sachpazidis, Rizou & Menary, 2008).

An effort in the maternity and prenatal care is the 'Prenatal Risk Calculation (PRC)'. PCR is a software solution based on a previously introduced system known as JOY. PCR and JOY work using chromosome data information (aneuploidies), through this analysis prenatal risk could detect symptoms such as Down syndrome and potential cancer cells on the product. The test performance between PCR and JOY gave higher significant results while detecting aneuploidies in the first trimester trial; testing alone, the test performance results of JOY were better than the results of PRC. PRC demonstrated to be a good tool to detect prenatal risk but it still needs to be improved (Hörmansdörfer et al., 2008).

A clinical decision support system on maternal care field was created and implemented for rural health care centers in Africa. The QUALMAT CDSS provides guidance for antenatal, delivery and post delivery care. This guidance is possible by incorporating features such as an orientation process based on set of routinely actions, algorithms to detect situations of concern, and electronic tracking of perinatal and postnatal care. CDSS is a java-based application that incorporates the World Health Organization (WHO) guidelines for pregnancy and childbirth care. The CDSS was first developed in English for the use in Ghana and consist of four parts: a user interface; an XML-database for patient data, a set of algorithms to screen entered values; and a set of training documents. Decision support is implemented by offering guidance trough routine action in maternal and perinatal care, detection of critical situations using clinical data and electronic partographs for observation on the progress of delivery up to 24 hours. This system requires an equipped site with a laptop computer. Staff members in charge receive general software and QUALMAT training and are left in charge of user administration. The implementation presented limitations in complex medical environments leading to a different conclusion than expected. Another challenging issue was the implementation of the system in a resource-poor environment, leading to hardware insufficiencies and user frustration (Blank et al., 2013).

In general, as we have seen in this section, a great deal of effort in applying IT to health systems is based on keeping records and monitoring patients through a network. However, little effort has been set to use mobile technologies for a better diagnostic in remote areas. One example of applying mobile and wireless computing in health remote health assistance is our previous work called ERPHA.

ERPHA (Emergency Remote Pre-Hospital Assistance) is an example of a IT solution based on mobile technologies to improve remote monitoring under emergency situations like car accidents. ERPHA is an Information Technology solution that enables the continuous monitoring of a patient´s condition during the pre-hospital period. ERPHA enhances the pre-hospital care quality by allowing early intervention of specialist physicians with key data such as video, audio and visualization of patient´s vital sings. ERPHA collects key health data form patient using body sensors that transfer their data to a mobile device (usually a smartphone) creating a body-sensor-network (BSN). The mobile device processes, displays and forwards the collected data to a hospital or medical center where a specialist physician can remotely assist paramedics in the diagnosis. Additionally, at the medical center the data sent by de mobile device is stored into a database for maintaining historical records of the patient. These records can be later used for identifying patterns for a more effective treatment or for classifying the severity of injuries. The mobile device can resend all collected data from the BSN plus video to a medical center where a physician can provide a better diagnostic of the patient being monitored. The BSN is built with Bluetooth-enabled sensors for vital sings such as ECG, stethoscope, pulse-oximeter, and blood glucose-meter. The mobile device has been implemented using smartphones running Windows Mobile and Android as operating systems. The mobile device currently transmits video, GPS location and data from the BSN to the hospital via Wi-Fi and 3G. Besides the smartphone a tablet can be used as alternate mobile device. At the hospital, the transmitted video, vital sign and patient information are stored and managed using dedicated database and video servers. The hospital front-end is implemented using Microsoft Visual Studio 2010 (ASP.NET) and Microsoft SQL Server 2008 R2. Further ERPHA details are available at (Muñoz, Avila, Lavariega, González, & Grote 2012).

3. RESEARCH METHODOLOGY

Based on a real case, we describe our research in the following sections. In the following description, some identities have changed to be anonymous. The intention is to highlight the improvement of healthcare quality and accessibility using wireless technology in a rural area.

Our research is in its initial state. A team of colleagues in the demographic area has already performed an evaluation study of the needs and requirement of the people in the selected rural area. From that study several projects were identified; some related to rainwater harvesting; dignified dwelling; reforestation and better use of natural resources; and of course, heath improvement. For health improvement we have identified as the key problem maternal and infant care.

In this initial part of the project we will develop, based on our in-site observations, an information technology solution for assisting the monitoring and evolution of pregnancy in the area.

Then, we will perform a pilot evaluation of the IT solution and make the required adjustments. As a result, we expect to see a progress in the quality of the information during pregnancy monitoring; an improvement in the quality of the health care services and eventually a downfall in the maternal and infant death indices.

4. DESCRIPTION OF THE PROJECT

Existing healthcare support systems have been proved to be efficient in the improvement of medical services. Most of these systems are applied in controlled environments like hospitals. Other systems are implemented to be used at home, where patients have access to such technologies and can follow the health recommendations that an expert or experts provide remotely. Also, as shown in the related work, aiming the healthcare problem in rural areas seems to be a growing concern, particularly in less developing countries such as Mexico, Peru, or Brazil in Latin America or Ghana in Africa. However, direct application of similar technologies would result in an inefficient solution for the Mexican communities included in the scope of this proposal. This is mainly because of the limited communication technology to which those rural areas have access. Our project is focused on the Magdalena Peñasco community, a rural area in the state of Oaxaca, Mexico. In that region, the communities lack of current communication systems such as Internet or Cellular Networks. Most of the time, the only communication service to which they have access is civil band radio communication.

4.1. Background

The current process for maternity-infant care attention in the community of Magdalena de Peñasco is a manual process. Because primary attention is performed by volunteers, enough documentation exists about the attention protocols to follow. However, it is hard to identify if everyone involved has a full knowledge of the steps to follow when immediate attention is required. Medical assistance, in particular Maternity-Infant assistance, is based in a hierarchy of levels of attention. Attention levels range from the most elemental home visit performed by a social worker (called Rural Volunteer Promoter or PRV) to the most equipped but expensive trip to the Zone Hospital at the capital of the state. In between the PRV and the Zone Hospital there are the Health House, the Rural Medical Unit (UMR), the Basic Services Hospital(HSB) and the Rural Hospital.

In order to understand what those levels of attention represent for anyone in the community a brief description of each level is given. The Social worker has a basic follow up equipment, accordingly to the Mexican Social Security Institute (IMSS). Health houses are a base for the social workers, vaccine campaigns, and have access to a basic medical kit. The UMR is conformed by a medicine practitioner or a general physician as well as an auxiliary worker. The HSB is considered similar to an UMR with some additional equipment such as an ambulance and a delivery room, although much of the information is not clearly defined. Only the Rural Hospital and Zone Hospital have all the basic services (pediatric, internal medicine, general surgery, and gynecology) with the difference that the Zone Hospital in Oaxaca also has more special services. However, Oaxaca´s Zone Hospital gives services to patients from the whole state and most of the time is over capacity.

In general terms, attention in the rural communities, in particular in Magdalena de Peñasco is very limited. Health services are hard to reach, personnel are sometimes undertrained and most of the time hospitals or health centers are overcapacity or can't cover the full needs of the community. In order to provide a better understanding, a case scenario is described.

4.2. Original Situation Scenario

This scenario illustrates in a fair amount the current state of maternity-infant attention in the community of Tlaxiaco. Names and fictitious characters have been developed to illustrate the case.

Maria is a voluntary Social Worker (or PVR) in the region of Chalcatongo; Rosa is a Mixtec woman that lives in a settlement 700m far from Chalcatongo. Rosa is 7 month pregnant, this is her fourth pregnancy; her children are 7, 4 and 2 years old. She is a healthy 36 years old woman. Her husband left 3 months ago to continue working in Los Angeles, California (USA); Maria lives 500m away from Rosa's home.

A Health House is 3km away from Rosa's home. UMR is 6km away from the Health House and 12km away from Rosa's. The closest HSB is 48km away. The orography of the zone makes travelling really slow and hard for all those distances.

As part of her duties as rural promoter, Maria performs a home visit to Rosa to check her pregnancy evolution. Maria following her basic training takes the recommended vital sings from Rosa such as blood pressure, cardiac rhythm, and belly size. However, Maria does not remember how to use properly the sphygmomanometer and is hard for her to interpret the attached instructions. Maria skips some measurements, mainly because the form where data is registered does not indicate them. Rosa has been working hard at home moving some heavy objects, and Maria does not know about that. Maria fills the form with normal data and proceeds to finish the evaluation. At that moment, Rosa begins to feel pain in her belly and turns pale. Maria interprets those symptoms as abnormal and proceeds to make Rosa rest while she seeks for help. Rosa's older son runs to the nearest home (100m away). A neighbor goes to the nearest Health House seeking for help, 20 minutes passed, and the place is closed. The neighbor goes to the nearest UMR, an extra 40min passed. Meanwhile, Rosa is feeling worse. People in the community find the kid and decide to help him by driving him to Rosa's home in order to take her to the nearest UMR. 1 hour and 15min has passed since the first symptom appeared on Rosa; she has not gotten any sort of expert medical attention yet. As situations gets worse, they decide to go straight to the HSB looking for better facilities and the possibility of having an ambulance. Thirty minutes of traveling hurt on Rosa's situation because of the ground conditions. Rosa's evaluation takes longer than expected because the doctor was not notified on time about the emergency. He wasn't ready to receive Rosa. Maria stayed and did not travel with Rosa, moreover the forms with information of Rosa's evaluation were missing. Therefore, there is no information that allows the doctor to make a smart decision. Rosa's critic situation forces her to be transferred to the hospital in Tlaxiaco. Fortunately, the ambulance was in good conditions, but still it takes 1.5 hours to take Rosa to Tlaxiaco. It was too late by then; unfortunately both Rosa and her baby die on arrival.

This case scenario illustrates that failing to communicate fast and efficiently is a critical factor to solve any emergency of this type on time and effectively. Also the incomplete information is a really big factor in the final outcome of the maternity-infant attention.

4.3. MAMICare System Description

We could mitigate the above-described problem, if we apply information technologies in a e-Health solution. The e-Health solution that is proposed aims to generate a positive impact in the community by improving the communication channels and offering the possibility of having reliable information about the patients at the time when it is most needed.

There are special characteristics in the highest needed rural areas that challenge the implementation of a simple healthcare solution. Currently, most of the monitoring is done by social workers without any special preparation and that belong to the same community. In the zone, there is no telecommunication infrastructure (Wi-Fi or cellular networks) - the most advanced technology is civil band radio. Due to the lack of sufficient communication technologies, the proposed solution is an asynchronous support system to assist the social workers in the monitoring process and the physician with reliable information. Also the system aims to work as a data center for patient's information.

MAMICare is the proposed system to cover three mayor setbacks currently present over rural communities in Mexico. First, the proper monitoring and control of the patient's evolution by storing adequate information and following up data required in basic maternity-infant care; second, the failure to detect risk situations on-time due to the lack of a proper knowledge under those circumstances; and finally, the communication gap within the rural communities in relation to the healthcare problem. MAMICare will cover those three issues under different use conditions. The eventual availability in the future of communication infrastructure in the different rural areas would make possible to extend the MAMICare functionalities to forward the recorded information in a live stream fashion to the nearest hospital or medical facility. This functionality provides an additional tool for the social worker by allowing a health professional to check on the patient and a remote physician to give complete feedback on time. Data in the MAMICare will be locally stored and used to properly follow up the patient's record. At the same time and when available, data will be shared to a centralized database in the community center in which data will be properly analyzed for statistics and in-depth knowledge of the illness under medical treatment. MAMICare will have a risk-condition assessment tool that will identify situations and alert the social worker of critical conditions.

MAMICare is integrated by two parts: MAMITa and MAMI Server, as illustrated in Figure 1, each will handle part of the previously described functionality. The first part (MAMITa) is a tablet device that will be used by the social worker or physician to record, store and analyze information of the patient. The MAMI Server is a system that allows wireless communications between the tablet (MAMITa) and the community center in which a database system will be implemented for the storage and administration of the data.

Figure 1. MAMICare overall architecture

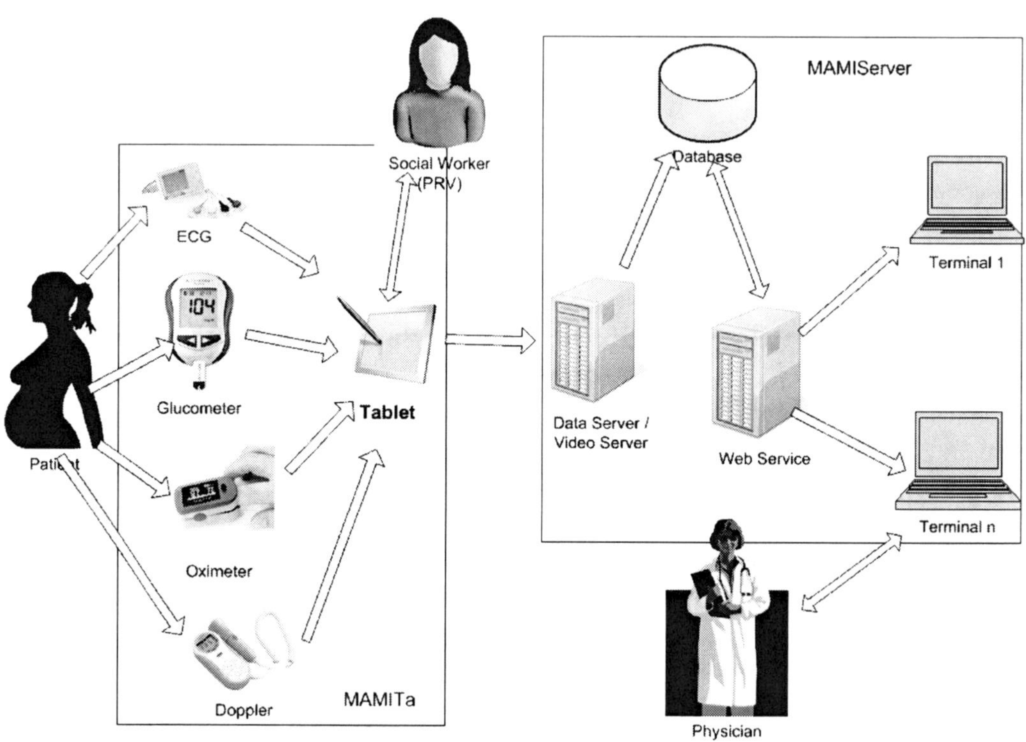

Figure 2. Social worker, patient interactions with the MAMITa through the use of devices

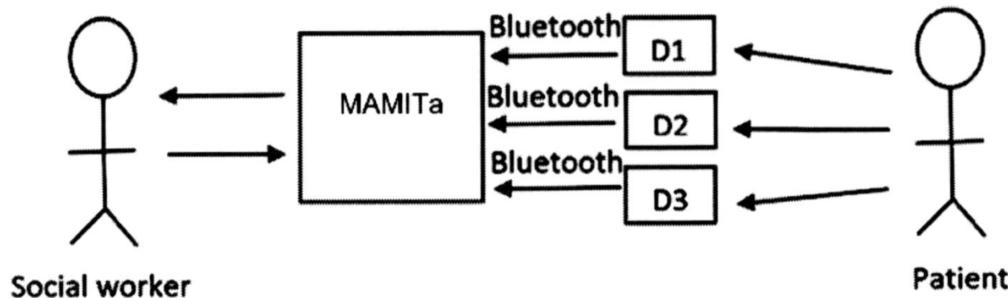

This paper focuses in the MAMITa part of the project; although MAMI Server may be briefly discussed it is only considered to be part of the long-term solution.

Following ERPHA architecture as a reference, the MAMITa system is a software solution that integrates different sensor devices (as shown in Figure 1) such as pulse-oximeter, ECG, Doppler, and glucometer. MAMITa is expected to keep valid track records of patients by aiding the social worker in her job through a visual interface. Such interface includes a step-by-step process to be followed in order to avoid any missing information. MAMITa will also include support video on how to use the sensors and follow the exploration protocols in order to avoid missing critical information. MAMITa will consist of a risk assessment tool that will alert if measurements are out of a healthy range and possibly become a risk situation for the patient. The application will incorporate the definition of system priorities to alert the social worker of any maternity-infant risk such as hypertension following norms and standards as the Mexican Official Norm NOM-007-SSA2-1993. This Mexican norm specifies prenatal, during and after labor attention for women and newborn children (Secretaria de Salud del Gobierno Mexicano, 1995). Also the WHO "Pregnancy, childbirth, postpartum and newborn care - A guide for essential practice" provides recommendations to guide health-care professionals in the treatment and management of women during their pregnancy, childbirth, postpartum period or any complications that may arise (World Health Organization, Department of Making Pregnancy Safer, 2006). When the system has been input with some conditions and considers a risk situation, MAMITa gives feedback to the PRV to communicate with and pass the system to the physician. The doctor is then informed by the system on the patient's current condition allowing him/her to make a smart decision by fully knowing all the details. As described in the original situation scenario, the patient, the social worker and the doctor are the ones that should be in direct contact with MAMITa system.

The proposed MAMITa solution includes a specific list of medical devices such as ECG (electrocardiogram), stethoscope, pulse-oximeter, and blood-glucose meter. Such devices will be synched with the tablet and used for the proper monitoring of the patient. Those devices are considered part of the basic medical kit included with the tablet; other devices will be selected in order to fulfill the requirements in the rural communities. Devices properly synched with MAMITa system allow the system to keep track of the patient's situation and at the same time to keep an electronic record of patient's health. Figure 2 illustrates the way in which MAMITa reads the patient measurements through the devices. Also it shows the way in which interaction occurs between the Social Worker, the patient and the device (D). System allows the social worker to input data as well as to receive readings and instructions from the system in order to aid in the process of recording information.

MAMITa interface allows interaction with multiple devices (D´s in Figure 2 and Figure 3). It is expected to use an internal database as well as an internal control layer that interacts with the view layer. View layer is in charge of communications and the tablet to be used is expected to have as well at least one of the Wi-Fi/3G/4G communication protocols that will be used for some external communication activities in a further stage of the project. All these are shown graphically in Figure 3.

While readings are being stored locally in the MAMITa, MAMITA Server complements the functionality by allowing communications between tablets and a data center. Local MAMITa data is synch with the community center database via Wi-Fi whenever communication is allowed or connection is achieved. This scenario happens

locally within a single health community center such as the Rural Hospital. MAMITa will be later extended to a wireless environment, when communications are allowed between medical centers. By allowing having patient's information centralized in one place the doctors or other social workers will have better accessibility to the patient's information without the original social worker or the tablet being required to travel. Storing the data will also allow further data processing for having statistics or applying algorithmic solutions that allow improving the risk assessment evaluation process.

Figure 4 illustrates the whole MAMICare system interactions. First, the MAMI Server in which different tablets from different patients are being synchronized and data is being centralized in order to be accessible from any workstation. Secondly, the MAMITa system in which medical measurements are input and stored locally in the tablet device.

Figure 5 shows the MAMICare system interactions in terms of the general architecture as proposed. The first part is an independent mobile system that interacts with a set of devices for data input. The second is a cloud service that provides communication between the mobile and server parts. The third part is a server application accessed via web from the hospitals, mainly for the use of the doctors.

Figure 3. Shows the MAMI Tablet (MAMITa) internal interface and communications

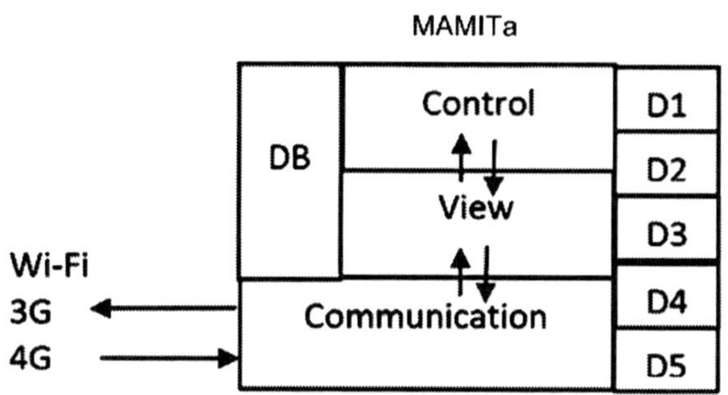

Figure 4. Full 2-part functionality of MAMI care project

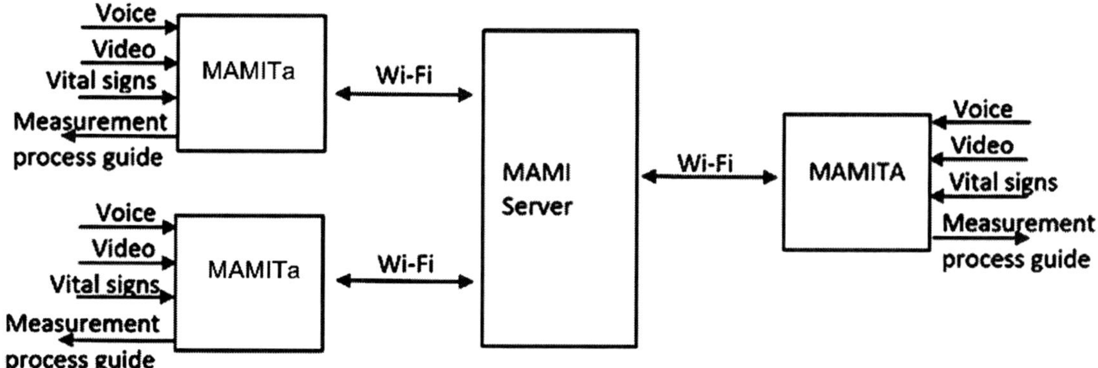

Figure 5. MAMICare system components interactions

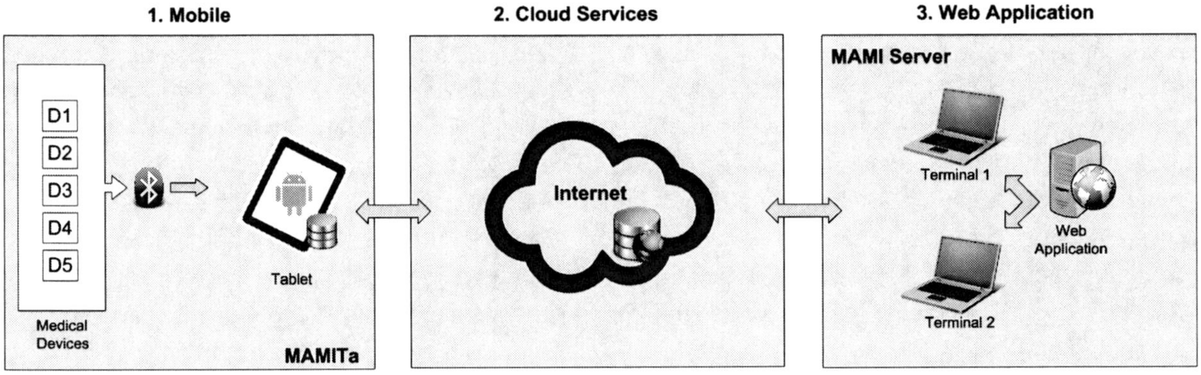

The described architecture allows not only to modularize the whole system for its development but also to generalize the system architecture. The proposed architecture shows a system that is easily adaptable, maintainable and mobile. The adaptability in the system will allow us to have a healthcare solution that even though is specialized in maternal attention could later be modified to assess different scenarios in which detection of critical conditions from a set of input measurements could be required. An example of this adaptability is available in a previous work from Muñoz, Avila and Lavariega (2012). In their research, a similar architecture for the mobile environment is applied to attend remote hospital emergencies.

For the short-term of this project, the Denis cheap CDMA 450/800 Mhz 7 inches Android 4.0 CDMA tablet has been defined as a base development environment due to its inclusion of the CDMA450 communications protocol which has been chosen by Mexican telephone company TELMEX (2008) to be used for expanding the communications services to the rural areas since 2007. However, now, while we are writing and reviewing this paper, there are no communication services yet in the rural area of our attention. The Denis CDMA tablet will also enable a later process of synchronizing the data with a central database, which will help to keep track of records of the patient's evolution.

It is important to highlight, that even though MAMICare is a full solution, having only MAMITa available does help to reduce the problems of data accuracy. Of course, current communication limitations still do not allow to have centralized data, but MAMITa still keeps valid track records of patients' information. While MAMI Server is unavailable, it is expected that MAMITa will be transported with the patient in case of an emergency; this allows the physician to have access to the patient's information and a proper assessment of conditions and a quick decision-making. In order to have a better understanding of the expected impact of this system, our original use-case situation will be exposed next, this time under the assumption that the MAMITa system is already implemented in the community.

4.4. Expected Impact of Health Information Technology Scenario

Considering the same characters, distances, orography and characteristics originally described in the original situation scenario. This time Maria has her full kit including the sensor devices and the MAMITa system.

During her scheduled visit to Rosa's home, Maria activates the MAMITa system. MAMITa guides her thoroughly during the metrics process. Maria uses the stethoscope as required by the system and data is stored in the system using wireless communication. MAMITa shows Maria a set of images/video on how to use the sphygmomanometer properly, the system receives the data and detects an abnormality in Rosa's health. MAMITa asks Maria to write down the anomaly in the form. Maria is asked by the system to make some follow up questions such as what her activities have been during the past days. MAMITa uses a microphone to record and store Rosa's description. Using a Doppler ultrasound, MAMITa stores data being sent by the device, in that moment the system detects another anomaly and asks the social worker to use her radio communication system to notify the Health House, UMR and HSB that a patient in critical situation has to be transferred to the HSB. One of the neighbors with vehicles comes to help move Rosa. Eight minutes later, Rosa is at the HSB, the physician practitioner in charge makes her diagnosis based on the tablet information. Data allows him to decide to move her to Tlaxiaco Hospital. In Tlaxiaco Rosa is timely attended; both Rosa and her baby are safe.

4.5. Expected Impact

As shown in the previous use cases, expected impact of implementing MAMICare in the rural areas include having truthful information and thus reducing diagnostic errors. The PVR will be better prepared to act under any circumstance. Another great advantage is the preservation of data. At the UMR, data could remain active from a few hours up to three days. In the Rural Hospital, data could remain relevant from one up to four days. Also inside the Hospital, communication and data transfer occurs immediately between tablets and workstations. MAMITa expects to reduce the time of capturing the medical records by giving proper instructions, as well as by having available truthful information that allows physicians and social workers to have the best possible scenario for decision-making and even highlighting any considered risk situation.

5. RESEARCH LIMITATIONS AND FUTHER STUDY ISSUES

As we mentioned before in our research methodology section, our work is based on observation of a real case, therefore there exists some limitations which can reduce our expected impact. First of all the communication issue: the lack of proper communication means is consider in the initial phase of MAMICare, but further versions depend on the availability of communication technologies in the region (WiFi, 3G, or 4G). Availability communication technology depends of federal agencies and findings, which are out of scope of influence. In addition, the adoption or rejection of MAMICare depends of the approval of the state and federal health agency. This approval however is not only based on the technical merit of our project, sometimes, political reasons have more impact that technical benefits. These findings and validity remain to be verified in additional/future research, that we will be reporting as the project evolves.

6. CONCLUSION

MAMICare System is a work in progress that is expected to make a positive impact once it is implemented in any of the rural areas in Mexico. Research demonstrates that MAMICare is a viable solution to the maternity-infant problem that is currently present among the rural community areas in the states of Chiapas, Oaxaca, and Guerrero. Also the use of electronic healthcare services makes possible to reduce attention issues associated with the main causes of death (hypertension, hemorrhages, and other complications of delivery) that are much higher in maternity-infant care. The MAMICare System is a two-part system to be developed both in the short, medium and long term. For the short term, the MAMITa – a tablet system to aid the social workers in the patient's assessment process will be developed. In the medium term MAMI Server should begin development with the possibility of being expanded to become a wireless system in the long-term, when such communication technology is made available in the communities.

ACKNOWLEDGMENT

We would like to acknowledge to Roberto Garza, Maria Castillo, and Carlos Cortina for their collaboration in this paper.

REFERENCES

Bates, D., & Gawade, A. (2003). Improving safety with information technology. *The New England Journal of Medicine*, *348*(25), 2526–2534. doi:10.1056/NEJMsa020847 PMID:12815139

Blank, A., Kaltschmidt, J., Krings, A., Sukums, F., Mensah, N., Haefeli, W., & Gustafsson, L. (2013). "Quality of prenatal and maternal care: Bridging the know-do gap" (QUALMAT study): An electronic clinical decision support system for rural Sub-Saharan Africa. *BMC Medical Informatics and Decision Making*, *13*(1), 44. doi:10.1186/1472-6947-13-44 PMID:23574764

Calman, N., Hauser, D., Lurio, J., Wu, W. Y., & Pichardo, M. (2012). Strengthening Public Health and Primary Care Collaboration Through Electronic Health Records. *American Journal of Public Health*, *102*(11), e13–e18. doi:10.2105/AJPH.2012.301000 PMID:22994274

Hörmansdörfer, C., Hillemanns, P., Schmidt, P., Scharf, A., Golatta, M., & Vaske, B. (2008). Preliminary analysis of the new 'Prenatal Risk Calculation (PRC)' software. *Archives of Gynecology and Obstetrics*, *279*(4), 1–5.

Jennett, P., Yeo, M., Scott, R., Hebert, M., & Teo, W. (2005). Delivery of rural and remote health care via a broadband Internet Protocol network - views of potential users. *Journal of Telemedicine and Telecare*, *11*(8), 419–424. doi:10.1258/135763305775013545 PMID:16356317

Macleod, B., Phillips, J., Stone, A., Walji, A., & Awoonor-Williams, J. (2012). The Architecture of a Software System for Supporting Community-based Primary Health Care with Mobile Technology: The Mobile Technology for Community Health (MoTeCH) Initiative in Ghana. *Online Journal of Public Health Informatics*, *4*(1). doi:10.5210/ojphi.v4i1.3910 PMID:23569631

Mougiakakou, S. G., Bartsocas, C. S., Bozas, E., Chaniotakis, N., Iliopoulou, D., Kouris, I., & Nikita, K. S. (2010). SMARTDIAB: A communication and information technology approach for the intelligent monitoring, management and follow-up of type 1 diabetes patients. *IEEE Transactions on Information Technology in Biomedicine*, *14*(3), 622–633. doi:10.1109/TITB.2009.2039711 PMID:20123578

Muñoz, D., Avila, A., Lavariega, J., González, A., & Grote, W. (2012) Emergency Remote Pre-Hospital Asssitance (ERPHA), Project Final Report at Latin America and Caribbean Collaborative ICT Research Federation.Retrieved from www.laccir.org

Sachpazidis, I., Rizou, D., & Menary, W. (2008). [Scopus database.]. *Broadband Health Care Network in Brazil and Peru.*, *1-5*, x.

Secretaria de Salud del Gobierno Mexicano. (1995). Norma Oficial Mexicana NOM-007-SSA2-1993, Atención de la mujer durante el embarazo, parto y puerperio y del recién nacido. Criterios y procedimientos para la prestación del servicio. Retrieved from www.salud.gob.mx/unidades/cdi/nom/007ssa23.html (available only in Spanish)

Teléfonos de México, S. A. B de C. V. (TELMEX). (2008). Comunicados 2008: Boletín Informativo. Retrieved from www.telmex.com/mx/corporativo/salaPrensa_ComPrensa2008_080117.89.html (available only in Spanish)

World Health Organization, Department of Making Pregnancy Safer. (2006). Pregnancy, childbirth, postpartum and newborn care - A guide for essential practice. Retrieved from www.who.int/reproductivehealth/publications/

World Health Organization, UNICEF, UNFPA and The World Bank. (2012). Trends in maternal mortality: 1990 to 2010 WHO, UNICEF, UNFPA and The World Bank estimates. Retrieved from www.who.int/reproductivehealth/publications

World Health Organization (WHO). (2006). Country Cooperation Strategy: at a glance – Mexico. Retrieved from www.who.int/countryfocus/cooperation_stratefy/briefs

This work was previously published in the International Journal of Healthcare Information Systems and Informatics (IJHISI), 9(4); edited by Joseph Tan, pages 32-43 copyright year 2014 by IGI Publishing (an imprint of IGI Global).

Chapter 18
The SHEEP Model:
Applying Near Miss Analysis

Deborah J. Rosenorn-Lanng
Royal Berkshire NHS Foundation Trust, UK

Vaughan A. Michell
University of Reading, UK

ABSTRACT

This chapter explains the development of a model, titled "SHEEP," to identify quality and safety factors relating to near misses. The model allows frequency of risk factors and their impact to be analysed at departmental or institutional levels, which enables a structured focusing of resources at an organisational level.

INTRODUCTION

As history unfolds, it seems often to be the case that only following a crisis that we gather sufficient inertia to set about initiating change. We suspect, and hope, that the Mid Staffordshire Report (QC, February 2013) will be one such turning point in healthcare. We wish to help initiate the new ideal of a 'learning culture with continuous improvement'.

While we invest large amounts of time and effort in investigating serious incidents, the learning points from near misses are often lost (Jeffs, Berta, Lingard, & Baker, 2012). The literature suggests near misses are ignored, covered up, lost in the reporting system or that some sort of quick fix is applied (Jeffs et al., 2012). In addition, the term 'near miss' is somewhat of a misnomer as nearly missing something implies hitting it. In

this chapter, we would like to propose a new term the 'nearly event'. This parallels more closely the nomenclature that includes 'never events'.

Currently we are not capturing the organisational learning from these 'nearly events'. Despite the undisputed frequency of medical errors, the methods of investigation are of varying standard and are often incomplete. With current investigation methods, there is little certainty that all the 'Reason-esque' layers of cheese (Reason, 2000) will have been identified. In other settings, Gawande (Gawande, 2007, 2010) and others (Hales, Terblanche, Fowler, & Sibbald, 2008) have shown us the benefits of a checklist rather then relying on the unprompted memory recall of the human mind. This checklist approach has not previously been applied to error investigation.

DOI: 10.4018/978-1-4666-8756-1.ch018

We propose the use of a new methodology linked to a factor model with the acronym SHEEP (Rosenorn-Lanng, 2014) that can be used to identify organisational learning actions from 'nearly events'. The frequency of risk factors and their impact can be analysed at a departmental or institutional level. This enables focusing of scarce resources in a cost effective manner at an organisational level, rather than knee jerk lurches of money and effort in an uncoordinated manner.

We believe that the structured factor model approach to 'nearly event' analysis will result in a fuller understanding of the multiple contributing factors. In particular, it will enhance patient safety by promoting better recall and understanding of specific human factors which are always present, but often ignored. The tool allows focused, solution-based allocation of resources to target problem areas (including attitudes, behaviours and culture) at local or organisational level (the latter via trend analysis). We believe the inclusion of human factors training routinely within a healthcare setting will deliver part of the essential culture change suggested in the Francis Report (QC, February 2013).

THE CONTEXT

The model is influenced by three contextual elements:

Limitations of Current Methods of Error Investigation in Nearly Events

The deployment of Root Cause Analysis (RCA), mini Root Cause Analysis, the 'quick fix', the 'reporting and black hole' phenomenon, denial, apathy and alas even the 'cover up' are among the current methods of error management (Jeffs et al., 2012). There is rarely time for RCA on nearly events. Even if an RCA is initiated, the standard of the output depends on the experience and training of those conducting the investigation. In health-

care, our investigative processes lag behind the rigour employed in the airline industry and other high reliability organisations, although attempts to bridge this gap are emerging (Bosma, Veen, & Roukema, 2011; Spiess, 2011).

RCAs are often seen in health use as 'uncontrolled case studies' (G, 2005) that provide a narrative report of interviews. RCAs in healthcare often lack the consistency applied in business RCAs using statistical 6 Sigma methods and other RCA tools such as interrelationship diagrams and reality trees (Dogget) to qualify and quantify potential causes (Carroll J, 2002). They are impacted by hindsight bias where obvious conclusions may be drawn when all the facts are present (AM, 2005) and imply there was one of few root causes rather than many combinations (Vincent, 2004). The focus on one-off initiatives (Wu AW, 2008) rarely link to, or use, other RCA evidence. RCA also fails to systematically include human factors, such as feelings and human dispositions, that often drive error impacting decisions (Wald H, 2001). Incorporating human factors in this way initiates safety positive culture change in line with key recommendations in the Francis Report (QC, February 2013) (1.152,1.176,1.180,1.184,1.185, 1.196).

Ignorance of the Discipline of Human Factors and Ergonomics within Healthcare

Whilst the Medical Protection Society rates human factors as responsible for 80% of litigation, these same human factors do not feature as fully in the action plans of how to remedy situations. RCA rarely includes human factors in its solution approach. Our model addresses this issue by enabling elicitation of these often ignored human factors within a framework. Whilst 'human factors' are well embedded within other industries such as aviation, it has been slow to be adopted into healthcare. The SHEL model (Edwards 1972, International Civil Aviation Organisation) and its derivative the

SHELL model (Hawkins 1975), were developed in aviation. Attempts were made to adopt this model into healthcare(Molloy, Feb 2005) but it was found that the aviation process models were not entirely applicable to healthcare settings. We have used grounded theory to ensure a healthcare focused model. This hope this organic approach to change (i.e. developed by healthcare for healthcare) will be more likely to embed effectively.

Lack of an Established Open Culture

Theories exist which suggest that a blame culture has detrimental effects on reporting levels and hence on patient safety (Mohr, Abelson, & Barach, 2002; Reason, 1998). It was originally thought that we should encourage a 'no blame' culture in its place. We prefer the terms 'open' culture and 'learning' culture. It implies that we can be honest when we make a mistake, but we will also be ready to embrace the learning that follows.

METHODS

The SHEEP factor model (Rosenorn-Lanng, 2014) was developed from factors identified from open questioning of over 250 human factors training course participants over 14 months. Respondents were drawn from all hospital staff (medical, nursing and non-clinical). Open questions were used to gather data about what human factors influence staff efficiency, patient safety and error (Denscombe, 2010).

A grounded theory approach was used as the most appropriate method to develop a structured model of the relevant factors (J. & A., 1990; Martin & Turner, 1986; Mills, Bonner, & Francis, 2006). This enabled an extensive range of themes and their relationships from varied participants to be elicited.

After each training session of appropriately 12 participants, the factors were analysed offline and structured into appropriate groups and duplicates removed. Axial coding involved investigating category relationships between the codes and established the primary groups based on accepted hospital norms rather than those in aviation (W Li, Liu, Li, & Yang, 2008; Mohr & Batalden, 2002). This data was then used as a starting point for an iterative review, adjustment and addition by follow on groups through 20 cycles until no new factors were contributed (although courses, data capture and review continues). Other offline work included iterative elective coding of the most significant categories based on feedback, followed by identification of logically related concepts to optimise the form and ease of recognition of the model.

The SHEEP(Rosenorn-Lanng, 2014) acronym was developed to enable easy memorisation of the categories. In addition as a metaphor, it alludes to the dangers of following blindly like sheep versus the imperative to adopt 'safety positive' behaviours.

- **S**ystem
- **H**uman interaction
- **E**nvironment
- **E**quipment
- **P**ersonal

The SHEEP (Rosenorn-Lanng, 2014) acronym represents the key categories: Systems, Human interaction, Environment, Equipment and Personal. An overview of each category is given in turn. Use of the SHEEP (Rosenorn-Lanng, 2014) factor model in nearly event analysis is then explained.

SYSTEMS AND HOW WE INTERACT WITH THEM

The 'Systems' Algorithm (Rosenorn-Lanng, 2014)

By *systems,* we refer to operational structures of information and organisation. These may be *informal,* i.e. socially driven, or *formal* constructs. These informal and formal norms are considered within the discipline of organisational semiotics (Li et al., 2008; Li, Liu, Li, & Yang, 2010). The informal or cultural aspects of behaviour underpin all that we do and form the largest influences within an organisation.

When considering errors, problems with information cannot be underestimated. In discussing organisational communication, we have defined the following terms: *information sets* relating to the information itself, *information systems* relating to structures where the information is stored, and *information flow* describing how information moves about.

Information Sets

Formal information sets include a sometimes bewildering array of protocols, guidelines, care pathways and care bundles. These can be produced *internally*, or by *external* groups, including international or national bodies and professional organisations. Within an organisation information sets may be produced in a structured way or can be instituted ad-hoc by local enthusiasts.

How we interact with an information set will depend on the information set itself, but also on the individual's personality, perception and cognitive ability. If the information set is hand written, there can be issues of legibility e.g. as seen in clinical notes. With any information set there are issues of the quality of the information. This involves accuracy of collecting the information, perhaps a degree of interpretation and processing/filtering and choice, and the correct recording of information. Recording information involves choosing which information, where to record it and in what format. The completeness of the information set is affected by many factors but key elements to consider include time to complete the task, familiarity, design of the raw set (e.g. amount of structure/prompts to aid recall), personality of the person completing the information and whether they are interrupted part way through the task.

Understanding the information set is again a multi-faceted issue. The information needs to be targeted at the most junior of users. In addition, it should be written in 'clean' language that is unambiguous (Grove, 1989). Length and complexity of a document are common barriers to successful understanding.

We consider a policy as an example of an information set. Having located the policy and understood it in the way it was intended, the next step is perhaps the most intriguing of all; whether someone chooses to follow it. There are times when it is deemed appropriate to *deviate from policy* (expert opinion, patient factors, policy out of date, new research) and other times when it is not (apathy, arrogance, recklessness) (Phansalkar et al., 2010; Reason, 1998). These deviations from policy can be termed violations. The previous suggestions could be viewed as a spectrum rather than discrete entities and there are further grey areas: *culture/informal norms* ('the way we do it here') and personality dependent choices. Whilst this degree of variation exists we will not achieve the safety levels of high reliability organisations (Carroll, 2002).

Information Systems

For the sake of this exercise we subdivide information systems into paper based and electronic systems. When interacting with a paper system the first critical step can be locating it (e.g. patient's notes). When interacting with an electronic system we face a different set of challenges. The first problem can be of adequacy of provision of stations on which to access the systems, the ease and design of their use and the adequacy of training in using the system. Some information systems are so hard to navigate that it is not possible to locate the policy, resulting in no guidance even when you search for it.

Information Flow

To achieve successful information flow or transfer, media choice is critical. The isolated written word (email or text) deprives us of aspects of communication involving body language and tone of voice resulting in increased chance of misinterpretation and yet the staff questioned revealed they felt 'consumed in an email culture'.

There is evidence that formalising information flow can make it more effective (Powell, 2007; "SBAR initiative to improve staff communication," 2005). Structured *handover* tools such as SBAR and RSVP can improve the chances of successful information transfer (Ascano-Martin, 2008; Guise & Lowe, 2006; Haig, Sutton, & Whittington, 2006). The same can be said for the introduction of a *formal briefing* (an example is the WHO checklist (Gawande, 2010)). The effectiveness of the tools however depends on how well the tools are embedded within the organisation. The successful introduction of a new tool or embracing a change of practice depends on many factors, one of which is *culture.*

HUMAN INTERACTION: HOW WE INTERACT WITH OUR PATIENTS AND EACH OTHER

Human Interaction Algorithm (Rosenorn-Lanng, 2014)

These interactions are sub-divided under 3 broad headings; those related to the *behaviours*, those related to the *team dynamic* and those related to interacting around a *task*.

Problems that resulted in errors in the first category were related to poor quality behaviours or poor quality communication.

Communication problems are reported to underlie the largest proportion of litigation and complaints. However the term 'communication' is used to refer to a large array of different processes. These include organizational information flow, as well as face to face information transfer. Communication is considered in component parts in the algorithm. Within the healthcare culture there is overuse of *abbreviations.* For example, PID: one person's personal identification data was another's pelvic inflammatory disease or project initiation document (Rosenorn-Lanng, 2014). Care is also needed with the use of *pronouns.* It is all too easy to misinterpret an instruction. 'Give it', 'I'm giving it now' are a couple of very short clips of the transcript of a drug error which occurred when one doctor was referring to one drug A but the second doctor was referring to drug B. This resulted in the inadvertent substitution of vincristine (Noble & Donaldson, 2010). Identification of the *correct patient* and performance of the *correct procedure* on the *correct site* relies on vital pieces of information being transferred accurately. Ambiguity, omission and inaccuracy of information transfer in these settings have resulted in never events. Task related issues arise around loss of *situational awareness*, poor *decision making* or a lack of *option generation.*

Examples of team problems follow:

Power distance is one of the dimensions described by Geert Hofstede (Hofstede, 2010) when describing the different aspects of organisational culture. A high power distance describes the tendency for people to accept the inequality of a steep hierarchy gradient. In societies with a low power distance, people strive for equality. Hofstede used the tools for inter-cultural comparisons across countries. The power distance index has been widely considered in aviation (MERRITT, 2000). We believe it is very applicable in a healthcare setting and we are not alone (Hanks, 2013).

Steep hierarchy seems entrenched in some sectors of the NHS and yet there is clear evidence from the SHEEP factor model (Rosenorn-Lanng, 2014) and the Bromiley case ("Bromiley Report verdict and corrected timeline,"), it is unhelpful in a patient safety setting and is contributing to error. It is vital that team members feel able to challenge the leader if they are making an error. This combination of *assertiveness s*kills within followership and *approachability* of the leader need to be present for a team to be safe.

A *flat hierarchy* can be just as problematic. Without clear leadership there is a lack of decision making, option generation, task allocation, co-ordination and the use of resources may be poor. In the setting of a naturally flat hierarchy (i.e. all staff present are of the same grade), a conversation should take place to establish a leader.

ENVIRONMENT AND HOW IT INFLUENCES US

Environment Algorithm (Rosenorn-Lanng, 2014)

Feedback suggested errors vary with environmental boundaries. The categories were defined as: *immediate environment* (i.e. within arm's reach)**,** *immediate vicinity* (taken as the space up until a door but not through it), a *department,* the *hospital/ unit/practice* where the department is located and the *external* places with which interaction may be required. The *location* of environments relative to each other is also relevant (e.g. theatre to ICU, emergency department to CT scanner).

The categories of a *static* environment were compared to one that is changing *(dynamic)* as there was a clear division in the responses. The dynamic changes included *changing location* (e.g. transferring a patient from emergency department to a ward or from a trolley to an operating theatre table) or that we are *interrupted* by something or someone coming into our environment and therefore altering it (Pereira et al., 2011).

If we consider the *physical* environment (e.g. lighting, temperature, noise levels) it is easy to think of examples which might make error more likely (e.g. at night on a ward when you can't see cyanosis, in a special care baby unit when it can be uncomfortably hot, in the middle of a poorly run cardiac arrest when everyone is talking at once and no-one is leading and co-ordinating activities (Montgomery, 2007)

The design of the space itself and the furniture and equipment within the space are important aspects of giving safe, high quality care. Theatre design is an interesting example, in particular, the site of pipeline gas installation within the theatre. The anaesthetist should be able to see the patient, the surgeon and theatre team and the monitor on the anaesthetic machine all at once (McIntyre, 1982). This is simply not possible with some theatre configurations and the pivotal element is the site of installation of the piped gases.

It is also important to consider task related examples; putting in a cannula or a urinary catheter on a ward. Standardisation of clinical areas make sit easier to locate equipment. By grouping items together (e.g. items for cannulation grouped together) and with a clear labelling system, it is easier to locate items quickly. Systems such as the Productive Ward (Improvement) series can aid with this type of formalised organisation of the environment. This approach is even more important under times of stress (high cognitive workload).

EQUIPMENT

Equipment Algorithm (Rosenorn-Lanng, 2014)

The term equipment is used in the very broadest sense to include all the machines/tools/objects of any sort that we interact with. This includes the more traditional medical equipment, instruments and administrative equipment but also drugs, blood products, implants, and inanimate consumables and non-consumables.

Errors can occur because they are inherent in the device, or because of human interaction with the device. There are generic issues across the categories with regards to availability, standardisation, maintenance and even cleaning (e.g. did the last person to put the device away report a fault or wipe the blood off it so it is ready to use next time?). Safety is an intrinsic consideration in the design phase of medical instruments. Based on the observed responses we note that further improvements need to be made to continue to introduce additional 'layers of cheese' according to the Reason model. On a patient monitor, for example, error risk can be related to the screen size, style of data presentation, graphical or analogue, colours, sweep speeds, specificity of alarms, button presses per task, attention to sound versus visual and the relationship of all of these and more to human cognitive ability and preferences (Boquet, Bushman, & Davenport, 1980; Kenny, 2011; Phansalkar et al., 2010; Westhorpe, 1994).

PERSONAL

Personal Algorithm (Rosenorn-Lanng, 2014)

We each have basic physiological requirements to eat, drink, sleep and empty our bladders. Studies and our responses clearly indicate that fatigue and stress significantly impair performance (Boult, 2005; "Health care worker fatigue and patient safety," 2011; Montgomery, 2007; Rogers, 2008). It is a frequent observation within the healthcare workforce that as caring professionals we will sacrifice our own well-being (meal break/drink/toilet stop) for the benefits of our patients. However, we need to consider that we are sacrificing our ability to concentrate with some of these decisions. Under this level of workload and self-sacrifice we are more likely to make a mistake. It is worth considering

Maslow's hierarchy of needs and its progression in this context (Kenrick, Griskevicius, Neuberg, & Schaller, 2010).

Questionnaire feedback highlighted that life events can also take a considerable toll on our ability to cognitively function and during such periods of our lives we need to increase our 'error awareness' and introduce extra checking behaviour to reduce error.

Job factors were also seen to influence safety. *High workload*, poor *job satisfaction* and poor *morale* are some of the factors that can result in higher incidence of errors (Carayon & Gurses, 2008; Endacott, 2012; Holden et al., 2011; Montgomery, 2007).

Knowledge of the part you have to play in human interaction begins with *self-awareness.* If you consider an iceberg analogy, personality is the part under the water and the part above the waterline represents behaviour. Whilst it is not possible to alter your personality, you can learn to modify your behaviour. By understanding yourself you can increase your self-awareness and move towards self-management.

Our *attitudes, behaviours and emotions* influence how we interact with patients and other staff. Following a 'negative' interaction, there is an increased chance of error (Darosa & Pugh, 2012; Shanafelt et al., 2010).

RESULTS: USING THE SHEEP SHEET (ROSENORN-LANNG, 2014)

The SHEEP sheet (Rosenorn-Lanng, 2014) can be used as to identify factors contributing to a 'nearly event', elicit inputs for trend analysis and to facilitate organisational learning.

In a subset pilot group, we found that using free recall of a significant incident, participants averaged 6 factors contributing to the error. By giving the group some brief training in the use of Ishikawa fish bone diagrams (Ishikawa, 1968) we increased the capture (mean 11) contributing factors. Using the SHEEP sheet the 'layers of cheese (Reason, 2000) identification' increased to a far higher number, sometimes as many as 70 factors with no training at all.

The vastly increased 'factor capture' would enable trend analysis, learning and organisational error prevention to be optimised.

The SHEEP sheet (Rosenorn-Lanng, 2014) has now been used by over 400 healthcare professionals of varying grades across professional and disciplinary groups mostly, but not exclusively, within secondary care. The average time for completion is under 10 minutes. The mean number of factors identified was 23.

STRATEGY FOR CHANGE

We would like to propose a change to 'nearly event' investigation and the initiation of organisational trend analysis of errors. The SHEEP (Rosenorn-Lanng, 2014) model encourages a shared mental model or provides a thinking framework.

By adopting the SHEEP sheet (Rosenorn-Lanng, 2014), patient safety will be influenced at several levels:

1. Promotes *better recall* by those involved in the 'nearly events' by using a framework ensuring more accurate capture of contributory factors.
2. The *ease of use*, with the SHEEP sheet (Rosenorn-Lanng, 2014) being completed in fewer than ten minutes, means it is more likely to be completed.
3. Raises awareness of and acknowledges the contribution of *human factors* to 'nearly events' and error. It provides a strong focus on maintaining an open or *learning culture*.

4. Helps highlight the need for *targeted preventative training*, rather than a reactive training response. Waiting until after the event is costly (to the patient and the organisation.) to rigorous statistical testing which could explore the likelihood of the differences being by chance or reason.
5. Identifies system, environmental, equipment, cultural issues and themes to be considered at *organisational level*. When used regularly it will help to identify 'nearly event' trends within the organisation before they happen. Supports the evolution of a local and potentially a national knowledge base of factors and trends.

CONCLUSION

We have produced a new methodology for 'nearly event' investigation which will allow the development of a dynamic database. Data mining will enable preventative trend analysis and organisational learning to reduce the cost and impact of errors. It can also be used to underpin factor retrieval in an RCA setting hence avoiding point solutions.

The SHEEP sheet (Rosenorn-Lanng, 2014) contains over 230 factors from over 400 healthcare workers. It has been developed using over 20 cycles of grounded theory from real healthcare experiences by healthcare workers. It is quick and easy to use. It is highly cost effective and evidence based.

Future plans include the development of an electronic version with the capability to evolve to suit changing health environments. This plasticity will allow continuous improvements of the model and the knowledge base. We envisage that this tool could be used to create a national database to enable comparison and optimisation of error performance.

REFERENCES

AM, D. (2005). Root cause analysis: A framework for tool selection. *Quality Management Journal*, *12*(4), 34.

Ascano-Martin, F. (2008). Shift report and SBAR: Strategies for clinical postconference. *Nurse Educator*, *33*(5), 190–191. doi:10.1097/01. NNE.0000334779.90395.67 PMID:18769315

Boquet, G., Bushman, J. A., & Davenport, H. T. (1980). The anaesthetic machine--A study of function and design. *British Journal of Anaesthesia*, *52*(1), 61–67. doi:10.1093/bja/52.1.61 PMID:7378231

Bosma, E., Veen, E. J., & Roukema, J. A. (2011). Incidence, nature and impact of error in surgery. *British Journal of Surgery*, *98*(11), 1654–1659. doi:10.1002/bjs.7594 PMID:21706475

Boult, M. (2005). Patient safety: The fatigue factor. *The Health Service Journal*, *115*(5962), 34–35. PMID:16032967

Carayon, P., & Gurses, A. P. (2008). Nursing workload and patient safety-A human factors engineering perspective. In R. G. Hughes (Ed.), *Patient safety and quality: An evidence-based handbook for nurses*. Rockville, MD: Academic Press.

Carroll, J. R. J., & Hatakenaka, S. (2002). Lessons learned from non-medical industries: Root cause analysis as culture change at a chemical plant. *Quality & Safety in Health Care*, *11*(3), 266–269. doi:10.1136/qhc.11.3.266 PMID:12486993

Darosa, D. A., & Pugh, C. M. (2012). Error training: Missing link in surgical education. *Surgery*, *151*(2), 139–145. doi:10.1016/j.surg.2011.08.008 PMID:22088811

Denscombe, M. (2010). *The good research guide for small scale social research projects* (4th ed.). London: Open University Press.

Dogget. (n.d.). *Root cause analysis: A framework for tool selection*. Academic Press.

Endacott, R. (2012). The continuing imperative to measure workload in ICU: Impact on patient safety and staff well-being. *Intensive Care Medicine*, *38*(9), 1415–1417. doi:10.1007/s00134-012-2654-5 PMID:22875337

G, A. (2005). Root cause analysis. *Psychiatric Bulletin*, *29*(2), 71 - 71.

Gawande, A. (2007). The checklist: If something so simple can transform intensive care, what else can it do? *New Yorker (New York, N.Y.)*, 86–101. PMID:18084821

Gawande, A. (2010). Checklists for success inside the OR and beyond: An interview with Atul Gawande, MD, FACS: Interview by Tony Peregrin. *Bulletin of the American College of Surgeons*, *95*(5), 24–27. PMID:21452644

Geert Hofstede, G. J. H. M. M. (2010). *Cultures and organizations: Software of the mind*. New York: McGraw-Hill.

Grove, D. P. B. I. (1989). *Resolving traumatic memories: Metaphors and symbols in psychotherapy*. New York: Irvington Publishers, Inc.

Guise, J. M., & Lowe, N. K. (2006). Do you speak SBAR? *Journal of Obstetric, Gynecologic, and Neonatal Nursing*, *35*(3), 313–314. doi:10.1111/j.1552-6909.2006.00043.x PMID:16700679

Haig, K. M., Sutton, S., & Whittington, J. (2006). SBAR: A shared mental model for improving communication between clinicians. *Joint Commission Journal on Quality and Patient Safety*, *32*(3), 167–175. PMID:16617948

Hales, B., Terblanche, M., Fowler, R., & Sibbald, W. (2008). Development of medical checklists for improved quality of patient care. *International Journal for Quality in Health Care*, *20*(1), 22–30. doi:10.1093/intqhc/mzm062 PMID:18073269

Hanks, S. D. (2013). *Recognizing healthcare's value in overcoming 'power distance'*. Retrieved from http://thocc.org/downloads/CL_Feb13.pdf

Health, C. W. F., & Safety, P. (2011)... *Sentinel Event Alert*, (48): 1–4.

Holden, R. J., Scanlon, M. C., Patel, N. R., Kaushal, R., Escoto, K. H., Brown, R. L., & Karsh, B. T. (2011). A human factors framework and study of the effect of nursing workload on patient safety and employee quality of working life. *BMJ Qual Saf*, *20*(1), 15–24. doi:10.1136/bmjqs.2008.028381 PMID:21228071

Ishikawa, K. (1968). *Guide to quality control*. Academic Press.

J., C., & A., S. (1990). Grounded theory research - Procedures, canons and evaluative criteria. *Zeitschrift fur Soziologie, 19*, 418-427

Jeffs, L., Berta, W., Lingard, L., & Baker, G. R. (2012). Learning from near misses: From quick fixes to closing off the Swiss-cheese holes. *BMJ Qual Saf, 21*(4), 287–294. doi:10.1136/bmjqs-2011-000256 PMID:22357777

Kenny, P. E. (2011). Alarm fatigue and patient safety. *Pa Nurse, 66*(1), 3, 22.

Kenrick, D. T., Griskevicius, V., Neuberg, S. L., & Schaller, M. (2010). Renovating the pyramid of needs: Contemporary extensions built upon ancient foundations. *Perspectives on Psychological Science*, *5*(3), 292–314. doi:10.1177/1745691610369469 PMID:21874133

Li, W., Liu, K., Li, S., & Yang, H. (2008). Normative modeling for personalized clinical pathway using organizational semiotics methods. In *Proceedings of International Symposium on Computer Science and Computational Technology*, (pp. 3-7). Academic Press.

Li, W., Liu, K., Li, S., & Yang, H. (2010). A semiotic multi-agent modeling approach for clinical pathway management. *Journal of Computers*, *5*(2). doi:10.4304/jcp.5.2.266-273

Martin, P., & Turner, B. (1986). Grounded theory and organizational research. *Journal of Behavioural Science*, *22*(2), 141–157. doi:10.1177/002188638602200207

McIntyre, J. W. (1982). Man-machine interface: The position of the anaesthetic machine in the operating room. *Canadian Anaesthetists' Society Journal*, *29*(1), 74–78. doi:10.1007/BF03007954 PMID:7055748

MERRITT, A. (2000). Culture in the cockpit: Do Hofstede's dimensions replicate? *Journal of Cross-Cultural Psychology*, *31*(3), 283–301. doi:10.1177/0022022100031003001 PMID:11543415

Mills, J., Bonner, A., & Francis, K. (2006). The development of constructivist grounded theory. *International Journal of Qualitative Methods*, *5*(1), 25–35.

Mohr, J. J., Abelson, H. T., & Barach, P. (2002). Creating effective leadership for improving patient safety. *Quality Management in Health Care*, *11*(1), 69–78. doi:10.1097/00019514-200211010-00010 PMID:12455344

Mohr, J. J., & Batalden, P. B. (2002). Improving safety on the front lines: The role of clinical microsystems. *Quality & Safety in Health Care*, *11*(1), 45–50. doi:10.1136/qhc.11.1.45 PMID:12078369

Molloy, G. J. O. B., & Ciarán, A. (2005). The SHEL model: A useful tool for analyzing and teaching the contribution of human factors to medical error. *Academic Medicine*, *80*(2), 152–155. doi:10.1097/00001888-200502000-00009 PMID:15671319

Montgomery, V. L. (2007). Effect of fatigue, workload, and environment on patient safety in the pediatric intensive care unit. *Pediatric Critical Care Medicine*, *8*(2Suppl), S11–S16. doi:10.1097/01.PCC.0000257735.49562.8F PMID:17496827

Noble, D. J., & Donaldson, L. J. (2010). The quest to eliminate intrathecal vincristine errors: A 40-year journey. *Quality & Safety in Health Care, 19*(4), 323–326. doi:10.1136/qshc.2008.030874 PMID:20211962

Pereira, B. M., Pereira, A. M., Correia Cdos, S., Marttos, A. C. Jr, Fiorelli, R. K., & Fraga, G. P. (2011). Interruptions and distractions in the trauma operating room: Understanding the threat of human error. *Rev Col Bras Cir, 38*(5), 292–298. doi:10.1590/S0100-69912011000500002 PMID:22124638

Phansalkar, S., Edworthy, J., Hellier, E., Seger, D. L., Schedlbauer, A., Avery, A. J., & Bates, D. W. (2010). A review of human factors principles for the design and implementation of medication safety alerts in clinical information systems. *Journal of the American Medical Informatics Association, 17*(5), 493–501. doi:10.1136/jamia.2010.005264 PMID:20819851

Powell, S. K. (2007). SBAR-It's not just another communication tool. *Professional Case Management, 12*(4), 195–196. doi:10.1097/01. PCAMA.0000282903.67672.fa PMID:17667779

QC. R. F. (2013). Report of the mid Staffordshire NHS foundation trust public inquiry. Academic Press.

Reason, J. (1998). Achieving a safe culture: theory and practice. *Work and Stress, 12*(3), 293–306. doi:10.1080/02678379808256868

Reason, J. (2000). Human error: Models and management. *BMJ (Clinical Research Ed.), 320*(7237), 768–770. doi:10.1136/bmj.320.7237.768 PMID:10720363

Report, B. (n.d.). *Verdict and corrected timeline.* Retrieved from http://www.chfg.org/resources/07_qrt04/Anonymous_Report_Verdict_and_Corrected_Timeline_Oct_07.pdf

Rogers, A. E. (2008). The effects of fatigue and sleepiness on nurse performance and patient safety. In R. G. Hughes (Ed.), *Patient safety and quality: An evidence-based handbook for nurses.* Rockville, MD: Academic Press.

Rosenorn-Lanng, D. (2014). *Human factors in healthcare.* Oxford, UK: Oxford University Press.

SBAR Initiative to Improve Staff Communication. (2005)... *Healthcare Benchmarks and Quality Improvement, 12*(4), 40–41. PMID:15915702

Shanafelt, T. D., Balch, C. M., Bechamps, G., Russell, T., Dyrbye, L., Satele, D., & Freischlag, J. (2010). Burnout and medical errors among American surgeons. *Annals of Surgery, 251*(6), 995–1000. doi:10.1097/SLA.0b013e3181bfdab3 PMID:19934755

Spiess, B. D. (2011). Human error in medicine: Change in cardiac operating rooms through the FOCUS initiative. *The Journal of Extra-Corporeal Technology, 43*(1), 33–38. PMID:21449238

Vincent, C. V. (2004). Analysis of clinical incidents: A window on the system not a search for root causes. *Quality & Safety in Health Care, 13*(4), 242–243. doi:10.1136/qshc.2004.010454 PMID:15289620

Wald, H. S. K. (2001). Root cause analysis. *Making Health Care Safer: A Critical Analysis of Patient Safety Practices, 51.*

Westhorpe, R. (1994). The anaesthetic machine and patient safety. *Annals of the Academy of Medicine, Singapore, 23*(4), 592–597. PMID:7979139

Wu, A. W. L. A., & Pronovost, P. J. (2008). Effectiveness and efficiency of root cause analysis in medicine. *Journal of the American Medical Association, 299*(6), 685–687. doi:10.1001/jama.299.6.685 PMID:18270357

This work was previously published in the Handbook of Research on Patient Safety and Quality Care through Health Informatics edited by Vaughan Michell, Deborah J. Rosenorn-Lanng, Stephen R. Gulliver, and Wendy Currie, pages 21-32 copyright year 2014 by Medical Information Science Reference (an imprint of IGI Global).

Chapter 19
A Systemic, Participative Design of Decision Support Services for Clinical Research

Alexandra Pomares Quimbaya
Pontificia Universidad Javeriana, Colombia

Rafael A. González
Pontificia Universidad Javeriana, Colombia

Wilson Ricardo Bohórquez
*Pontificia Universidad Javeriana, Colombia &
Hospital Universitario San Ignacio, Colombia*

Oscar Muñoz
*Pontificia Universidad Javeriana, Colombia &
Hospital Universitario San Ignacio, Colombia*

Olga Milena García
Hospital Universitario San Ignacio, Colombia

Dario Londoño
*Pontificia Universidad Javeriana, Colombia &
Hospital Universitario San Ignacio, Colombia*

ABSTRACT

Development of IT-based services to support decision-making in healthcare should be guided by the following considerations: rigor, relevance, user-centered participation and inclusion of the best practices for IT-based service systems. In this paper, the balance between rigor and relevance is achieved by following the design science research methodology; user-centered participation is tackled from the socio-technical tradition in information systems; best practices considered in the planning, design and implementation of the services are informed by the MOF framework. Moreover, and considering the premise that these pillars should holistically converge, this research has been approached from a systemic stance where iterative, participative, socio-technical activities have allowed the effective collaboration between information systems researchers, clinical researchers, medical staff and administrative hospital personnel. This paper argues for a move towards enhancing systemic, participative, design-centered service systems engineering by reporting a case which applies these concepts for providing decision-support services, enabled by data and text mining techniques, to contribute to clinical research and administration by being able to search electronic health records where narrative text hides meaningful information that would otherwise require a time-consuming human revision of these records.

DOI: 10.4018/978-1-4666-8756-1.ch019

1. INTRODUCTION

IT in healthcare has had a prominent place within applied information systems research and has a strong tradition, ranging from the very deeply technical and algorithmic – such as classic and modern uses of artificial intelligence and expert systems (Gresh, Rabenhorst, Shabo, & Slavin, 2002; Lisboa, 2002; McCauley & Ala, 1992) – to more socio-technically minded interventions – such as the use of Checkland's Soft Systems Methodology mostly within the context of the UK's NHS (e.g. Kalim, Carson, & Cramp, 2004, 2006). Despite the progress, real impact has not been felt significantly where it matters most. As Hesse and Shneiderman (2007) argue, it has probably been a matter of not asking the right questions: rather than focusing on what technology can do, we should be focusing on what people can do. This follows a general trend in information systems which pays attention to user-centered, participative design (Carroll & Rosson, 2007; Mao, Vredenburg, Smith, & Carey, 2005) as well on situated, context-dependent uses of technology (Orlikowski, 2000). The popularization of many user-oriented information technologies has shown that user experience and involvement in the design, appropriation and evolution of IT exceed consumer electronics and applications and are indeed morally and pragmatically desirable for information systems development in general (McCarthy & Wright, 2004).

This suggests that the development of IT-based services to support decision-making in healthcare should be guided by the following considerations: rigor, relevance, user-centered participation and inclusion of the best practices for IT-based service systems. These requirements are not mutually exclusive but dependent on each other. As such, this paper will present the ongoing development of a set of decision-support services for clinical research, based on a socio-technical, systemic, design-centered approach. The balance between rigor (transparency, validation, formalism, system-

atic use of existing knowledge) and relevance (utility, novelty) is achieved by following the design science research methodology (Hevner, March, Park, & Ram, 2004). User-centered participation is tackled from the socio-technical tradition in information systems (Stahl, 2007). Some best practices considered in the planning, design and implementation of the services are informed by the MOF framework (Pultorak, 2008). Moreover, and considering the premise that these pillars should holistically converge, this research has been approached from a systemic stance where iterative, participative, socio-technical activities have allowed the effective collaboration between information systems researchers, clinical researchers, medical staff and administrative hospital personnel.

Through this effort, we have been able to obtain meaningful findings in terms of the technical contribution that data and text mining can have for decision-support in clinical research and hospital administration as well as to explore the integration of participative mechanisms and IT service systems best practices into the growing body of work around development of artifacts through a design science research perspective. In sum, this paper argues for a move towards enhancing systemic, participative, design-centered service systems engineering. It does so by reporting a case which applies these concepts for providing decision-support services, enabled by data and text mining techniques, to contribute to clinical research and administration by being able to search electronic health records where narrative text hides meaningful information that would otherwise require a time-consuming human revision of these records.

One of the main sources for supporting decision-making in hospitals has been the creation and use of electronic health records (EHR), a rich source of data when properly exploited. Nonetheless, in practice, the use of EHR is more complex due in part to the lack of having considered the three pillars of rigor, relevance and user-centeredness.

Often, healthcare professionals are invited (or forced) to adapt to the systems that keep track of patient records, rather than having the system support the professionals in their activities. Of course, striking that balance is not easy, but neglecting it creates problems, such as the tendency to use open text fields to input information that should otherwise be input into structured fields. This narrative approach to recording patient information fits many healthcare practices but unfortunately does not exactly match the logic and technologies offered by current decision-support systems.

One specific approach that has garnered increased attention within the healthcare domain has been data mining (Bellazzi & Zupan, 2008; Windle, 2004). Through the various technologies that can be used for data mining, clinical research and practice can be considerably improved and new patterns can be extracted to help with diagnosis, treatment, and cost-benefit analysis, among others. However, as stated above, when data mining relies on electronic health records, the use of narrative text, makes traditional data mining approaches limited. This paper discusses the design of a support tool for clinical research (at a first stage) and administrative decision-making (at a second stage), using data mining technologies and considering the restrictions imposed by a dataset that is not structured and relies on narrative text.

This paper is structured as follows. Section 2 describes the research methodology to go onto Section 3, which presents related works surrounding the use of data mining techniques for patient identification and visualization of electronic health records. Section 4 then presents some of the potential uses of these techniques in supporting decision making both for clinical research and health administration. Section 5 goes on to present the proposal of system, dubbed DISEarch, to be used for patient identification using health records from a university hospital information system. Some early results of the prototype are discussed in Section 6, and then some conclusions and future work are mentioned in Section 7.

2. RESEARCH METHODOLOGY

This research follows a design science research philosophy (Hevner et al., 2004), which has gained increasing support from information systems researchers, given its open goal of providing a framework for research that is both relevant and rigorous. The tension between these often conflicting aspects is dealt with through a design-centered paradigm, where the relevance of solving real-world problems is achieved through a specific design, which in Herbert Simon's tradition is no less than problem-solving itself, i.e. design is problem-solving as it fills the gap between a present situation and a desired one (Simon, 1996). In addition, design also involves the use of applicable knowledge which becomes embedded in the design process and product, thus being rigorous insofar as this knowledge is applied transparently and systematically. As a result, design science research offers a tripartite framework, relevance-design-rigor, onto which this paper further elaborates the recommendation that the core design be participative in nature, making it more relevant, as the beneficiaries (be they users, beneficiaries or customers) become co-designers. It is in the multi-disciplinary interaction between this research group and an information systems research group that a user-centered participative design has been followed. Together with the participation of other potential users, a prototype has been developed as a proof of concept of the underlying data (text) mining models and algorithms and as a source of medical validation with respect to the quality of the results.

The research approach has followed a problem-initiated process, guided by a three-cycle design science research approach (see Hevner, 2007), as shown in Figure 1. An initial relevance cycle has been used to identify requirements, potential users, associated processes (both for clinical research and for administrative purposes), existing technology (the hospital's information system, the underlying databases, the users' capabilities),

Figure 1. Research cycles, adapted from Hevner (2007)

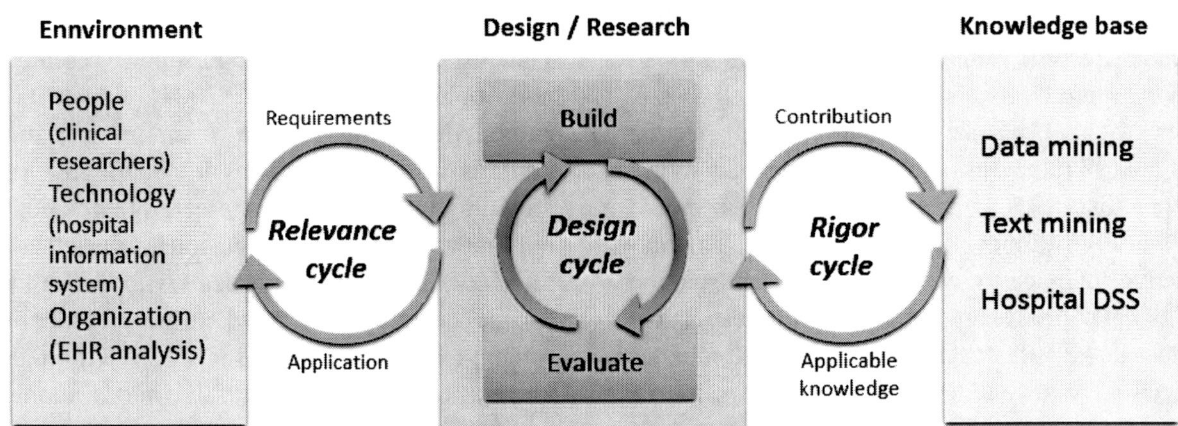

as well as identifying other hospitals that, given similar technologies, could also benefit from the resulting artifact. A rigor cycle has helped uncover the applicable knowledge by doing a literature. Although it could appear as if the rigor cycle follows after the relevance cycle, in reality both cycles have moved mostly in parallel. This simultaneous cycling through rigor and relevance is desirable and natural, since by uncovering requirements the researchers have been led to revise and refine the search space within the knowledge base. Conversely, and given the fact that the initial problem was ill-defined and thus still open, as applicable knowledge is found and shared with the medical researchers, this feeds back on the relevance cycle, by making explicit the possibilities offered by existing methods, tools and technologies.

Once the relevance and rigor cycles have offered sufficiently clear requirements and applicable knowledge, they meet inside a design cycle, which iterates between actual design and continued evaluation. This process is akin to classic information systems design, where initial mockups, forms and flow charts are built, refined and evaluated both from a technical point of view and from a potential user's point of view, until these preliminary models can be codified, following a traditional data mining process. Inspired by

CRISP-DM (Shearer, 2000), understanding the business is followed by understanding the data, after which such data is prepared (to make it amenable for treatment by data mining techniques), models are created to process the data and finally the solution is evaluated and deployed. As can be seen, this data mining process fits naturally within the design science research approach and simply gives it a specific flavor.

Evaluation, as stated above, is an iterative process in parallel with the design and refinement of the data mining models and the resulting software prototype. The aim has been to use a test copy of the hospitals EHR database in order to produce the required results and then sharing such results with the complete research team so that evaluation is carried out not only from an information systems (data mining) point of view, but crucially from a medical perspective as well. Final validation of the resulting artifact is achieved by using the prototype as a proof of concept and analyzing the results so that the desired EHRs are found with precision and recall criteria, or in clinical terms, with enough sensitivity and specificity. The EHRs to be found respond to the requirements, which stem from the following research question.

The main problem and research question has been how to identify patients associated with a specific diagnosis within the set of electronic health records contained in the hospital information system. Though at first this may seem a straightforward question amenable to treatment through simple database queries, the complexity of an actual diagnostic process (for instance, the fact that it is not a point in time, but the result of several events) and the aforementioned nature of the data (unstructured narrative text) make using queries limited and indeed impractical. For example, one may query the system for patients whose EHR contains "diabetes" in a specific field for diagnosis, but very often the diagnosis is not contained in this field in such a clear-cut fashion. Moreover, extending the query to other fields does not solve the problem because the narrative is nuanced and dynamic (one could find, for instance, "discard diabetes").

Having access to the list of patients with an identified diagnosis is useful given that it is the basis for many of the clinical research studies being carried out by the chronic disease research group involved in this project, but of course of other groups as well. Furthermore, this data is also invaluable for administrative purposes in assessing fitness to treatment protocols, costs and patient distributions.

According to Hevner (2007), design science research goes through relevance, rigor and design cycles. This cyclical nature also emphasizes the fact that the cycles are connected. One should thus expect that being inside the "design cycle" still will require a connection and parallel advancement in rigor (by continuously revising knowledge applicable to the design) and in relevance (by clarifying and getting feedback fro the real problem environment). This is the way this research has proceeded in general, given its iterative and participative nature. However, the paper structure benefits from a following a more linear model of design science research, as proposed by (Peffers, Tuunanen, Rothenberger, & Chatterjee, 2007). Accordingly, the rest of this paper presents the problem (Section 2) and related solutions (Section 3) first and subsequently the design of the artifact (Section 4) and its evaluation and validation (Section 6) are explained.

3. RELATED WORKS

Today, healthcare organizations are carrying out significant efforts to correctly include the use of information technologies and collect data in an electronic format, for example in Electronic Health Records. Nonetheless, such accumulation of data has overcome the capacity of healthcare organizations to use this data in profitable ways and support business decisions. In order to truly leverage digital clinical data to its full potential, investment in Healthcare Analytics solutions must be carried out. Ferranti et al. (2010) state: "hospitals have lagged in adopting thoughtful analytical approaches that would allow operational leaders and providers to capitalize upon existing data stores… We believe that such active investment in health analytics will prove essential to realizing the full promise of investments in electronic clinical systems".

Healthcare analytics is increasingly supported by data mining strategies and their associated techniques. In order to uncover the evolution of these strategies, this section discusses the results of a literature review focused on identifying some of the main contributions, institutions and authors centered on this topic. Subsequently, the second part of this section describes some outstanding recent contributions for the improvement of medical data visualization to support healthcare analytics, offering a view of their strengths and opportunities for improvement that have been taken into consideration in designing the proposal brought forward in this paper.

The development of tools, techniques and models for identifying (that is, searching and retrieving EHR according to a specific information need) and analyzing (that is, looking for patterns, classifying or processing EHR for decision making) electronic health records in the last thirty years has been studied through systematic queries in the Scopus database using keywords related to patient, medical or health records, coupled to data preparation, data classification, data and text mining, prioritization, and decision or regression trees. Iteratively, different queries have been used in order to refine the coverage and relevance of the results. In addition, since medical data is particularly sensitive, anonymization, data protection and privacy protection have also been coupled to EHR.

Although the main goal of this research is centered on data mining (and related) strategies for clinical research, most of the work found is aimed at aiding in diagnosis and contributing to effectiveness analysis of particular treatments (or drugs), whether from a medical or an economic point of view. There are few contributions directly related to identifying or analyzing a set of health records for which a specific diagnosis has already been registered for use in clinical research on that specific disease, and given a context in which such diagnosis is hidden in free or narrative text, as described elsewhere in this paper.

By looking at some of the most cited papers, it can be seen that, for instance in (Gaspar et al., 1997), cited 774 times at the time of query, patient records are partitioned according to their being treated with radiation therapy, in order to estimate the effectiveness of the treatment through decision trees. However, as pointed out, these patient records have already been identified as belonging to the interest group, prior to the study. Furthermore, the actual analysis is purely statistical in nature and although most data mining techniques are indeed statistics-based, in building the model proposed in this research, the interest is on techniques supported directly by software. In (Highet, Forrest, Ballow, & Schentag, 1999), cited 45 times, a similar contribution is related this time to determining the effectiveness of an antibiotic through regression analysis.

Another important project, more closely related to informatics or computer science techniques, can be seen in (Burbidge, Trotter, Buxton, & Holden, 2001), with 265 citations. This time it deviates from the clinical or medical domain into chemistry (drug research), by reporting a data mining algorithm which, through machine learning, can be used to predict the effect of a particular drug, according to its chemical composition. A similar effort is found in (Kroes et al., 2004), except this time the emphasis is on predicting the toxicity of the compound.

Moreover, the work presented in (Suppes et al., 2005), cited 176 times, report on algorithms that are used in decision making support for treating bipolar disorder; in this case, given the disorder, certain treatment protocols are designed. For the purposes of the present work, the opposite would be more appropriate; that is, tracing the compliance with a given treatment protocol on a set of patients that have to be identified as having been diagnosed with a given disease – the idea would then be to extract treatment patterns from the identified set and then comparing those patterns to the already established protocol.

One of many cases found reporting a cost-benefit analysis is presented in (Hill et al., 2000), cited 156 times. This time related to using prophylactic antiemetic therapy for reducing postoperative nausea and vomiting. Similarly, (Adams, Gregor, Kertesz, & Valberg, 1995), with 124 citations, evaluates the effectiveness of carrying out a hemocromatosis test in blood donors in order to demonstrate the economic benefit of doing so for a national health system.

One paper potentially more closely related to the purpose of this paper's contribution is (Hess, Abbruzzese, Lenzi, Raber, & Abbruzzese, 1999), cited 130 times. Their work is aimed at classifying patients into specific groups, according to a set of medical variables. The difference lies in that the starting set of patient records is already known to be diagnosed with unknown primary carcinoma, while our work starts one step behind: identifying patients diagnosed with a specific condition from a complete set of records of diverse patients. Furthermore, Hess et al. only consider quantitative, structured variables, while our work considers also unstructured narrative text.

In terms of the sources of these related works, something worth noting is that they are mostly originating in hospitals, medical centers and pharmaceutical labs. Few of the results are explicitly affiliated to collaboration between hospitals and universities or between university hospitals and other departments (especially those related to computer science).

Other recent contributions explore the analysis of narrative texts to identify special associations as in the case of (Iyer, Harpaz, Lependu, Bauer-Mehren, & Shah, 2013) which analyzes drug-event associations based on the identification of drug mentions in clinical notes. Another work presents CLIX (Clinithink, s. f.), an engine that analyzes medical narrative texts and transforms them into structured content based on a specific standard code like SNOMED CT, ICD-9, ICD-10, among others. Although in both cases the input is narrative text contained in a medical record and the output is a structured content, they cannot act, by themselves, as a decision support system that can improve the work of clinical research and administration. However, these works can be useful to enrich a decision support system.

In sum, a detailed exploration of relevant works suggests that there have been many contributions to patient identification using data mining techniques and that these have been growing rapidly. However, recalling the introduction of this paper, there is still work to be done in order to generalize these works into decision-support tools to be used widely for clinical research and health administration. Significantly, it has been found that the majority of works are aimed at sets of data for which a diagnosis, disease or condition has already been determined. In other words, the population for study has already been defined. There is a clear opportunity to contribute works that support the preceding stage; that is, we have found that in practice most clinical research group and health administration must go through a time-consuming, labor-intensive, statistically supported, iteratively queried process of determining patients for study.

4. IMPROVING DECISION-MAKING FOR CLINICAL RESEARCH AND HEALTH ADMINISTRATION

As the previous section discusses, electronic health record systems (EHR) have improved the access to patient information by health care providers. They are a rich source of knowledge widely used to improve health care activities such as diagnostic and treatment definition. In addition, they have been also used to enhance health research processes and administrative tasks in health institutions; however, their use for these purposes is limited due to different factors such as confidentiality, heterogeneity of information and incompleteness of medical data. As a consequence, most of decision-making in health sector does not take full advantage of the vast source of information from EHR because of the difficulty of obtaining the adequate information at the right moment. This section aims to analyze how can be improved the decision making process specifically for clinical research and health administration using as a source of information EHR.

The problems around decision-making were studied in a general hospital in Bogotá, Colombia. This hospital has a main information system called SAHI that includes modules to manage the Electronic Health Record, Contracts, Human Resources, Client Service, Budgeting, Purchases and Supply, etc. This system allows physicians to obtain the EHR of each patient during the medical attention; however, their use for research purposes has been limited due to the fact that important information is stored in narrative texts, intended for human beings that are difficult to search and analyze automatically. One of the common requirements of medical research is to find the medical records of patients that have been diagnosed with a specific disease. This task that should be easily done using classical queries (e.g. using SQL) is very time-consuming. This is because diagnosis is frequently hidden in narrative texts (e.g. medical notes, progress notes), hindering the possibility of automatically detecting relevant records and requiring the participation of an expert in the analysis. Similarly, the administration of the Hospital frequently requires analyzing costs and efficiency of medical treatments. Even if some of this information is well structured, as medications and laboratory orders, the complete sequence of events related to a patient is hidden in narrative texts. In summary, the main requirement of this hospital decision support system is to recognize which medical records are useful for clinical and administrative research, taking into account all the information in the EHR, including the one that is in narrative texts. Particularly, the decision support system must support biomedical research and quality analysis and service delivery.

Currently, the processes for assessing adherence to international recommendations and in general to evaluate medical decisions include long term activities of analysis of EHR. Figure 2 illustrates a classic EHR analysis process from the point of view of data requirements. As it can be seen an important and currently time-consuming task is the exploration and identification of relevant EHR. IT staff members are the owners of the EHR and they are frequently a bottleneck during research projects. In addition, the effort to validate the relevance of the provided EHR implies time between five and forty minutes for reading each one of the attentions of patients. Providing a facility

to obtain these EHR automatically will improve process time metrics. In addition, providing visual analysis of the relevant EHR enriches the quality of the decision process due to the improvement of user empowerment.

5. DISEARCH: A SYSTEM FOR ELECTRONIC MEDICAL RECORD ANALYSIS

This section describes the decision support system created in order to support the requirements of clinical research and health administration, mentioned in the previous section, using as a source of information EHR. The main principle of this system called DISearch is to combine the analysis of structured and unstructured information contained in EHR to enhance decision-making.

Considering the main users of DISEArch are medical doctors, during the development of this system the definition of functionalities and the user interface were made using a participatory design approach. In this approach users cooperate with designers and developers during the different phases of the project. The design followed an evolutionary cycling where the system was discussed mainly from a clinical and practical point of view rather than a technical perspective.

Figure 2. EHR analysis process

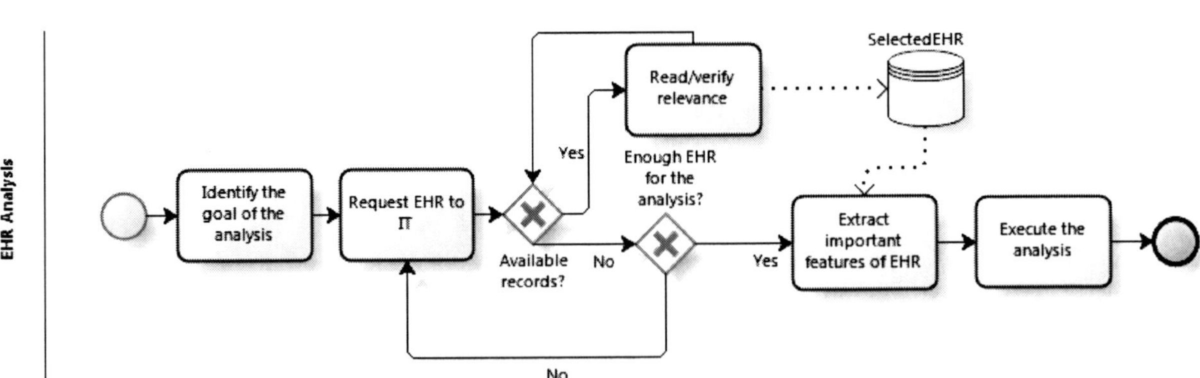

In what follows, this section presents the general architecture of the system and explains in detail its main components.

5.1. DISEArch Architecture

The architecture of DISEArch is illustrated in Figure 3. The principle of the system is to provide different capabilities of visualization and analysis to enhance biomedical research as well as quality and services delivery analysis.

The components are divided in three layers. The components of the Data Layer are in charge of store all the information used or generated by the system. The Knowledge base component manages the relevant taxonomies and definitions required to analyze EHR. For instance, it stores the taxonomies of diseases and medications that are used to categorize a record. The DISEarch database stores all the temporal results and the analysis results obtained by the components of the business level. The Electronic Health System component represents the database of the Hospital Information System that contains the EHR. Even if this last component is external, DISEArch contains all the information required to extract the EHR from it.

The Business Layer components contain the main capabilities of the decision system. The *Extraction Manager* is responsible for extracting the set of medical records according to the pre-selection defined by the users (e.g. gender, age, date). This is the only component that interacts directly with the *Electronic Health System* component, and contains the logic for wrapping the schema of the original source of health records. In addition, when it is required, this component launches an anonymization service that assures the de-identification of identifiers and seudo-identifiers from EHR. The *Analysis Engine* is in charge of analyzing the structured and non-structured elements of EHR to identify and prioritize which of them are useful for a specific study (e.g. descriptive study). The *Knowledge Engine* goal is to extract knowledge from different points of view. First, the *LifeLine Generator* presents a

Figure 3. DISEArch architecture

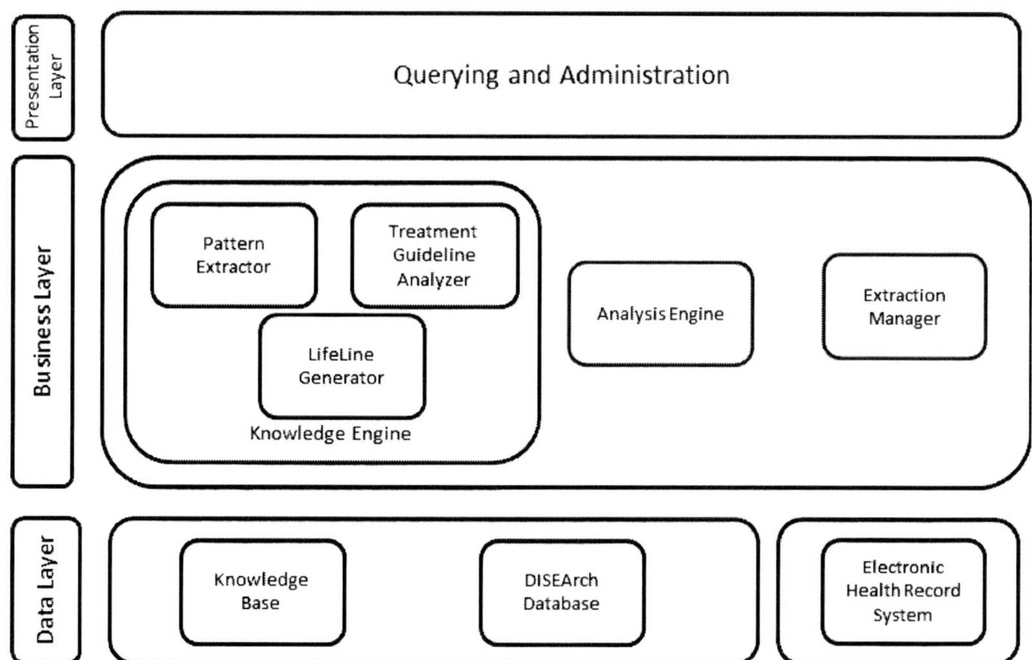

360-degree view of a patient visualizing all the events where he/she has been involved. The event extraction includes the identification of events that were written in narrative text as well as those that are well structured. The second component is the *Pattern Extractor*; this component applies data mining techniques over a set of EHR to obtain natural clusters, association rules and sequence patterns. The *Treatment Guideline Analyzer* allows structuring a disease treatment guideline and comparing it to a specific medical record or a group of medical records. Using this component a medical institution may know at what level its patients follow the recommended treatment guideline. This component is especially important for quality and service delivery analysis.

Finally, the presentation layer contains the graphical user interface to query the different components of the business layer.

5.2. Prototype

DISEArch architecture was developed in Java language using different libraries to improve the analysis of EHR, specially the narrative texts. The components implemented in DISEArch 1.0 are presented in Figure 4.

In the Presentation Layer, the researcher can describe the characteristics of the EHR that he/she is interested on using the EHR analysis form. As presented in Figure 5, this form allows specifying the characteristics of the EHR

Figure 4. DISEArch prototype

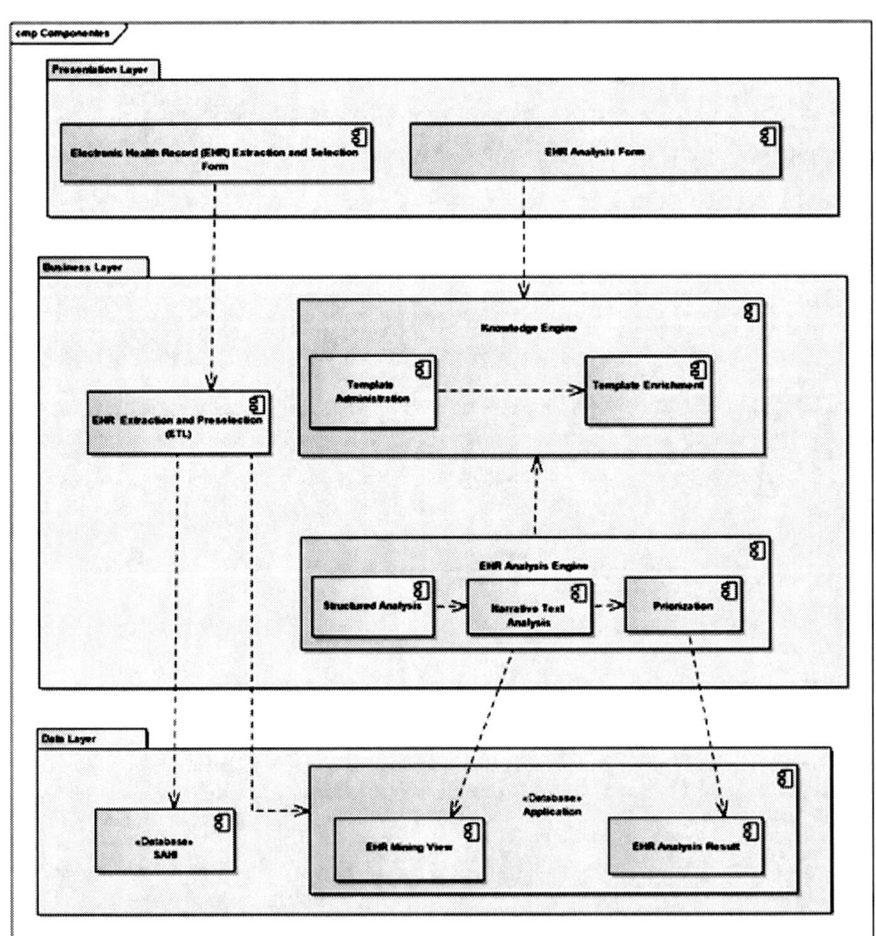

Figure 5. DISEArch presentation

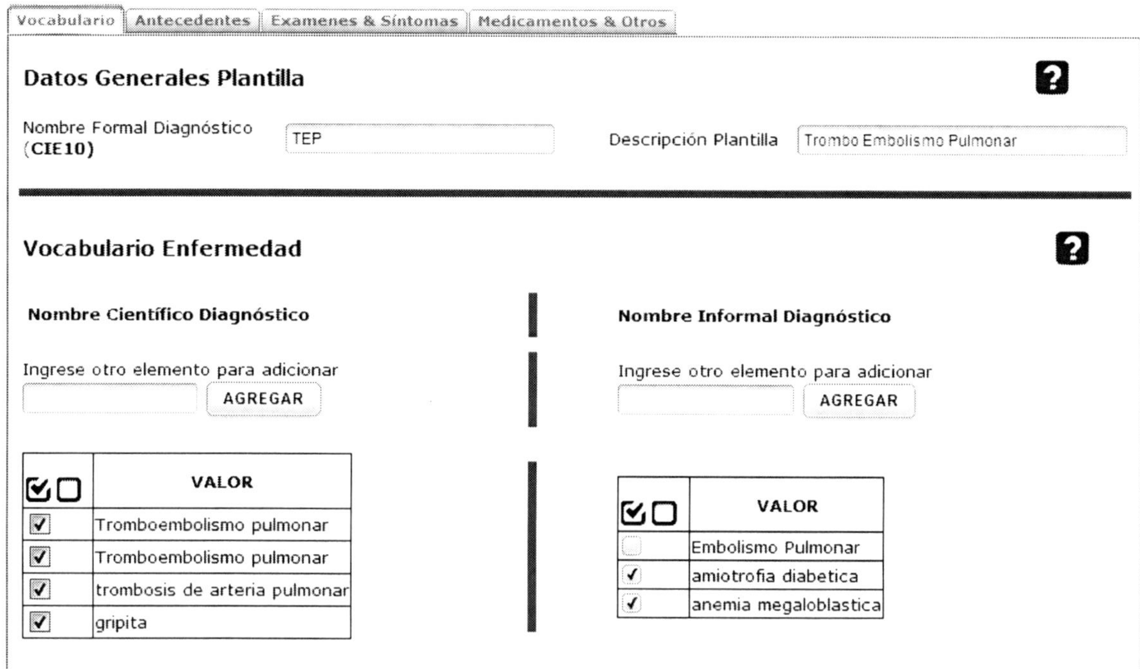

required for the analysis like the vocabulary of the disease, the related lab exams, etc. The Knowledge Engine handles the knowledge base that allows the enrichment of the description of the disease defined in the EHR analysis form. This enrichment increases the definitions made by the researcher adding synonyms or related words to the initial description.

The Extraction and Pre-selection component is in charge of the extraction and initial preprocessing of medical records from the EHR system. This component is parameterized according to the characteristics of the system and extracts the records according to the definition of initial parameters, such as date of admission, gender or age of patients. This component was built using the analysis services of SQL Server 2008.

The EHR Analysis Engine is the core of the analysis. It uses natural language processing to analyze EHR. It implements Stemming using Porter Stemmer algorithm, simple string tokenization, sentence splitting, POS tagging using Probabilistic Part-of-Speech Tagging Using Decision Trees (Schmid, 1994) for annotating text with part-of-speech and lemma information and finally gazetteer lookup using regular expressions. This component has a coordinator that calls each of the search engines. The Narrative Text Analysis is in charge of the analysis of natural language and was developed using the GATE API (Cunningham et al., 2011). This API enables the inclusion of all the language processing functionality within DISEArch. In addition, we use Tree tagger (Schmid, 1994), a Pearl implementation which provides tokenization and Part of the Speech tagger.

The Structured Analysis Engine is in charge of searching the disease over the structured attributes. Finally, the Prioritization component integrates the results using the semantic rules and prioritizes the set of records.

6. RESULTS

One of the main results of this project is the reduction of time and the improvement of the accuracy in the results of retrospective medical research. The design as proposed and implemented in the DISEArch software prototype proves to be useful to promote a systematic approach to query EHR including an important portion of narrative texts. These characteristics aim to fill the gap found during the analysis of the evolution of tools, techniques and models related to EHR analysis in the last thirty years. This section presents first the evaluation method followed to demonstrate this improvement; the second part illustrates the limitations that were found in DISEArch during this evaluation.

6.1. Evaluation Results

The aim of this project is to allow the hospital administrators and medical researchers to recognize the utility of the information contained in EHR to improve quality of service and research processes. To evaluate this goal we developed a process to measure the utility of the system, the quality of the results (in terms of the accuracy of obtained records) and the efficacy of the system to change the related processes.

The team that carried out the evaluation combined medical doctors, students of medical specializations and the university hospital IT staff. For evaluation purposes, three diseases were selected as case studies: diabetes mellitus, heart failure and pulmonary hypertension. These diseases were selected taking into consideration their common characteristic of being chronic diseases. This alone makes the use and evaluation of the system easier to analyze, because it is more likely that such patients have continued visits to the hospital, thus making their EHRs a richer source of data. In addition, those diseases also exhibit differences related to their ease of detection, their prevalence and incidence proportions, which helps in triangulating the evaluation results.

The utility and quality of results were measured using the EHR from the SAHI system. During the first phase a group of medical doctors analyzed manually 400 EHR selected randomly from pa-

tients in the department of Internal Medicine. From this analysis we obtained three sets of EHR, each one with the patients with the selected diseases. In essence, this is used as the control dataset, obtained with the current manual method for obtaining EHRs related to a disease.

The second phase consisted in the use of DIS-EARch by a group of medical doctors specialized in each one of the diseases. They described the diseases using DISEArch and ask for the relevant EHR. The utility was measured evaluating the consistency of the manual selection results with respect to the selected EHR by DISEArch. Considering that DISEArch generates a list of prioritized EHR, in order to compare it with the control dataset, we set three partitions within the results: EHRs with a score between 70% and 100% are in the set A, EHR with a score between 40% and 69% are in the set B and those EHR with a score below 40% are in the set C. The hypothesis of the process developed by DISEArch is that set A should contain mostly EHR of patients with the disease; set B should include patients whose EHR match some literals of the disease query, but not necessarily have the disease, in this case the user must analyze the findings of DISEArch to make a decision; and set C contain primarily EHR with some coincidences, but with a low probability of having the disease.

The comparison of DISEArch results with respect to the manual analysis is presented in Figures 6, 7 and 8. The x axe represents partitions according to DISEArch results; the y axe represents the percentage of EHR. The set % Yes means the EHR was classified manually as Yes, The set %No means the EHR was classified manually as No.

As expected by the hypothesis of DISEArch, the EHR in set A correspond to patients with the analyzed disease. This fact was true for prevalent diseases like Heart Failure and Diabetes Mellitus.

On the contrary, Pulmonary Hypertension had another behavior; in this case the ratio of Yes and No founded was similar. The analysis of the result details for this disease revealed that most of the percentage of *No* EHR in partition A

Figure 6. Heart failure comparison

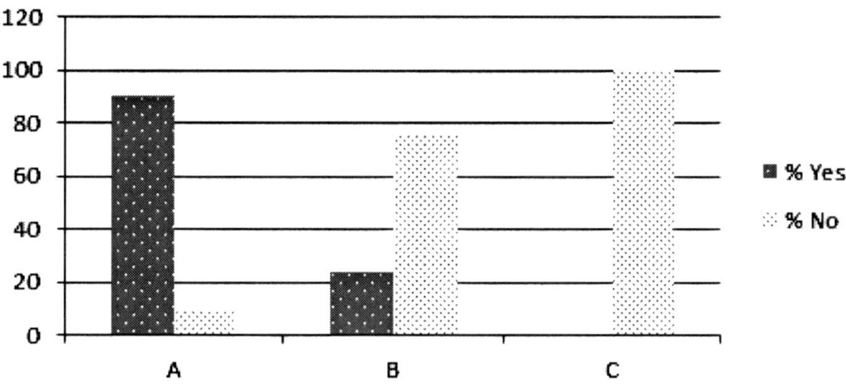

Figure 7. Pulmonary hypertension

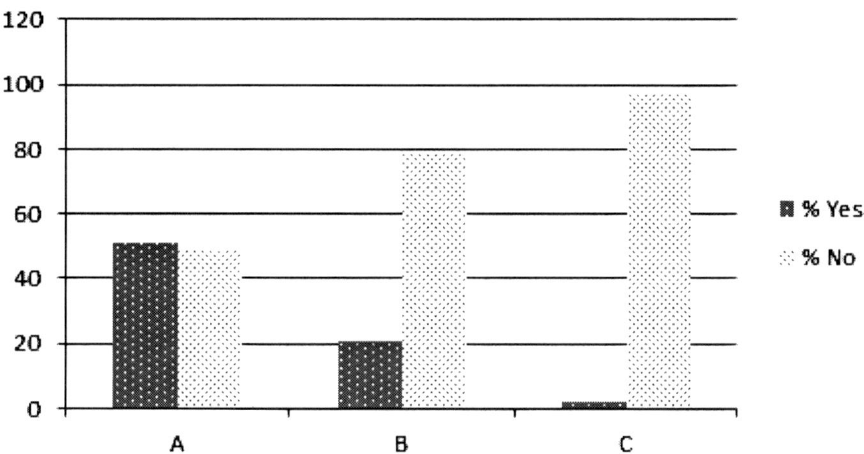

Figure 8. Diabetes mellitus comparison

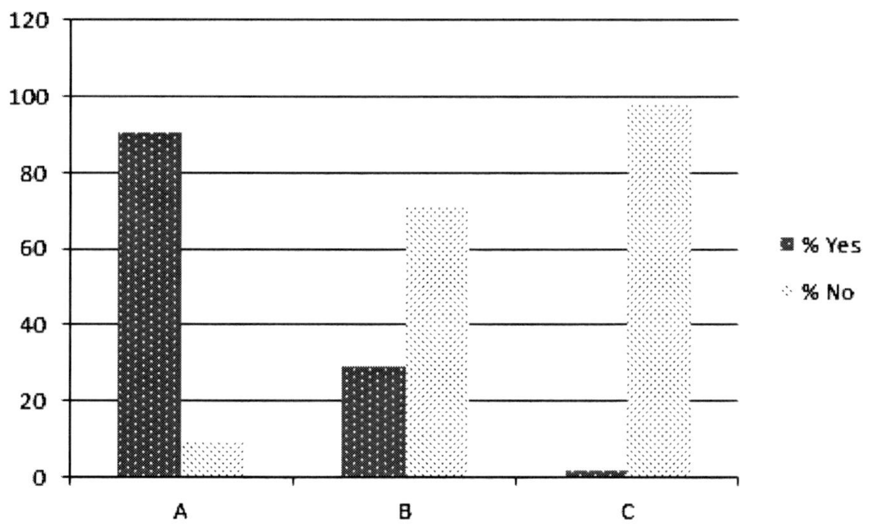

are from patients who have had a lot of related and confirmatory tests, but were never diagnosed with the disease. This fact allowed us to conclude that uncommon diseases require the analysis of the result details to select or discard an EHR for the analysis.

With respect to Partitions B and C, the results were as expected; EHR in Partition C can be discarded most of the times, except for those analyses that required being exhaustive. Finally, Partition B requires the analysis of DISEArch result details in order to identify the set of relevant EHR. Even if this implies an effort, the number of details that should be analyzed is not representative with respect to the original amount of data.

These results prove the utility of DISEArch to identify the EHR required for the analysis. However, even if lower, the not-matching results in partition B were analyzed to identify what kind of coincidences they have.

Medical doctors analyzed once again all the events associated with the "problematic" EHRs. The new analysis identified that there are patients with an early stage of a disease and because of that the manual analysis determined it was not relevant; however, the evolution of the patient would probably end in a Heart Failure diagnosis. According to the doctors, neither the medical doctor that did the early analysis, nor DISEarch were wrong: the difference was the level of evolution that each one of them aimed to use to identify EHR. This is worth

noting because neither the manual process nor DISEArch are free from error. In fact, as discussed in an evaluation meeting, some medical doctors view the situation as if each individual actually carries all diseases potentially in him or her, and if we lived long enough we would all eventually develop the diseases. As such, selecting patients will always leave out some that could have been included and it is a human decision whether to include those with borderline conditions.

The other set of EHR analyzed correspond to patients with a large number of service records (visits, tests, hospitalizations, etc). Some of these included early medical statements discarding the disease, but more recent ones confirmed its presence. These cases represent a great challenge to DISEArch because the analysis involves a new variable of analysis that initially was not taken into account; the next section develops this issue further.

The efficacy of the system to renew the process of analysis was measured comparing the previous (manual) process with the new (DISEarch-supported) one, and the effects it has in time invested and user empowerment. Figure 9 illustrates the new process. In this new process the final user is not dependent on IT staff, avoiding the bottleneck that this implied; In addition, Table 1 illustrates improvements on the time required for the analysis of EHR.

Figure 9. EHR Analysis Process with DISEArch

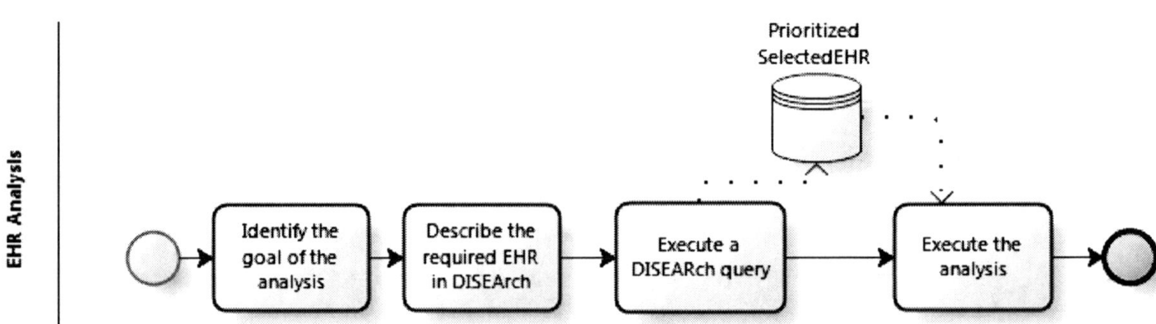

Table 1. DISEarch time performance

	Manual Process	**DISEArch**
Number of EHR	1350	400
Time required	166 hours	10 minutes

6.2. Implications for IT-Based Service Systems (ITSS)

In order to assure that the new system would deliver the expected results, the project followed the guidelines of the MOF framework (Pultorak, 2008). The *Plan, Deliver, Operate and Manage* phases of the IT service lifecycle allowed us to bring together information and people; however, in some of these phases we had to take important decisions that worth mentioning.

During the Plan phase, the formation of the project team was extremely time consuming because of the misalignment between the IT area and the legal and human resources department. Even if these problems were solved, for new projects it will be essential to do a pre-analysis of the financial structure of the project to prevent time consumption in administrative tasks.

Considering this project followed a participatory design approach, during the Manage phase we needed to take into account an open strategy for change management. In this strategy we defined formal mechanisms to register required changes on the system, but an open participatory mechanism to evaluate the consequences on time and effort to deliver these changes. IT analysts worked together with final users to prioritize changes according to the effects it will have on the improvement of the business value. In such a way, we avoided frequent iterations that will impact project time.

Since the initial problem on this project was ill-structured, the Envision function of the Deliver phase did not include a clearly documented vision and scope of the project. Nevertheless, the fact that the project followed a participatory design approach allowed to reduce the risks of this shallow original definition.

6.3. Discussion

In fact, a long term goal of this research is to gradually improve the quality of patient treatments based on formal evidence gathered through the specific analysis of each disease, especially chronic diseases.

The process used to design and create DISEArch followed an integration of rigor and relevance reinforced through user experience and involvement during the design that enabled the appropriation and evolution of the information system created. This approach demonstrates the value of participatory design to enrich the requirements phase during all the process to assure the quality of the final design and the fulfillment of user expectations. However, the drawback of the approach is the high time consumed to undertake the process, particulary during the design of the user interface. This may not be a disadvantage but the evidence that time typically used for this activity was considerably lower than required.

7. CONCLUSION AND FUTURE WORK

This paper presents a health decision-support system called DISEArch that allows the identification and analysis of relevant EHR for decision-making. It uses structured and non-structured data, and provides analytical as well as visualization facilities over individual or sets of EHR. DISEArch proves to be useful to empower researchers during analysis processes and to reduce considerably the time required to obtain relevant EHR for a study. Technically speaking, the main novel contribution of DISEArch is its ability to analyze multiple EHRs simultaneously prioritizing the most relevant to improve decision making, using a hybrid approach that combines text mining techniques and structured analysis. Contrary to other related works, DISEARch provides a complete set of components that can be used to manage, visualize and analyze EHRs. From a methodological point of view, this work represents a successful case of using participative, design-centered service systems engineering to produce a rigorous and relevant solution in the health care domain.

This work opens important research issues. Among them, the extension of DISEARch design to include temporal analysis over events of EHR with the same diagnosis. This kind of analysis involves the recognition of events from narrative texts and the application of time series analysis to identify temporal patterns. Such event-based patterns should contribute to matching actual treatment against proposed protocols and guidelines, open up traceability for a clinical and administrative use, and provide alternative views on health records that can enhance daily medical practice. In addition, the use of text mining techniques for creating abstract summaries of EHR in DISEArch is promising. The combination of such techniques with the analysis of semantic distance between EHR should also be further developed.

Future research also involves the use of our proposal in other medical institutions leading probably to other analysis requirements and technical issues related to other hospital information systems.

Probably the most important research perspective we consider is the further use of participatory design for the enrichment of health decision-making system. It is complex but necessary to strike a balance and generate a fruitful discussion from very different sets of expertise. As with any information systems project, a conversation needs to be put in place to realize the full potential that IT-based systems offer for people, in this case within the medical domain. It is a mutual learning experience that requires constant translations, frequent prototype discussions, grounding of new IT-based support in current practices and clear identification of existing problems and future opportunities that are opened up in order to enrich the momentum of the project, enlarge the community of early adopters and guaranteeing the continued financial, scientific and administrative support for the project from management stakeholders. Our experience is very positive and we intend to further pursue this approach and extract lessons learned for similar projects.

ACKNOWLEDGMENT

This work is part of the project entitled "Identificación semiautomática de pacientes con enfermedades crónicas a partir de la exploración retrospectiva de las historias clínicas electrónicas registradas en el sistema SAHI del Hospital San Ignacio" funded by Hospital Universitario San Ignacio and Pontificia Universidad Javeriana.

REFERENCES

Adams, P. C., Gregor, J. C., Kertesz, A. E., & Valberg, L. S. (1995). Screening blood donors for hereditary hemochromatosis: Decision analysis model based on a 30-year database. *Gastroenterology*, *109*(1), 177–188. doi:10.1016/0016-5085(95)90283-X PMID:7797016

Bellazzi, R., & Zupan, B. (2008). Predictive data mining in clinical medicine: Current issues and guidelines. *International Journal of Medical Informatics*, *77*(2), 81–97. doi:10.1016/j.ijmedinf.2006.11.006 PMID:17188928

Burbidge, R., Trotter, M., Buxton, B., & Holden, S. (2001). Drug design by machine learning: Support vector machines for pharmaceutical data analysis. *Computers & Chemistry*, *26*(1), 5–14. doi:10.1016/S0097-8485(01)00094-8 PMID:11765851

Carroll, J. M., & Rosson, M. B. (2007). Participatory design in community informatics. *Design Studies*, *28*(3), 243–261. doi:10.1016/j.destud.2007.02.007

Clinithink, C. (n.d.). CLiX is the leading NLP solution for healthcare and extracts the meaning from unstructured clinical narrative. *Clinithink*. Retrieved November 27, 2013, from http://clinithink.com/info/product-info/clix-engine/

Cunningham, H., Maynard, D., Bontcheva, K., Tablan, V., Aswani, N., Roberts, I., … Others. (2011). *Text Processing with GATE (Version 6)*. University of Sheffield Department of Computer Science.

Ferranti, J. M., Langman, M. K., Tanaka, D., McCall, J., & Ahmad, A. (2010). Bridging the gap: Leveraging business intelligence tools in support of patient safety and financial effectiveness. *Journal of the American Medical Informatics Association*, *17*(2), 136–143. doi:10.1136/jamia.2009.002220 PMID:20190055

Gaspar, L., Scott, C., Rotman, M., Asbell, S., Phillips, T., & Wasserman, T. et al. (1997). Recursive Partitioning Analysis (RPA) of prognostic factors in three Radiation Therapy Oncology Group (RTOG) brain metastases trials. *International Journal of Radiation Oncology, Biology, Physics*, *37*(4), 745–751. doi:10.1016/S0360-3016(96)00619-0 PMID:9128946

Gresh, D. L., Rabenhorst, D. A., Shabo, A., & Slavin, S. (2002). PRIMA: A case study of using information visualization techniques for patient record analysis. In IEEE Visualization, 2002. VIS 2002 (pp. 509–512). doi:10.1109/VISUAL.2002.1183817

Hess, K. R., Abbruzzese, M. C., Lenzi, R., Raber, M. N., & Abbruzzese, J. L. (1999). Classification and regression tree analysis of 1000 consecutive patients with unknown primary carcinoma. *Clinical Cancer Research*, *5*(11), 3403–3410. PMID:10589751

Hesse, B. W., & Shneiderman, B. (2007). eHealth Research from the User's Perspective. *American Journal of Preventive Medicine*, *32*(5SUPPL.), S97–S103. doi:10.1016/j.amepre.2007.01.019 PMID:17466825

Hevner, A. R. (2007). A Three Cycle View of Design Science Research. *Scandinavian Journal of Information Systems*, *19*(2), 39–64.

Hevner, A. R., March, S. T., Park, J., & Ram, S. (2004). Design science in information systems research. *Management Information Systems Quarterly*, *28*(1), 75–105.

Highet, V. S., Forrest, A., Ballow, C. H., & Schentag, J. J. (1999). Antibiotic dosing issues in lower respiratory tract infection: Population-derived area under inhibitory curve is predictive of efficacy. *The Journal of Antimicrobial Chemotherapy*, *43*(90001SUPPL. A), 55–63. doi:10.1093/jac/43.suppl_1.55 PMID:10225573

Hill, R. P., Lubarsky, D. A., Phillips-Bute, B., Fortney, J. T., Creed, M. R., Glass, P. S. A., & Gan, T. J. (2000). Cost-effectiveness of prophylactic antiemetic therapy with ondansetron, droperidol, or placebo. *Anesthesiology*, *92*(4), 958–967. doi:10.1097/00000542-200004000-00012 PMID:10754614

Iyer, S. V., Harpaz, R., Lependu, P., Bauer-Mehren, A., & Shah, N. H. (2013). Mining clinical text for signals of adverse drug-drug interactions. *Journal of the American Medical Informatics Association: JAMIA*. doi:10.1136/amiajnl-2013-001612

Kalim, K., Carson, E., & Cramp, D. (2004). The role of soft systems methodology in healthcare policy provision and decision support. In *Conference Proceedings - IEEE International Conference on Systems, Man and Cybernetics* (Vol. 6, pp. 5025–5030). doi:10.1109/ICSMC.2004.1400989

Kalim, K., Carson, E. R., & Cramp, D. (2006). An illustration of whole systems thinking. *Health Services Management Research*, *19*(3), 174–185. doi:10.1258/095148406777888116 PMID:16848958

Kroes, R., Renwick, A. G., Cheeseman, M., Kleiner, J., Mangelsdorf, I., & Piersma, A. et al. (2004). Structure-based thresholds of toxicological concern (TTC): Guidance for application to substances present at low levels in the diet. *Food and Chemical Toxicology*, *42*(1), 65–83. doi:10.1016/j.fct.2003.08.006 PMID:14630131

Lisboa, P. J. G. (2002). A review of evidence of health benefit from artificial neural networks in medical intervention. *Neural Networks*, *15*(1), 11–39. doi:10.1016/S0893-6080(01)00111-3 PMID:11958484

Mao, J.-Y., Vredenburg, K., Smith, P. W., & Carey, T. (2005). The state of user-centered design practice. *Communications of the ACM*, *48*(3), 105–109. doi:10.1145/1047671.1047677

McCarthy, J., & Wright, P. (2004). *Technology as Experience*. Cambridge, MA: The MIT Press.

McCauley, N., & Ala, M. (1992). The use of expert systems in the healthcare industry. *Information & Management*, *22*(4), 227–235. doi:10.1016/0378-7206(92)90025-B

Orlikowski, W. J. (2000). Using Technology and Constituting Structures: A Practice Lens for Studying Technology in Organizations. *Organization Science*, *11*(4), 404–428. doi:10.1287/orsc.11.4.404.14600

Peffers, K., Tuunanen, T., Rothenberger, M., & Chatterjee, S. (2007). A Design Science Research Methodology for Information Systems Research. *Journal of Management Information Systems*, *24*(3), 45–77. doi:10.2753/MIS0742-1222240302

Pultorak, D. (2008). Mof - Microsoft Operations Framework: V4.0 (3Rev Ed.). Van Haren Publishing.

Schmid, H. (1994). Probabilistic Part-of-Speech Tagging Using Decision Trees. Presented at the Proceedings of International Conference on New Methods in Language Processing, Manchester, UK.

Shearer, C. (2000). The CRISP-DM Model: The new blueprint for data mining. *Journal of Data Warehousing*, *5*(4), 13–22.

Simon, H. A. (1996). *The Sciences of the Artificial (Vol. Third)*. Cambridge, MA: MIT Press.

Stahl, B. C. (2007). ETHICS, Morality and Critique: An Essay on Enid Mumford's Socio-Technical Approach. *Journal of the Association for Information Systems*, *8*(9), 479.

Suppes, T., Dennehy, E. B., Hirschfeld, R. M. A., Altshuler, L. L., Bowden, C. L. Jr, & Calabrese, J. R. et al. (2005). The Texas Implementation of Medication Algorithms: Update to the algorithms for treatment of bipolar I disorder. *The Journal of Clinical Psychiatry*, *66*(7), 870–886. doi:10.4088/JCP.v66n0710 PMID:16013903

Windle, P. E. (2004). Data mining: an excellent research tool. *Journal of Perianesthesia Nursing: Official Journal of the American Society of PeriAnesthesia Nurses / American Society of PeriAnesthesia Nurses*, *19*(5), 355–356.

This work was previously published in the International Journal of Information Technologies and Systems Approach (IJITSA), 7(2); edited by Manuel Mora, pages 20-40 copyright year 2014 by IGI Publishing (an imprint of IGI Global).

APPENDIX A

Compliance with Design Science Research Guidelines

In Hevner et al (2004), seven guidelines are proposed to be addressed by all design science research in order for it to be complete and effective. As a reflective assessment of the present work, we provide a table indicating where and how this research addresses each of the guidelines (See Table 2).

Table 2. Design science observations

Design Science Guideline	Observation On How it is Followed in this Research
Design as an artifact	The product of design is always an artifact, which in information systems may be classified as either a concept, model, method or instantiation. This paper describes the way in which a model is developed to enable identifying and prioritizing electronic health records (EHRs). This model is instantiated in a particular software system which contributes to decision support in clinical research.
Problem relevance	In striking a balance between rigor and relevance, all design science research in information systems, creates a technical artifact to solve a business problem; in this case, the problem is how to identify and prioritize EHRs to aid decision-making in clinical research, where the EHRs contain unstructured text which holds significant but hidden information.
Design evaluation	Section 6 in this article describes the evaluation carried out to test the quality and efficacy of the model, as instantiated in a first software system prototype, showing a significant improvement in efficiency, when compared to the current process as well as better accuracy in the results.
Research contributions	Transparent description of the process behind this research is intended to provide design process knowledge related to the method, procedures and overall participative aspects of this project in order for similar problem settings to be treated in a similar fashion. It is precisely through the integration of data and text mining techniques, together with participative, iterative design cycles that this project was able to articulate medical and informatics expertise resulting in a decision support artifact for clinical research. In the same vein, describing the resulting model, its architecture and its application domain, this paper is able to contribute design product knowledge, extending the solution space for similar scenarios within medical informatics and decision-support information systems, especially when the problem data involves unstructured text.
Research Rigor	On the other side of relevance, a sound design science research project should also be rigorous. In this Project, rigor is anchored in the systematic study and incorporation of applicable knowledge, as described in Section 3. This rigor is followed through by employing an ordered design process and executing several tests on the resulting system.
Design as a search process	Having a systemic, iterative approach guiding the design process enabled the construction of an artifact that does not merely employ useful knowledge and existing data and text mining techniques and tools, but also configures them and creates a user experience in tune with the exiting technological, organizational and user capabilities, increasing the chance of its acceptance beyond the already mentioned technical quality and effectiveness attributes embedded in the system.
Communication of Research	The early stages of this project have already been shared with the academic community in conferences and book chapters. However, in line with design science research, it has been also presented in professional (in this case clinical research) contexts and innovation forums, enabling the research team to find not only valuable feedback and insights, but also potential partners for further deployment and extensions.

APPENDIX B

System Development Process

The development process conducted for creating DISEArch follows an iterative approach. The main feature of this approach is the system construction through iterations allowing the system to be gradually refined. This process promotes a permanent communication with final users, who play an important role on the evaluation of the iteration progress.

As illustrated in Figure 10, in order to assure the robustness of the system, the first phase consists of the abstract specification, which objective is to specify the general characteristics of the system and design its global architecture. During this specification the team decides the number and the objective of each one of the iterations.

An iteration is developed based on an initial technical design that ensures it will fit in the general architecture. Then, it is delivered to the medical part of the team for being evaluated. If the evaluation result is successful, the next iteration is developed until the whole system is suitable for the users. In case of having a problem with an iteration, its design is refined and the changes are developed to begin a new evaluation process.

Figure 10. EHR analysis process with DISEArch

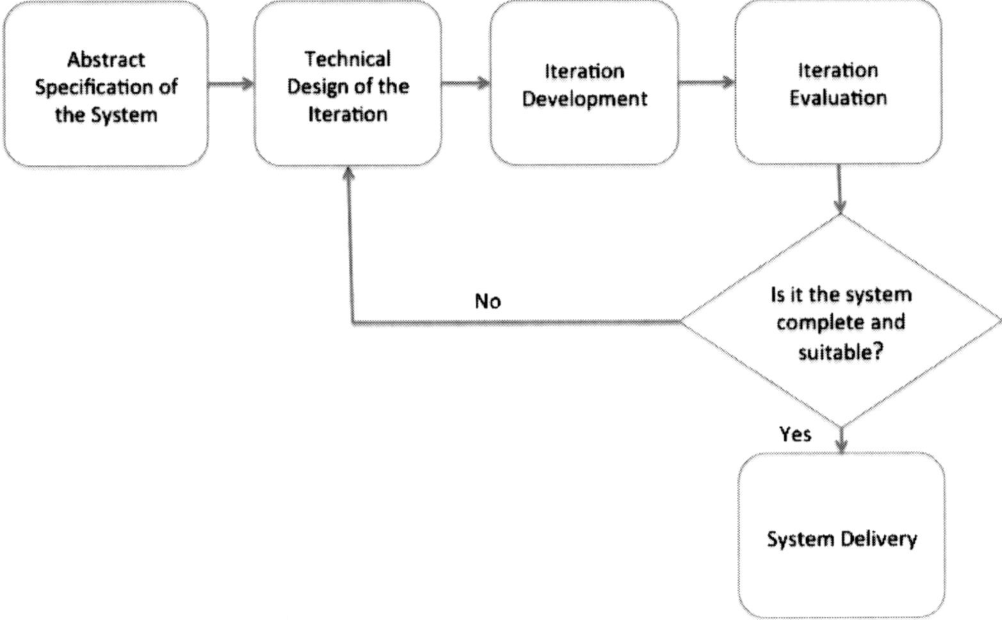

Chapter 20

To Adopt or Not to Adopt:
A Perception–Based Model of the EMR Technology Adoption Decision Utilizing the Technology–Organization–Environment Framework

Colleen Schwarz
University of Louisiana at Lafayette, USA

Andrew Schwarz
Louisiana State University, USA

ABSTRACT

For several decades the information systems field has studied the individual-level decision to adopt Information Technology (IT) with the primary goal of making it easier for organizations to derive value out of IT by increasing their effective and efficient use of the deployed IT. While the topic of non-adoption has been discussed within the literature, the focus in previous work has been upon the perceptions of the individual towards the innovation (or a micro-level of analysis), neglecting the broader context within which the adoption/non-adoption decision takes place (or a macro-level of analysis). However, what about situations in which there is institutional pressure influencing an adoption decision? This paper posits that institutional pressure external to an organization may alter the directionality and outcome of the decision. This study adopts the Technology-Organization-Environment framework to examine the context of a physician's decision about whether or not to adopt Electronic Medical Record (or EMR) technology. It reports on a multiple state study within the United States that examines the technology, organization, and environmental factors that discriminate between adopters and non-adopters.

1. INTRODUCTION

For several decades the information systems field has studied the individual-level decision to adopt Information Technology (IT) with the primary goal of making it easier for organizations to derive value out of IT by increasing their effective and efficient use of the deployed IT (Viswanath Venkatesh, Thong, & Xu, 2012). This line of work has resulted in a broad set of theories including

DOI: 10.4018/978-1-4666-8756-1.ch020

the Unified Theory of Acceptance and Use of Technology (UTAUT) (Venkatesh, Morris, Davis, & Davis, 2003; Venkatesh et al., 2012), the Task-Technology Fit (TTF) (Goodhue & Thompson, 1995), the Perceived Characteristics of Innovations (PCI) (Moore and Benbasat, 1991), and others (Schwarz & Chin, 2007). While these adoption theories seek to explain how and why users adopt technology, little is known about the behavior of non-adoption.

While the topic of non-adoption has been discussed within the literature (Bhattacherjee and Hikmet, 2007; Lapointe & Rivard, 2005; Schwarz, Schwarz, & Cenfetelli, 2012), the focus in previous work has been upon the perceptions of the individual towards the innovation (or a micro-level of analysis), neglecting the broader context within which the adoption/non-adoption decision takes place (or a macro-level of analysis). The micro-level focus on individual-level adoption (as exemplified by UTAUT) focuses upon how an individual perceives an innovation and the role of this perception on the decision regarding whether or not to adopt the innovation. We expect that in many technology adoption contexts this view will adequately address the key factors influencing adoption. However, what about situations in which there is institutional pressure influencing an adoption decision? We posit that institutional pressure external to an organization may alter the directionality and outcome of the decision. Specifically, in situations in which there is strong institutional pressure, we postulate that organizational and environmental considerations (or macro-level factors) will be significantly stronger than innovation-level perceptions (or micro-level factors) in the adoption decision.

In this study, we adopt the Technology-Organization-Environment framework to examine the context of a physician's decision about whether or not to adopt Electronic Medical Record (EMR) technology. Given the pressure from the United States government for physicians nationwide to adopt EMR technology and that the adoption and implementation of EMR technology was ranked as the top concerns for physicians (Gregg 2013), we will examine the impact of this institutional pressure upon the adoption decision, theorizing that this pressure has shifted the salient factors away from the innovation (or micro) level to the organizational and environmental (or macro) level. Thus, we highlight a gap in the literature, namely, a lack of understanding of the relationship between the environmental considerations, the organizational structure, and the individual level attitudes and decisions regarding the adoption/non-adoption decision of the individual.

2. THEORETICAL DEVELOPMENT

2.1. The Technology-Organization-Environment Framework

While many theories exist to explain adoption behavior, few of our approaches examine macro-level influences on micro-level behaviors. One notable exception is the Technology-Organization-Environment (or T-O-E) framework proposed by Tornatzky and Fleischer (1990). According to the T-O-E framework (Figure 1), there are three elements that influence the adoption decision: the organizational context, the technological context, and the environmental context. Within each of these contexts are specific constructs that dictate whether or not an innovation is adopted.

Originally proposed at the firm level, T-O-E has been utilized as a broad framework utilized to study both individual and organizational level adoption decisions. As summarized in Table 1, the framework has been employed across a variety of contexts, including e-business (Lin & Lin, 2008; T. Oliveira & Martins, 2010; Kevin Zhu, Kraemer, & Xu, 2003; Zhu & Kraemer, 2005; Zhu, Kraemer, & Xu, 2006), ERP (Pan & Jang, 2008), Knowledge Management Systems (Lee, Wang, Lim, & Peng, 2009), e-commerce (Liu, 2008; Oliveira & Martins, 2009; Teo, Rangana-

Figure 1. Technology organization environment framework

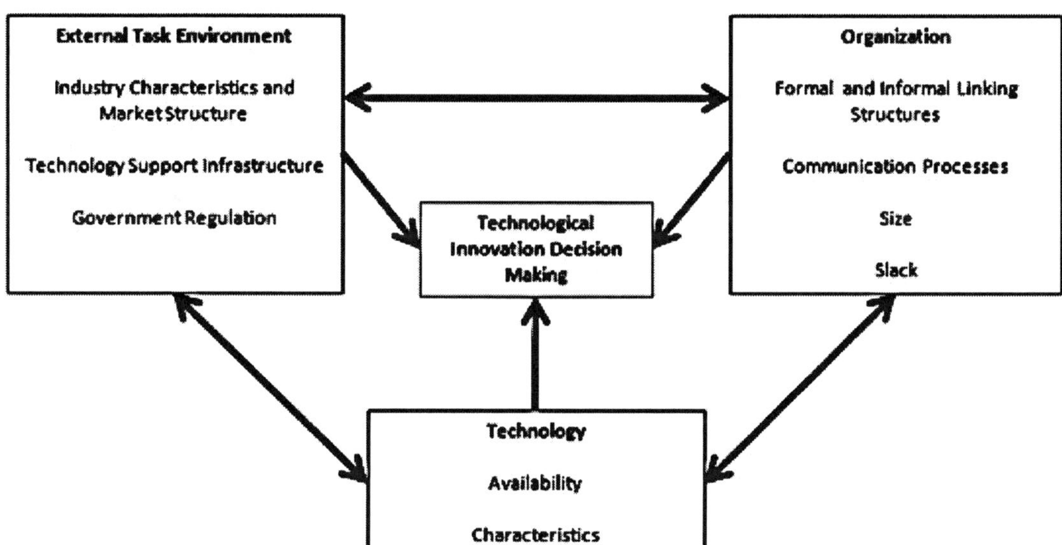

than, & Dhaliwal, 2006), EDI (Kuan & Chau, 2001), and open systems (Chau & Tam, 1997). Moreover, as our review of the literature reveals, constructs within the elements have been conceptualized using a variety of theoretical lenses in order to understand various aspects of each of the environments.

However, the framework is not without critiques. As Baker (2012) notes "the majority of the theoretical development that has taken place related to the TOE framework has been limited to enumerating the different factors that are relevant in various adoption contexts" (p. 237). Nonetheless, we posit that the framework provides a valuable lens with which to view technology adoption, although it has not been employed in a cumulative tradition in expanding and employing the model. Thus, we argue that there are two gaps in the literature in previous research that has utilized the T-O-E framework that we seek to overcome: (1) A lack of theoretical consistency with the original constructs and (2) A lack of understanding the framework in different environmental settings.

The first gap in the literature with the T-O-E framework that we identify is with the constructs that were originally identified. We argue that the strength of the framework, namely that it is broad in defining the three contexts has also contributed to the difficulty of the development of a cumulative research stream in this area, namely that there has been little theoretical consistency in the implementation of the constructs. Our analysis of Table 1 highlights that, within each of the dimensions, there has been little consistency in how the technology, organization, and environmental contexts have been enacted, thus contributing to minimal evolution of the theory since the framework was proposed. Specifically, the original T-O-E framework enumerated specific dimensions within each of the contexts (i.e. availability and characteristics within the technology context; formal and informal linking structures, communication processes, size, and slack within the organizational context; and industry characteristics and market structure, technology support infrastructure, and government regulation within the environmental context), yet none of the literature within Table 1 addressed all of the dimensions within each of these contexts. To overcome this limitation, we start by utilizing the original definitions of the constructs and include

Table 1. Review of previous literature utilizing the T-O-E framework

Article	Technology Factors	Organization Factors	Environment Factors	Context
(Chau & Tam, 1997)	Perceived Benefits; Perceived Barriers; Perceived importance of compliance to standards, interoperability, and interconnectivity	Complexity of IT infrastructure; satisfaction with existing systems; formalization of system development and management	Market uncertainty	Open systems
(Kuan & Chau, 2001)	Perceived Direct Benefits; Perceived Indirect Benefits	Perceived Financial Cost; Perceived Technical Competence	Perceived Industry Pressure; Perceived Government Pressure	EDI
(Lee et al., 2009)	Organizational IT competence; KMS characteristics	Top management commitment; hierarchical organizational structure	With external vendors; among internal employees	Knowledge Management Systems
(Lin & Lin, 2008)	IS infrastructure; IS expertise	Organizational compatibility; expected benefits of e-business	Competitive pressure; trading partner readiness	e-business
(Liu, 2008)	Support from technology; human capital; potential support from technology	Management level for information; firm size	User satisfaction; e-commerce security	e-commerce development level
(Oliveira & Martins, 2009)	Technology readiness; technology integration; security applications	Perceived benefits of electronic correspondence; IT training programs; access to the IT system of the firm; internet and e-mail norms	Internet competitive pressure; web site competitive pressure; e-commerce competitive pressure	Internet Web site E-commerce
(Oliveira & Martins, 2010)	Technology readiness; technology integration; security applications	Perceived benefits of electronic correspondence; IT training programs, access to the IT system of the firm; internet and e-mail norms	Web site competitive pressure	E-business
(Pan & Jang, 2008)	IT Infrastructure; technology readiness	Size; perceived barriers	Production and operations improvement; enhancement of products and services; competitive pressure; regulatory policy	ERP
(Teo et al., 2006)	Conceived as inhibitors, namely: unresolved technical issues; lack of IT expertise and infrastructure; lack of interoperability	Conceived as inhibitors, namely: difficulties in organizational change; problems in project management; lack of top management support; lack of e-commerce strategy; difficulties in cost-benefit assessment	Conceived as inhibitors, namely: unresolved legal issues; fear and uncertainty	Deployment of B2b e-commerce
(Zhu, Kraemer, & Xu, 2003)	IT infrastructure; e-business know-how	Firm scope, firm size	Consumer readiness; competitive pressure; lack of trading partner readiness	E-business
(Zhu & Kraemer, 2005)	Technology competence	Size; international scope; financial commitment	Competitive pressure; regulatory support	E-business
(Zhu et al., 2006)	Technology readiness; technology integration	Firm size; global scopes; trading globalization; managerial obstacles	Competition intensity; regulatory environment	E-business

every dimension included within the contexts of the framework to guide the development of our research model.

The second gap in the literature with the T-O-E framework that we identify is the limited environmental settings that have been utilized to understand the adoption decision. Our review of the literature reveals that no prior work has examined the T-O-E framework within the context of heavy institutional pressure, instead focusing upon volitional decisions made by adopting firms. None of the technologies that were previously studied were mandated by an external institution. We postulate that heavier institutional pressure will alter the salience of environmental factors, while simultaneously altering the influence of the technology and organizational contexts. Specifically, we could speculate that institutional pressure from the environment could be more significant in driving adoption, while assessments of the technology might be less salient. Nonetheless, without understanding this environmental context, this postulation remains a gap in our understanding of adoption. To overcome this gap in the literature, we applied the T-O-E framework within a context that is currently undergoing significant institutional pressure – the adoption of Electronic Medical Records.

2.2. Empirical Context: EMR Adoption

Strong institutional pressure is being exerted for physicians to adopt Electronic Medical Record (EMR) technology in the United States of America. The American Recovery and Reinvestment Act (ARRA) of 2009 invested nearly $20 billion to facilitate the widespread adoption and use of health information technology (HIT) (Blumenthal, 2009). This funding provides incentives for physicians who are early adopters of interoperable HIT, but it also enacts penalties in future years for physicians not demonstrating "meaningful use" of EMRs (Miller, 2011). In IT adoption theory, these pressures would be deemed coercive (in the case of the payments/penalties) and mimetic (in the case of interoperable network technologies among physician organizations). The *macro-level*, institutional theory applied to technology adoption clearly identifies these pressures (Robey & Boudreau, 1999; Scott, 1987; Van de Ven, 2005). Interestingly, although physicians are knowledgeable about these incentives and are aware of the potential penalties for non-adoption, they have been slow to adopt the technology (DesRoches et al., 2008). As of 2013, only 48% of office-based physicians had adopted an EMR systems that at least met the criteria for a basic system (Hsiao and Hing 2014). Moreover, some states' adoption rates were as low as 21% (Charles, King, Patel, & Furukawa, 2013; Hsiao & Hing, 2014). These results suggest that institutional theory drivers (i.e. coercive pressures) were attempted with policy imperatives but they were inadequate to motivate adoption as expected.

Consistent with end user IT adoption research exemplified in UTAUT's performance expectancy construct, one reason identified through research for the low EMR adoption rate is that some physicians question the value of EMRs. According to the 2010 National Progress Report on eHealth, a majority (55%) of respondents believe the value of health IT is not widely understood. Moreover, *The Wall Street Journal* has found that some physicians are skeptical about the ability of EMRs to improve productivity or patient care, and that there is an even greater challenge to determine how to get doctors to "meaningfully use" the systems (Hobson, 2011) once they are implemented. As Sarah Corley, the chief medical officer at NextGen Healthcare, noted, many "hospitals have underestimated how hard it can be to get full participation by staff" (Hobson, 2011).

Research into EMRs is eclectic and spans many disciplines, including public health, sociology, business, epidemiology, economics, and strategy (Fichman, Kohli, & Krishnan, 2011). With performance expectancy as the most salient driver of adoption (V. Venkatesh et al., 2003) in combination with the pervasive assumption that EMRs provide numerous benefits once adopted, one would predict high adoption rates. However, research has found that the potential adopters, particularly smaller, private practices, are not adopting at levels that would be expected considering the overall high performance expectancy (Reardon & Davidson, 2007). On the contrary, early findings have provided a variety of rationales for non-adoption of the technology (as we have summarized in Table 2). Therefore, we posit that other factors must be influencing the adoption decision, such as macro-level considerations. For example, financial considerations which are not included in traditional adoption models could be causing organizations to pause or struggle in their decision (Reardon & Davidson, 2007). This study seeks to determine the impact of macro-level factors on the adoption decision.

2.3. A Perception-Based Model of the EMR Technology Adoption Decision Using the Technology-Organization-Environment Framework

Based upon the T-O-E framework, we propose a model of EMR adoption. This model includes the technology context, the organization context, and the environmental context. In our adaptation of T-O-E, we theorize that each of these contexts are perceived – that the physician possesses an awareness of the role of each of these factors, but that this awareness is focused upon two different levels of analysis. From the vantage point of the physician, we theorize that the technology context are micro-level perceptions – perceptions based upon the narrowly targeted area of the specific technology under consideration. In contrast, we theorize that the organization and environmental perceptions are macro-level perceptions – percep-

Table 2. Review of previous literature within EMR

Level of Analysis (Most Closely Associated IS Theory Rationale)	Factor	Studies
Macro-Level: (Diffusion of Innovations)	Financial barriers	(Anderson, 2007; Ash & Bates, 2005; Bates, Ebell, Gotlieb, Zapp, & Mullins, 2003; DesRoches et al., 2008; Gans, Kralewski, Hammons, & Dowd, 2005; Miller & Sim, 2004; Reardon & Davidson, 2007; Simon et al., 2007)
Micro-Level: (UTAUT: Effort Expectancy)	EMR technology factors	(DesRoches et al., 2008)
Micro-Level: (UTAUT: Facilitating Conditions)	Organizational factors (within hospital or practice)	(Burt & Sisk, 2005; Simon et al., 2007)
Macro-Level: (Institution Theory: Normative Pressure)	Lack of standards between EMR systems	(Bates et al., 2003; Simon et al., 2007)
Micro-Level: (UTAUT: Moderators)	Physician characteristics	(DesRoches et al., 2008)
Micro-Level: (UTAUT: Performance Expectancy)	Perceived loss of productivity and time with the patient	(Ash & Bates, 2005; DesRoches et al., 2008; Gans et al., 2005)
Micro-Level: (UTAUT: Effort Expectancy)	Concerns over ability to use the EMR system	(Gans et al., 2005; Miller & Sim, 2004; S. R. Simon et al., 2007)]
Micro-Level: (UTAUT: Effort Expectancy & Performance Expectancy)	Incompatibility with physician work flow	(Miller & Sim, 2004)

tions that are outside of the scope of the technology, but that play a role in the EMR adoption decision. Each of these three contexts is discussed next.

3. THE TECHNOLOGY CONTEXT

The technology context includes micro-level assessments made by physicians in considering their EMR adoption decision. The technology context includes two components: the *characteristics* and *availability* of the technology (Tornatzky & Fleischer, 1990). Within our context, we theorize the technology context as the perceived characteristics and the perceived availability of an EMR technology. Perceived characteristics focus upon how the actors in the firm perceive the technology (an internally-oriented assessment), while the perceived availability is focused upon whether there are viable solutions available in the marketplace (an externally-oriented assessment).

We contextualize the characteristics of the technology as the perceived attributes of the EMR technology. While a robust set of theories (e.g. UTAUT, PCI, TTF, et al) define a broad set of potential factors, we selected quality, an attribute that has been touted to be a key characteristic in the adoption of EMR systems (Øvretveit, Scott, Rundall, Shortell, & Brommels, 2007; Shekelle, Morton, & Keeler, 2006). Within the IS adoption community, systems quality has been found to be a key driver of IS usefulness (Saeed & Abdinnour-Helm, 2008), with the argument that a technology that offers a high quality experience will be perceived as being useful and, by extension, will be used more (Davis, 1993). The importance of perceived systems quality has been codified within the DeLone and McLean model of success (DeLone & McLean, 1992) and has been demonstrated to be important in both a pre and post-adoption context (Nelson, Todd, & Wixom, 2005). Extending these arguments, we posit that systems quality will also influence the likelihood of adoption for a physician of an EMR technol-

ogy. These arguments lead us to the following hypothesis:

Hypothesis 1a: Higher levels of perceived quality of EMR technology will positively affect the likelihood of EMR adoption.

The second technology context is the availability of the technology, described as the extent of a firm's technical opportunities in the external marketplace. Research into human behavior (under the umbrella of economics and behavioral finance) has examined the individual's difficulty in making decisions under complex market conditions. For example, Heiner (1983) suggests that an individual will make sub-optimal decisions in a marketplace that is overly complex for the consumer (further supported by the formal processing model of De Palma, Myers, and Papageorgiou (1994)). Theoretically, the roots of market complexity affecting human behavior can be traced back to the argument of bounded rationality (March, 1978; Simon, 1955). Despite the empirical evidence outside of IS for market complexity influencing human choice, to our knowledge, little work has examined the impact of market complexity on adoption. We theorize that if a physician, due to bounded rationality, perceives the EMR vendor marketplace to be complex, he/she will not adopt an EMR system. This logic leads us to the following hypothesis:

Hypothesis 1b: Higher levels of perceived availability of EMR technology will positively affect the likelihood of EMR adoption.

4. THE ORGANIZATION CONTEXT

The organization context includes macro-level assessments made by physicians in considering their EMR adoption decision. The organization context includes four components: formal and informal linking structures; communication processes;

size and slack. Overall, the organization context includes the processes, structures, and profile of the organization that will facilitate the adoption of the innovation. The focus of the organization context is how the actors in the firm perceive these aspects of the organization (Tornatzky & Fleischer, 1990).

The first component of the organization context is *formal and informal linking structures*. These structures are the processes that exist external to the firm in order to facilitate scanning the environment for information about needs and opportunities for technological change and to process and transfer the information so that it can support decisions about adoption. We contextualize formal and informal linking structures as the formal relationships and structures that facilitate the flow of data about patients from other hospital and practices to the physician. Researchers and practitioners have long recognized the need for organizations to integrate data both internal and external to the firm (Goodhue, Quillard, & Rockart, 1988; Goodhue, Wybo, & Kirsch, 1992), with these external sources providing a mechanism through which physicians learn about EMR systems. We therefore theorize that it is through these relationships that a physician discovers information about EMR solutions. This leads us to the following hypothesis:

Hypothesis 2a: Higher levels of data integration with other practices and hospitals will positively affect the likelihood of EMR adoption.

The second component of the organization context is *communication processes*. While the formal and informal linking structures are external to the firm, communication processes are the business processes internal to a firm that refer to how the information about a new technology diffuses through an organization. The focus is upon whether organizations create conditions conducive to the initiation and continued use of an innovation. We contextualize communication processes as the business processes within firms that facilitate the sharing of information. Considerations of information flow are not necessarily new to the IS discipline, yet the focus has been mainly within the context of an Enterprise Resource Planning (or ERP) solution. Previous research within ERP has argued that information flow is crucial in order to facilitate success (Scott, 2003). If the physician perceives that an EMR will facilitate information sharing[1], then we theorize that the conditions are conducive to the adoption of the innovation. This leads us to the following hypothesis:

Hypothesis 2b: Higher levels of data integration within a practice or hospital will positively affect the likelihood of EMR adoption.

The third component of the organization is the size of the firm. The nature of how to evaluate the size of a firm is a debated subject, with scholars lacking consensus on the appropriate measurement. However, T-O-E argues that size refers to the amount of work done in an organization, with previous studies demonstrating that organizational size influences the adoption of technological innovations (Damanpour, 1992; Hage, 1980; Kimberly & Evanisko, 1981). We contextualize size as the number of patients seen, arguing that a physician who sees more patients will be more likely to adopt an EMR so as to better control the workflow in the practice. This leads us to the following hypothesis:

Hypothesis 2c: Higher number of patient visits per day will positively affect the likelihood of EMR adoption.

The fourth component in the organization is the slack. The T-O-E framework distinguishes two types of slack resources, namely the financial and human resources. The presence of financial slack affords an organization with the ability to adopt an innovation and integrate the technology into the firm. It has been found to be a significant driver of adoption (Aiken & Hage, 1971; Miller & Friesen, 1982). Moreover, it is the least absorbed form of slack and the easiest to redeploy (Greve, 2003; Miller, 2003). In our context, we theorize that the availability of financial resources provides the physician with the means to adopt an EMR solution, while non-adopters will lack the financial slack to do so. This leads us to the following hypothesis:

Hypothesis 2d: Higher levels of financial slack will positively affect the likelihood of EMR adoption.

The other slack type involves human resources. Within the context of T-O-E, human resource slack refers to specialized and skilled human resources that are rare and absorbed (Mishina, Pollock, & Porac, 2004). Specifically, as Voss, Sirdeshmukh, and Voss (2008) demonstrates, human resource slack is absorbed because "the resources are tied up in the organization's current operations" (p. 151). In our context, we theorize that the availability of physicians and staff with more free time (or slack) will provide the users with the ability to learn the EMR software. Thus, the presence of human resource slack will give the physician the capability to adopt an EMR solution, while non-adopters will not have the slack to adopt. This leads us to the following hypothesis:

Hypothesis 2e: Higher levels of human resources slack will positively affect the likelihood of EMR adoption.

5. THE ENVIRONMENTAL CONTEXT

The environmental context includes macro-level assessments made by physicians in considering their EMR adoption decision. The environmental context includes three components: the industry characteristics and market structure; the technology support infrastructure; and government regulation (Tornatzky & Fleischer, 1990). These three components place adoption pressure upon a firm in unique manners and depend upon the specific situation in which the organization is situated. We will review and discuss each component next.

The first component of the environmental context is the industry characteristics and market structure, which refers to differences in competitive and market conditions. We theorize that these differences materialize in the form of mimetic pressure. Mimetic pressure "exist[s] when an organization imitates the actions of other structurally equivalent organizations because these organizations occupy a similar economic network position in the same industry" (Sherer, 2010). Institutional theory suggests that the imitation behavior enables an actor to reduce search costs and is typically more prevalent when questions of relative advantage are present (Shi, Shambare, & Wang, 2008; Son & Benbasat, 2007; Teo, Wei, & Benbasat, 2003; Urgin, 2009). Given the concerns over the advantages that derive from EMR systems by physicians and the high degree of search costs with EMR technology, we therefore theorize that the presence of mimetic pressure will lead a physician to adopt an EMR system. Specifically, we suggest that a positive perception of mimetic pressure will lead to adoption, while a negative view will lead a physician to reject an EMR system. It is the presence of this pressure that leads us to the following hypothesis:

Hypothesis 3a: Higher levels of adoption by other physicians and hospitals that offer services similar to the physician will positively affect the likelihood of EMR adoption.

The second component of the environmental context is the technology support infrastructure within the environment. The technology support infrastructure refers to the constraints or opportunities that a firm must take into account when developing its' technology acquisition strategy, depending upon labor costs, skills of the available labor force, and access to suppliers of technology-related services. According to the theory of situational normality, when an individual believes that the environment in which a product is purchased is in proper order, then success in acquiring and being satisfied with a product is likely because the situation in the purchasing environment is normal or favorable (Baier, 1986; Garfinkel, 1963; Lewis & Weigert, 1985). In our context, we postulate that a physician who believes that the vendors offering products within the marketplace are in proper order will be more likely to adopt an EMR system. Drawing from previous work (McKnight, Choudhury, & Kacmar, 2002), physicians who possess positive views towards situational normality believe that, in general, vendors offering EMR systems are competent, benevolent, and have integrity. In our context, however, we selected one of these three dimensions: whether the physician perceives that there is a vendor who is capable of meeting customer needs (McKnight et al., 2002) in the marketplace. Thus, we theorize that adopters will have a more positive assessment of vendors than non-adopters, leading us to the following hypothesis:

Hypothesis 3b: Higher levels of perceived positive assessments of EMR vendors will positively affect the likelihood of EMR adoption.

The third component of the environmental context is government regulation. Government regulation refers to the pressure imposed upon firms to induce a search for technical alternatives to current practice. In our context, we theorize that government regulation refers to the pressure from state and federal governments to adopt EMR technology, which equates to coercive pressures. Coercive pressures are defined as formal or informal pressures exerted by other organizations upon which they are dependent (DiMaggio & Powell, 1983; Son & Benbasat, 2007). Drawing upon institutional theory, we therefore posit that

institutions with which physicians are dependent can coercively exert pressure upon him/her in order to influence adoption. By linking re-imbursement rates for performing services with a physician's EMR adoption decision, both government and insurance companies are relying upon formal, financial pressure to influence adoption. We therefore theorize that these forms of coercive pressure will lead a physician to adopt an EMR system. Specifically, we postulate that a positive perception of coercive pressure will lead to adoption, while a negative view will lead a physician to reject an EMR system. It is the presence of this pressure that leads us to the following hypothesis:

Hypothesis 3c: Higher levels of perceived government regulation will positively affect the likelihood of EMR adoption.

6. RESEARCH MODEL

Based upon our theoretical development, we propose the research model in Figure 2.

7. RESEARCH METHOD

7.1. Item Development

With a proposed research model, we will now discuss the development of our research items. Based upon the definitions of our constructs, we created items to measure the constructs identified. Where possible, we utilized previously published scales to measure each construct. In Table 3, we have outlined the construct, the definition of the construct, the items employed to measure each construct (for both adopters and non-adopters), and the source of the measurement. The dependent variable (i.e. the adoption/non-adoption decision) was based upon whether or not the physician was currently using (i.e. made the decision to adopt)

Figure 2. Proposed research model

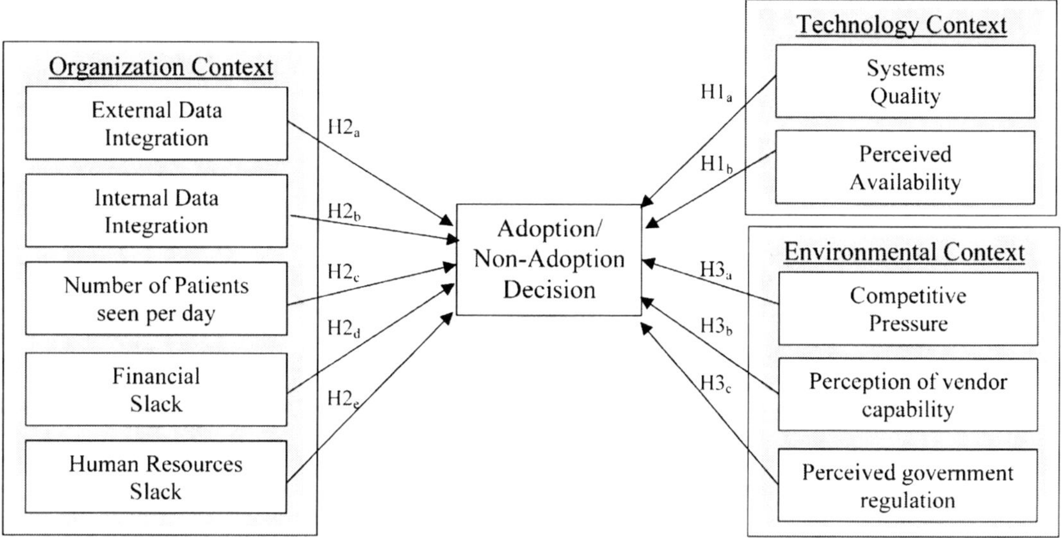

or not currently using (i.e. made the decision not to adopt) an EMR system. The dependent variable was thus binary – with 0 being non-adoption and 1 being adoption.[2]

7.2. Sample

In order to test our research model, a survey was conducted with physicians within four regions of the United States, each representing differing levels of EMR adoption. We began by analyzing the adoption of EMR technology by state, focusing upon the adoption of a basic EMR system (based upon the report issued by the Robert J. Woods Foundation (2012)). We divided the adoption rates into four groups through a systematic analysis of the adoption rate. First, we divided the states into two groups – those above the mean (20 states) and those below the mean (30 states). Then, within each of the two groups, we divided the groups again. This approach resulted in four groups: Low adoption rate (15.9% to 28.2%), low to medium adoption rate (28.4% to 33.3%), medium to high adoption rate (33.9% to 40.4%), and high adoption rate (41.2% to 60.9%). We then selected one state from each group to analyze in this study and contacted state medical societies to offer an opportunity to be included in the study. Thus, we collected data from physicians within each of these four groups.

Each state in America has its own medical society, which is a voluntary association that provides advocacy and education for physicians within the state. By working with medical societies we have access to a more comprehensive group of physicians, including physicians from various hospitals, rural physicians, physicians across a wide range of specialties, and physicians in private practice, who may otherwise be difficult to locate. We have blinded the specific state names and will refer to each state by its adoption rate. The adoption rates were as follows: the low adoption rate state: 25.8%; low to medium: 31.1%; medium to high: 37%; and high: 54.5%. Table 4 presents the number of respondents from each state included in the study.

For three of the four states, the medical society for the state distributed the survey to the membership utilizing an e-mail invitation distributed by the leadership of the organization.

Table 3. Research items

Construct		Definition	Non-Adopter Items	Adopter	Source
Technology Characteristics					
Systems Quality		User perceptions of the quality of the EMR system (Nelson et al., 2005)	Overall, I would give the quality of EMR systems a high rating	Overall, I would give the quality of my EMR system a high rating	Nelson et al. (2005)
Perceived availability		The degree to which a physician perceives the vendor marketplace to be too complex	The EMR marketplace has too many systems		New item
Organization Characteristics					
External data integration		The degree to which a physician is concerned that other organizations they need to share information with will be unable to integrate with their EMR systems	At this point in time, EMR systems will facilitate the sharing of information between physicians from different practices/hospitals	At this point in time, my EMR system facilitates the sharing of information between physicians from different practices/ hospitals	Adapted from Nelson et al. (2005)
Internal data integration		The degree to which a system facilitates the combination of information from various sources internal to the firm (Nelson et al., 2005)	EMR systems effectively combine data from different areas of my practice	My EMR system effectively combines data from different areas of my practice	Adapted from Nelson et al. (2005)
Patients seen		An indicator of organizational size; measured as the number of patients seen per day	During your last full week of work, approximately how many patients did you see?		New item
Financial Slack		The extent to which a physician perceives the total cost of an EMR system to be reasonable and should be afforded financial slack	All things considered, the total cost of an EMR system is reasonable considering what you receive	All things considered, the total cost of my EMR system was reasonable considering what I received	New item
Human Resources Slack	Physicians [R]	The extent to which the human resources would be tied up in the organization's operations to engage the new EMR solution (extending Voss et al. (2008))	The time that it will take for me to learn how to use an EMR is significant	The time that it took for me to learn how to use my EMR is significant	New item
	Staff [R]		The time that it will take for my staff to learn how to use an EMR is significant	The time that it took for my staff to learn how to use my EMR is significant	

continued on following page

Table 3. Continued

Construct		Definition	Non-Adopter Items	Adopter	Source
Environmental Characteristics					
Competitive Pressure		The prevalence of a practice in the focal organization's industry that have adopted an EMR solution (Scott, 1987)	What is the extent of EMR adoption by physicians in your area that offer services similar to yours? (None have adopted: 7 - All have adopted)		New item
Perception of vendor capability		The extent to which EMR vendors are competent (i.e. the vendors can do what the physician needs) (McKnight et al., 2002)	Most EMR vendors do a capable job of meeting customer needs	My EMR vendor does a capable job of meeting customer needs	McKnight et al. (2002)
Perceived government regulation	Federal government	Formal penalties exerted on organizations by other organizations upon which they are dependent. In our case, we define these organizations as the state and federal government (Scott, 1987).	Penalties from the federal government for not adopting an EMR by the deadline will play a critical role in whether or not I adopt an EMR	Penalties from the federal government for not adopting an EMR by the deadline played a critical role in my EMR adoption decision	New item
	State government		Penalties from the state government for not adopting an EMR by the deadline will play a critical role in whether or not I adopt an EMR	Penalties from the state government for not adopting an EMR by the deadline played a critical role in my EMR adoption decision	New item

Note: The [R] indicates that an item is reverse coded

Table 4. Profile of four state contexts

State	Non-Adopter	Adopter	Total
Low Adoption Rate	34	86	120
Low to Medium Adoption Rate	20	66	86
Medium to High Adoption Rate	35	106	141
High Adoption Rate	45	155	200
Total	134	413	547[3]

In the medium to high adoption rate state, the researchers were provided with a one-time use of e-mail addresses from the medical society database, but no contact information was included with this list. In each of the four states, an initial invitation to participate was distributed, along with a follow-up reminder. All physicians were given two weeks to complete the survey.

The invitation directed the respondents to a web-based survey containing our research items. Non-adopters and adopters were distinguished based upon their answer to whether or not their practice (or hospital) had adopted an EMR system. Based upon the answer to this question, respondents were provided with either the non-adopter or adopter items.

8. PROFILE OF RESPONDENTS

The respondents were varied in their background and experience, and they tended to be older. The average age of our respondents was 55.4, with an average time in medicine of 23.5 years. Sixty six

Table 5. Profile of respondents

Gender	%	Payment Source	Average Percent
Male	72	Medicare	34.6
Female	23	Medicaid	20
Decline	5	Insurance	44.2
		Patient	12
		Other	21.5

percent (66%) worked in private practice, 31% worked in a hospital, with the remainder working for other healthcare organizations. In Table 5, we profile our respondents more in depth. A majority of our physicians were male (72%) and insurance was the primary driver of their payment mix (44%). A wide variety of specialists (almost 200 different specialties) were included in our study.

9. RESEARCH ANALYSIS

Given that our dependent variable was binary (adoption/non-adoption), we selected binary logistic regression for our analysis. We specified each of the items in Table 3 as independent variables, with our dependent variable defined as whether or not the physician had adopted the technology. We also included one control variable – the state in which the physician operated, so as to control for geographic location. The results are displayed in Table 6.

The results indicate that there were seven significant factors in predicting the adoption of EMR technology, namely perceived quality (0.490), competitive pressure (0.455), financial slack (0.408), and penalties from the federal government (0.377). These results signify that if a physician perceives EMR systems to be of high quality and

Table 6. Results of binary logistic regression analysis

Variable	B	S. E.	Wald	Df	Sig.	Exp(B)
Systems Quality	**.490**	**.113**	**18.662**	**1**	**.000**	**1.633**
Competitive pressure	**.455**	**.094**	**23.631**	**1**	**.000**	**1.576**
Financial Slack	**.408**	**.127**	**10.348**	**1**	**.001**	**1.504**
Perceived government regulation: federal	**.377**	**.105**	**12.835**	**1**	**.000**	**1.457**
HR Slack: Doctor [R]	.094	.172	.300	1	.584	1.099
External Data Integration	.023	.093	.063	1	.802	1.024
Number of Patients seen per day	-.001	.000	1.565	1	.211	.999
HR Slack: Staff [R]	-.069	.184	.141	1	.707	.933
Perception of vendor capability	-.160	.120	1.771	1	.183	.853
Internal Data Integration	**-.222**	**.088**	**6.383**	**1**	**.012**	**.801**
Perceived Availability [R]	**-.231**	**.093**	**6.236**	**1**	**.013**	**.794**
Perceived government regulation: state	**-.292**	**.115**	**6.463**	**1**	**.011**	**.747**
State			1.005	3	.800	
State (1)	-.306	.330	.857	1	.355	.736
State (2)	-.236	.328	.519	1	.471	.790
State (3)	.234	15684.701	.000	1	1.000	1.264
Constant	17.760	15026.184	.000	1	.999	51674851.385

Note: Bolded items refer to the factors that are significant at the level of $p < 0.05$

[R] refers to items that were reverse coded

reasonably priced, another physician similar to him/her adopts an EMR, and the penalties from the federal government are perceived as significant, then a physician is likely to adopt an EMR. Furthermore, perceptions regarding the effectiveness of the integration of the EMR technology within the firm differentiate between adopter and non-adopter physicians of EMR technology (-0.222). Furthermore, if the marketplace is viewed as too complex, then the physician is more likely to not adopt the EMR (-0.231). Moreover, in contrast to the significant impact of federal government penalties, if penalties are from the state, the physician is less likely to adopt the technology (-0.292).

Beyond the interpretation of the beta weights, logistic regression offers the opportunity to determine the extent to which the independent variables can be utilized to discriminate between the two categories. In Table 7, the "observed column" indicates the number of individuals who were within each category (i.e. 134 non-adopters and 413 adopters). The "predicted" column displays the number of individuals who were classified into each category, with the numbers in bold indicating the number that were *correctly* classified. As the results in Table 7 indicate, the independent variables are able to correctly categorize adopters 92.5% of the time and non-adopters 49.3%, for an overall correct percentage of 81.9%. Therefore, these results demonstrate a significant ability to predict the adoption decision.

The results of the classification table indicate that the factors from the Technology-Organization-Environment framework are able to classify adopters at a higher rate than non-adopters. While the

model was able to correctly classify non-adopters only half the time, it provides the ability to correctly classify adopters in over 90% of cases.

The factors that are most significant in predicting adoption can be found in Figure 3, with the significant factors highlighted. Our results demonstrate that systems quality, competitive pressure, financial slack, perceived government regulation, internal data integration, and perceived availability contribute to the EMR adoption decision, while the other factors are non-significant.

10. DISCUSSION

Physicians are currently under heavy institutional pressure from both federal and state government to adopt EMR technology. The presence of this strong external pressure provided us with an opportunity to examine how external environmental pressure influences the adoption/non-adoption decision. Utilizing the T-O-E framework, we specified and studied constructs that assess the technological, organizational, and environmental contexts.

Our results indicate that each context exerts significant pressure on the adoption decision. Specifically, the technological factors of quality and availability, the environmental factors of competitive pressure and government regulation, and the organizational factors of financial slack and effective internal integration[4] are all significant drivers of adoption. Thus, by expanding our view of the factors influencing the adoption decision, we discovered that users want not only a high quality, reasonably priced systems but they also want the

Table 7. Classification table

	Observed	Predicted		
		Non-Adopters	Adopters	Percentage Correct
Non Adopters	134	**66**	68	49.3
Adopters	413	31	**382**	92.5
Overall Percentage	547			81.9

Figure 3. Results: Research model

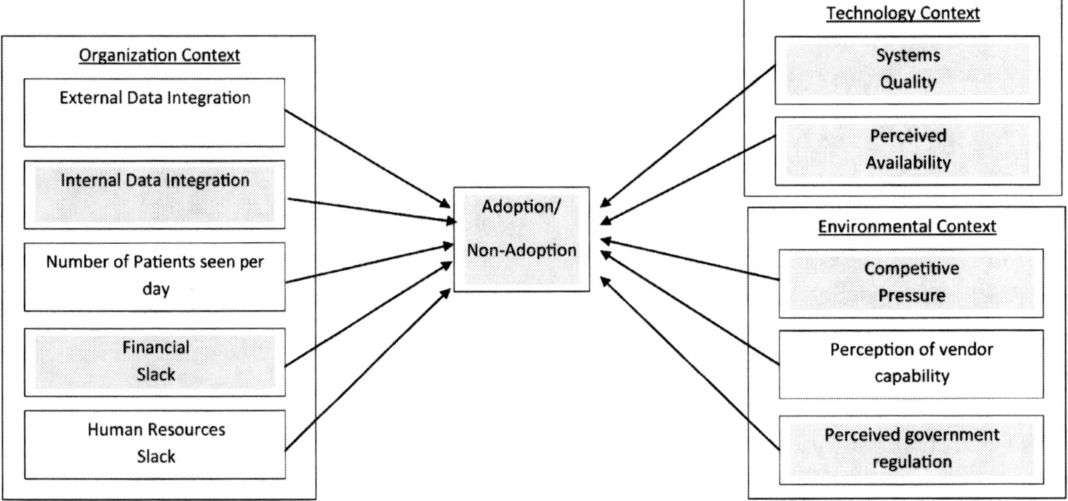

system to integrate effectively with other areas of the organization. Moreover, users are influenced by the extent to which competitors have adopted new technology, and they desire more availability of these systems in the marketplace. Government regulation, both from the state and federal government, has also been effective in inducing adoption. Therefore, this study demonstrates the importance of incorporating macro level factors when studying the adoption decision in a context with heavy institutional pressure.

The environmental pressures materialized not from the institutions that are currently seeking to pressure adoption (namely the federal and state governments), but more significantly from other physicians. Competitive pressure was a stronger factor in influencing adoption than either of these two key institutions. This finding suggests that additional work is necessary to understand the nexus of competitive and institutional pressures in organizational decision making. Furthermore, the positive beta weight for penalties from the federal government and the negative for penalties from the state government demonstrate that physicians want EMR adoption to be handled as a component of a broader national HIT strategy

as opposed to a more limited statewide initiative. Our findings indicate that driving this initiative at a more localized level is not an approach favored by physicians, and may result in lower adoption rates.

Moreover, the findings indicate that while users desire the system to combine data within their organization, they are not concerned about whether the system shares data across different organizations. As internal compatibility is typically a requirement for new technology now, users have developed an expectation that any new IT will seamlessly integrate into the organization. However, integration across organizations is not yet the norm, and users have not developed expectations that technology should be able to seamlessly integrate data between external entities. Thus, users are pragmatic about the limitations of current technology, and they are willing to wait for inter-organizational integration. We posit that users especially in a medical context realize that if a complex technology like the one necessary for external data integration is not yet established and stable, then utilization of it may cause more problems than it may fix. Instead, they desire the more mature and stable technology and do not yet need the untested cutting-edge technology.

When examining slack, we included two forms of slack, namely financial slack and human resources slack. While financial slack was found to influence adoption, human resources slack was unrelated to adoption. Thus, while physicians wanted to see a reasonable cost for the technology, the amount of time it would take to learn the new system was not a factor in their adoption decision. One may surmise that if the physician and his/her staff are spending their time learning the new system, then they have less time to see patients and make money to pay for the new system. However, this finding indicates that physicians believe that it will not take an inordinate amount of time to learn the new system, and that the value of the system is greater than the monetary cost.

11. LIMITATIONS

Our work, however, does not come without limitations. First, we have limited our study to four states within the United States. By utilizing a theoretically-based sampling technique, we seek to overcome this limitation by altering the influence of the environment (a chief motivation for the current study). Furthermore, as most previous EMR studies were conducted within one state or one hospital context, we posit that this study represents a broader study of adoption. Next, we were unable to calculate an accurate response rate for our physicians. However, the medical societies indicated to us that the response rate we received was typical. Third, while the original Technology-Organization-Environmental framework included reciprocating relationships between the constructs, we instead opted to focus upon the direct effects. This decision was made in order to focus attention upon our main constructs and the ability of these factors to explain the adoption/non-adoption decision. Finally, while we have included formal and informal linking relationships as one, we encourage other researchers to examine these two separately to determine their impact (including the

role of social contagion). Despite these limitations, the work has some important implications for both researchers and practitioners.

12. IMPLICATION FOR RESEARCHERS AND PRACTICE

For researchers, these findings demonstrate that adoption researchers needs to move beyond simple models that are focused upon micro-level factors to incorporate the broader context under which the adoption decision occurs. In the motivation for our work, we enumerated two limitations of prior work: (1) A lack of consistency in understanding the constructs within the T-O-E framework and (2) Not utilizing the framework where environmental considerations differ. By returning to the original framework, we proposed a model that was theoretically consistent with the original theory. While we recognize that contextualization is necessary, we urge other researchers to draw upon the richness of the original theory and to refine the theory rather than simply utilizing its' broad nature to amalgamate current theoretical approaches under an umbrella framework.

Our second critique was that the environment would influence the adoption decision. Our results validate this critique. However, our findings also demonstrate that the mechanisms that underpin institutional theory are more nuanced – namely that the institutions that seek to put pressure upon organizations may not be the most salient in influencing that behavior. In our context, one would expect that the penalties from the government (the institution seeking to encourage adoption) would be the strongest in influencing the adoption behavior, but in reality it was the competitive pressure that had the most significant impact. The chasm between the institution exerting the pressure and the institution having the most significant impact is an interesting and exciting area of research that we urge others to pursue.

Beyond our critiques, our findings provide a pathway for future research in three main areas. The first is in the domain of non-adoption. Our finding that our factors could only classify half of the non-adopters correctly indicates that more work is necessary in order to understand the behavior of non-adoption. An attempt to understand only the enablers (or positively valenced factors) in the adoption decision in the context of non-adoption does not enable us to adequately understand why a physician (or user) choses to not adopt a technology. According to Inhibitor Theory, inhibitors are worthy of their own investigation (Cenfetelli & Schwarz, 2011), and we urge other researchers to pursue this line of study.

Second, while we have organized our sample into two groups based upon the adoption decision, we acknowledge that the differences in organizational structure and the resulting impact on control may also influence the adoption decision. Thus, a physician in private practice may have control over the adoption decision, while in a hospital, a physician may tend to have less control over (or input into) the decision. We urge adoption researchers to begin to understand the organizational variables that can explain differences between organizational contexts as a mechanism to begin to understand the complexity of the adoption and non-adoption decision.

The third implication for future research is for researchers who are interested in the intersection between technology, organization, and environment. We first urge other researchers to use this framework to begin to understand the intersection of these factors. We argue that the focus on the IT artifact has come at the expense of understanding the organizational artifact and the impact of the environment. The T-O-E framework is designed to incorporate these often-overlooked contexts to provide insights into the broader role of the organization and environment in the adoption decision. We encourage others to utilize this lens to understand how varying organizational and environmental contexts influence the adoption decision.

For our colleagues-in-practice, our model demonstrates that with an understanding of seven factors, we can predict the adoption/non-adoption decision correctly 82% of the time. For physicians and EMR providers, quality and internal data integration are the two practice-focused factors that are salient. For policy makers, we urge careful consideration of the role of penalties, the availability of financial slack, and the presence of pressure from other physicians in order to influence the adoption decision.

13. CONCLUDING THOUGHTS

In conclusion, understanding the adoption/non-adoption decision is an important research and organizational-level topic that merits further investigation. In our study, we examined the impact of institutional pressure upon the adoption decision, examining whether the pressure escalates the salient factors away from the innovation (or micro) level to the organizational and environmental (or macro) level of analysis. We have discovered that there is some evidence that this is occurring; specifically, when heavy institutional pressure is present, environmental and organizational factors do matter. However, this shift towards the macro-level should not diminish micro-level factors. Instead, it presents an opportunity for the incorporation of both sets of factors in a more comprehensive examination of the decision to adopt or not to adopt.

ACKNOWLEDGMENT

This work was funded in part through a grant from the Physicians Foundation.

REFERENCES

Aiken, M., & Hage, J. (1971). The organic organization and innovation. *Sociology*, *5*(1), 63–82. doi:10.1177/003803857100500105

Anderson, J. G. (2007). Social, ethical and legal barriers to e-health. *International Journal of Medical Informatics*, *76*(5), 480–483. doi:10.1016/j.ijmedinf.2006.09.016 PMID:17064955

Angst, C. M., Agarwal, R., Sambamurthy, V., & Kelley, K. (2010). Social contagion and information technology diffusion: The adoption of electronic medical records in US hospitals. *Management Science*, *56*(8), 1219–1241. doi:10.1287/mnsc.1100.1183

Ash, J. S., & Bates, D. W. (2005). Factors and forces affecting EHR system adoption: Report of a 2004 ACMI discussion. *Journal of the American Medical Informatics Association*, *12*(1), 8–12. doi:10.1197/jamia.M1684 PMID:15492027

Baier, A. (1986). Trust and antitrust. *Ethics*, *96*(2), 231–260. doi:10.1086/292745

Baker, J. (2012). *The technology–organization–environment framework Information Systems Theory* (pp. 231–245). Springer. doi:10.1007/978-1-4419-6108-2_12

Bates, D. W., Ebell, M., Gotlieb, E., Zapp, J., & Mullins, H. (2003). A proposal for electronic medical records in US primary care. *Journal of the American Medical Informatics Association*, *10*(1), 1–10. doi:10.1197/jamia.M1097 PMID:12509352

Bergkvist, L., & Rossiter, J. R. (2007). The predictive validity of multiple-item versus single-item measures of the same constructs. *JMR, Journal of Marketing Research*, *44*(2), 175–184. doi:10.1509/jmkr.44.2.175

Bhattacherjee, A., & Hikmet, N. (2007). Physicians' resistance toward healthcare information technology: A theoretical model and empirical test. *European Journal of Information Systems*, *16*(6), 725–737. doi:10.1057/palgrave.ejis.3000717

Blumenthal, D. (2009). Stimulating the Adoption of Health Information Technology. *The New England Journal of Medicine*, *360*(15), 1477–1479. doi:10.1056/NEJMp0901592 PMID:19321856

Burt, C. W., & Sisk, J. E. (2005). Which physicians and practices are using electronic medical records? *Health Affairs*, *24*(5), 1334–1343. doi:10.1377/hlthaff.24.5.1334 PMID:16162581

Cenfetelli, R. T., & Schwarz, A. (2011). Identifying and Testing the Inhibitors of Technology Usage Intentions. *Information Systems Research*, *22*(4), 808–823. doi:10.1287/isre.1100.0295

Charles, D., King, J., Patel, V., & Furukawa, M. F. (2013). *Adoption of Electronic Health Record Systems among US Non-federal Acute Care Hospitals: 2008-2012.*. ONC Data Brief.

Chau, P. Y. K., & Tam, K. Y. (1997). Factors Affecting the Adoption of Open Systems: An Exploratory Study. *Management Information Systems Quarterly*, *21*(1), 1–24. doi:10.2307/249740

Damanpour, F. (1992). Organizational size and innovation. *Organization Studies*, *13*(3), 375–402. doi:10.1177/017084069201300304

Davis, F. D. (1993). User acceptance of information technology: System characteristics, user perceptions and behavioral impacts. *International Journal of Man-Machine Studies*, *38*(3), 475–487. doi:10.1006/imms.1993.1022

De Palma, A., Myers, G. M., & Papageorgiou, Y. Y. (1994). Rational choice under an imperfect ability to choose. *The American Economic Review*, 419–440.

DeLone, W. H., & McLean, E. R. (1992). Information systems success: The quest for the dependent variable. *Information Systems Research, 3*(1), 60–95. doi:10.1287/isre.3.1.60

DesRoches, C. M., Campbell, E. G., Sowmya, R. R., Rao, S. R., Donelan, K., & Ferris, T. G. et al. (2008). Electronic health records in ambulatory care–a national survey of physicians. *The New England Journal of Medicine, 359*(1), 50–60. doi:10.1056/NEJMsa0802005 PMID:18565855

DiMaggio, P. J., & Powell, W. W. (1983). The iron cage revisited: Institutional isomorphism and collective rationality in organizational fields. *American Sociological Review, 48*(2), 147–160. doi:10.2307/2095101

Drolet, A. L., & Morrison, D. G. (2001). Do we really need multiple-item measures in service research? *Journal of Service Research, 3*(3), 196–204. doi:10.1177/109467050133001

Fichman, R. G., Kohli, R., & Krishnan, R. (2011). The Role of Information Systems in Healthcare: Current Research and Future Trends. *Information Systems Research, 22*(3), 419–428. doi:10.1287/isre.1110.0382

Foundation, R. J. W. (2012). Health Information Technology in the United States: Driving Toward Delivery System Change, 2012. 2013, from http://www.rwjf.org/content/dam/farm/reports/reports/2012/rwjf72707

Gans, D., Kralewski, J., Hammons, T., & Dowd, B. (2005). Medical groups' adoption of electronic health records and information systems. *Health Affairs, 24*(5), 1323–1333. doi:10.1377/hlthaff.24.5.1323 PMID:16162580

Garfinkel, H. (1963). A conception of and experiments with" trust" as a condition of concerted stable actions. *The production of reality: Essays and readings on social interaction*, 381-392.

Goodhue, D. L., Quillard, J. A., & Rockart, J. F. (1988). Managing the data resource: A contingency perspective. *Management Information Systems Quarterly, 12*(3), 373–392. doi:10.2307/249204

Goodhue, D. L., & Thompson, R. L. (1995). Task-technology fit and individual performance. *Management Information Systems Quarterly, 19*(2), 213–236. doi:10.2307/249689

Goodhue, D. L., Wybo, M. D., & Kirsch, L. J. (1992). The impact of data integration on the costs and benefits of information systems. *Management Information Systems Quarterly, 16*(3), 293–311. doi:10.2307/249530

Greve, H. R. (2003). A behavioral theory of R&D expenditures and innovations: Evidence from shipbuilding. *Academy of Management Journal, 46*(6), 685–702. doi:10.2307/30040661

Hage, J. (1980). *Theories of Organizations: Form, Process, and Transformation*. Wiley New York.

Heiner, R. A. (1983). The origin of predictable behavior. *The American Economic Review, 73*(4), 560–595.

Hobson, K. (2011). Getting Docs to Use PCs. *The Wall Street Journal Online*.

Hsiao, C.-J., & Hing, E. (2014). *Use and Characteristics of Electronic Health Record Systems Among Office-based Physician Practices* (pp. 2001–2012). United States: US Department of Health and Human Services, Centers for Disease Control and Prevention, National Center for Health Statistics.

Kimberly, J. R., & Evanisko, M. J. (1981). Organizational innovation: The influence of individual, organizational, and contextual factors on hospital adoption of technological and administrative innovations. *Academy of Management Journal, 24*(4), 689–713. doi:10.2307/256170 PMID:10253688

Kuan, K. K. Y., & Chau, P. Y. K. (2001). A Perception-Based Model for EDI Adoption in Small Businesses Using a Technology-Organization-Environment Framework. *Information & Management*, *38*(8), 507–521. doi:10.1016/S0378-7206(01)00073-8

Lapointe, L., & Rivard, S. (2005). A Multilevel Model of Resistance to Information Technology Implementation. *Management Information Systems Quarterly*, *29*(3), 461–492.

Lee, O. K., Wang, M., Lim, K. H., & Peng, Z. (2009). Knowledge management systems diffusion in Chinese enterprises: A multistage approach using the technology-organization-environment framework. [JGIM]. *Journal of Global Information Management*, *17*(1), 70–84. doi:10.4018/jgim.2009010104

Lewis, J. D., & Weigert, A. (1985). Trust as a social reality. *Social Forces*, *63*(4), 967–985. doi:10.1093/sf/63.4.967

Lin, H. F., & Lin, S. M. (2008). Determinants of e-business diffusion: A test of the technology diffusion perspective. *Technovation*, *28*(3), 135–145. doi:10.1016/j.technovation.2007.10.003

Liu, M. (2008). Determinants of e-commerce development: An empirical study by firms in Shaanxi, China. *International Conference on Wireless Communications, Networking and Mobile Computing*, 2008. doi:10.1109/WiCom.2008.2143

March, J. G. (1978). Rationality, ambiguity, and the engineering of choice. *The Bell Journal of Economics*, *9*(2), 587–608. doi:10.2307/3003600

McKnight, D. H., Choudhury, V., & Kacmar, C. (2002). Developing and validating trust measures for e-commerce: An integrative typology. *Information Systems Research*, *13*(3), 334–359. doi:10.1287/isre.13.3.334.81

Miller, C. (2003). Hidden in plain sight: Understanding nonprofit capital structure. *The Nonprofit Quarterly*, *10*(1), 1–7.

Miller, D., & Friesen, P. H. (1982). Innovation in conservative and entrepreneurial firms: Two models of strategic momentum. *Strategic Management Journal*, *3*(1), 1–25. doi:10.1002/smj.4250030102

Miller, R. H., & Sim, I. (2004). Physicians' use of electronic medical records: Barriers and solutions. *Health Affairs*, *23*(2), 116–126. doi:10.1377/hlthaff.23.2.116 PMID:15046136

Miller, R. K. (2011). *Healthcare Business Market Research Handbook*. Loganville, GA: Richard K. Miller and Associates.

Mishina, Y., Pollock, T. G., & Porac, J. F. (2004). Are more resources always better for growth? Resource stickiness in market and product expansion. *Strategic Management Journal*, *25*(12), 1179–1197. doi:10.1002/smj.424

Moore, G. C., & Benbasat, I. (1991). Development of an instrument to measure the perceptions of adopting an information technology innovation. *Information Systems Research*, *2*(3), 192–222. doi:10.1287/isre.2.3.192

Nelson, R. R., Todd, P. A., & Wixom, B. H. (2005). Antecedents of Information and System Quality: An Empirical Examination Within the Context of Data Warehousing. *Journal of Management Information Systems*, *21*(4), 199–235.

Oliveira, T., & Martins, M. F. (2009). Determinants of Information Technology Adoption in Portugal. Paper presented at the *International Conference on e-Business*.

Oliveira, T., & Martins, M. F. (2010). Firms Patterns of E-Business Adoption: Evidence for the European Union- 27. *The Electronic Journal of Information Systems Evaluation*, *13*(1), 47–56.

Øvretveit, J., Scott, T., Rundall, T. G., Shortell, S. M., & Brommels, M. (2007). Improving quality through effective implementation of information technology in healthcare. *International Journal for Quality in Health Care*, *19*(5), 259–266. doi:10.1093/intqhc/mzm031 PMID:17717038

Pan, M. J., & Jang, W. Y. (2008). Determinants of the adoption of enterprise resource planning within the technology-organization-environment framework: Taiwan's communications. *Journal of Computer Information Systems*, *48*(3), 94–102.

Petrescu, M. (2013). Marketing research using single-item indicators in structural equation models. *Journal of Marketing Analytics*, *1*(2), 99–117. doi:10.1057/jma.2013.7

Reardon, J. L., & Davidson, E. (2007). An organizational learning perspective on the assimilation of electronic medical records among small physician practices. *European Journal of Information Systems*, *16*(6), 681–694. doi:10.1057/palgrave.ejis.3000714

Robey, D., & Boudreau, M. C. (1999). Accounting for the contradictory organizational consequences of information technology: Theoretical directions and methodological implications. *Information Systems Research*, *10*(2), 167–185. doi:10.1287/isre.10.2.167

Saeed, K. A., & Abdinnour-Helm, S. (2008). Examining the effects of information system characteristics and perceived usefulness on post adoption usage of information systems. *Information & Management*, *45*(6), 376–386. doi:10.1016/j.im.2008.06.002

Schwarz, A., & Chin, W. (2007). Looking forward: Toward an understanding of the nature and definition of IT acceptance. *Journal of the Association for Information Systems*, *8*(4), 4.

Schwarz, A., Schwarz, C., & Cenfetelli, R. T. (2012). A Profile of Rejecters of Electronic Medical Record Technology. Paper presented at the *Americas Conference on Information Systems*.

Scott, W. R. (1987). The Adolescence of Institutional Theory. *Administrative Science Quarterly*, *32*(4), 493–511. doi:10.2307/2392880

Scott, W. R. (2003). *Organizations: Rational, Natural and Open Systems*. NJ: Prentice Hall.

Shekelle, P., Morton, S. C., & Keeler, E. B. (2006). Costs and Benefits of Health Information Technology. *Evidence Reports/Technology Assessments*, 132.

Sherer, S. A. (2010). Information Systems and Healthcare XXXIII: An Institutional Theory Perspective on Physician Adoption of Electronic Health Records. *Communications of the Association for Information Systems*, *26*(1), 7.

Shi, W., Shambare, N., & Wang, J. (2008). The adoption of internet banking: An institutional theory perspective. *Journal of Financial Services Marketing*, *12*(4), 272–286. doi:10.1057/palgrave.fsm.4760081

Simon, H. A. (1955). A behavioral model of rational choice. *The Quarterly Journal of Economics*, *69*(1), 99–118. doi:10.2307/1884852

Simon, S. R., Kaushal, R., Cleary, P. D., Jenter, C. A., Volk, L. A., & Poon, E. G. et al. (2007). Correlates of electronic health record adoption in office practices: A statewide survey. *Journal of the American Medical Informatics Association*, *14*(1), 110–117. doi:10.1197/jamia.M2187 PMID:17068351

Son, J.-Y., & Benbasat, I. (2007). Organizational Buyers' Adoption and Use of B2B Electronic Marketplaces: Efficiency- and Legitimacy-Oriented Perspectives. *Journal of Management Information Systems*, *24*(1), 55–99. doi:10.2753/MIS0742-1222240102

Teo, H. H., Wei, K. K., & Benbasat, I. (2003). Predicting Intention To Adopt Interorganizational Linkages: An Institutional Perspective. *Management Information Systems Quarterly*, *27*(1), 19–49.

Teo, T. S., Ranganathan, C., & Dhaliwal, J. (2006). Key dimensions of inhibitors for the deployment of web-based business-to-business electronic commerce. *IEEE Transactions on Engineering Management, 53*(3), 395–411. doi:10.1109/TEM.2006.878106

Tornatzky, L. G., & Fleischer, M. (1990). *The Processes of Technological Innovation.* Lexington, MA: Lexington Books.

Urgin, J. C. (2009). The Effect of System Characteristics, Stage of Adoption, and Experience on Institutional Explanations for ERP Systems Choice. *Accounting Horizons, 23*(4), 365–389. doi:10.2308/acch.2009.23.4.365

Van de Ven, A. H. (2005). Running in Packs to Develop Knowledge-Intensive Technologies. *Management Information Systems Quarterly, 29*(2), 365–377.

Venkatesh, V., Morris, M. G., Davis, G. B., & Davis, F. D. (2003). User Acceptance of Information Technology: Toward a Unified View. *Management Information Systems Quarterly, 27*(3), 425–478.

Venkatesh, V., Thong, J. Y. L., & Xu, X. (2012). Consumer acceptance and use of information technology: Extending the unified theory of acceptance and use of technology. *Management Information Systems Quarterly, 36*(1), 157–178.

Voss, G. B., Sirdeshmukh, D., & Voss, Z. G. (2008). The Effects of Slack Resources and Environmentalthreat on Product Exploration and Exploitation. *Academy of Management Journal, 51*(1), 147–164. doi:10.5465/AMJ.2008.30767373

Wanous, J. P., & Reichers, A. E. (1996). Estimating the reliability of a single-item measure. *Psychological Reports, 78*(2), 631–634. doi:10.2466/pr0.1996.78.2.631

Zhu, K., & Kraemer, K. L. (2005). Post-Adoption Variations in Usage and Value of E-Business by Organizations: Cross-Country Evidence from the Retail Industry. *Information Systems Research, 16*(1), 61–84. doi:10.1287/isre.1050.0045

Zhu, K., Kraemer, K. L., & Xu, S. (2003). Electronic business adoption by European firms: A cross-country assessment of the facilitators and inhibitors. *European Journal of Information Systems, 12*(4), 251–268. doi:10.1057/palgrave.ejis.3000475

Zhu, K., Kraemer, K. L., & Xu, S. (2006). The Process of Innovation Assimilation by Firms in Different Countries: A Technology Diffusion Perspective on E-Business. *Management Science, 52*(10), 1557–1576. doi:10.1287/mnsc.1050.0487

ENDNOTES

[1] We acknowledge that physician may have concerns with data integration regarding potential problems with data security and potential power differentials that could come as a result (Angst, et al 2010).

[2] The issue of single-item versus multiple-item constructs is debated within the measurement community, with proponents on both sides of the issue (Petrescu, 2013). However, we have selected single item constructs for contextual reasons, namely that in the case of long and complicated surveys, for hard to reach populations (such as physicians), single item scales are appropriate and justifiable without a loss in reliability or validity (Wanous and Reichers, 1996; Drolet and Morrison, 2001; Bergkvist and Rossiter, 2007).

[3]   Due to the privacy concerns of the medical societies, the link to the web-based survey was distributed by the medical society to their membership database. As membership in a medical society is not restricted to just physicians, an accurate number of practicing physicians (the target population) within the database is unknown or was not provided. While the medical societies indicated to us that the response rate we received was typical, an actual response rate was unable to be calculated.

[4]   While the negative beta weight for internal data integration may appear counter-intuitive, we theorize that this finding was due to the word "effectively" in our research item. We suggest that physicians were responding over skepticism that an EMR solution would *effectively* integrate their firm, not about the overall goal of integration per se. We encourage additional research into this factor.

This work was previously published in the Journal of Organizational and End User Computing (JOEUC), 26(4); edited by Tanya McGill, pages 57-79 copyright year 2014 by IGI Publishing (an imprint of IGI Global).

Chapter 21
Review of the Consumer Perspective Framework for Healthcare Applications

Eh Eh Tin
University of Tasmania, Australia

Elizabeth Cummings
University of Tasmania, Australia

Elizabeth Borycki
University of Victoria, Canada

ABSTRACT

Cummings, Borycki, and Roehrer (2013) developed a Consumer Perspectives Framework that identified a range of consumer-related issues and concerns that should be considered when downloading and using healthcare applications for mobile phones. The framework identifies data-related issues with mobile applications, such as ownership, location, completeness, corporate use, storage, and privacy. This chapter documents research undertaken in confirming the Consumer Perspectives Framework. Finally, the authors propose a method by which the Consumer Perspectives Framework can be implemented for use by consumers prior to downloading healthcare applications.

INTRODUCTION

The ubiquity of mobile phone accessibility around the world is increasing. Worldwide the number of mobile phones in use grew from fewer than 1 billion in 2000 to around 6 billion in 2012. Recent estimates conclude that over 75% of the world's population have access to a mobile phone (World Bank, 2012). Globally, there has been a rapid rise in the use of smart phones by consumers with over 1 billion Smart Phones subscribers (Approximately 30% of smartphone users are likely to use wellness apps by 2015, (Bjornland, Goh, Haanæs, Kainu, & Kennedy, 2012) with more than 30 billion mobile applications being downloaded in 2011 (World Bank, 2012).

DOI: 10.4018/978-1-4666-8756-1.ch021

Along with this increase in penetration, there has been a significant increase in the development and deployment of mobile software applications across multiple computing platforms (e.g. smart phones, tablets and laptops). The most popular of these include Apple's iOS and Google's Android software. Both were designed for use with touch screen mobile devices such as iPhones. Today, there are a plethora of differing types of software applications that have been made available for use with the iOS and Android platforms. Software applications written for mobile or smart phones serve a range of purposes and uses, including; business, financial, educational, entertainment, gaming, lifestyle, health and fitness, news, music, photography, productivity, reference, graphics and design, developer tool, medical and health care consumer applications.

More recently, there has emerged significant interest in health care applications written for mobile phones. Mobile phone software applications are of particular interest because of their ability (in some cases) to improve lifestyle habits in well individuals and improve health outcomes in the chronically ill (Katz, Mesfin, & Barr, 2012).

In conjunction with this there has emerged a significant growth in the number of consumers that are downloading these health specific software applications for self-use (Kay, Santos, & Takane, 2011). Research suggests that mobile phone users use differing types of software applications in conjunction with their smart phones and their use of specific software applications may be role dependent. For example, research has found that physicians and other health care professionals tend to use mobile health applications that differ from those used by patients or members of the general public. Physicians and health professionals are more likely to use mobile software applications that provide them with access to references to health care information (e.g. guidelines, information found in journal articles). These applications provide information to health professionals (i.e. they allow health profession-

als to review evidence-based research) that can be used in their clinical decision making. Unlike health care consumers that input data into mobile health applications, health professionals are less likely to employ mobile applications in the process of collecting data about patients. This may be because health professionals may perceive there to be privacy and security issues associated with collecting, transmitting and storing patient data via a mobile device (Jones, Hook, Park, & Scott, 2011). As well, mobile phone applications present a potential risk for public health as some software applications have been questioned in regards to their clinical efficacy and other such software applications have been noted to induce technology-induced errors. Technology induced errors are errors made by software/hardware users that "arise from the: design and development of a technology; implementation and customisation of a technology; and interactions between the operation of a new technology and the new work processes that arise from the technology's use" (Borycki & Kushniruk, 2008).

Therefore, even as some software applications have been shown to improve consumer health and wellness, there have emerged concerns about the quality of these applications, the privacy and confidentiality of the information captured by these software applications (Spiekermann & Lorrie, 2009) and the ability of the technology to introduce technology-induced errors (Borycki & Kushniruk, 2008). This has led to calls by some researchers to achieve a balance between patient safety and innovation in mobile application development with the intent that no harm should occur to the general public (Barton, 2012) and for a deep integration of consumers' perspectives into the development of applications. More user centric applications for Smart Phones are needed (Jones et al., 2011).

This has led some researchers to develop frameworks that can aid consumers and health professionals to better understand and make decisions regarding the use of the technology. For example, researchers such as Cummings, Borycki and Roehrer (2013) have identified a number of issues that should be considered by consumers and health professionals when considering using these applications. In their work they developed a consumer perspective framework that identifies the relation between the use of health related consumer software applications and privacy, confidentiality and safety of the applications. The framework describes a method that can be used by consumers to evaluate health related applications before purchasing the software for use with a mobile or smart phone. The framework can be used by consumers as an aid to selecting the right health related software applications for their own personal use. Therefore, in order to better understand how these mobile software applications are being used as well as some of the issues that have arisen in recent years, the authors have conducted a review of the literature and a review of a range of free iOS applications in relation to the Consumer Perspective Framework.

CONSUMER PERSPECTIVES FRAMEWORK

The potential benefits of mobile software applications in assisting consumers in obtaining, managing and maintaining healthy lifestyles is evident. For example, the ability to incorporate Global Positioning Systems (GPS) and location tracking into a mobile software application provides additional opportunities for health and lifestyle maintenance as well as community-based data collection that can be used in public health surveillance (Aanensen, Huntley, Feil, al-Own, & Spratt, 2009). However, there continue to be a number of risks associated with the use of these technologies – they include issues in and around confidentiality of citizen information and security risks associated with using the technology.

Many of these mobile software applications are easy to purchase on the WWW so consumers can easily buy this technology for use. Therefore, the burden of assessing where the technology is appropriate rests with the individual consumer. To date there have been few published frameworks that can help consumers evaluate software for issues and risks associated with its use. One such framework that can be used by consumers and health professionals to assess their mobile device software is the *Consumer Perspectives Framework* by Cummings et al. (2013).

Cummings et al.'s (2013) *Consumer Perspectives Framework* allows the consumer or health professional to consider (for their personal use) mobile health care applications and helps the consumer to determine if the mobile health care application is appropriate for them. The framework emphasises some key aspects of mobile application use that should be considered by consumers in relation to health and lifestyle prior to purchase (see Table 1). In the framework mobile phones and their associated applications are reviewed in context of data and software issues. Data issues include storage and privacy, ownership, corporate use, location, and completeness. Software issues include accessibility, clinical effectiveness, credibility, information quality, and consumer usage.

In relation to the category of data issues, storage and privacy refer to ensuring the privacy of data is not violated and that it is stored in a secure manner. Ownership refers to who claims or maintains ownership of the data that is collected and stored through use of the software application. Corporate use is related to ownership but refers to the use of data by the application developer for their own purposes that are not necessarily evident at the

Table 1. Consumer Perspectives Framework

Data Issues	Software Issues
Storage and privacy	Accessibility
Ownership	Clinical effectiveness
Corporate use	Credibility
Location	Information quality
Completeness	Consumer usage

Source: Cummings et. al. (2013)

time of collection or storage. Location relates to the actual location at which data is stored, which can be an issue if data crosses national borders. Completeness relates to the completeness of the data that is collected.

Software issues are the other main category described in the consumer perspectives framework. This includes such things as accessibility which refers to the ability to easily identify and access reliable applications. Clinical effectiveness refers to whether there is evidence of the effectiveness of the app. Information quality relates to the quality and accuracy of information and advice provided through the software and consumer usage refers to the motivation behind a consumer's use of the application. Each of these issues needs to be considered by consumers when purchasing mobile health care applications.

METHOD

During January 2013, a broad literature search was conducted using ProQuest and Web of Knowledge using the following key words; Storage and Privacy, Ownership, Corporate Use, Location, and Completeness, Accessibility, Clinical Effectiveness, Credibility, Information quality, Consumer Usage, and mobile app*. We chose to focus our search on consumer medical, health and fitness applications used on mobile phones as this is the focus of the *Consumer Perspectives Framework*. Following this, the abstracts of articles focusing on the above outlined key areas that were published after 2006 were reviewed by two individuals trained in health informatics. Articles post 2006 were used as this is the timeframe for the rise in the use of mobile phones and subsequent increase

Figure 1. Literature search method

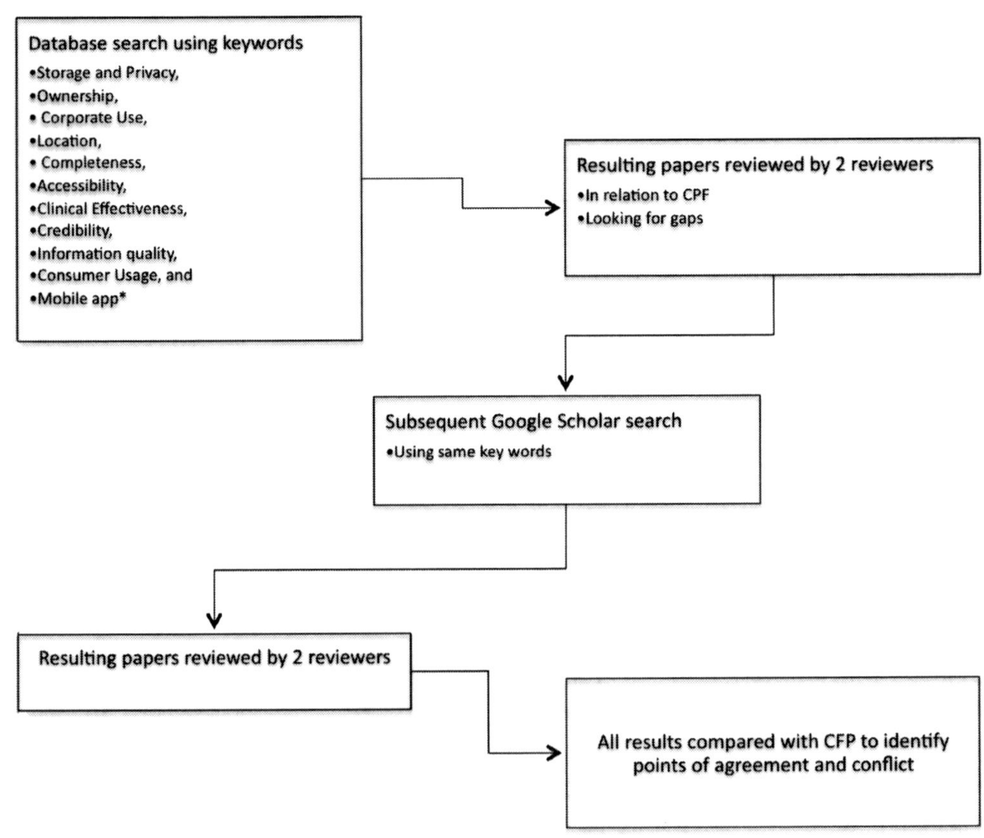

in the development of mobile applications. Articles that met the following criteria were reviewed more fully for their quality and within the context of Cummings and colleagues' framework:

- Articles that described the use of mobile phone applications in relation to consumers in the community;
- Articles outlined the issues with mobile phone applications in relation to consumers in the community; and
- Articles where mobile phone application use was not prescribed by a medical practitioner.

Grey literature, including web based publications, were sourced from a Google search to supplement the original search and ensure completeness.

RESULTS

Forty articles were returned. Eighteen articles met our criteria and were read. As each article was read the researchers developed a table (see Table 2) that describes the articles more fully (i.e. author name, year of publication, sample, setting, methods and key findings). From our review of the literature using the lens of the Cummings et al. framework we identified several themes that emerged and are in keeping with the Consumers Perspectives Framework (see Table 2).

In our review of the literature we found that few researchers fully address the elements of the Consumer Perspectives Framework. This may indicate that few consumers are aware that mobile software applications have issues associated with their use or that consumers may have little interest in understanding the technology. More research is needed to understand the underlying reasons for this phenomenon. However, there were also some concerns noted in the literature that were outside the expectations of the framework. A broader dis-

cussion in relation to the literature highlights and a number of considerations will be discussed in the next section. The authors begin by discussing those aspects of the literature review that validate the framework.

Storage and Privacy

Computing activities such as data collection, storage and processing may lead to an invasion of privacy and may raise privacy concerns among consumers (Spiekermann & Lorrie, 2009). Most mobile applications require interaction with internal or external systems to produce expected results. A recent study found that integrated personal health records (PHRs) can have a huge impact upon patient care, leading to transformational changes in health care delivery as well as self-care by patients (Detmer, Bloomrosen, Raymond, & Tang, 2008). Electronic exchange of personal health information is a major concern for the public. Survey research suggests that consumer concerns about confidentiality and security issues still remain where technology is concerned (Detmer et al., 2008). With the rise in popularity of Smart Phone applications (with varying functions) among medical practitioners, clinicians, medical students and patients, there has also arisen an increased concern about patient privacy (Mosa, Yoo, & Sheets, 2012). This indicates that high use of mobile applications by those working in the health sector and by the general public will also lead to increased awareness of sharing patient and personal information via mobile applications.

Privacy has become a major concern for individuals. Survey research suggests that people are very concerned about privacy especially in the U.S where the majority of people say there is no reasonable level of consumer privacy protection and this allows companies to share personal information inappropriately (IAPP, 2011; Spiekermann & Lorrie, 2009; Whitaker, 2008). The key things consumers want from their health privacy include

Table 2. Consumer Perspective Framework related literature example

		Literature	Comment
Data Issues	Storage and Privacy	Spiekermann and Lorrie (2009)	A framework for privacy friendly systems was discussed: the framework provides the two designs for systems development through the use of privacy by policy and privacy by architecture.
		Croll (2011)	How data is used affects its value. The main concern for application consumers is the inappropriate use of their personal data.
	Ownership	Spiekermann and Lorrie (2009)	Secondly use of data by third parties was discussed by various literature. Some users prefer their online data should not be available to any third party. An increasing majority of US citizens say that existing laws and organizational practices do not provide a reasonable level of consumer privacy protection and that companies share personal information inappropriately.
	Corporate Use	Whitaker (2008)	The key things consumers want from their health privacy include trust, quality of service, transparency and respect.
		IAPP (2011)	Cases for misused information are discussed.
	Location	None found	
	Completeness	HIMSS (2012)	Suggest that instead of completeness, it would be more general to say as *usability* which covers usability issues including completeness. Usability is the effectiveness, efficiency and satisfaction with which specific users can achieve a specific set of tasks in a particular environment.
Software Issues	Accessibility	Luxton, McCann, Bush, Mishkind, and Reger (2011)	More research is needed to provide data on the usability and clinical effectiveness of Smartphone technology in the behavioural health field.
	Clinical Effectiveness	Gustafson et. al. (2011)	It is too early to generalize about the usefulness applications especially for non-evaluated applications.
		Gerdes and Ohrstrom (20110	Although methods exist to evaluate software credibility there is still a need for more measurements and evaluation (e.g., further refinement as well as empirical support informing us about issues of system credibility).

trust, quality of service, transparency and respect (Whitaker, 2008). The consumer perspective framework suggests there are data issues relevant to storage and privacy of a consumer's data stored on their Smart Phones or remotely on servers. Location based software applications may even collect consumers' data to identify a customer's location for accuracy. However, some businesses or application developers fail to notify users of how sensitive data are stored. There are two main approaches towards ensuring the privacy of consumers' data. They are privacy by policy and privacy by architecture (Spiekermann & Lorrie, 2009). In the future application developers will need guidance, where the design and development of mobile applications, is concerned.

Ownership of the Data

Acquiring ownership of data in the digital age is quite a challenge as there is no physical possession of collected data to establish a boundary of ownership. Data storage and processing are required as part of many smartphone applications (Barton, 2012; Detmer et al., 2008; Laakko, Leppanen, Lahteenmaki, & Nummiaho, 2008; Mosa et al., 2012; Ng, Sim, & Tan, 2006; Perrig, Stankovic, & Wagner, 2004; Shi & Perrig, 2004; Spiekermann & Lorrie, 2009). However, Smart Phones have limited capabilities for storing and processing data so they may require external storage and processing power (Laakko et al., 2008). Data that flows out of users' devices may be accessible by third parties in various ways and may be used for many purposes. Consumers need to understand how secure the security mechanism build is in the type of Smart Phone they are using as well as the level of security being considered in application development. Nowadays many software applications utilise centralised storage for easy access to data and interoperability between different Smart Phone platforms.

The privacy-by-policy approach focuses on the implementation of the notice and choice principles of fair information practices, while the privacy-by-architecture approach minimises the collection of identifiable personal data and emphasises anonymisation and client-side data storage and processing (Spiekermann & Lorrie, 2009). A number of studies have investigated individuals' privacy concerns (Brown & Muchira, 2004) and there are seven areas of activity that cause concerns (Smith, Milberg, & Burke, 1996): collection and storage of extensive amounts of personal data, unauthorised secondary use by the collecting organisation, unauthorised secondary use by an external organisation with whom personal data has been shared, unauthorised access to personal data, e.g., identity theft or snooping into records, errors in personal data, whether deliberately or accidentally created, poor judgment through decisions made automatically based on incorrect or partial personal data, and a combination of personal data from separate databases to create a combined and thus more comprehensive profile for a person.

Corporate Use

According to Cummings et al. (2013), corporate use and access to data collected by and entered into a mobile software application should be considered an important issue by consumers and health professionals who are reviewing mobile software applications and making decisions about using them. Here, the researchers identified that some mobile software applications developed by

some corporations were collecting data about the users and it was unclear how the data was being used. In the research literature few publications described this potential consumer/health professional concern. In addition, there was little research that described how such data were used by corporations (if it was collected). Instead, much of the dialogue in the literature focused on the importance of maintaining the privacy of consumer data (see earlier section above). There were a few case studies that were published in the literature and described the misuse of information collected by mobile devices (IAPP, 2011). More research is needed in this area to determine if health care consumers and health professionals are concerned about health data being collected by corporations and to what extent the corporate analysis of that data (e.g. for marketing purposes) is a concern for consumers.

Location

Cummings and colleagues (2013) suggested that location based information collected by mobile devices and their software should be a concern for health care consumers and health professionals. Here, the researchers suggested that some consumers or health professionals do not want their location to be tracked on a daily or ongoing basis. In reviewing the literature focusing on the ability of mobile devices to continually provide information about the location of an individual, there was little literature that specifically identified location as an important type of data that health care consumers were concerned about reporting to an organisation or to other individuals.

It is interesting and worthy to note, that new mobile software applications are being developed that allow health care consumers to provide information about their location and the type of activity they are engaging in. In the case of these applications, such software not only report on the location of the individual, but on other individuals that they are tracking or others who may be in the same area or region of a park, city block etc. Such software applications allow individuals to track each other's locations. Such tracking may provide some individuals with incentives to continue engaging in an activity or to find other individuals who are engaging in a similar activity at the same time. For example, a jogger may wish to know if his or her friends are also jogging and where they are located so they can jog to that persons location and then jog as a group rather than an individual. The ability to track the location of individuals can turn a solitary physical activity into a group-based one and this may motivate some individuals to exercise more often. More research is needed to determine if disclosure of location is a concern for those who use these types of applications and if such disclosure of location in conjunction with a physical activity can lead to greater physical activity by those using such applications.

Completeness

Completeness of the mobile software application is another aspect of the Cummings framework that needs to be considered. Completeness can be defined as having all the necessary or appropriate parts (Oxford University Press, 2013). In the research literature, completeness is linked to the usability of mobile software. Here, researchers such as Kushniruk et al. (2005) have suggested that all software needs to be efficient, effective, enjoyable, safe and learnable in order for it to be usable. Tied to this is the ability of the mobile software to collect all information that is needed to provide feedback to the user, but at the same time to be usable. Research is needed to identify those mobile phone interface designs that balance the need to collect sufficient information for the software application to act as a true aid to the health care consumer while at the same time be easy to use or usable so the software application's design is not a barrier to its full use. More research will be needed to understand the nature of this balance between clinical effectiveness, completeness and usability.

Accessibility

Accessibility is degree to which an application is available to as many people as possible. There are two aspects to this: firstly, it is related to how easy it is to access and download applications, and secondly, it relates to the ability to be accessed and used by all people irrespective of ability or disability. Currently there is a lack of interoperability between mobile application platforms and so applications need to be developed for specific platforms (Cummings et al., 2013; Qiang, Yamamichi, Hausman, & Altman, 2011). To maximise the benefits and potential power of health and wellbeing applications as tools for assisting consumers take control it is necessary to create an open-source platform that can be used across operating systems (Qiang et al., 2011)

Clinical Effectiveness

Clinical Effectiveness or the ability of the mobile software application to improve a patient's clinical outcomes is an important area of research. In the framework, Cummings and colleagues (2013), identify that it is important for all mobile software applications to be reviewed in terms of their clinical effectiveness. Here, a consumer or health professional should ask the question; will the mobile phone software improve my health outcomes? (e.g. help me reduce my weight if I am obese, help me control my blood glucose levels if I have diabetes). In recent years there have been a number of studies have attempted to determine if such mobile software can lead to improvements in health outcomes. Some researchers have found that some mobile software, when targeted to a specific aspect of a disease and when designed to be usable and easy to integrate into an individual's life, can effectively improve health outcomes in that individual. Yet, this is not the case for all software. Here, consumers and health professionals need to be cognisant that some software does not provide clinically effective interventions that could improve a person's health outcomes. As well, poorly designed software that is neither usable nor easily used in the context of one's lifestyle may not be clinically effective. There is a need to for future research to fully describe how mobile phone software can be clinically effective and what consumers should look for to determine if the software they are purchasing leads to better health outcomes.

Credibility

Cummings and colleagues (2013) identify that mobile software credibility should be considered from a consumer perspective. Credibility can be defined as the quality of being trusted and believed in (Oxford University Press, 2013). Over the past several years, there have been numerous research publications that have documented the importance of obtaining information from a credible source when looking for information on the world wide web. Internationally, the credibility of health information remains a significant concern that many countries and individuals continue to struggle with when assessing information found on websites. Many government and health care organisations provide credible information for consumers to review and use in their health care journeys. For example, the government of the United States provides information on the National Institutes of Health website for health professionals and consumers. The information is developed by individuals who have a health care background and specialist expertise in varying health care conditions and diseases. Health care organisations such as the Canadian Lung Association also provide information to health care consumers about specific lung disease to help them not only learn about the disease but to identify health care resources in their community. As well, there are several tools that can be used by consumers to assess the quality of information published on a website and there are organisations that certify the quality of information on a given health care website.

There is a range of organisations that offer health care consumers the ability to purchase health care software. Many of these organisations guarantee the quality of the software itself, but may not guarantee the credibility of the corporation that developed the software. Some health care consumers may find this confusing. Future research may involve developing and testing tools that can help health care consumers evaluate the credibility of mobile phone software.

Information Quality

Information quality and credibility are linked together in some of the mobile software literature. Interestingly, information quality remains a concern even when considered in the context of mobile applications. There is concern about the clinical effectiveness of mobile software applications, the credibility of the organisations who produce these technologies and also the quality of the information provided or produced by these devices. In the research literature a key theme has emerged where information quality is considered in the context of mobile software applications. The key theme in this area is the need for education for consumers about the importance of information quality and how information quality should be assessed by consumers when considering using such applications (AHIMA, 2007). As some researchers suggest, it is possible to gather large quantities of low quality data as easily as high quality data and care is required for consumers to understand the difference (Chhablani et al., 2012; Luxton et al., 2011; Palmier-Claus et al., 2012). If consumers understand this issue they will give careful consideration to quality of the information presented and gathered by mobile software applications. Future research will need to attend to the need to develop tools that will help consumers assess the quality of the information provided by software applications as well as the quality of the information gathered by these applications to ensure consumers are fully supported in their health care related decision making.

CONCLUSION

In summary research has shown that mobile software applications can help health care consumers to self-manage their health and wellness (Barton, 2012). There has been some demonstration that mobile applications can lower costs and improve the quality of health care. It is also believed that mobile applications can change behaviour to increase the prevention of diseases and combined these can improve long term health outcomes (Qiang et al., 2011).

There is however a paucity of data on the actual impact of m-health services and this has led to challenges for policymakers and governments in regulating the industry. Qiang et al. (2011) suggest that strategies for regulation of the industry should focus on the health care system's most urgent needs.

Katz et al. (2012) find that in relation to chronic disease management there are certain challenges that mobile applications may be successful in addressing, namely improving patient skills and self-management techniques. However, there is a need for improved quality assurance in relation to mobile health applications. Currently approximately 95% of all health related applications are consumer only products and many are not based upon rigorous research and so the outcome from their use is not well researched.

FUTURE RESEARCH DIRECTIONS

Although the research in the area of mobile phone software has advanced considerably, there remain a number of gaps. For example, there is a need to understand how consumers view continuous connectivity. Some health care consumers do not want to be continuously connected to their health care software, preferring to turn it on and off when needed and only in times where they need their health related decision making supported. Other consumers may wish to be continually monitored by their mobile phone application. In addition to this researchers have identified that it is challenging for mobile phone technologies to continuously monitor health and physiologic status as there may be a need for continuous connectivity. Issues such as limited battery life and variability in mobile signalling continue to affect continuous monitoring. As well, many mobile health applications will not function without continuous data exchange with an external server via the Internet. Maintaining such a continuous connection may be challenging due to limited wireless connectivity in some locations and due to the cost of maintain such as connection.

More recently, the safety of mobile software applications has emerged as an issue. Many software applications used in medical diagnosis or treatment have had their safety called into question. Researchers have identified that some software features and functions may introduce new types of errors (i.e. technology-induced errors). In the upcoming years, governments will be introducing new regulations and safety standards to prevent harm arising from technologies used by health care consumers and health care providers in treating patients. Research is needed to better understand how the safe and unsafe features and functions of the technology.

In keeping with our previous work, we found that security was identified by researchers as being important to consider when purchasing mobile health applications (Jones et al., 2011). However, we noted that utilising wireless sensor networks along with health care applications brings a new dimension to mobile phone use – a dimension that requires a well-design security mechanism (Ng et al., 2006). This includes fast authentication for sensor nodes and efficient key distribution in a large network (Ng et al., 2006). Resource constraints sometimes bring challenges as they may be difficult to embed in a multi-layer security solution (Ng et al., 2006) to protect against data leaks. There are many key aspects to ensuring digital traffic flows within mobile health care applications. Many mobile phone software applications that utilise sensor networks are vulnerable to security breaches. Therefore, a secure sensor network that maintains data aggregation, secure group management, secure routing, resilience to node compromise, availability, integrity and authentication, confidentiality and privacy, and key establishment and trust set-up is key to ensuring the security of mobile software applications (Perrig et al., 2004; Shi & Perrig, 2004).

Currently mobile applications are developed for single operating systems and need to then be redeveloped if there is a requirement to use on another operating system. This can lead to issues with interoperability. Additionally, medical, and health and fitness applications are more regularly incorporating external devices for data collection. These devices need to be interoperable with the mobile operating systems. Research will be needed in this area. Some of this work will need to include standards. There are variety of international standards that provide specifications for services, products and best practices. The standards can be accessed by category from the International Standards Organisation (ISO) website and there is a variety of standards available for software developers. Mobile applications development is an emerging area of software developer practice where the ISO has not fully developed standards covering mobile application development. As mobile devices and their applications are becoming more and more consumers focused, application developers are forced to overcome issues through the use of appropriate practices. Research on standards involving mobile devices and mobile health care software will need to be undertaken. Choosing the right health care application requires certain knowledge that encompasses the development of Smart Phones applications. Not all application developers consider notifying the applications consumers of how data entered into the applications will be processed. The consumer perspective framework is a starting point that would guide consumers to better decide and choose the application with limited security risks.

REFERENCES

Aanensen, D., Huntley, D., Feil, E., Al-Own, F., & Spratt, B. (2009). EpiCollect: Linking smartphones to web applications for epidemiology, ecology and community data collection. *PLoS ONE*, *4*(9), e6968. doi:10.1371/journal.pone.0006968 PMID:19756138

AHIMA. (2007). *Statement on Quality Healthcare Data and Information*. Retrieved 10 Jan 2013, from http://library.ahima.org/xpedio/groups/public/documents/ahima/bok1_047492.pdf

Barton, A. J. (2012). The regulation of mobile health applications. *BMC Medicine*, *10*(46). PMID:22569114

Bjornland, D., Goh, E., Haanæs, K., Kainu, T., & Kennedy, S. (2012). *The Socio-Economic Impact of Mobile Health*. The Boston Consulting Group.

Borycki, E. M., & Kushniruk, A. W. (2008). Where do Technology-Induced Errors Come From? Towards a Model for Conceptualizing and Diagnosing Errors Caused by Technology. In A. W. Kushniruk & E. M. Borycki (Eds.), *Human, Social, and Organizational Aspects of Health Information Systems* (pp. 148–166). Hershey, PA: IGI Global. doi:10.4018/978-1-59904-792-8.ch009

Brown, M., & Muchira, R. (2004). Investigating the Relationship between Internet Privacy Concerns and Online Purchase Behavior. *Journal of Electronic Commerce Research*, *5*(1), 62–70.

Chhablani, J., Kaja, S., & Shah, V. (2012). Smartphones in ophthalmology. *Indian Journal of Ophthalmology*, *60*(2), 127–131. doi:10.4103/0301-4738.94054 PMID:22446908

Croll, A. (2011). *Who Owns Your Data?* Retrieved 17 December, 2012, from http://mashable.com/2011/01/12/data-ownership/

Cummings, E., Borycki, E. M., & Roehrer, E. (2013). Issues and considerations for healthcare consumers using mobile applications. *Studies in Health Technology and Informatics, 183*, 227–231. PMID:23388288

Detmer, D., Bloomrosen, M., Raymond, B., & Tang, P. (2008). Integrated Personal Health Records: Transformative Tools for Consumer-Centric Care. *BMC Medical Informatics and Decision Making, 8*(45). PMID:18837999

Gerdes, A., & Øhrstrøm, P. (2011). The role of credibility in the design of mobile solutions to enhance the social skill-set of teenagers diagnosed with autism. *Journal of Information. Communication and Ethics in Society, 9*(4), 253–264. doi:10.1108/14779961111191057

Gustafson, D., Boyle, M., Shaw, B., Isham, A., McTavish, F., & Richards, S. et al. (2011). An E-Health Solution for People with Alcohol Problems. *Alcohol Research & Health, 33*(4), 327–337. PMID:23293549

HIMSS. (2012). *Selecting a Mobile App: Evaluating the Useability of Medical Applications.* Retrieved 17 December, 2012, from http://www.yumpu.com/en/document/view/10378687/himssguidetoappusabilityv1mhimss

IAPP. (2011). *US Privacy Enforcement Case Studies Guide.* Retrieved 17 December, 2012, from https://www.privacyassociation.org/media/pdf/certification/CIPP_Case_Studies_0211.pdf

Jones, J., Hook, S., Park, S., & Scott, L. (2011). *Privacy, security and interoperability of mobile health applications.* Paper presented at the 6th International Conference on Universal Access in Human-Computer Interaction. New York, NY.

Katz, R., Mesfin, T., & Barr, K. (2012). Lessons from a community-based mHealth diabetes self-management program: It's not just about the cell phone. *Journal of Health Communication, 17*(1), 67–72. doi:10.1080/10810730.2012.650613 PMID:22548601

Kay, M., Santos, J., & Takane, M. (2011). mHealth: New horizons for health through mobile technologies. Geneva, Switerland: World Health Organization.

Kushniruk, A., Triola, B., Borycki, E., Stein, B., & Kannry, J. (2005). Technology Induced Error and Usability: The Relationship Between Usability Problems and Prescription Errors When Using a Handheld Application. *International Journal of Medical Informatics, 74*(7-8), 519–526. doi:10.1016/j.ijmedinf.2005.01.003 PMID:16043081

Laakko, T., Leppanen, J., Lahteenmaki, J., & Nummiaho, A. (2008). Mobile Health and Wellness Application Framework. *Methods of Information in Medicine, 47*(3), 217–222. PMID:18473087

Luxton, D., McCann, R., Bush, N., Mishkind, M., & Reger, G. (2011). mHealth for mental health: Integrating smartphone technology in behavioral healthcare. *Professional Psychology, Research and Practice, 42*(6), 505–512. doi:10.1037/a0024485

Mosa, A. S. M., Yoo, I., & Sheets, L. (2012). A Systematic Review of Healthcare Applications for Smartphones. *BMC Medical Informatics and Decision Making, 12*(67). PMID:22781312

Ng, H. S., Sim, M. L., & Tan, C. M. (2006). Security issues of wireless sensor networks in healthcare applications. *BT Technology Journal, 24*(2), 138–144. doi:10.1007/s10550-006-0051-8

Ozdalga, E., Ozdalga, A., & Ahuja, N. (2012). The Smartphone in Medicine: A Review of Current and Potential Use Among Physicians and Students. *Journal of Medical Internet Research, 14*(5), e128. doi:10.2196/jmir.1994 PMID:23017375

Palmier-Claus, J., Ainsworth, J., Machin, M., Barrowclough, C., Dunn, G., & Barkus, E. et al. (2012). The feasibility and validity of ambulatory self-report of psychotic symptoms using a smartphone software application. *BMC Psychiatry, 12*, 72. doi:10.1186/1471-244X-12-172 PMID:22759565

Perrig, A., Stankovic, J., & Wagner, D. (2004). Security in wireless sensor networks. *Communications of the ACM, 47*(6), 53–57. doi:10.1145/990680.990707

Qiang, C. Z., Yamamichi, M., Hausman, V., & Altman, D. (2011). *Mobile Applications for the Health Sector*. Washington, DC: ICT Sector Unit, World Bank.

Savitz, E. (2012). 5 Ways Mobile Apps Will Transform Healthcare. *CIO Network: Insights and Ideas for Technology Leaders*. Retrieved 10 Jan 2013, from http://www.forbes.com/sites/ciocentral/2012/06/04/5-ways-mobile-apps-will-transform-healthcare/

Shi, E., & Perrig, A. (2004). Designing secure sensor networks. *IEEE Wireless Communications, 11*(6), 38–43. doi:10.1109/MWC.2004.1368895

Smith, J., Milberg, S., & Burke, S. (1996). Information Privacy: Measuring Individuals' Concerns about Organizational Practices. *Management Information Systems Quarterly, 20*(2), 167–196. doi:10.2307/249477

Spiekermann, S., & Lorrie, F. C. (2009). Engineering privacy. *IEEE Transactions on Software Engineering, 35*(1), 67–82. doi:10.1109/TSE.2008.88

Whitaker, J. (2008). *Health Privacy: What Consumers Want*. Retrieved 17 December 2012, from http://www.privacy.org.au/Papers/HealthInfoPrivacy-081110.pdf

World Bank. (2012). *Information and Communications for Development 2012: Maximizing Mobile*. Washington, DC: World Bank.

ADDITIONAL READING

Bjornland, D., Goh, E., Haanæs, K., Kainu, T., & Kennedy, S. (2012). The Socio-Economic Impact of Mobile Health: The Boston Consulting Group

Katz, R., Mesfin, T., & Barr, K. (2012). Lessons from a community-based mHealth diabetes self-management program: It's not just about the cell phone. *Journal of Health Communication, 17*(1), 67–72. doi:10.1080/10810730.2012.650613 PMID:22548601

Kay, M., Santos, J., & Takane, M. (2011). mHealth: New horizons for health through mobile technologies. Geneva, Switerland: World Health Organization

Qiang, C. Z., Yamamichi, M., Hausman, V., & Altman, D. (2011). *Mobile Applications for the Health Sector*. Washington, DC: ICT Sector Unit, World Bank.

KEY TERMS AND DEFINITIONS

Accessibility: The ability to easily identify and access reliable applications.

Clinical Effectiveness: The presence/absence of evidence of the effectiveness of an application.

Completeness: The completeness of the data that is collected.

Consumer Perspective Framework: A simple framework that assists mobile app consumers to determine if a specific mobile health care application is appropriate for their needs.

Consumer Usage: The motivation behind a consumer's use of the application.

Corporate Use: Refers to the use of data by the application developer for their own purposes that are not necessarily evident at the time of collection or storage.

Credibility: The quality of being trusted and believed in.

Health Apps: Software that claim to provide health related information or services via mobile devices.

Information Quality: The quality and accuracy of information and advice provided through the software.

Location: The actual location at which data is stored.

Mobile Applications (Apps): Software designed for use on mobile or handheld devices.

Ownership: Who claims or maintains ownership of the data that is collected and stored during use of an application.

This work was previously published in Social Media and Mobile Technologies for Healthcare edited by Mowafa Househ, Elizabeth Borycki, and Andre Kushniruk, pages 1-15 copyright year 2014 by Medical Information Science Reference (an imprint of IGI Global).

Chapter 22
Incorporating Usability Testing into the Development of Healthcare Technologies

Shilo H. Anders
Vanderbilt University, USA

Judith W. Dexheimer
Cincinnati Children's Medical Center, USA

ABSTRACT

The use of mobile devices in healthcare is increasing in prevalence and poses different constraints for use than traditional desktop computing. This chapter introduces several usability testing methods that are appropriate for use when designing and developing mobile technologies. Approaching the development of mobile technologies through a user-centered approach is critical to improve the interaction and use of the hardware and software that is implemented on a mobile platform in healthcare. User-centered design adds value by getting feedback about functionality, design, and constraints that need to be built into the system prior to its completion. Future work in this domain will require further tailoring and use of novel usability methods to evaluate and improve the design of mobile healthcare technologies.

INTRODUCTION

Standard mobile devices function frequently as more than just as cellular telephones, and include additional functionality such as email, Internet access, and application. Mobile technology is pervasive throughout the culture of the United States. As of 2012, approximately 326 million mobile devices are used (CTIA: The Wireless Association, 2012) with a wireless penetration of greater than 100%. (CTIA: The Wireless Associa-tion, 2012) It leads from the saturation of mobile technology, that it will become very important not just in personal but also in professional settings.

The goal of this chapter is to provide an understanding of how the user-centered design process can be incorporated into the design and development of mobile applications. Especially as applications evolve to provide individuals with targeted and just-in-time interventions tailored to incorporate an individual's specific healthcare needs. In this chapter, we will discuss

DOI: 10.4018/978-1-4666-8756-1.ch022

the importance and strategies for implementing usability testing, and more broadly human factors engineering, into mobile healthcare technology design and development. We will discuss what user-centered design entails, why it is important to use when developing mobile Health IT, how it can be incorporated into system design and development, and finally we will discuss common barriers to the implementation of a user-centered design process and how these may be overcome. We will include an example of a mobile Health IT system that incorporated usability testing into its development process.

BACKGROUND

Mobile devices and associated technologies are transforming clinical healthcare systems, communication between patients and clinicians, and the utilization of personal health information. Advances in integrating mobile technology with the Internet, cloud computing, and clinical data systems provide unparalleled abilities to monitor, support, and motivate just-in-time clinical and patient-centered health decision-making. Examples of the potential of mobile technology transforming healthcare systems include providing low-cost, real-time means for assessing disease, behavior, environmental toxins, metabolites and other physiological variables, as well as integrating multiple sources of data from movement, images, social interactions, to inform health behaviors and healthcare decisions. With the increasing popularity of technologies, new issues arise that involve not just the accuracy of the medical advice but also the user's interaction with the system. It is important to involve the users in the design and implementation of any electronic system, but it is also important to ensure the system is well designed.

Mobile healthcare (mHealth) technology has the potential to bring data and contextually appropriate support to patients, clinicians and research-ers in ways never before possible but only if they are efficient, effective and easy to use. Mobile technology encompasses cellular telephones and tablet computers. In two US surveys, approximately 90% of adults reported using mobile phones with 61% of them using smartphones (Sterling, 2013), and approximately one third of adults have a tablet computer. (Pew Internet & American Life Project & Zickuhr, June 2013) Mobile devices have the ability to store reams of information in a small, convenient and lightweight device that is highly portable for easy communication or reference. Devices are frequently wireless enabled that allow a user to access wireless or cellular networks. The devices have the potential to provide both data stored on the device along with external data that can be accessed through network, like cloud-based computing. This provides a mountain of information and support at each users almost instantaneous disposal.

What are some of the issues with using mobile devices and why are they difficult to use?

While the portability of mobile devices is valuable for the availability of information, the devices have some issues that hinder their usability. The security of mobile devices should be considered. Several key factors are important to consider including password protection, requiring 2-step authentication, and ensuring secure wireless transmissions. Devices are electronic and therefore users must be mindful of being charged, being available, as well as knowing where to find the appropriate data. If the data is available externally, network connectivity is an issue to overcome, especially in clinical care when immediate access may be necessary. Software included on mobile devices must be user-friendly and optimized to be viewed and digested on significantly smaller screens than may be currently used. Mobile devices are frequently small to optimize portability, which leads to a lessening of screen size. With this limited viewing area software needs to consider what is optimal to display, when it needs shown and how to display it.

Human factors engineering has been used to evaluate systems, design and evaluate new technology, analyze adverse events and catastrophic accidents. (Cook, Render, & Woods, 2000; Evans et al., 1998; Raschke et al., 1998; Reason, 1995; Salvendy, 2006) Health information technology (Health IT) intended for mobile technologies faces a unique set of challenges that are not a relevant to other platforms. In addition, Health IT design for a specific audience, be it clinicians or patients must accommodate multiple and diverse users; many, often complex tasks, and various contexts of use (e.g. at home, or in multiple locations throughout the hospital. Human factors engineering is a recognized approach to effectively address mobile Health IT design challenges because it is predicated on an empirical understanding of users, tasks, and contexts of use to design and test products rather than the developers perceptions of what users can, want and are capable of doing (Nielsen, 1993; Preece, 1995; Vicente, 2004). Specifically user-centered design, will allow for the development of technology that is useful, well designed and easy to use. This approach to mobile technology design has a demonstrable track record of useful and usable designs (Weinger, Gardner-Bonneau, & Wiklund, 2011), although it's emergence in mobile technologies has been limited (Mulvaney, Anders, Smith, Pittel, & Johnson, 2012). The human factors engineering approach is promoted in ISO standards for design and evaluation, FDA requirements for medical devices, and key publications (American National Standards Institute & Association For the Advancement of Medical Instrumentation, 2009; International Organization for Standardization, 2006, 2007, 2010). For example, a recent AHRQ report stated the Health IT projects should 'engage human factors experts in the design team' and use a user-centered design methodology; thus far this approach has seen minimal use in the development of Health IT products (Agency for Healthcare Research and Quality, 2011). Low adoption rates, abandonment, workarounds, and use errors are testaments to this failure (Patterson et al., 2005; Wong et al., 2003).

In summary, mobile technologies hold great promise and potential to change how we engage, monitor and communicate about our health and health management. Mobile technologies have reached wide-spread use and will continue to be integrated in personal and professional settings. In order to sustain and improve the software design for mHealth, a recognized approach to design and evaluation is human factors engineering. is an approach that will be discussed further.

USER-CENTERED DESIGN FOR MOBILE TECHNOLOGIES

The design of user-centered sustainable mobile health IT requires a targeted and iterative approach. We will leverage the depth and breadth of current usability frameworks from the literature as they apply to mobile technologies in healthcare. Using current literature and authors' experience with usability in mobile technologies, we will systematically present usability aspects to consider during design including: 1) target user characteristics, 2) contexts, and 3) functional tasks in which technology will ultimately be used.

What is User-Centered Design (UCD)?

User-centered design (UCD) is an approach to the development of products, devices, or systems to be used to complete tasks efficiently, effectively, safely and satisfactorily by their intended users (International Organization for Standardization, 2010). This relies heavily on the application of knowledge about human physiology and behavior which is then applied to the design context.

The UCD approach is a rigorous set of methods in which to improve the design of systems including software/hardware, people, and process. For UCD, the system to be developed includes the mobile technology, people that will ultimately use that technology and the environment in which it will be used to achieve desired results (Woods & Hollnagel, 2006). For computer science often the software and hardware are typically the focus for system design, while UCD practitioners focus on the people and their interactions with the software and hardware. A core characteristic of UCD that differentiates it from other technology design processes is that the users are involved in the design of the technology throughout the development of the project. When considering mHealth technologies, future users should help shape the key information requirements and needs for the project since viewing space is limited. As the development cycle continues, users may provide additional requirements and feedback on usability aspects with early prototypes. This is especially true if they are able to use them in practice. Another characteristic of UCD is iterative and multiple approaches to the development of a mobile technology may be taken. In fact, it is likely that UCD practitioners will use a number different methods to aid in design requirement development and evaluation. Prior to a UCD evaluation, clear goals and outcomes should be

defined. For example, the focus of an evaluation may be to determine how best to represent a key pieces of information that practitioners require for their decision-making. The usability evaluation would what to test to criterion, which may be as defuse as the user could accomplish the task, or a specific time allocation may be specified.

Effective UCD (or redesign) depends on an in-depth understanding of the individuals that will ultimately use the mobile technology and its ability to integrate into the IT development cycle (Mayhew, 1999). Figure 1 shows a notional architecture for how this integration could occur. For UCD the initiating step in Health IT design requires a thorough understanding of frontline work and the perspective of health providers or patients and their caregivers depending on who will use the technology (it might be both!) and how that prospective might be obtained (Weinger, et al., 2011; Wiklund & Wilcox, 2005). This knowledge drives specific design requirements, which are then incorporated into the user interface (UI) design concepts. UCD includes the development of multiple alternative designs, followed by

Figure 1. Ideal user-centered design process integrated with software development process

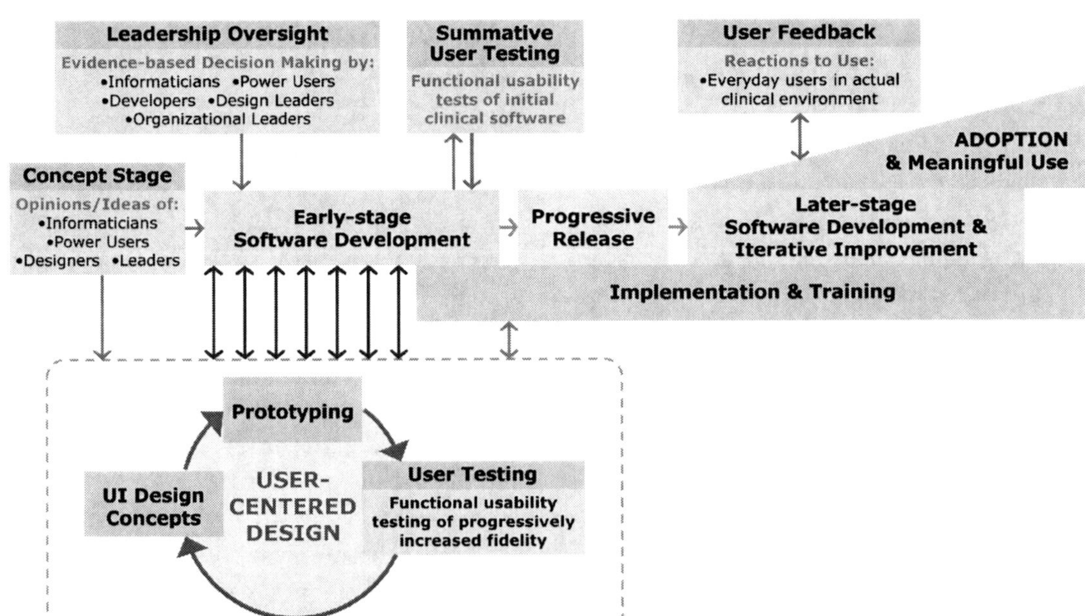

the development of higher fidelity prototypes in which these potential solutions are then evaluated through user testing. User testing may initially be informal and prior to deploy a summative usability evaluation of the designed system would ideally be conducted. Design evaluation then assesses whether users' needs were met as well as considers the contextual factors related to success or failure, and factors that will facilitate or prevent generalizability beyond the initial deployment site (Shilo Anders, Woods, Patterson, & Schweikhart, 2008; Wong, et al., 2003). After initial system implementation, facilitating and gathering user feedback is way to incorporate user driven changes into future system iterations.

Why is UCD Important?

Including UCD in the development process provides insight to better understand how to design a product that fits with what people want, need and desire. It also promotes the approach that one size does not fit all, and helps developers to identify any incorrect assumptions about particular healthcare user groups and the tasks that they would like to be able to complete. Thus, UCD helps to create products that are easier to use with increase efficiency, reliability while decreasing frustration and costs associated with learning the mobile technology (Nielsen, 1993). Many health IT tools have been designed and implemented without UCD influence and have experienced low adoption rates, abandonment and use errors (Eysenbach, 2005; Haggstrom et al., 2011; Zayas-Caban & Dixon, 2010). UCD also promotes the development of a maximum amount for flexibility to help prevent potentially unsafe workarounds (Patterson, Cook, & Render, 2002). Finally, the UCD process allows individuals to evaluate and be involved in the actual design of the product or systems which may ease implementation burdens, increase user appeal and satisfaction (McCurdie et al., 2012), and provide individual champions in various hospital settings (Kortum & Safari Technical Books., 2008).

Approaches to UCD

UCD methodologies are varied in approach and can be modified according to the needs and challenges that a particular mobile technology is trying to achieve. The table lists the methodologies most utilized by UCD practitioners that are applicable to mHealth. Three of the ones that the authors have used most are subsequently described in more detail.

Card Sort

The card sort method is most utilized early in the UCD process, often prior to any interface design development. The researcher will create a number of paper cards that include the information to be included in the interface. This may consist of information such as physiological data, clinician notes, or information that is relevant. The number of cards depends on the amount of information that the system is being designed for, but the more cards the longer it will take to complete the card sort. For mobile technologies the card sort provides a way to parse and constrain the information that is to be grouped into specific displays. Additionally, this can be completed in individual or group settings. Individuals sort the cards into groups that make sense to them, then the participants are asked to talk through why they sorted the information in the way that they did. Other questions may address the lack of key pieces of information that should be included or additional ways in which they may sort information based on specific constraints or knowledge (e.g. clinicians may sort information differently with various patient diagnoses.) Across individuals patterns of information sets or groups can be found which can be used for the design of the system. The card helps to ensure that the information is organized in a manner that is consistent and logical for the individuals that will use the system.

For example, a project conducted by the authors involved using a card sort methodology to group

Table 1. Summary of methodologies for UCD in mobile technology development

Methods	Definition
Card Sort	A technique that consists of individuals that will be users combining information found on cards in ways that make sense to them.
Expert evaluations	Review of the product or system by which a UCD or human factors expert preferably in conjunction with a product user (e.g. Heuristic evaluation).
Focus Groups	A skilled moderator leads 6-12 users in a discussion about a system or mobile technology. The moderator elicits answers to qualitative questions about use practices or envisioned system use.
Paper and pencil evaluations	Individual aspects of the user interface or system design are shown drawn on paper. The user is asked questions about how to operate and interact with the interface to accomplish task requirements.
Surveys	Questions about use and feedback about a system are generated and presented in a consumer friendly format. Traditional survey development involves validating the survey prior to wide-spread dissemination.
Cognitive Walk-through	A UCD professional leads a individual through actual user tasks. The user talks about their goals, feedback about the user interface and performance challenges.
Formative Usability Evaluation	Involves the development of problem statements or test objectives that are representative of the tasks that users engage. The user completes tasks where performance measures are collected. The outcome is improvement recommendations.
Summative Usability Evaluation	Test of the system just prior to implementation that usually involves the user performing tasks that test hypotheses. The user performs task unaided and any issues with the interface are noted, so improvements can be made.

Sources: (Dumas & Redish, 1999; Rubin, 1994; Wiklund & Wilcox, 2005)

physiological variables for ICU patients. The nurses that were asked to participate in the study grouped the variables according to how they monitored their patients and ordered the information by importance. The subsequent information display, while not specifically designed for a mobile platform grouped functional information together, which could be opened individually and ultimately displayed on a mobile platform. The subsequent design was further usability tested using numerous methods and culminated in a summative usability evaluation (S. Anders et al., 2012).

In mobile technology design, the use of the card sort affords the development of interfaces that group information in ways that make sense to the users. This can also help to constrain and put information on interfaces that assist in meeting the goals of the system thus minimizing extraneous information. For clinicians the card sort may contribute to the design of interfaces that provide the necessary information at a glance rather than having to navigate through multiple interfaces where data must then be synthesized. The limited screen size can be a detriment to ease of use of the system. When doing the card sort for mobile technologies it will be instrumental to limit the groupings to a manageable number that can easily be displayed on the interface. Additionally, in the mobile environment the researcher may also ask the user to consider a number of different situations for use (at home versus in the hospital) as this may influence the grouping of information.

Cognitive Walk-Through

A cognitive walk-through is a UCD method that involves the user and a moderator walking through the interface and subsequent user interaction of a mock-up or functioning prototype. The user talks out loud has he/she goes through the interface, explaining what they think a specific button, graphic or text means and how it links to other parts of the proposed system. This approach assists designers in helping to understand where there are uncertainties embedded in the interface that are likely to result in user confusion and errors.

As the user walks through the interface they will provide feedback about their likes and potential improvements. Additionally, the user may suggest including information that was not previously considered as integral to the system and conversely information that is extraneous. The cognitive walk-through may be completed rapidly and iteratively with small incremental changes being made to the interface when participants suggest similar changes or encounter similar barriers. The walkthrough is conducted on an individual basis and may be conducted with prototype interfaces that are displayed as paper printouts. Conversely it may also be utilized with interfaces that are in production or close to production.

In a project involving the development of a mobile application to assist busy outpatient clinicians this method was employed to garner feedback from busy clinicians with minimal time available. The research team developed prototype interfaces that were printed and taken to users to provide feedback using this method (Figure 2). Participants were asked to walk through the elements in the interface and the expectation of how that element should behave was captured. After hearing feedback from a minimum of three users, the team improved upon the interface taking the user feedback into account (Figure 3). As can be seen in the figures below, over five iterations with a total of fifteen clinicians the interface changed dramatically to more accurately embody the clinicians work in their environment (i.e. high volume clinics). It should be noted that initially this project was not specifically focused on designing for a mobile platform, however after initial feedback from clinicians the research team decided to include this in the requirements and platform flexibility

Figure 2. Interface prior to numerous cognitive walk-through iterations

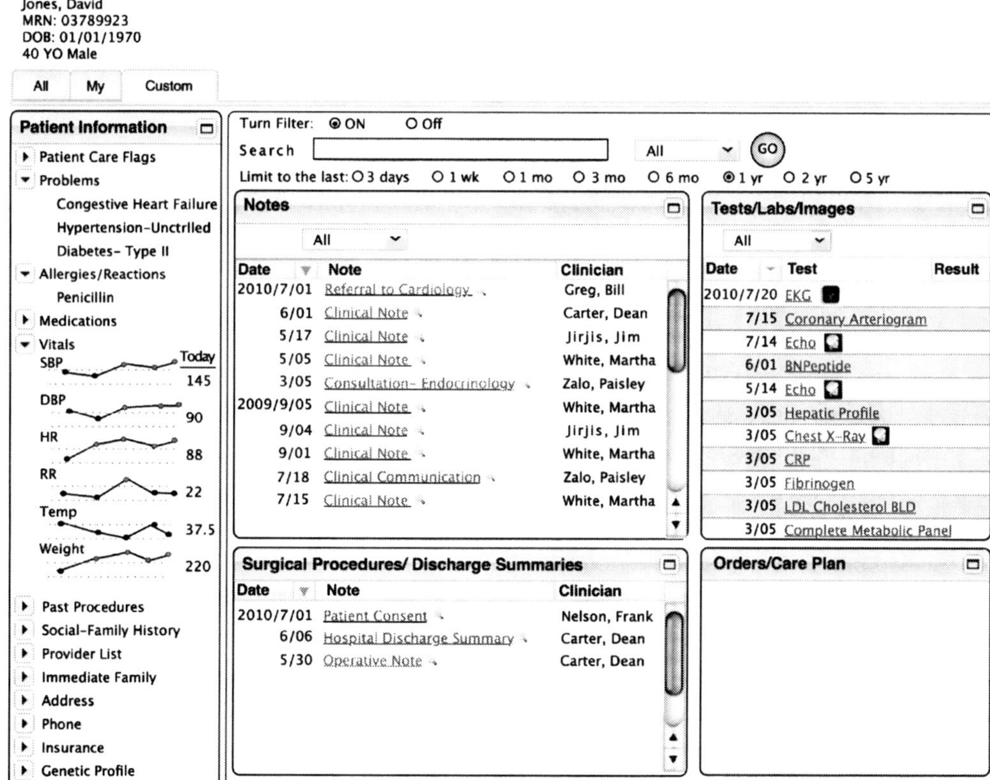

Figure 3. Interface after numerous cognitive walkthroughs

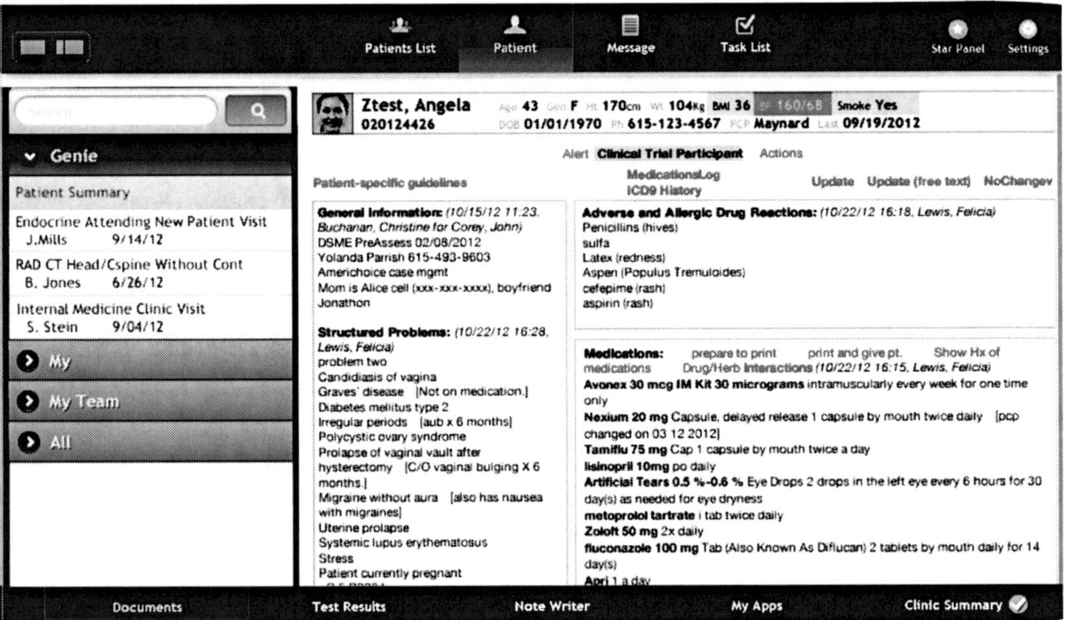

became a key aspect of the design for subsequent iterations of the cognitive walkthrough.

For mobile technologies the cognitive walk-through is a quick and efficient way in which to gather feedback from users that can easily be incorporated into the design. If using paper print-outs comments can be directly annotated onto the interface and there are numerous outlines for the various mobile technologies available. Online software exists in which prototypes may be tested in this manner and some even allow the user to enter comments into the interface. This is convenient if the population one wants to talk with are at a distance. Thus remote evaluations may be an alternative approach, and technologies exist in which these session may be video and audio recorded. The walk-through approach may be complicated if a prototype is use and the researcher and participant are both attempting to view the same interface. Finally, it may behoove the researcher and user to walk-through the interface in the context of use, such that potential issues with information viewing while on the go, sharing in the context of a visit or even connectively issues may be revealed.

Summative Usability Evaluation

A summative usability evaluation is an individual session involving a working prototype or beta version of the software, just prior to release. In the UCD process this is the final step before product implementation and if the UCD process is implemented, minimal use errors and user frustrations should exist. A total of 5-12 users will interact with the product completing the tasks that the functions of the product support. The researchers will create a realistic environment in which that practitioners will use the system although a usability lab setting may be utilized as well. The scenarios that each participant will work through should be representative of a set of tasks. Use errors, frustration, incomplete tasks and time on task are usually included in the evaluation that may be based on hypotheses about the system. In some cases, two diverse products are evaluated and compared for usability.

In a project that illustrates this type of evaluation, 19 nurses and 3 anesthesia providers utilized one of two patient identification devices for blood verification to complete a series of scenarios (S. Anders et al., 2011). The goal of the project was to assist hospital leadership in deciding which technology to implement, thus the focus was on user satisfaction, use errors (e.g. did the provider give inappropriate blood products), and efficiency of use. The results revealed that both products had usability issues that included a lack of feedback to the user, limited information about required subtasks and lack of visibility about system state and limitation. These handheld devices both led to user frustration and workarounds during actual use.

Summative usability evaluations of mobile technologies especially when scenario driven can reveal usability issues and process errors that were previously unknown. The difficulty is in adequately capturing these events. If the scenario is in situ with a mobile device the UCD team may not notice the error or misstep unless special consideration is taken that captures the actual interface as the user is interacting with it.

In conclusion UCD methods have been and should continue to be applied to mHealth technology development. Special considerations regarding the viewing area and context of use should be considered when testing this technology. The next section presents a variety of barriers and challenges to incorporating UCD into the development process and recommendations to overcome these issues.

Challenges of Incorporating UCD into Development and Recommendations

Incorporating UCD into the Health IT design framework can be a daunting task. Some of the challenges that the authors have faced in doing this are described below as well as how these were overcome. Further, the challenges are illustrated through generalized examples that relate not only to mobile devices, but also to social medial and hospital systems.

The most commonly cited challenges to including of a UCD process into the design and development of mobile technologies are presented below.

1. The UCD process will add more time than developers have allotted for project completion.

Overcoming this challenge involves the persistence and flexibility on the part of both the UCD team and the IT development process. The early that the UCD team can become involved in the development of the system, the easier it will be to incorporate these processes into the development cycle. UCD members should consider attending IT development meetings, especially if an agile software development cycle is used. Ideally the interface design should be ahead of the development team and be testing functionality prior to it being developed in the system. Countless redesigns of systems have occurred because UCD was not included in the system development process (Eysenbach, 2005; Haggstrom, et al., 2011; Zayas-Caban & Dixon, 2010).

2. There are not enough resources to include UCD.

Investment in UCD on the front end leads to greater user satisfaction, ease of use and sustained use. Depending on what you are designing, there may be room to creatively include UCD in the design process. Additionally, UCD processes can be as involved or minimally included as necessary and dependent upon what is being designed. Formal usability evaluations may not be necessary or desirable for some products, and some methods may be conducted with as few as three participants with minimal time involved. A mobile application may include UCD with minimal effort or incorporated into larger studies or as projects for students.

3. Limited access to users.

In mHealth, users can be highly varied and are usually all very busy; this seems to be especially true with clinicians. For UCD approaches to involve a number of participants the research must consider alternative ways to involve users. Having an advocate that regularly interacts with the users of interest to be your advocate may help to get time with users. Additionally, especially with physicians, alternative times, offering incentives, and limiting the amount of time that you are requesting can also help to get users. Finally, when the UCD team meets with the user they should be quick, direct and willing to visit at nontraditional times. For example, cognitive walk-throughs can use paper printouts and in 15 minutes get useful feedback about the interface, provided that questions are succinct and the interfaces included are not all possible options.

4. No expertise in UCD processes.

In this case, seek outside help and find the expertise that is needed. The IT department at a large academic medical center knew that implementing a UCD approach to its technology development was important. Thus, they sought and formed a relationship with UCD experts at the medical center that were conducting research in this area. The collaboration has been beneficial to both parties and to the users that are now using the products.

FUTURE RESEARCH DIRECTIONS

This chapter highlights the need for a UCD in mobile healthcare technology development and briefly describes some of the common methods. Currently UCD in healthcare organizations has been minimally incorporated in the development of technologies, although there are exceptions (Russ et al., 2012). Furthermore, applying UCD to mHealth has the potential to improve both the functionality and use of the mobile devices and their related applications.

To incorporate UCD into the design and implementation of new systems, an organizational change is required for adoption and integration. Including UCD requires extra time, planning, and money during the design phase of a project. While this investment will ultimately pay off, in user satisfaction and adoption of the technology, the importance of considering these design elements must be a priority to the organization. No application is created or used solely on it's own. Integration between devices and systems should be considering during the design, as should the integration between users of a system. If users are happy with the mHealth application, they are more likely to use it and suggest it to other interested users.

There is minimal research available in the literature regarding the impact of mobile health technologies on practice (Divall et al, 2013). Given the healthcare providers desire for hand-held devices, it is inevitable that more healthcare decisions and information will come from mobile devices. Future research should focus on the design, functionality, and availability of information through mHealth devices. Important topics such as connectivity, security, and accessibility should be addressed in both the literature and considered through the design process.

CONCLUSION

With the increase in mobile devices in everyday use and healthcare specifically, the importance of design is increasing. Overall the chapter used the framework of usability engineering to help capture how efforts to translate scientific evidence into clinical practice could be more successful. This chapter provides a human-centered design focus to the mobile health technical and intellectual literature. User-centered design can improve the functionality and use of applications on mobile devices. There is currently a dearth of information in the literature about using mobile devices for healthcare, future work should focus on employing usability methods in the design and evaluation of applications aimed to improve clinician performance and improve clinical care.

REFERENCES

Agency for Healthcare Research and Quality. (2011). Improving Consumer Health IT Application Development: Lessons from Other Industries-Background Report (AHRQ Publication No. 11-0065-EF). Rockville, MD: AHRQ.

American National Standards Institute & Association For the Advancement of Medical Instrumentation. (2009). ANSI/AAMI HE75, 2009 Ed. - Human factors engineering - Design of medical devices. Arlington, VA: American National Standards Institute.

Anders, S., Albert, R., Miller, A., Weinger, M. B., Doig, A. K., Behrens, M., & Agutter, J. (2012). Evaluation of an integrated graphical display to promote acute change detection in ICU patients. *International Journal of Medical Informatics*, *81*(12), 842–851. doi:10.1016/j. ijmedinf.2012.04.004 PMID:22534099

Anders, S., Miller, A., Joseph, P., Fortenberry, T., Woods, M., Booker, R., & France, D. (2011). Blood product positive patient identification: Comparative simulation-based usability test of two commercial products. *Transfusion*, *51*(11), 2311–2318. doi:10.1111/j.1537-2995.2011.03185.x PMID:21599676

Anders, S., Woods, D. D., Patterson, E. S., & Schweikhart, S. (2008). Shifts in Functions of a New Technology over Time: An Analysis of Logged Electronic Intensive Care Unit Interventions. *Proceedings of the Human Factors and Ergonomics Society Annual Meeting, 52*(12), 870-874.

Cook, R. I., Render, M., & Woods, D. D. (2000). Gaps in the continuity of care and progress on patient safety. *British Medical Journal*, *320*(7237), 791–794. doi:10.1136/ bmj.320.7237.791 PMID:10720370

CTIA. The Wireless Association. (2012). *Wireless Quick Facts: Year-End Figures*. Retrieved September 30, 2013, from http://www.ctia.org/ advocacy/research/index.cfm/aid/10323

Divall, P., Camosso-Stefinovic, J., & Baker, R. (2013). The use of personal digital assistants in clinical decision making by health care professionals: A systematic review. *Health Informatics Journal*, *19*(1), 16–28. doi:10.1177/1460458212446761 PMID:23486823

Dumas, J. S., & Redish, J. (1999). *A practical guide to usability testing* (Rev. ed.). Norwood, NJ: Intellect Books.

Evans, R. S., Pestotnik, S. L., Classen, D. C., Clemmer, T. P., Weaver, L. K., Orme, J. F. Jr, & Burke, J. P. (1998). A computer-assisted management program for antibiotics and other antiinfective agents. *The New England Journal of Medicine*, *338*(4), 232–238. doi:10.1056/NEJM199801223380406 PMID:9435330

Eysenbach, G. (2005). The law of attrition. *Journal of Medical Internet Research*, *7*(1), e11. doi:10.2196/jmir.7.1.e11 PMID:15829473

Haggstrom, D. A., Saleem, J. J., Russ, A. L., Jones, J., Russell, S. A., & Chumbler, N. R. (2011). Lessons learned from usability testing of the VA's personal health record. *Journal of the American Medical Informatics Association*, *18*(Suppl 1), i13–i17. doi:10.1136/amiajnl-2010-000082 PMID:21984604

International Organization for Standardization. (2006). *ISO 9241-110:2006 Ergonomics of human-system interaction -- Part 110: Dialogue principles*. Geneva, Switzerland: ISO.

International Organization for Standardization. (2007). [*Medical devices -- Application of usability engineering to medical devices*. Arlington, VA: AAMI.]. *IEC, 62366*, 2007.

International Organization for Standardization. (2010). *ISO 9241-210:2010 Ergonomics of human-system interaction -- Part 210: Human-centred design for interactive systems*. Geneva, Switzerland: ISO.

Kortum, P., & Safari Technical Books. (2008). *HCI beyond the GUI design for haptic, speech, olfactory and other nontraditional interfaces*. San Francisco: Morgan Kaufmann.

Mayhew, D. J. (1999). *The usability engineering lifecycle: A practitioner's handbook for user interface design*. San Francisco: Morgan Kaufmann Publishers. doi:10.1145/632780.632805

McCurdie, T., Taneva, S., Casselman, M., Yeung, M., McDaniel, C., Ho, W., & Cafazzo, J. (2012). mHealth consumer apps: The case for user-centered design. *Biomedical Instrumentation & Technology*, 49–56. doi:10.2345/0899-8205-46. s2.49 PMID:23039777

Mulvaney, S. A., Anders, S., Smith, A. K., Pittel, E. J., & Johnson, K. B. (2012). A pilot test of a tailored mobile and web-based diabetes messaging system for adolescents. *Journal of Telemedicine and Telecare*, *18*(2), 115–118. doi:10.1258/jtt.2011.111006 PMID:22383802

Nielsen, J. (1993). *Usability engineering*. Boston: Academic Press.

Patterson, E. S., Cook, R. I., & Render, M. L. (2002). Improving patient safety by identifying side effects from introducing bar coding in medication administration. *Journal of the American Medical Informatics Association*, *9*(5), 540–553. doi:10.1197/jamia.M1061 PMID:12223506

Patterson, E. S., Doebbeling, B. N., Fung, C. H., Militello, L., Anders, S., & Asch, S. M. (2005). Identifying barriers to the effective use of clinical reminders: Bootstrapping multiple methods. *Journal of Biomedical Informatics*, *38*(3), 189–199. doi:10.1016/j.jbi.2004.11.015 PMID:15896692

Pew Internet & American Life Project, & Zickuhr, K. (2013, June). *Tablet Ownership 2013*. Retrieved September 30, 2013, from http://pewinternet.org/Reports/2013/Tablet-Ownership-2013.aspx

Preece, J. (1995). *Human-computer interaction*. Wokingham, UK: Addison-Wesley Pub. Co.

Raschke, R. A., Gollihare, B., Wunderlich, T. A., Guidry, J. R., Leibowitz, A. I., Peirce, J. C., & Susong, C. (1998). A computer alert system to prevent injury from adverse drug events: Development and evaluation in a community teaching hospital. *Journal of the American Medical Association*, *280*(15), 1317–1320. doi:10.1001/jama.280.15.1317 PMID:9794309

Reason, J. (1995). Understanding adverse events: human factors. *Quality in Health Care*, *4*(2), 80–89. doi:10.1136/qshc.4.2.80 PMID:10151618

Rubin, J. (1994). *Handbook of usability testing: How to plan, design, and conduct effective tests*. New York: Wiley.

Russ, A. L., Weiner, M., Russell, S. A., Baker, D. A., Fahner, W. J., & Saleem, J. J. (2012). Design and implementation of a hospital-based usability laboratory: Insights from a Department of Veterans Affairs laboratory for health information technology. *Joint Commission Journal on Quality and Patient Safety*, *38*(12), 531–540. PMID:23240261

Salvendy, G. (2006). *Handbook of human factors and ergonomics* (3rd ed.). Hoboken, NJ: John Wiley. doi:10.1002/0470048204

Sterling, G. (2013). *Pew: 61 Percent in US Now Have Smartphones.* Retrieved September 30, 2013, from http://marketingland.com/pew-61-percent-in-us-now-have-smartphones-46966

Vicente, K. J. (2004). *The human factor: Revolutionizing the way people live with technology.* New York: Routledge.

Weinger, M. B., Gardner-Bonneau, D., & Wiklund, M. E. (2011). *Handbook of human factors in medical device design.* Boca Raton, FL: CRC Press.

Wiklund, M. E., & Wilcox, S. B. (2005). *Designing usability into medical products.* Boca Raton, FL: Taylor & Francis/CRC Press. doi:10.1201/9781420038088

Wong, D. H., Gallegos, Y., Weinger, M. B., Clack, S., Slagle, J., & Anderson, C. T. (2003). Changes in intensive care unit nurse task activity after installation of a third-generation intensive care unit information system. *Critical Care Medicine, 31*(10), 2488–2494. doi:10.1097/01.CCM.0000089637.53301.EF PMID:14530756

Woods, D. D., & Hollnagel, E. (2006). *Joint cognitive systems: Patterns in cognitive systems engineering.* Boca Raton, FL: CRC/Taylor & Francis. doi:10.1201/9781420005684

Zayas-Caban, T., & Dixon, B. E. (2010). Considerations for the design of safe and effective consumer health IT applications in the home. *Quality & Safety in Health Care, 19*(Suppl 3), i61–i67. doi:10.1136/qshc.2010.041897 PMID:20959321

ADDITIONAL READING

Anders, S., Albert, R., Miller, A., Weinger, M. B., Doig, A. K., Behrens, M., & Agutter, J. (2012). Evaluation of an integrated graphical display to promote acute change detection in ICU patients. *International Journal of Medical Informatics, 81*(12), 842–851. doi:10.1016/j.ijmedinf.2012.04.004 PMID:22534099

Anders, S., Miller, A., Joseph, P., Fortenberry, T., Woods, M., Booker, R., & France, D. (2011). Blood product positive patient identification: comparative simulation-based usability test of two commercial products. *Transfusion, 51*(11), 2311–2318. doi:10.1111/j.1537-2995.2011.03185.x PMID:21599676

Bevan, N. (2001). International standards for HCI and usability. *International Journal of Human-Computer Studies, 55*(4), 533–552. doi:10.1006/ijhc.2001.0483

Carayon, P. (2010). Human factors in patient safety as an innovation. *Applied Ergonomics, 41*(5), 657–665. doi:10.1016/j.apergo.2009.12.011 PMID:20106468

Chaudhry, B., Wang, J., Wu, S., Maglione, M., Mojica, W., Roth, E., & Shekelle, P. G. (2006). Systematic review: impact of health information technology on quality, efficiency, and costs of medical care. *Annals of Internal Medicine, 144*(10), 742–752. doi:10.7326/0003-4819-144-10-200605160-00125 PMID:16702590

Eysenbach, G. (2011). CONSORT-EHEALTH: improving and standardizing evaluation reports of Web-based and mobile health interventions. *Journal of Medical Internet Research, 13*(4), e126. doi:10.2196/jmir.1923 PMID:22209829

Grudin, J. (1994). Computer-supported cooperative work: history and focus. *IEEE Computer, 27*(5), 19–26. doi:10.1109/2.291294

Hicks, J., Ramanathan, N., Kim, D., Monibi, M., Selsky, J., Hansen, M., & Estrin, D. (2010). *AndWellness: an open mobile system for activity and experience sampling.* Paper presented at the Wireless Health 2010, San Diego, California.

Hollnagel, E., & Woods, D. A. (2005). *Joint cognitive systems: foundations of cognitive systems engineering.* Boca Raton, FL: CRC Press. doi:10.1201/9781420038194

Johnson, C. W. (2006). Why did that happen? Exploring the proliferation of barely usable software in healthcare systems. *Quality & Safety in Health Care, 15*(Suppl 1), i76–i81. doi:10.1136/qshc.2005.016105 PMID:17142614

Karsh, B. T. (2004). Beyond usability: designing effective technology implementation systems to promote patient safety. *Quality & Safety in Health Care, 13*(5), 388–394. doi:10.1136/qshc.2004.010322 PMID:15465944

Karsh, B. T., Weinger, M. B., Abbott, P. A., & Wears, R. L. (2010). Health information technology: fallacies and sober realities. *Journal of the American Medical Informatics Association: JAMIA, 17*(6), 617–623. doi:10.1136/jamia.2010.005637 PMID:20962121

Kientz, J. A., Choe, E. K., Birch, B., Maharaj, R., Fonville, A., Glasson, C., & Mundt, J. (2010). *Heuristic evaluation of persuasive health technologies*. Paper presented at the Proceedings of the 1st ACM International Health Informatics Symposium, Arlington, Virginia, USA.

Kjeldskov, J., Skov, M., Als, B., & Høegh, R. (2004). Is It Worth the Hassle? Exploring the Added Value of Evaluating the Usability of Context-Aware Mobile Systems in the Field. In S. Brewster & M. Dunlop (Eds.), *Mobile Human-Computer Interaction - MobileHCI 2004* (Vol. 3160, pp. 61–73). Springer Berlin Heidelberg. doi:10.1007/978-3-540-28637-0_6

Koppel, R., Metlay, J. P., Cohen, A., Abaluck, B., Localio, A. R., Kimmel, S. E., & Strom, B. L. (2005). Role of computerized physician order entry systems in facilitating medication errors. *Journal of the American Medical Association, 293*(10), 1197–1203. doi:10.1001/jama.293.10.1197 PMID:15755942

Kushniruk, A. (2002). Evaluation in the design of health information systems: application of approaches emerging from usability engineering. *Computers in Biology and Medicine, 32*(3), 141–149. doi:10.1016/S0010-4825(02)00011-2 PMID:11922931

Middleton, B., Bloomrosen, M., Dente, M. A., Hashmat, B., Koppel, R., Overhage, J. M., & Zhang, J. (2013). Enhancing patient safety and quality of care by improving the usability of electronic health record systems: recommendations from AMIA. *Journal of the American Medical Informatics Association: JAMIA, 20*(e1), e2–e8. doi:10.1136/amiajnl-2012-001458 PMID:23355463

Miller, R. A., & Gardner, R. M. (1997). Recommendations for responsible monitoring and regulation of clinical software systems. American Medical Informatics Association, Computer-based Patient Record Institute, Medical Library Association, Association of Academic Health Science Libraries, American Health Information Management Association, American Nurses Association. *Journal of the American Medical Informatics Association: JAMIA, 4*(6), 442–457. doi:10.1136/jamia.1997.0040442 PMID:9391932

Mulvaney, S. A., Anders, S., Smith, A. K., Pittel, E. J., & Johnson, K. B. (2012). A pilot test of a tailored mobile and web-based diabetes messaging system for adolescents. *Journal of Telemedicine and Telecare, 18*(2), 115–118. doi:10.1258/jtt.2011.111006 PMID:22383802

Nemeth, C. P. (2004). *Human factors methods for design: making systems human-centered*. Boca Raton, Fla.: CRC Press. doi:10.1201/9780203643662

Nielsen, J. (1993). *Usability engineering*. Boston: Academic Press.

Nilsen, W., Kumar, S., Shar, A., Varoquiers, C., Wiley, T., Riley, W. T., & Atienza, A. A. (2012). Advancing the science of mHealth. *Journal of Health Communication, 17*(Suppl 1), 5–10. doi:1 0.1080/10810730.2012.677394 PMID:22548593

Patterson, E. S., Cook, R. I., & Render, M. L. (2002). Improving patient safety by identifying side effects from introducing bar coding in medication administration. *Journal of the American Medical Informatics Association: JAMIA, 9*(5), 540–553. doi:10.1197/jamia.M1061 PMID:12223506

Rubin, J. (1994). *Handbook of usability testing: how to plan, design, and conduct effective tests.* New York: Wiley.

Saleem, J. J., Patterson, E. S., Militello, L., Anders, S., Falciglia, M., Wissman, J. A., & Asch, S. M. (2007). Impact of clinical reminder redesign on learnability, efficiency, usability, and workload for ambulatory clinic nurses. *Journal of the American Medical Informatics Association: JAMIA, 14*(5), 632–640. doi:10.1197/jamia. M2163 PMID:17600106

Saleem, J. J., Russ, A. L., Sanderson, P., Johnson, T. R., Zhang, J., & Sittig, D. F. (2009). Current challenges and opportunities for better integration of human factors research with development of clinical information systems. *Yearbook of Medical Informatics*, 48–58. PMID:19855872

Shneiderman, B. (2011). Tragic errors: Usability and electronic health records. *Interaction, 18*(6), 60–63. doi:10.1145/2029976.2029992

Svanaes, D., Alsos, O. A., & Dahl, Y. (2010). Usability testing of mobile ICT for clinical settings: methodological and practical challenges. *International Journal of Medical Informatics, 79*(4), e24–e34. doi:10.1016/j.ijmedinf.2008.06.014 PMID:18789753

Svanaes, D., & Seland, G. (2004). *Putting the users center stage: role playing and low-fi prototyping enable end users to design mobile systems.* Paper presented at the Proceedings of the SIGCHI Conference on Human Factors in Computing Systems ACM, Vienna, Austria.

Weinger, M. B., Gardner-Bonneau, D., & Wiklund, M. E. (2011). *Handbook of human factors in medical device design.* Boca Raton, FL: CRC Press.

KEY TERMS AND DEFINITIONS

Card Sort: A data collection method that involves sorting and categorizing data so that it makes sense to the participant.

Cognitive Walk-Through: Method of data collection, where a participant is shown the candidate interface and asked to think aloud as they interact with the interfaces.

Health Information Technology: Area of information technology that involves the design, development, and use of information systems and tools for the healthcare industry.

Human Factors Engineering: The study of fitting the cognitive abilities and human body dimensions to the design of equipment and devices.

Mobile Healthcare Technology: Easily portable tools or applications that are pertain to well-being and management of illness.

Usability: How easy a system or technology is to use. Usability typically refers to how the efficiently, effectively, and error free a user interaction with a system is.

User-Centered Design: A process of system/ tool development that emphasizes the involvement of who will be the user and is iterative.

This work was previously published in Social Media and Mobile Technologies for Healthcare edited by Mowafa Househ, Elizabeth Borycki, and Andre Kushniruk, pages 32-47 copyright year 2014 by Medical Information Science Reference (an imprint of IGI Global).

Chapter 23
Development of a Methodological Approach for Data Quality Ontology in Diabetes Management

Alireza Rahimi
*University of New South Wales, Australia &
Isfahan University of Medical Sciences, Iran &
SWSLHD General Practice Unit, Australia*

Nandan Parameswaran
University of New South Wales, Australia

Pradeep Kumar Ray
University of New South Wales, Australia

Jane Taggart
*University of New South Wales Australia, &
SWSLHD General Practice Unit, Australia*

Hairong Yu
University of New South Wales, Australia

Siaw-Teng Liaw
*University of New South Wales, Australia &
SWSLHD General Practice Unit, Australia*

ABSTRACT

The role of ontologies in chronic disease management and associated challenges such as defining data quality (DQ) and its specification is a current topic of interest. In domains such as Diabetes Management, a robust Data Quality Ontology (DQO) is required to support the automation of data extraction semantically from Electronic Health Record (EHR) and access and manage DQ, so that the data set is fit for purpose. A five steps strategy is proposed in this paper to create the DQO which captures the semantics of clinical data. It consists of: (1) Knowledge acquisition; (2) Conceptualization; (3) Semantic modeling; (4) Knowledge representation; and (5) Validation. The DQO was applied to the identification of patients with Type 2 Diabetes Mellitus (T2DM) in EHRs, which included an assessment of the DQ of the EHR. The five steps methodology is generalizable and reusable in other domains.

DOI: 10.4018/978-1-4666-8756-1.ch023

1. INTRODUCTION

Improving data quality (DQ) in health organizations can improve quality of decisions and support better policy, strategies, and evidence-based patient care. DQ can be defined in terms of its *fitness for purpose* (Wang, 1998). The most frequently used DQ dimensions are *accuracy, completeness, consistency, correctness* and *timeliness* (S. T. Liaw et al., 2013). Research in DQ has tended to focus on the identification of generic quality characteristics that are applicable in a wide range of domains (Wand & Wang, 1996).

In the field of healthcare, data is collected routinely and may be used for research. It is becoming apparent that the quality of routinely collected data is not as good as it should be for many research applications. It is still not clear how DQ can be expressed in the context of fitness for purpose. Reference terminologies and ontologies have been used to specify DQ thus influencing data collection and analysis (Brown, Warmington, Laurence, & Prevost, 2003). They also act as benchmarks for assessing DQ (S. Liaw, Taggart, Dennis, & Yeo, 2011). An ontological approach can play a major role in the assessment of DQ and specification of fitness for purpose of a dataset (S. T. Liaw, et al., 2013; Rahimi, Liaw, Ray, Taggart, & Yu, 2014).

Building robust ontologies for DQ in healthcare helps automation of data extraction from the Electronic Health Records (EHRs) into clinical data warehouses; assessment and management of the quality of big data so that they are fit for purposes such as research, quality improvement, health information exchange and sharing; management of controlled vocabularies and optimizing semantic interoperability; curation of data for use by human users and applications such as electronic decision support systems; mining of data to discover relationships between the concepts; discovery of new knowledge; and finally reuse of knowledge in the management of chronic diseases (Wand & Wang, 1996).

In the biomedical informatics literature, ontologies have been described as collections of formal, machine process-able and human interpretable representation of the entities, and the relations among those entities, within a definition of the application domain (Rubin et al., 2006). Pipino (2002) proposed the most widely accepted definition, where he considers ontologies as an explicit specification of a conceptualization (Pipino, Lee, & Wang, 2002). Ontology provides a vocabulary of terms, their meanings and relationships to be used in various application contexts (Borst, 1997). This allows intelligent software agents to act more meaningfully in spite of differences in concepts and terminology.

We have previously described and discussed an ontology based approach (S. T. Liaw, et al., 2013; Rahimi, et al., 2014) to assessing the completeness, correctness and consistency (the 3Cs of DQ) of data and datasets. This approach is helpful in modeling the domain and representation of data and metadata requirements to identify diabetes on the data set from the University of NSW electronic Practice Based Research Network (ePBRN). This study used the dataset of 927 active patients from a general practice participating in the ePBRN, hereafter referred to as the General Practice Unit (GPU) dataset.

The ePBRN DQ research and development has focused on the 3Cs of DQ for ongoing ontology-based work to better define and address DQ, examine the issues and challenges for the network of data extraction and linkage, and semantic interoperability of large data sets (S. Liaw, et al., 2011). The ontology based approach can assist the terminology management and decision support to identify and classify different types of diabetes (S. Liaw, et al., 2011). This approach is also helpful in developing automated techniques and tools to extract and semantically link data elements (and concepts) in large data sets derived from multiple EHRs.

The objective of this study is to develop a methodology for the systematic construction of a Data Quality Ontology (DQO), use the ontology to identify patients with Type 2 Diabetes Mellitus (T2DM) in an EHR, and assess the quality of data and its impact on the accuracy of identification.

The paper is organized as follows. Section 2 details the background. Section 3 describes the methodology and different steps in the development of the DQO for T2DM and the materials and tools used for the work. Section 4 discusses perspectives expected from this work. Section 5 draws conclusions from this work.

2. BACKGROUND

DQ is a complex idea with many dimensions, often overlapping conceptually (Devillers, Bedard, Jeansoulin, & Moulin, 2007; Nimmagadda, Nimmagadda, Dreher, & Ieee, 2008; Wand & Wang, 1996) with completeness, accuracy, correctness, consistency and timeliness being the most commonly used dimensions. Liaw et al (2010) developed a framework for extrinsic (e.g. representation) and intrinsic (e.g. correctness and consistency) concepts of data elements, and fitness for purpose (e.g. completeness) of data set for research and clinical purposes. Talaei-Khoei et al (2011) examined the consistency and completeness of data in healthcare settings, reporting that these issues may result in disruption for practitioners (Talaei-Khoei, Solvoll, Ray, & Parameshwaran, 2011, 2012).

A previous literature review showed the understanding of DQ, as a multidimensional concept applied to the data elements (intrinsic DQ) and the set of data elements (extrinsic DQ) is progressing (S. T. Liaw, et al., 2013). Ontological approaches are emerging and theoretically important to address the complex relationships among overlapping concepts in this domain (Rahimi, et al., 2014).

The literature on the specification of DQ is fragmentary, lacks a comprehensive approach and is poorly evaluated (Rahimi, et al., 2014). A few other studies have examined ontology based approaches to support data consistency and accuracy (O-Hoon, Jung-Eun, Hong-Seok, & Doo-Kwon, 2008). However, no research was found that formally and systematically assessed the association between ontologies for DQ and fitness for purpose in various contexts. There are also few comparative and evaluative studies on assessment of DQ or that compared ontological and non-ontological approaches to representing knowledge in clinical information systems (Nimmagadda, et al., 2008).

The recent literature review (Rahimi, et al., 2014) also suggested that compared to non-hierarchical data models, there may be more advantages and benefits in the use of ontologies to solve semantic clinical issues and improve the validity and reliability of data retrieval, collection, storage, extraction and linkage algorithms and tools. Formal ontological approaches enable systematic development of automated, valid and reliable methods to assess and manage data and semantic interoperability issues (Lee et al., 2009; Valencia-Garcia, Fernandez-Breis, Ruiz-Martinez, Garcia-Sanchez, & Martinez-Bejar, 2008; Verma et al., 2009; Verma, Kasabov, Rush, & Song, 2008). The expressiveness of ontology-based models can facilitate accuracy and precision compared to non-ontology models and approaches (Esposito, 2008a, 2008b; Preece, Missier, Ernbury, Jin, & Greenwood, 2008).

Current ontological approaches are poorly evaluated, with few comparative studies in chronic disease management or DQ assessment or management. The challenges to the development and validation of ontology-based models to assess and manage DQ include methodological immaturity, immature knowledge base, lack of tools to support ontology-based design of information systems, evaluation of ontological approaches, and engagement of users in design and implementations (Rahimi, Liaw, Ray, & Taggart, 2012; Rahimi, et al., 2014). There have also been several attempts to define ontology evaluation metrics and provide practical techniques to evaluate ontological approaches (in terms of flexibility, scalability and reusability) against non-ontology based models (Cur & #233, 2012; Maragoudakis, Lymberopoulos, Fakotakis, Spiropoulos, & Ieee, 2008). There is a lack of valid and reliable DQ assurance (D. Arts, De Keizer, & Scheffer, 2002; D. G. Arts, Bosman, de Jonge, Joore, & de Keizer, 2003; Peleg, Keren, & Denekamp, 2008) to ensure fitness for a range of uses by consumers, patients, health providers and professionals.

The significance of this work emanates from the fact that DQ research has been identified as a priority in medical informatics. Dixon (2011) and Huaman (2009) in their review of literature identified research in the quality of clinical data as a critical informatics research priority (Dixon, McGowan, & Grannis, 2011; Huaman et al., 2009). The authors cited DQ research as necessary for improving health care through the translation of research findings into practice (S. Liaw, et al., 2011), national deployment of EHRs (Dixon, et al., 2011; Huaman, et al., 2009), and development of the National Health Information Network (NHIN) (Richesson & Krischer, 2007).

A recent review (Rahimi, et al., 2014) demonstrated a lack of comprehensive studies on the use of ontology-based tools to assess and manage DQ so that data sets are fit for purpose in healthcare and chronic disease management (CDM). This paper reports on a rich methodological approach to develop a DQO, using the identification of patients with T2DM as a case study to illustrate the important issues, focusing on fitness for purpose along the lines presented in Section 3.

3. A METHODOLOGY FOR DATA QUALITY ONTOLOGY (DQO)

In this section, we present the details of a 5 step methodology to develop a DQO for application in the domain of Diabetes Mellitus. The DQO was applied to the identification of patients with Type 2 Diabetes Mellitus (T2DM) in an EHR. The validation of the DQO examined the technical aspects of the model and its accuracy in identifying patients with T2DM.

The purpose and scope of DQO is to identify, in this case, diabetic patients using three core attributes namely Reason for Visit (RFV), Pathology (Path) tests results such as Hemoglobin A1c (HbA1C), Blood Sugar Level (BSL) and Random Blood Glucose (RBG), and medication (Rx) in the GPU dataset. We first determined the scope of the domain, and purpose of the task that the DQO is to be fit for. The ePBRN has selected completeness, correctness, and consistency as the core DQ metrics for demographic and clinical data collected from disparate EHRs, and even within an individual EHR. We now briefly discuss the three core dimensions of DQ.

- **Completeness:** Completeness refers to the extent to which information is not missing and when available it is of sufficient breadth and depth for the task at hand (Kahn, Strong, & Wang, 2002). In our domain, this requirement means the availability of at least one record for the main patient attributes of RFV, Rx, Path and risk factors to identify Type 2 Diabetes mellitus. At the clinical level, completeness could mean that it include the availability of all information required to make a clinical decision about diabetes. Thus, each patient must have at least 1 record in one of the target attributes which consist of RFV, Path and Rx (S. Liaw, et al., 2011).

- **Correctness:** Correctness refers to data for each attribute being free of any errors (Pipino, et al., 2002) that is, each valid and appropriate clinical record must have the correct unit of measurements and must be within the acceptable clinical ranges. For instance, 'diabetes' is a correct value for the attribute RFV, and there are no errors in the way it has been written. Any other type of value for RFV is incorrect. For pathology tests and risk factors, correct ranges lie between the minimum and the maximum range of ePBRN data while respecting the Australian National Guidelines for T2DM ("Diabetes Management in General Practice Guidelines for Type 2 Diabetes ", 2012). A datum that lies outside this range is considered incorrect. Similarly, for medication, it would be incorrect if there were other attributes recorded for the script and the script name was missing.

- **Consistency:** Consistency refers to representing data values of the attributes following the same schema and format (Kahn, et al., 2002). It includes values and physical representation of data (Wand & Wang, 1996). External consistency uses a uniform data type, format and standard terminology (S. Liaw, et al., 2011) based on the Systematized Nomenclature of Medicine - Clinical Terms Australian version (SNOMED CT-AU) (McBride, Lawley, Leroux, & Gibson, 2012). Internal consistency uses a standard adopted specially for practice. For example, the following issues are relevant: Do doctors record diabetes type 2 the same way or does each doctor record it differently? Also, for internal consistency, at the first level, how are the attributes being recorded? An ePBRN question is whether different GPs and general practices record diabetes the same way? For external consistency, each term e.g. RFV used is externally consistent if it can be coded with or mapped to the same concepts in SNOMED CT-AU.

Based on the analysis of currently available techniques and commonly adopted conceptual steps (Corcho, Fernandez, & Gomez, 2003; Fernandez, 1999; Hadzic, Dillon, & Dillon, 2009; Kuziemsky & Lau, 2010; Pinto, 2004), we used a five stages methodology to create our ontology to identify T2DM in an EHR and assess DQ of the resulting register (See Figure 1): (1) Knowledge acquisition; (2) Conceptualization of the domain to create DQO; (3) Semantic modeling; (4) Knowledge representation; and (5) Validation

Figure 1. Five stages approach for the development of DQO

Stages		Knowledge acquisition	Conceptualization	Semantic modeling	Knowledge representation	Validation
• Main task		• Determain and collect the scope of the domain	• Finalize hierarchical conceptual model	• Ontology design	• Run DQO over the big dataset	• Measure Sensitivity and Specificity of the SPARQL queries
• Representation		• Textual	• Textual	• Technical	• Technical	• Textual
• Outcome		• Represent all assumptions and implicit notions	• Ontology domain and health professionals needs	• Formal model of DQO, revisions, feedbacks, extentions	• Map DQO and ePBRN database/Query and infere data	• Show accuracy of the model

of SPARQL query results and comparison with manual results as our research gold standard.

3.1. Knowledge Acquisition

In this step, we acquired knowledge about the domain and its scope with information from the domain experts and relevant published works. The techniques used include: brainstorming, interviews, questionnaires, text analysis, and inductive techniques (Pinto, 2004).

3.1.1. Patient Data Audit

An audit carried out on 7 patient data tables in the ePBRN included the following attributes: *Patients*, *Prescription*, *Diagnosis*, *Measure*, *Family History*, *Consultation* and *Patient Referral*. Data collected included: medical information (such as Reason for visit, Medication, Pathology test results), and information about patients' demographics (such as Date of Birth, History, Status and Sex). The ePBRN patient data audit formed the source of the clinical (user) vocabulary for the ontology.

3.1.2. GPs and Nurses Consensus Meetings

Two types of practice experience data were collected: clinician meetings and clinical observations. Clinician meetings involved one of the authors (AR) attending three meetings with 4 clinicians (2 physicians, 1 nurse and 1 data manager). The clinician meetings took place over 3 months and involved developing different models of diabetes management practices as well as discussion of conceptual models of diabetes management. Data from the clinician meetings provided a large volume of data which were useful in the design of our ontology. In those meetings there were also discussions about system design considerations for the computer-based diabetes assessment tool. Clinical observations involved the same author (AR) spending 44 hours performing qualitative observation and documentation of diabetes management themes on the clinical flowchart. Those observations were crucial for understanding the clinical workflow.

3.1.3. Literature Review

A literature review on the automation of identifying diabetes patients, diabetes management, and chronic disease management was carried out. Researching the literature brought in current evidence on diabetes management such as mechanisms for the assessment and management of diabetes, conceptual models on diabetes management and educational resources for primary and secondary care, assessment, diagnosis and management of different types of diabetes. Moreover, the conceptualization of diabetes assessment and management was drawn from evidence-based guidelines based on the Australian National Guidelines for T2DM ("Diabetes Management in General Practice Guidelines for Type 2 Diabetes ", 2012). Also, the SNOMED CT-AU standard guided the specification of the data and domains in the DQO. The research literature was valuable for contextualization of the ontological concepts and the clinical practices. Current published medical ontologies included the Human Diseases Ontology (DO) (Hadzic & Chang, 2004), Infectious Diseases Ontology (IDO) (Cowell & Smith, 2010), Galen (Rector & Rogers, 2005), and Gene Ontology (GO) (Pan Du et al., 2009). While these are comprehensive and essential models to draw on to develop the DQO prototype, they are not focused on diabetes specifically.

3.2. Conceptualization

In this step, we identified the key concepts and relationships in the domain and defined terms used to represent these concepts and relationships. Conceptualization denotes the process of turning raw knowledge into clearly established concepts that can be used to create a DQO. It typically includes the identification of the concepts and their relationships within the diabetes domain, taking advice from domain experts.

3.2.1. Task

In the current application, the conceptual model was developed through the results of an exhaustive literature review, ePBRN patient data audit, and GPs and nurses meetings.

3.2.2. Output

The final consensus meeting of our research team identified 68 concepts to comprehensively model the domain of diabetes management. Table 1 shows the categories (along with subcategories) of concepts in four different layers and the concepts relevant to each category.

For example, in the hierarchical conceptual model for *Mechanism* (which is the main class in diabetes management), there are 7 subclasses consisting of *Billing, Assessment, Review, Prescription, Referral, Advise,* and *Order.* Similarly, the subcategory *Order* includes subclasses *Medication, Imaging* and *Blood test.*

3.3. SEMANTIC MODELING

Semantic modeling refers to formalizing the domain ontology. This ontology and the defined rules generate logical inferences and control the relevant objects such as the patient with a diagnosis of diabetes mellitus (DM) and their related properties.

3.3.1. Task

In this stage we systematically transform the conceptual models into a formal model through the development of hierarchies and relationships and thus removing any ambiguities in the meanings of the concepts. The semantic model for a concept includes a set of attributes and its relationships

Table 1. Categories of collected concepts in four different layers

Main Categories	Subcategories	Relevant Concepts
Actor	Organization	Research Institution, University
	Person	Doctor, Nurse, Patient, Specialist
Context	Problem	Disease
	Setting	Primary care, Secondary care
Impact	Disease Indicator Control	HbA1c, random and fasting glucose levels
	Patients Satisfaction	Patient satisfaction questionnaires
	Quality of Life	QOL questionnaires
Mechanism	Advise	Lifestyle advice
	Assessment	Diagnosis, Family history, Risk Factor
	Billing	Services and supplies
	Consultation	Type of consultations
	Order	Imaging, Medication, Pathology tests
	Prescription	Medication
	Referral	Endocrinologist or general
	Review	Diabetes cycle of care

with other concepts that characterize the meaning of the concept. The DQO used previously reported definitions of the 3Cs of DQ (S. Liaw, et al., 2011).

3.3.2. Output

The formalized ontological model was developed using the Protégé 4.3 ontology editing tool (Gennari et al., 2003) and (Min et al., 2009) with frames as the representational construct. In Protégé, a reference terminology such as SNOMED CT-AU can be flexibly used with the Australian CIS used in this study; OntopPro (Rodrıguez-Muro, Kontchakov, & Zakharyaschev, 2013) can be used as an Ontology-based Data Access (OBDA) plug-in for Protégé for querying, inferring and mapping of DQO and the dataset used; and logic ontology reasoners provide automated support for reasoning tasks in ontology and instance checking and they include Pellet, Racer, Quest as the most popular and effective semantic reasoning engines (Huang, Li, & Yang, 2008).

In Table 1, Column 1 describes the main classes and Columns 2 and 3 their subclasses in the DQO. The output of this stage is a formalized ontology consisting of 4 main classes (*Actor, Content, Mechanism and Impact*) and 51 subclasses (Figure 2) with 8 object properties and 15 data properties. Figures 3 and 4 provide some illustrations to show the formalization of DQO developed (the hierarchical model and the relations) using the ontology tools and the definition of objects and properties. Protégé was used to add more terms to describe properties and classes within the diabetes domain, viz., relations between classes (e.g. disjointness such as PrimaryCare disjoint_with SecondaryCare), cardinality (e.g. *exactly one*), equality, richer typing of properties, characteristics of properties (e.g. functional for PatientUUID), and enumerated classes (e.g. MaritalStatus that has several characteristics such as single, married, divorced and widowed).

We have specified which classes are disjoint, so that an object cannot be an instance of more than one of these. It ensured consistency in DQO. Figure 3, defines (at this stage) object properties and relationships between different classes and subclasses. Careful modeling of object properties in Protégé helped to achieve all patients' data requirements. As figure 4 shows, the constraints presented by data properties in Protégé 4.3 are mainly capturing (a) the correctness of valid clinical records in ePBRN (for example, range for HbA1C is between 3.0 and 20 mmol/L), and (b) consistency of patients' data.

The end product of this stage is a semantic data model that has been defined as classes, sub-classes and their relationships to assist in identifying diabetic patients by Protégé 4.3 (Chen, Lu, & Liu, 2007). Our formalized ontology consist of 8 object properties, 15 data properties, 68 concepts and 14 major themes in 4 main classes comprising *Actor, Content, Mechanism* and *Impact* for improved identification of T2DM patients. Two ontology reasoners (Pellete 3.2.0, HermiT 1.3.6) (Huang, et al., 2008) were also applied to check internal consistency of the T2DM ontology and

Figure 2. The Ontology hierarchical conceptual model with data properties

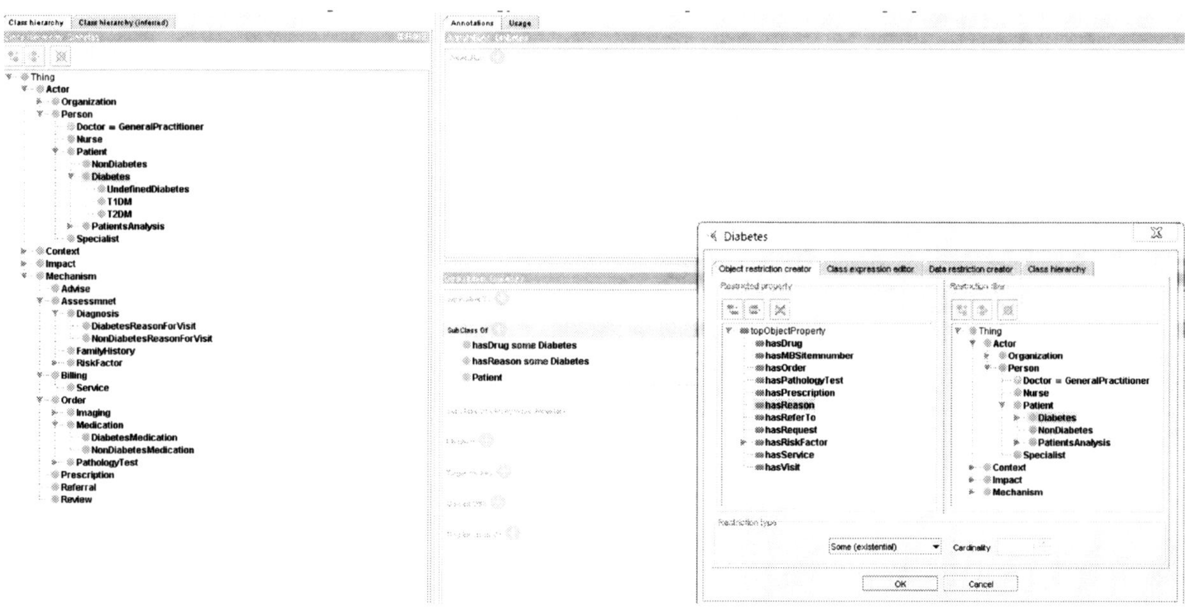

Figure 3. A sample of object property to show how as an example "hasT2DMRFV" can link two joint classes with together

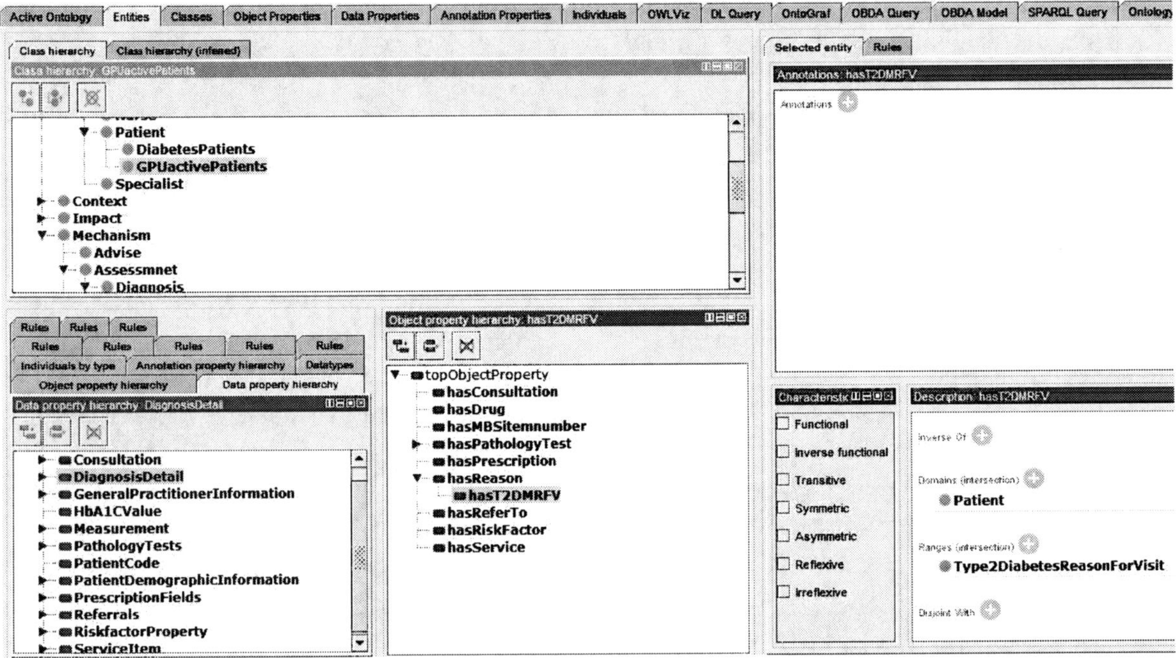

Figure 4. The data property tab to define various data ranges, types and values for each class

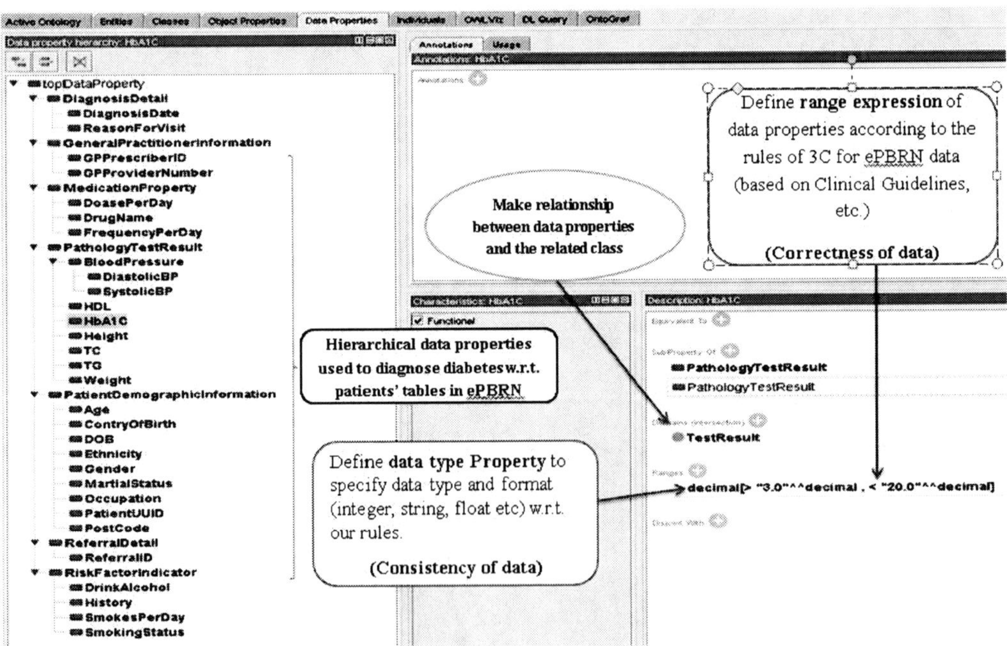

the reasoners found no logical inconsistencies in our ontology.

In Figure 5, we show that the ontology can be mapped onto the SNOMED CT-AU Ontology (SCAO) which has more than 300,000 concepts (Yu, Liaw, Taggart, & Rahimi, 2013).

3.4. Knowledge Representation

In this step, we developed an ontology model initially to represent the domain broadly. The necessary general concepts were included first, followed by the addition of the necessary constraints. For the Diabetes Mellitus domain, we added the constraints required to assess the DQ of the exracted data.

3.4.1 Task

This stage implemented the formalized ontology over the clinical data set extracted from a specific general practice participating in the ePBRN. This data set is a subset of the ePBRN data repository. The DQO has been implemented first to represent

the domain broadly. We used it to describe the necessary general concepts from the diabetes management point of view and then added constraints for lower datasets from the database in order to meet our DQ goals.

3.4.2. Output

To implement the DQO over the test data set, data was formalized using Microsoft SQL Server 2008 R2 and OntopPro (Rodrıguez-Muro, et al., 2013) as a plug-in for Protégé 4.3. The semantic query language Simple Protocol and Resource Description Framework Query Language (SPARQL), and the reasoner (Quest) (Rodrıguez-Muro & Calvanese, 2012) were then used. We additionally installed drivers to connect the test (relational) database and DQO using Protégé 4.3 preferences tab. Database connections were established using the Java Data Base Connectivity Framework (JDBC) (Calvanese et al., 2009). In this case, Quest and OntopPro used MS JDBC Driver for SQL Server to connect to the GPU data set. This required JDBC parameters; we

Figure 5. The 'Context' as an example class hierarchy shows expanded in a Protégé screenshot. The annotation associated with the subclass "Type 2 diabetes mellitus" describes semantic relationship of this subclass with the reference terminology SNOMED CT-AU

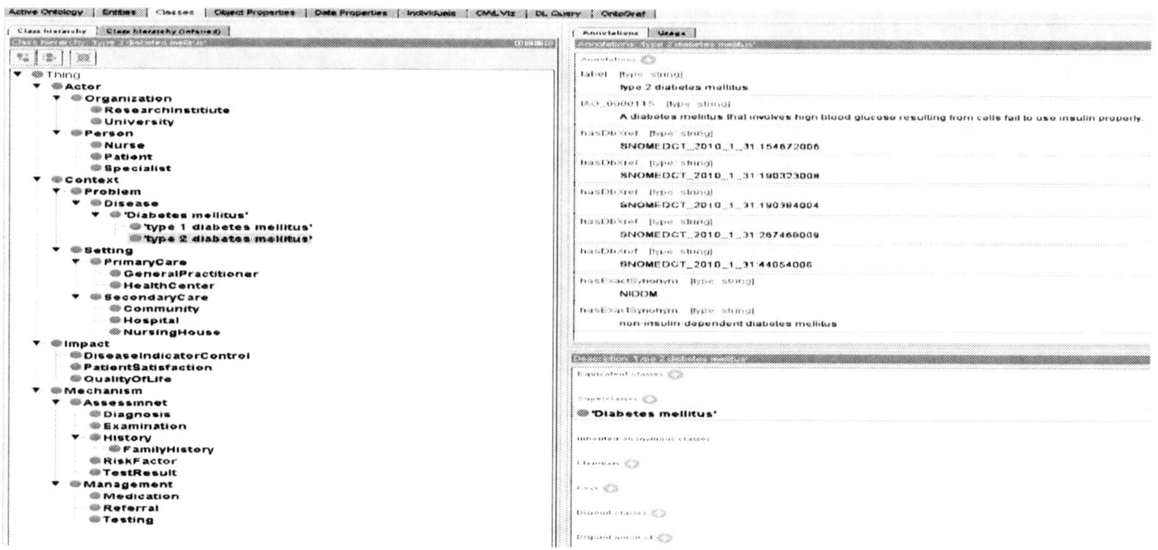

Figure 6. DQO OBDA tab to define JDBC connection parameters

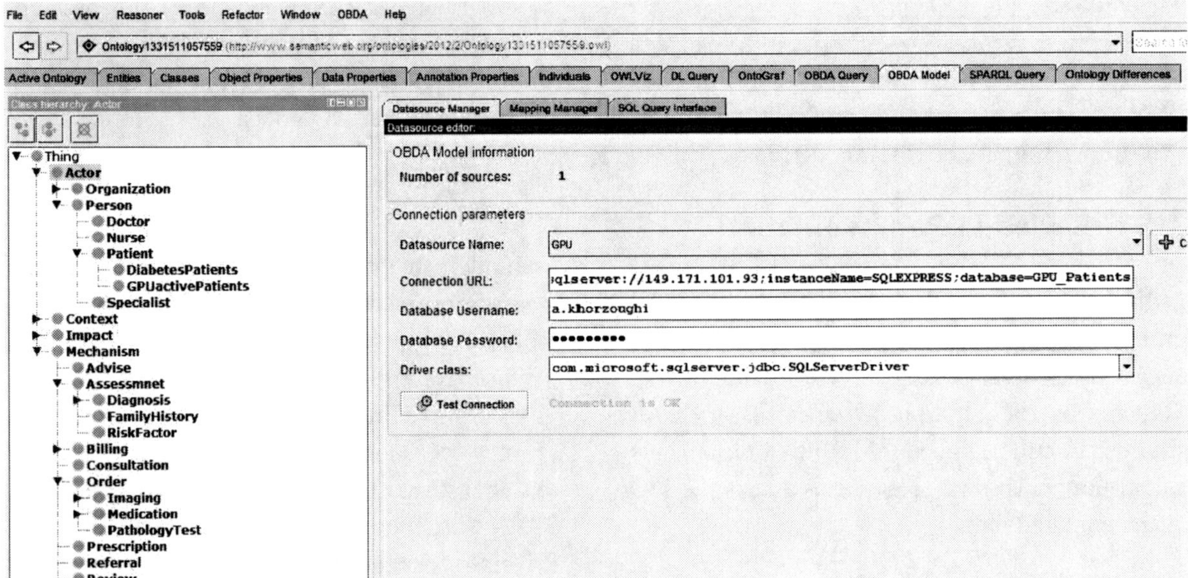

defined 4 parameters: Driver class, JDBC URL, username and password (Figure 6).

Once mappings were created, the plug-in was used to generate Resource Description Framework (RDF) triples for use with OntopPro to query the test dataset, without any imports. A mapping axiom was used to generate RDF triples, and one set of RDF triples for each result row was returned by the source query. The triples were created by replacing the place holders in the target with the values from the row. Each mapping must also contain one or more mapping axioms. A mapping axiom is defined with a source and a target, where the source is an arbitrary SQL query over the database and the target is a triple template that contains placeholders that reference column names mentioned in the source query.

In Figure 7, we defined the requirements for the following examples:

Example-1: Query for active Patients.
Example-2: Query for all Patients with the T2DM Reason Item.

Example-3: Use object property to join two tables using Patient_UUID as a unique identifier and identify active patients with T2DMRFV

3.4.2.1. Step 1: Analysis of sources and targets

From DQO, we needed to map the following entities:

- Classes, i.e., Patient and Diagnosis.
- Data properties, i.e., PatientID and ReasonItem.
- Object properties, i.e., hasT2DMRFV

Analyzing our database we find that the following tables can be used to create mappings for these classes and properties: i.e., ePBRN_Active_Patient and ePBRN_DIAGNOSIS. We can see that there is a one to one correspondence between the entities stored in the tables and the classes we wanted to map. Likewise, the columns Patient_UUID from ePBRN_Active_Patient table and REASON from ePBRN_DIAGNOSIS can be

Figure 7. Mapping the Diagnosis table with the ontology model

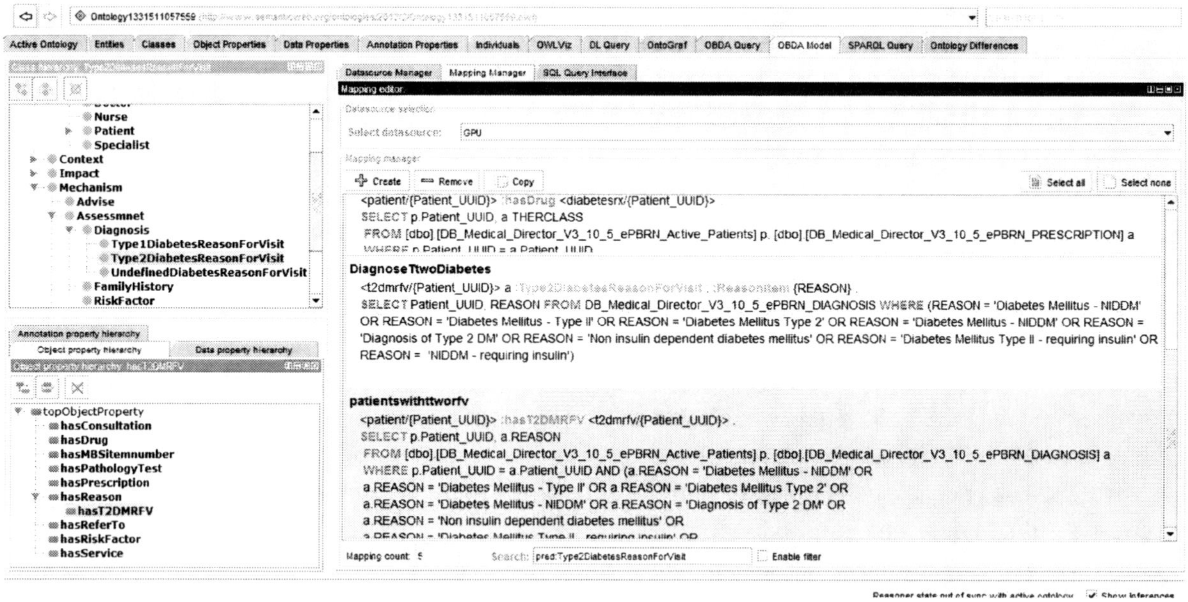

used for the data properties. To create the Uniform Recourse Identifiers (URIs) for those entities we could use Patient_UUID as a unique-identifier for these tables.

3.4.2.2. Step 2: Mappings and Queries

The tables were analyzed using the following mappings:

- Example-1: Query for all active Patients.
  Source: SELECT Patient_UUID FROM ePBRN_Active_Patients
  Target: <patient/{Patient_UUID}> a:GPUactivePatients.
- Example-2: Query for all active Patients with the T2DM Reason Item.
  Source: SELECT Patient_UUID, REASON FROM ePBRN_DIAGNOSIS WHERE (REASON = 'Diabetes Mellitus - NIDDM' OR REASON = 'Diabetes Mellitus - Type II' OR REASON = 'Diabetes Mellitus Type 2' OR REASON = 'NIDDM' OR REASON = 'Diagnosis of Type 2 DM' OR REASON = 'Non-insulin dependent diabetes mellitus' OR REASON = 'Diabetes Mellitus Type II - requiring insulin' OR REASON = 'NIDDM - requiring insulin')
  Target: <t2dmrfv/{Patient_UUID}> a:Type2DiabetesReasonForVisit ;:ReasonItem {REASON}.
- Example-3: Use object property to show how it joins two tables using Patient_UUID as a unique identifier and identify active patients with T2DMRFV
  Source: SELECT 'Patient_UUID' as pid, 'Patient_UUID' as t2dmrfv.
  FROM ePBRN_PATIENT_V1, ePBRN_DIAGNOSIS
  WHERE ePBRN_PATIENT_V1.Patient_UUID = ePBRN_DIAGNOSIS.Patient_UUID
  Target: <t2dmrfv/{Patient_UUID}> a:Type2DiabetesReasonForVisit ;:ReasonItem {REASON}.

All mappings required for our criteria to identify T2DM patients were thus complete. Indeed in our knowledgebase, the ABox, associated with instances of ontology classes or properties, was populated through OntopPro. The TBox, related to conceptual terminologies, was built using Protégé. Therefore, once mappings have been created, we were able to use the plug-in to generate RDF triples and use them with OntopPro to query the GPU dataset, without any imports.

Semantic queries were formulated in SPARQL according to requirements from domain experts, and were run using QUEST, a query engine and ontology reasoner. SPARQL used relevant objects, such as T2DM diagnosis, medications and pathology test results, singly and in combination, to construct queries for the identification of patients with T2DM. The sensitivity and specificity of the SPARQL query, and therefore the implementation of the T2DM ontology, were measured (Rahimi, Liaw, Taggart, Ray, & Yu, in-press). The SPARQL queries were validated using SQL over an artificial dataset of 100 patients schematically similar to the ePBRN dataset.

3.5. Validation

In this step, the quality of the DQOwas assessed as to the correctness and validity of the knowledge encoded in the ontology. The validation of the ontology involves verifying whether the meaning of the concepts and their relationships faithfully model the real world for which the ontology was created. This validation is essential to ensure that the ontology based approach and the DQO developed is fit for purpose.

3.5.1. Task

The DQO was tested for its compliance to the requirements domain experts, DQ attributes (3Cs), and accuracy in identifying patients with T2DM over a data set extracted from the EHR of a small general practice participating in the ePBRN. The methodology used was to compare the cases of T2DM identified by the DQO with the saes identified by a manual audit of the EHR from which the data was extracted (GPU dataset). We audited the EHR information of all 908 active patients (i.e. those who have attended the practice at least 3 times in the past 2 years) using a specific template to ensure that we understood all the reasons why the patient might or might not be a T2DM patient. This accuracy the DQO methodology has been reported in another paper (Rahimi et al., in-press) The following section (outputs) uses information reported in this paper to highlight the compliance of the technical components of the DQO methodology to the requirements of the domain experts and DQ attributes.

3.5.2. Outputs

Explicit and unambiguous queries, using patterns, disjunctions and conjunctions, were built in SPARQL to identify patients with T2DM. The constraints presented by object properties in Protégé 4.3 were used to set up relationships between classes. SPARQL was also used to apply data properties to assess DQ in the patient's attributes. For example, constraints presented by data properties were used to capture: (a) the correctness of valid clinical records in ePBRN (e.g., correct value for HbA1C is $=>7\%$); and (b) consistency of patients' data (e.g. all T2DM patients with uniform, data type and standard value of HbA1C).

Semantic queries in SPARQL were verified by clinicians in the research team (JT, STL) to ensure that they complied with the requirements of the domain experts previously consulted. The DQ requirements were also verified for its fit for identification of T2DM. Once this was verified, and the queries were run through QUEST, the query engine and OWL reasoner.

The query results met all our expectations regarding the identification of T2DM patients and the assessment of the DQ of the data set (Rahimi

Table 2. Part of a SPARQL query using 3 patients' attributes to identify patients with T2DM

Diabetes' attributes	Sample of SPARQL query using combined patients' attributes
T2DM RFV and Rx and abnormal pathology tests	SELECT DISTINCT ?pid WHERE {{?pid a:GPUactivePatients. ?pid:hasT2DMRFV ?r. ?r:ReasonItem ?reason. FILTER(?reason = "Diabetes Mellitus - Type II"^^xsd:String ‖ ?reason = "Diabetes Mellitus - NIDDM"^^xsd:String ‖ ?reason = "Diagnosis of Type 2 DM"^^xsd:String ‖ ?reason = "Diabetes Mellitus Type II - requiring insulin"^^xsd:String ‖ ?reason = "Diabetes Mellitus - Type II"^^xsd:String ‖ ?reason = "Diabetes Mellitus Type 2"^^xsd:String ‖ ?reason = "NIDDM - requiring insulin"^^xsd:String ‖ ?reason = "Non insulin dependent diabetes mellitus"^^xsd:String ‖ ?reason = "NIDDM"^^xsd:String ‖ ?reason = "Diabetes Mellitus - NIDDM"^^xsd:String)} UNION {?pid a:GPUactivePatients. ?pid:hasT2DMHistory ?h. ?h:Condition ?history. FILTER(?history = "Diabetes Mellitus - NIDDM"^^xsd:String ‖ ?history = "Diabetes Mellitus - Type II"^^xsd:String ‖ ?history = "Non insulin dependent diabetes mellitus"^^xsd:String ‖ ?history = "NIDDM"^^xsd:String ‖ ?history = "Diagnosis of Type 2 DM"^^xsd:String ‖ ?history = "Diabetes Mellitus Type II - requiring insulin"^^xsd:String ‖ ?history = "Diabetes Mellitus Type 2"^^xsd:String ‖ ?history = "NIDDM - requiring insulin"^^xsd:String)} UNION {?pid a:GPUactivePatients. ?pid:hasDrug ?d. ?d:TherapyClass ?rx. FILTER(?rx = "HDI"^^xsd:String ‖ ?rx = "HDO"^^xsd:String ‖ ?rx = "HDI"^^xsd:String ‖ ?rx = "ODB"^^xsd:String ‖ ?rx = "HD"^^xsd:String ‖ ?rx = "HDOA"^^xsd:String ‖?rx = "HDOD"^^xsd:String ‖ ?rx = "ODU"^^xsd:String)} UNION {?pid a:GPUactivePatients. ?pid:hasRepeatDrug ?r. ?r:TherapyClass ?rerx. FILTER(?rerx = "HDI"^^xsd:String ‖ ?rerx = "HDO"^^xsd:String ‖ ?rerx = "HDI"^^xsd:String ‖ ?rerx = "ODB"^^xsd:String ‖ ?rerx = "HD"^^xsd:String ‖ ?rerx = "HDOA"^^xsd:String ‖?rerx = "HDOD"^^xsd:String ‖ ?rerx = "ODU"^^xsd:String)} UNION {?pid a:GPUactivePatients. ?pid:hasT2DMPathologyTest ?p. ?p:TestName ?test. ?p:ResultTest ?result. FILTER(?test = "HbA1C"^^xsd:String && ?result >= "6.5"^^xsd:Integer ‖ ?test = "GLUCOSE PLASMA FASTING"^^xsd:String && ?result >= "7.0"^^xsd:Integer ‖ ?test = "GLUCOSE Random"^^xsd:String && ?result >= "11.1"^^xsd:Integer ‖ ?test = "Glucose Fasting"^^xsd:String && ?result >= "7.0"^^xsd:Integer)}}

et al 2014, in press). For example in Table 2 it can be seen how a semantically flexible approach uses different object and data properties as well as relevant classes to combine different T2DM attributes (RFV, Rx and Path) for the identification of T2DM patients. The first level of completeness of patients' DQ requirements can be achieved by carefully modeling object properties.

Table 2 presents a part of the novel SPARQL query results for a different level of identification of Type 2 diabetic patients. SPARQL queries only referred to classes, object properties and data properties to combine main diabetes criteria for the identification of diabetes semantically. The DQO-based query, partly shown in Table 2, identified 105 T2DM using T2DM RFVs, Rx and Path. The query was implemented over the data set using SQL Server 2008 R2. The accuracy of the DQO-based query, as compared to the manual validation as the benchmark, is summarized in Table 3. The manual of the EHR that the T2DM RFV was scattered across a number of tables (PAST_HISTORY_TABLE, DIAGNOSIS_Table) and in the progress notes as text unstructured data. Where the RFV were recorded in a structured field, the semantic SPARQL queries identified them accurately. This was similar for the other attributes used to identifdiabetes T2DM (usingRX and Path).

The Sensitivity and Specificity of the DQO-based queries implemented in SPARQL were calculated and compared with the accuracy of the manual audit. Patients identified as T2DM by the DQO based query and manual audit are true positives (TP); those identified by DQO based query as T2DM but not on manual audit are false positives (FP); the reverse are false negatives (FN); and patients not identified

Table 3. Accuracy of the model developed (Rahimi, et al., in-press)

	RFV	Medication	Pathology tests	All attributes
Sensitivity	100%	96.55%	15.6%	97.67%
Specificity	99.88%	98.97%	98.92%	99.18%

as T2DM by both DQO based query and manual audit are true negatives (TN). Sensitivity, defined as TP/ (TP + FP) denotes the ability of the system to accurately identify all those patients who are T2DM patients. Specificity, defined as TN/ (FN+TN) measures the model's accuracy in identifying the proportion of all patients without T2DM who are not included in the dataset. As Table 3 suggests, identification of T2DM using Path data was not as accurate as that using RFV or Rx.

This reflects inaccurate Path data due to change in the units for reporting of HbA1c results. However, this level of inaccuracy was acceptable for our purpose as confirmed by the very small relative deterioration of the accuracy (Sensitivity and Specificity were 97.67% and 99.18%, respectively) when calculated for the combination of RFV, Rx and Path. The completeness and correctness of the RFV and Rx data compensated for the poor completeness and correctness of the Path data in the DQO-based approach. The manual EHR audit suggested that the accuracy of the algorithm was determined by DQ issues such as unavailability of data due to non-documentation or documented in the wrong place, problems with data extraction, encryption and data management errors. The multi-attribute ontological approach to defining a T2DM case, can compensate for poor DQ in one or more of the component attributes and therefore not lose the overall accuracy.

4. DISCUSSION

This paper presented a semantic knowledge management approach for identifying T2DM and assessed its DQ using: (a) knowledge acquisi-tion techniques to derive diabetes management strategy from the results obtained in our literature review and evidence-based resources; (b) a con-ceptualization process to develop a hierarchical data model; (c) a knowledge model to transfer the conceptual model to the formal model with the help of knowledge management tools; (d) knowledge representation techniques to map the data set into the DQO, using OntoPro; and (e) manual validation to confirm the accuracy of the DQO based approach.

The DQO based approach to identify T2DM patients can be modular and generic, enabling the development of intelligent software agents (A. H. Ghapanchi & Aurum, 2011; Amir Hos-sein Ghapanchi & Aurum, 2012) to act in vari-ous semantic contexts to identify patients with a range of diseases (Mabotuwana & Warren, 2009), support decision making in health care (Lezcano, Sicilia, & Rodríguez-Solano, 2011), and conduct audit, evaluation and research on patients with other chronic diseases (Pathak, Kiefer, Bielinski, & Chute, 2012a, 2012b; Pathak, Kiefer, & Chute, 2012).

4.1. Usefulness of the Ontological Based Approach for DQ Specification

As we presented in the Conceptualization and Se-mantic modeling section, the ontology based model is particularly useful to enable quick development and testing so that feedback can be cycled back into the development process. For example, the ontology classes and data properties guide research team to ensure fields, records, tables and relationships in the database are appropriately presented.

The ontology-based approach can therefore access and manage the quality of data in a way that is generalizable and reusable, to examine the issues and challenges in data extraction, linkage and semantic interoperability (S. T. Liaw, et al., 2013; Rahimi, et al., 2014).

The DQO based approach implemented here corroborates the belief that ontological approaches have theoretical and practical advantages in developing automated methods for identifying patients with chronic diseases, guiding clinical care, and quality improvement and research (Buranarach, Chalortham, Chatvorawit, Thein, & Supnithi, 2009; Chalortham, Buranarach, & Supnithi, 2009; Colombo et al., 2010; Coltell et al., 2004).

4.2. Applicability of the ontology based approach for DQ specification

The suggested ontology based approach can accurately specify metadata for DQ specification and assessment for particular clinical domains. In the semantic modeling stage, it has been shown that DQ can be expressed by constraints and axioms to cope with DQ specification. For example, as we demonstrated in the semantic modeling section, class attributes (data properties) have been defined to capture correctness and consistency of valid clinical records. The ePBRN team has created the rules for quality metrics (3Cs), using Australian National T2DM diagnosis and management Guidelines and SNOMED CT-AU (S. Liaw, et al., 2011; Rahimi, et al., 2012; Yu, et al., 2013) to:

- Define data properties.
- Use uniform data types and formats (e.g. integer, string, and real) for each variable (for Internal Consistency).
- Define uniform data format for each concept (e.g. for Assessment sub-class, hasHbA1C is selected as the property of the class, decimal is selected as the type and a value v where $3 <= v$ and $v >= 20$ is entered for Correctness)

- Select standard label for each entity (e.g. use type 2 diabetes mellitus instead T2DM for External Consistency).

The knowledge management tools, such as Protégé, allows specifications of properties of classes, such as disjoint, so that an individual (or object) cannot be an instance of more than one of the specified classes. This leads to more consistency and correctness, as well as enable an assessment of data set completeness.

In addition to accuracy, a DQO based application to enable automated assessment of patients' data can also be flexible and applicable to other chronic diseases such as COPD and other areas such as population health. Therefore, our model can support other studies that it is applicable to information retrieval and analysis (Valencia-Garcia, et al., 2008), intelligent data mining (seeking concepts and relationships) (Chen, et al., 2007), discover new knowledge, and reuse knowledge for decision support systems and patient decision aids (Abidi, 2011). Our approach fills current gap in the application and applicability of ontological models to assess and manage quality of information in EHRs.

4.3. Evaluation of DQO Methodology

Our methodology confirmed that the validation of an ontology should and can be done through its use in a concrete application (e.g. the identification of T2DM) (Kuziemsky & Lau, 2010; Rahimi, et al., in-press). The development and deployment of ontologies must include evaluation metrics. Our previous literature reviews have shown that the ontological approach to develop DQ is poorly validated (S. T. Liaw, et al., 2013; Rahimi, et al., 2014) and identified the most common criteria to assess validity of ontologies and data models are Flexibility, Reusability and Scalability (Rahimi, et al., 2014).

The DQO based approach can add more axioms and constraints to the concepts based on the specific purposes of DQ assessment and management. The ontology based approach is more flexible than the non-ontological and non-semantic techniques for solving semantic interoperability and technological issues derived from poor DQ (Gangemi, Catenacci, Ciaramita, & Lehmann, 2006; Gilbert & Ddembe, 2008; Pannarale et al., 2012). It also has the flexibility of being applicable to and therefore reusable in other domains (Gilbert & Ddembe, 2008; Pinto, 2004).

As shown in the Knowledge Representation stage, the DQO approach mapped a small part, a unique general practice with 908 active patients, from the larger ePBRN data repository. This demonstrates the scalability of the ontology based approach (Cur & #233, 2012).

4.4. Comparison of DQO and Non-Ontological Approaches in CDM

The proposed methodological approach particularly in the Conceptualization and Semantic Modeling stages reveals that the ontology based approach contains more explicit semantic information compared to non-semantic and non-ontological approaches. Hence, for DQ specification, as opposed to non-ontological approaches, an ontology is a formal, explicit specification of a shared conceptualization that provides a vocabulary of terms, their meanings and relationships to be used in various application contexts so that intelligent agents can act in spite of differences in terminology and their meanings (Pinto, 2004). They enable the modeling of the domain and representation of information requirements to specify the context in collaborative environments (Ganguly, Ray, & Parameswaran, 2005). DQ models and ontologies are being developed to enable the application of ontology-based tools for automated specification, assessment and management of DQ (Ganguly, et al., 2005; Ying, Wimalasiri, Ray, Chattopadhyay, & Wilson, 2010).

5. CONLUSION

The ontology-based approach to DQ assessment and management in the context of type 2 diabetes mellitus identification has been examined. The traditional five stage methodology - knowledge acquisition, conceptualization, semantic modeling, knowledge representation, and validation was successfully used to develop the DQO. This semantic mechanism to purposefully capture patient data from EHRs is flexible, generalizable and potentially reusable in other domains. The accuracy was validated by a manual audit of active patients from the EHR. This approach can address the challenges in automated data extraction, linkage and assessment of the quality of routinely collected data in EHRs.

ACKNOWLEDGMENT

The authors would like to thank the ePBRN research team for their previous and ongoing contributions in this study.

REFERENCES

Abidi, S. R. (2011). *Ontology-based knowledge modeling to provide decision support for comorbid diseases*. Paper presented at the The 19th European Conference in Artificial Intelligence. Retrieved from http://www.scopus.com/inward/record. url?eid=2-s2.0-79952016090&partnerID=40& md5=d6e8e7441e3e9118fa395e5fc0b77b95

Arts, D., De Keizer, N., & Scheffer, G. J. (2002). Defining and Improving Data Quality in Medical Registries: A Literature Review, Case Study, and Generic Framework. *Journal of the American Medical Informatics Association, 9*(6), 600–611. doi:10.1197/jamia.M1087 PMID:12386111

Arts, D. G., Bosman, R. J., de Jonge, E., Joore, J. C., & de Keizer, N. F. (2003). Training in data definitions improves quality of intensive care data. *Critical Care (London, England)*, *7*(2), 179–184. doi:10.1186/cc1886 PMID:12720565

Borst, W. N. (1997). *Construction of Engineering Ontologies*. Enschede, NL: University of Tweenty.

Brown, P., Warmington, V., Laurence, M., & Prevost, A. (2003). Randomised crossover trial comparing the performance of Clinical Terms Version 3 and Read Codes 5 byte set coding schemes in general practice. *BMJ (Clinical Research Ed.)*, *326*(7399), 1127. doi:10.1136/bmj.326.7399.1127 PMID:12763986

Buranarach, M., Chalortham, N., Chatvorawit, P., Thein, Y., & Supnithi, T. (2009). An Ontology-based Framework for Development of Clinical Reminder System to Support Chronic Disease Healthcare. Retrieved from http://text.hlt.nectec. or.th/ontology/sites/default/files/reminder_is-bme09_cr_0.pdf

Chalortham, N., Buranarach, M., & Supnithi, T. (2009). Ontology Development for Type II Diabetes Mellitus Clinical Support System. Retrieved from http://text.hlt.nectec.or.th/ontology/sites/default/files/CRdm2css_0.pdf

Chen, X. H., Lu, J., & Liu, Z. Y. (2007). Assistance ontology of quality control for enterprise model using data mining. In M. Helander, M. Xie, M. Jaio, & K. C. Tan (Eds.), *2007 Ieee International Conference on Industrial Engineering and Engineering Management*, Vols 1-4 (pp. 602-606). doi:10.1109/IEEM.2007.4419260

Colombo, G., Merico, D., Boncoraglio, G., De Paoli, F., Ellul, J., & Frisoni, G. et al. (2010). An ontological modeling approach to cerebrovascular disease studies: The NEUROWEB case. *Journal of Biomedical Informatics*, *43*(4), 469–484. doi:10.1016/j.jbi.2009.12.005 PMID:20074662

Coltell, O., Arregui, M., Perez, C., Domenech, M. A., Corella, D., & Chalmeta, R. (2004). *Building an ontology on genomic epidemiology of cardiovascular diseases*. Orlando: Int Inst Informatics & Systemics.

Corcho, O., Fernandez, M., & Gomez, A. (2003). Methodologies, tools and languages for building ontologies. Where is their meeting point? *Data & Knowledge Engineering*, *46*(1), 41–64. doi:10.1016/S0169-023X(02)00195-7

Cowell, L. G., & Smith, B. (2010). The Infectious Disease Ontology. In S. V. (Ed.), Infectious Disease Informatics (Vol. Chapter 19, pp. P373-395). New York: Springer

Cur, O. (2012). Improving the Data Quality of Drug Databases using Conditional Dependencies and Ontologies. *J. Data and Information Quality*, *4*(1), 1–21. doi:10.1145/2378016.2378019

Devillers, R., Bedard, Y., Jeansoulin, R., & Moulin, B. (2007). Towards spatial data quality information analysis tools for experts assessing the fitness for use of spatial data. *International Journal of Geographical Information Science*, *21*(3), 261–282. doi:10.1080/13658810600911879

Diabetes Management in General Practice Guidelines for Type 2 Diabetes (2012). In D. A. a. R. A. C. o. G. Practitioners (Ed.), (Seventeenth edition 2011/12 ed., Vol. 2011/12): Diabetes Australia.

Dixon, B., McGowan, J., & Grannis, G. (2011). *Electronic Laboratory Data Quality and the Value of a Health Information Exchange to Support Public Health Reporting Processes*. Paper presented at the AMIA 2011 Annual Symposium Improving Health: Informatics and IT Changing the World.

Esposito, M. (2008a). Congenital Heart Disease: An ontology-based approach for the examination of the cardiovascular system. In I. Lovrek (Ed.), *Knowledge - Based Intelligent Information and Engineering Systems, Pt 1* (Vol. 5177, pp. 509–516). Proceedings. doi:10.1007/978-3-540-85563-7_65

Esposito, M. (2008b). *An ontological and non-monotonic rule-based approach to label medical images*. Los Alamitos: Ieee Computer Soc.

Fernandez, M. (1999). *Overview Of Methodologies For Building Ontologies.* Paper presented at the IJCAI-99 workshop on Ontologies and Problem-Solving Methods (KRR5), Stockholm, Sweden.

Gangemi, A., Catenacci, C., Ciaramita, M., & Lehmann, J. (2006). *Modelling ontology evaluation and validation.* Paper presented at the Proceedings of the 3rd European conference on The Semantic Web: research and applications. doi:10.1007/11762256_13

Ganguly, P., Ray, P., & Parameswaran, N. (2005). Semantic Interoperability in Telemedicine through Ontology-Driven Services. *Telemedicine Journal and e-Health, 11*(3), 8. doi:10.1089/tmj.2005.11.405 PMID:16035934

Gennari, J. H., Musen, M. A., Fergerson, R. W., Grosso, W. E., Eriksson, H., & Noy, N. F. et al. (2003). The evolution of Protege: An environment for knowledge-based systems development. *International Journal of Human-Computer Studies, 58*(1), 89–123. doi:10.1016/S1071-5819(02)00127-1

Ghapanchi, A. H., & Aurum, A. (2011, 4-7 Jan. 2011). *Measuring the Effectiveness of the Defect-Fixing Process in Open Source Software Projects.* Paper presented at the System Sciences (HICSS), 2011 44th Hawaii International Conference on.

Ghapanchi, A. H., & Aurum, A. (2012). The impact of project capabilities on project performance: Case of open source software projects. *International Journal of Project Management, 30*(4), 407–417. doi:10.1016/j.ijproman.2011.10.002

Gilbert, M., & Ddembe, W. (2008). A Flexible Approach for User Evaluation of Biomedical Ontologies. *International Journal of Computing and ICT Research, 2*(2), 62–74.

Hadzic, M., & Chang, E. (2004). Role of the ontologies in the context of grid computing and application for the human disease studies. *Semantics of a Networked World: Semantics for Grid Databases, 3226*, 316–318. doi:10.1007/978-3-540-30145-5_22

Hadzic, M., Dillon, D. S., & Dillon, T. S. (2009). *Use and Modeling of Multi-agent Systems in Medicine.*

Huaman, M. A., Araujo-Castillo, R. V., Soto, G., Neyra, J. M., Quispe, J. A., & Fernandez, M. F. et al. (2009). Impact of two interventions on timeliness and data quality of an electronic disease surveillance system in a resource limited setting (Peru): A prospective evaluation. *BMC Medical Informatics and Decision Making*, 9. PMID:19272165

Huang, T., Li, W., & Yang, C. (2008). *Comparison of Ontology Reasoners: Racer, Pellet, Fact++* Paper presented at the American Geophysical Union, Fall Meeting 2008.

Kahn, B. K., Strong, D. M., & Wang, R. Y. (2002). Information quality benchmarks: Product and service performance. *Communications of the ACM, 45*(4), 8. doi:10.1145/505248.506007

Kuziemsky, C., & Lau, F. (2010). A four stage approach for ontology-based health information system design. *Artificial Intelligence in Medicine, 50*(3), 133–148. doi:10.1016/j.artmed.2010.04.012 PMID:20510592

Lee, C. S., Wang, M. H., Acampora, G., Loia, V., Hsu, C. Y., & Ieee. (2009). *Ontology-based Intelligent Fuzzy Agent for Diabetes Application.* New York: Ieee.

Lezcano, L., Sicilia, M.-A., & Rodríguez-Solano, C. (2011). Integrating reasoning and clinical archetypes using OWL ontologies and SWRL rules. *Journal of Biomedical Informatics, 44*(2), 343–353. doi:10.1016/j.jbi.2010.11.005 PMID:21118725

Liaw, S., Taggart, J., Dennis, S., & Yeo, A. (2011). *Data quality and fitness for purpose of routinely collected data – a general practice case study from an electronic Practice-Based Research Network (ePBRN)*. Paper presented at the AMIA 2011 Annual Symposium Improving Health: Informatics and IT Changing the World.

Liaw, S. T., Rahimi, A., Ray, P., Taggart, J., Dennis, S., & de Lusignan, S. et al. (2013). Towards an ontology for data quality in integrated chronic disease management: A realist review of the literature. *International Journal of Medical Informatics*, *82*(1), 10–24. doi:10.1016/j.ijmedinf.2012.10.001 PMID:23122633

Mabotuwana, T., & Warren, J. (2009). An ontology-based approach to enhance querying capabilities of general practice medicine for better management of hypertension. *Artificial Intelligence in Medicine*, *47*(2), 87–103. doi:10.1016/j.artmed.2009.07.001 PMID:19709865

Maragoudakis, M., Lymberopoulos, D., Fakotakis, N., Spiropoulos, K., & Ieee. (2008). A Hierarchical, Ontology-Driven Bayesian Concept for Ubiquitous Medical Environments- A Case Study for Pulmonary Diseases *2008 30th Annual International Conference of the Ieee Engineering in Medicine and Biology Society, Vols 1-8* (pp. 3807-3810). New York: Ieee.

McBride, S. J., Lawley, M. J., Leroux, H., & Gibson, S. (2012). Using Australian medicines terminology (AMT) and SNOMED CT-AU to better support clinical research. *Studies in Health Technology and Informatics*, *178*, 144–149. PMID:22797033

Min, H., Manion, F. J., Goralczyk, E., Wong, Y. N., Ross, E., & Beck, J. R. (2009). Integration of prostate cancer clinical data using an ontology. *Journal of Biomedical Informatics*, *42*(6), 1035–1045. doi:10.1016/j.jbi.2009.05.007 PMID:19497389

Nimmagadda, S. L., Nimmagadda, S. K., Dreher, H., & Ieee. (2008). Ontology based data warehouse modeling and managing ecology of human body for disease and drug prescription management *2008 2nd Ieee International Conference on Digital Ecosystems and Technologies* (pp. 465-473).

O-Hoon., C., Jung-Eun, L., Hong-Seok, N., & Doo-Kwon, B. (2008). *An Efficient Method of Data Quality using Quality Evaluation Ontology*. Paper presented at the Third 2008 International Conference on Convergence and Hybrid Information Technology.

Pan Du, P., Feng, G., Flatow, J., Song, J., Holko, M., & Kibbe, W. et al. (2009). From disease ontology to disease-ontology lite: Statistical methods to adapt a general-purpose ontology for the test of gene-ontology associations. *Bioinformatics (Oxford, England)*, *25*(12), i63–i68. doi:10.1093/bioinformatics/btp193 PMID:19478018

Pannarale, P., Catalano, D., De Caro, G., Grillo, G., Leo, P., & Pappada, G. et al. (2012). GIDL: A rule based expert system for GenBank Intelligent Data Loading into the Molecular Biodiversity Database. *BMC Bioinformatics*, *13*(Suppl 4), S4. doi:10.1186/1471-2105-13-S4-S4 PMID:22536971

Pathak, J., Kiefer, R. C., Bielinski, S. J., & Chute, C. G. (2012a). Applying semantic web technologies for phenome-wide scan using an electronic health record linked Biobank. *J Biomed Semantics*, *3*(1), 10. doi:10.1186/2041-1480-3-10 PMID:23244446

Pathak, J., Kiefer, R. C., Bielinski, S. J., & Chute, C. G. (2012b). Mining the human phenome using semantic web technologies: A case study for Type 2 Diabetes. *AMIA... Annual Symposium Proceedings / AMIA Symposium. AMIA Symposium*, *2012*, 699–708. PMID:23304343

Pathak, J., Kiefer, R. C., & Chute, C. G. (2012). Using semantic web technologies for cohort identification from electronic health records for clinical research. *AMIA Summits Transl Sci Proc, 2012*, 10–19. PMID:22779040

Peleg, M., Keren, S., & Denekamp, Y. (2008). Mapping computerized clinical guidelines to electronic medical records: Knowledge-data ontological mapper (KDOM). *Journal of Biomedical Informatics, 41*(1), 180–201. doi:10.1016/j.jbi.2007.05.003 PMID:17574928

Pinto, H. S., & Martins, J. P. (2004). Ontologies: How can They be Built? *Knowledge and Information Systems, 6*(4), 441–464. doi:10.1007/s10115-003-0138-1

Pipino, L., Lee, Y. W., & Wang, R. Y. (2002). Data quality assessment. Association for Computing Machinery. *Communications of the ACM, 45*(4), 211–218. doi:10.1145/505248.506010

Preece, A., Missier, P., Ernbury, S., Jin, B., & Greenwood, M. (2008). An ontology-based approach to handling information quality in e-Science. *Concurrency and Computation, 20*(3), 253–264. doi:10.1002/cpe.1195

Rahimi, A., Liaw, S., Ray, P., & Taggart, J. (2012). *Developing an ontology for data quality in chronic disease management.* Paper presented at the the 24th European Medical Informatics Conference.

Rahimi, A., Liaw, S., Ray, P., Taggart, J., & Yu, H. (2014). Ontological specification of quality of chronic disease data in EHRs to support decision analytics: A realist review. *Decision Analysis, 1*(5), 31.

Rahimi, A., Liaw, S. T., Taggart, J., Ray, P., & Yu, H. (in-press). Validating an ontology-based algorithm to identify patients with Type 2 Diabetes Mellitus in electronic health records.

Rector, A., & Rogers, J. (2005). *Ontological & practical issues in using a description logic to represent medical concepts: experience from GALEN Tech rep CS* (Vol. 35, pp. 1–35). Manchester, England: School of Computer Science, University of Manchester.

Richesson, R. L., & Krischer, J. (2007). Data standards in clinical research: Gaps, overlaps, challenges and future directions. *Journal of the American Medical Informatics Association, 14*(6), 687–696. doi:10.1197/jamia.M2470 PMID:17712081

Rodrıguez-Muro, M., Kontchakov, R., & Zakharyaschev, M. (2013). OBDA with Ontop. *Proc. of the OWL Reasoner Evaluation Workshop.*

Rubin, D. L., Lewis, S. E., Mungall, C. J., Misra, S., Westerfield, M., & Ashburner, M. et al. (2006). National Center for Biomedical Ontology: Advancing biomedicine through structured organization of scientific knowledge. *OMICS: A Journal of Integrative Biology, 10*(2), 185–198. doi:10.1089/omi.2006.10.185 PMID:16901225

Talaei-Khoei, A., Solvoll, T., Ray, P., & Parameshwaran, N. (2011). Policy-based Awareness Management (PAM): Case study of a wireless communication system at a hospital. *Journal of Systems and Software, 84*(10), 1791–1805. doi:10.1016/j.jss.2011.05.024

Talaei-Khoei, A., Solvoll, T., Ray, P., & Parameshwaran, N. (2012). Maintaining awareness using policies; Enabling agents to identify relevance of information. *Journal of Computer and System Sciences, 78*(1), 370–391. doi:10.1016/j.jcss.2011.05.013

Valencia-Garcia, R., Fernandez-Breis, J. T., Ruiz-Martinez, J. M., Garcia-Sanchez, F., & Martinez-Bejar, R. (2008). A knowledge acquisition methodology to ontology construction for information retrieval from medical documents. *Expert Systems: International Journal of Knowledge Engineering and Neural Networks*, *25*(3), 314–334. doi:10.1111/j.1468-0394.2008.00464.x

Verma, A., Fiasché, M., Cuzzola, M., Iacopino, P., Morabito, P., & Kasabov, N. (2009). Ontology based personalized modeling for type 2 diabetes risk analysis: An Investigated Approach. In C. S. Leung, M. Lee, & J. H. Chan (Eds.), *ICONIP 2009, Part II* (pp. 360–366). Berlin: Springer-Verlag.

Verma, A., Kasabov, N., Rush, A., & Song, Q. (2008, 2008). *Ontology based personalized modeling for chronic disease risk analysis: an integrated approach*. Paper presented at the The 15th international conference on Advances in neuro-information processing

Wand, Y., & Wang, Y. (1996). Anchoring Data Quality Dimensions in Ontological Foundations. *Communications of the ACM*, *36*(11), 86–95. doi:10.1145/240455.240479

Wang, R. Y. (1998). A product perspective on total data quality management. *Communications of the ACM*, *41*(2 (Feb)), 58–65. doi:10.1145/269012.269022

Ying, W., Wimalasiri, J., Ray, P., Chattopadhyay, S., & Wilson, C. S. (2010). An Ontology Driven Multi-Agent Approach to Integrated e-Health Systems [IJEHMC]. *International Journal of E-Health and Medical Communications*, *1*(1), 28–40. doi:10.4018/jehmc.2010010103

Yu, H., Liaw, S., Taggart, J., & Rahimi, A. (2013). *Using Ontologies to Identify Patients with Diabetes in Electronic Health Records*. Paper presented at the Proceedings of the 12th International Semantic Web Conference and the 1st Australasian Semantic Web Conference, Sydney, Australia.

Chapter 24

Anomaly Detection in Medical Wireless Sensor Networks using SVM and Linear Regression Models

Osman Salem
University of Paris Descartes, France

Alexey Guerassimov
University of Paris Descartes, France

Ahmed Mehaoua
University of Paris Descartes, France, Centre National de la Recherche Scientifique (CNRS), LaBRI, France

Anthony Marcus
Florida Atlantic University, USA

Borko Furht
Florida Atlantic University, USA

ABSTRACT

This paper details the architecture and describes the preliminary experimentation with the proposed framework for anomaly detection in medical wireless body area networks for ubiquitous patient and healthcare monitoring. The architecture integrates novel data mining and machine learning algorithms with modern sensor fusion techniques. Knowing wireless sensor networks are prone to failures resulting from their limitations (i.e. limited energy resources and computational power), using this framework, the authors can distinguish between irregular variations in the physiological parameters of the monitored patient and faulty sensor data, to ensure reliable operations and real time global monitoring from smart devices. Sensor nodes are used to measure characteristics of the patient and the sensed data is stored on the local processing unit. Authorized users may access this patient data remotely as long as they maintain connectivity with their application enabled smart device. Anomalous or faulty measurement data resulting from damaged sensor nodes or caused by malicious external parties may lead to misdiagnosis or even death for patients. The authors' application uses a Support Vector Machine to classify abnormal instances in the incoming sensor data. If found, the authors apply a periodically rebuilt, regressive prediction model to the abnormal instance and determine if the patient is entering a critical state or if a sensor is reporting faulty readings. Using real patient data in our experiments, the results validate the robustness of our proposed framework. The authors further discuss the experimental analysis with the proposed approach which shows that it is quickly able to identify sensor anomalies and compared with several other algorithms, it maintains a higher true positive and lower false negative rate.

DOI: 10.4018/978-1-4666-8756-1.ch024

1. INTRODUCTION

With the continual growth in expected duration of the average human lifetime (Kumar & Lee, 2012), the rise in population and number of elderly persons has led to inflated healthcare costs and shortage of professionals able to provide the care and treatment necessary to satisfy this increase in demand.

Today, healthcare professionals and caregivers are very interested in remote monitoring of elderly people and patient vital signs, as well as their surrounding environment. These requirements have sparked enormous interest in the utilization of Wireless Sensor Networks (WSNs).

Scientists and researchers have developed networks of wireless sensors, known as Wireless Body Area Networks (WBANs), which are composed of a set of small miniaturized sensors with wireless transmission capabilities, and may be externally attached or implanted. These devices are used to continuously gather physiological signals from patients or elderly people at home or in hospitals, and transmit collected data to a Local Processing Unit (LPU).

The LPU (e.g., smart phone, tablet, etc.) has superior processing power, batteries with increased energy resources and greater transmission range and bandwidth than the individual WBAN nodes. LPUs must be robust and able to process received measurements in real time, and raise medical alarms for caregivers upon sensing the deteriorating health state of patients to quickly react by taking appropriate actions (Otto, Milenkovi, Sanders, & Jovanov, 2005). Data may also be transmitted by the LPU to remote databases (DB) for storage and long term analysis.

WBANs have several advantages such as enabling doctors to monitor specific attributes of patients regardless of location, improving diagnosis accuracy and efficiency, and reducing the overall cost of health care by permitting doctors to constantly monitor patient health.

WBAN may also improve the chances of discovering diseases which further reduces risk and impacts the lifespan of individuals on a global scale. In this paper, we look to increase the usefulness of WBAN systems used in the healthcare industry by creating an application which is capable of "intelligently" discerning between patient health irregularities and sensor node failure.

There exist many medical WBAN systems which are publicly available for purchase including MICAz, MICA2, Tmote Sky, TelosB, IRIS, Imote2, and Shimmer. These types of WBANs are used to monitor and collect various physiological parameters of individuals such as Heart Rate (HR), pulse, oxygen saturation (SpO2), Respiration Rate (RR), Body Temperature (BT), ElectroCardioGram (ECG), ElectroMyoGram (EMG), Blood Pressure (BP), Blood Glucose Levels (BGL), Galvanic Skin Response (GSR), etc.

The ECG sensor, for example, is connected to three electrodes each of which is attached to the patients' chest for real time monitoring of the heart. Another type of sensor, the pulse oximeter, using infrared light and a photo sensor, simply clips to a patient finger and measures the pulse and blood oxygenation ratio (SpO2). While it may seem simplistic, the SpO2 sensor may detect asphyxia, insufficient oxygen (hypoxia), pneumonia and other blood oxygen related anomalies. The average human SpO2 ratio naturally exceeds 95%, but when this ratio drops below 90%, the pulse oximeter will trigger an alarm due to possible lung problems or respiratory failure. Prior to the assistance of these types of WBAN sensors, healthcare providers were reliant on big, expensive machines which were in short supply and required that the patient is observed directly while situated at the location of the machine.

The use of WBANs has been extended to monitor patients diagnosed with chronic illnesses and cognitive disorders such as Parkinson's, Diabetes, Alzheimer's, Asthma, and Epilepsy. WBANs have proven to be great assets to both patients and healthcare providers in that they have reduced the costs associated with healthcare by solving problems such as overcapacity in hospitals, excessive waiting or sojourn times and the required number of nurses and doctors on call. WBANs also allow greater mobility for monitored individuals while constantly gathering and transmitting critical physiological data to their associated healthcare providers which may be useful for situations that require the long-term monitoring of a patient's recovery after leaving the hospital or assessing the impact of a patient's rehabilitation.

While WBANs have numerous advantages, their disadvantages range from poor reliability to the high susceptibility of security attacks after deployment. For us to exploit the strengths while reducing the probability of any weaknesses occurring, we must first look at what these weaknesses are in more detail so that we may find some means of mitigation. WBAN sensor nodes are prone to both hardware and software issues such as impaired components, sensor calibration, battery exhaustion or dislocation.

The sensor readings are themselves both unreliable and inaccurate (Ko, et al., 2010; Wang, Fang, Xing, & Chen, 2011; Zhang, et al., 2012), resulting from constrained hardware resources including reduced processing power, limited memory and energy resources, and transmission range. Individual sensor data gathering and transmission is also prone to several types of irregularities such as interference, noise, sensor misplacement, sweating patients, exhausted energy resources and external hacks and malevolent attacks such as data injection, modification or replay attacks that indirectly affect the LPU. This may lead to unexpected results, faulty alarms and diagnosis, and a reduction in public trust of these systems.

As a result, high false alarm rate and faulty measurements directly influence the public credibility of WBANs especially where dependability is exceedingly important as in the medical domain (Sahoo, 2012). If, for example, a pulse oximeter sensor is incorrectly attached or external fluorescent light radiates to the infrared sensor, erroneous measurements may result. In Chipara, Lu, Bailey, and Roman (2010), the authors found that the first source of unreliability in medical WSNs was the sensing components as opposed to some other problems (i.e. network failure, data transfer).

Nodes transmitting erroneous data have a negative impact on the accuracy of the gathered data which may have an effect on the patients' diagnosis. This may, in turn, lead to life threatening situations where emergency personnel receive false alarms based on node faults for a code blue. As a result, it becomes an extremely important task to detect erroneous measurements at the node level and differentiate between patient anomalies and node faults to minimize false alarms. Both patient anomalies and node faults produce abnormal measurements and require that each should be detected with the highest accuracy possible. We may only achieve this using an anomaly detection mechanism to recognise and extract abnormal patterns and correlations in the data and to differentiate between sick individuals and faulty sensors.

Anomaly based systems (Jurdak, Wang, Obst, & Valencia, 2011) typically look for irregular patterns in the data received from sensors as opposed to signature based intrusion detection systems where signatures are required to detect attacks. Signatures are neither available nor easy to write for healthcare monitoring applications. However, anomalies are defined as deviations from a dynamically updated normal model from the sensed data. Therefore an anomaly based detection approach is more adequate for WBANs given the absence of attack signatures. It is also important to note that anomaly based systems face challenges related to the training phase as it is difficult to find normal data in order to establish an appropriate normal profile.

Several anomaly-based detection techniques for sensor fault identification and isolation have been proposed and applied (Liu, Cheng, & Chen, 2007; Jurdak, Wang, Obst, & Valencia, 2011; Miao, Liu, He, Liu, & Papadias, 2011; Chen

& Juang, 2012). These distributed techniques identify anomalies at the node level to prevent transmission of irregular values and reduce energy consumption. Using these distributed methods typically requires additional resources not found in most sensor node hardware. As a result, their accuracy is lower than centralized approaches which utilize a global representation for spatial-temporal analysis. To ensure reliable operation and accurate diagnosis, correlations between physical parameters, which exist in time and space, must be exploited in order to detect and extract irregular measurements. Usually, there is no spatial or temporal correlation among monitored attributes for faulty measurements.

Our primary focus in this paper is the detection of anomalous measurements in medical WBANs. We propose a novel machine learning based approach to detect abnormal values. First we use Support Vector Machine (SVM) (Bishop, 2006) to detect abnormal records, and when detected, we apply linear regression (Witten, Frank, & Hall, 2011) to pinpoint abnormal sensor measurements in an abnormal record. However, physiological attributes are heavily correlated, and changes occur typically in at least two or more parameters, e.g. in Atrial Fibrillation (AF) & Asthma, the heart rate and respiration rate increase simultaneously.

Our solution will increase the reliability of medical WBANs used for monitoring patients. Its primary task is to detect and extract anomalies in the WBAN data and, once found, differentiate between irregular patient vital signs and defective sensor measurements. Additionally, we seek to minimize false alarms triggered by anomalous sensors data.

The rest of this paper is organized as follows. In section 2, we review related work on anomaly detection and machine learning algorithms used in medical WSN. Section 3 briefly reviews SVM and linear regression used in our detection system. The proposed approach is presented in section 4. In section 5, we present our results from experimental evaluation, where we conduct a performance analysis of the proposed solution with real patient data. Finally, section 6 concludes the paper with a discussion of the results and plans for future work.

2. RELATED WORK

With the population of mankind ever increasing, medical facility vacancies are difficult to find, frustratingly lengthy waiting lines clogging emergency rooms, and the demand for doctors and staff seems to never be satisfied. These shortages result in the inability for many individuals to receive the care they needed. Due in part to the excessive congestion caused by many outpatients requiring minimal attention in these facilities and the evolution of WSN and smart devices, a new market was created for remote patient monitoring using small, wearable sensor systems. Researchers and scientists have worked hard to satisfy this demand, creating many novel systems which may alleviate, to some degree, the overcrowding issues for medical staff and healthcare facilities.

Novel architectures for monitoring patients, both in house and remotely, have been designed, developed and deployed in real world environments. One such system, MEDiSN (Ko, et al., 2010), CodeBlue (Malan, Fulford-jones, Welsh, & Moulton, 2004; Havard Sensor Networks Lab, 2013), LifeGuard (Montgomery, et al., 2004), AlarmNet (Wood, et al., 2006), Medical MoteCare (Navarro, Lawrence, & Lim, 2009), Vital Jacket (Cunha, et al., 2010). Some comprehensive survey studies of medical applications using WSNs are available in (Alemdar & Ersoy, 2010; Grgic, Žagar, & Križanovic, 2012). All of these systems are plagued with similar problems such as limited energy, faulty sensor hardware, and wireless transmission failure. As these networks often are responsible for monitoring a patient's livelihood, many researchers have created methods of autonomous fault detection for WSN and WBAN.

Authors in Zhang, Meratnia, and Havinga (2010) present a comprehensive analysis of modern fault and outlier detection techniques for WSNs. They present a comparative guideline detailing the steps necessary to appropriately select the best technique suitable for the characteristics of the data set. Several types of irregular readings have been captured and extracted from medical WSN data including single spikes, long duration spikes resulting from noisy environments, and continuously anomalous line fluctuations. To simplify the classification of WSN sensor fault types, the authors in Sharma, Golubchik, and Govindan (2010) categorize faulty measurements into short faults, faults resulting from noise and constant faults.

WSNs are plagued by a variety of issues that may endanger their functionality which stem from lack of quality and poor reliability (Zhang, Meratnia, & Havinga, 2010; Ying-xin, Xiang-guang, & Jun, 2011; Zhang, et al., 2012). Some of the more prevalent issues include hardware and software errors and faults, interference, widely variable environment dependent noise, dropped and lost packets, inconsistencies, and damaged sensors. New anomaly detection schemes for WSNs have been proposed which locate, extract, and classify atypical deviations in collected data to reduce false alarms generated as a result of faulty sensor measurements.

Authors in Banerjee, Xie, and Agrawal (2008) propose an algorithm to identify faulty sensors using the minimum and the maximum boundaries of the monitored parameters. Measurements which exceed the threshold of these boundaries are classified as inconsistent or outliers. Furthermore, medical WBAN systems may not assume all patients have the same attribute boundary intervals, as the min-max threshold values are dependent on an individuals' physiological characteristics including sex, age, weight, height, stress, and health condition.

Investigation and further study of machine learning algorithms for supervised classification and data mining algorithms for clustering has led to additional inspiration for our research team. Machine learning algorithms including Naïve Bayes (NB) (Yang, Dinh, & Chen, 2010), Bayesian Network (BN) (Farruggia, Giuseppe, & Ortolani, 2011), decision tree (C4.5) (Cheng, Xu, Pei, & Liu, 2010), Neural Networks (NN) (Bishop, 2006), K-Nearst Neighbor (KNN) (Bishop, 2006), Self-Organizing Map (SOM) (Siripanadorn, Hattagam, & Teaumroong, 2010) and Support Vector Machine (SVM) (Bishop, 2006) generate a variety of mathematical models based on correlational statistics from a training data set which are then applied to classify test instances as either normal or abnormal.

Several regression algorithms have been used in medical WBANs to build a model generated from time series data such as AutoRegression (Curiac & Volosencu, 2012), Least Square Error (Li, 2010), Non-seasonal Holt-Winters (Li, 2010). The authors in Xiaozhen, Hong, and Tong (2011) apply linear regression for missing data prediction and the experimental results validate their success, claiming low prediction errors. Another such project which applies logistic regression modelling (Huang, Jiang, Zhang, & Gao, 2010) evaluates the reliability of large scale industrial WSNs utilizing a static threshold. In Cheng, Xu, Pei, and Liu (2010) based on the J48 (decision tree) algorithm, the authors propose a large scale WSN diagnostic methodology which merges local classifier models into a single network spanning tree, responsible for the accuracy of the method and representative of the whole network.

To monitor an individual's physical activity, the authors in Yang, Dinh, and Chen (2010) use SunSpOT sensors attached to the thighs. Naïve Bayes is used to calculate values from the data to determine body position (i.e. sitting, standing, lying down, and walking). In a similar project which uses logistic regression (Choi, Ahmed, & Gutierrez-Osuna, 2012), a system is described which claims to use heart rate variability measurements to differentiate mental stress states from relaxation states.

In recent years SVM classification has become a more popular selection partially due to its simplistic numerical comparison for data classification and is often found to be the optimum solution for specific context. Several modern SVM based approaches have been proposed (Zhang, Meratnia, & Havinga, 2009; Rajasegarar, Leckie, Bezdek, & Palaniswami, 2010; Xu, Hu, Wang, & Zhang, 2012) for anomaly detection in WSNs. Furthermore, many non-linear versions (kernel based) of SVM have been investigated to find the optimum hyperplane that encompasses the majority of normal data in training phase. Once established, any data point landing outside the hyperplane boundary is classified as abnormal.

Often a major challenge in machine learning is that accurate model generation requires a training data set which has the classes labelled for each instance. The training data frequently requires close attention by researchers which must conduct extensive experiments to determine applicable pre-processing and balancing algorithms. We refer to Bishop (2006) for more details about these classification methods. Many attempts to resolve these challenges in training data set for machine learning led to methods of unsupervised learning or data mining.

Data mining algorithms group similar instances from the data into a single cluster and label smaller size clusters containing less than a given percentage of the total values, as abnormal. Some of the most popular and widely applied data mining algorithms include (Bishop, 2006) K-means, hierarchical clustering, Fuzzy C-means and GMM (Theodoridis, Pikrakis, Koutroumbas, & Cavouras, 2010). One challenge facing these clustering methods is that they assume anomalous data, which typically occurs much less frequently, is easily distinguished from normal data. We refer to Abduvaliyev, Pathan, Zhou, Roman, and Wong, (2013) for comprehensive classification of various detection techniques.

In Zhang, et al. (2010) a novel Outlier Detection and Countermeasure Scheme (ODCS) based on k-means, K-Nearest Neighbours (K-NN), static threshold and transmission frequency. K-NN is unsuitable for WSNs as it is computationally expensive and requires large amounts of memory space to store the training data as opposed to classification methods which discard the training data after building the model. Authors in Xie, Hu, Han, and Chen (2012) proposed a KNN-based anomaly detection method based on hyper-grid which has lower computational complexity than K-NN for WSNs. An unsupervised approach for anomaly detection in WSNs, Siripanadorn, Hattagam, and Teaumroong (2010) combines multiple models such as Discrete Wavelet Transform (DWT) and Self-Organizing Map (SOM). In this case, the DWT is used to reduce the size of input data for SOM clustering.

The authors in Liu, Cheng, and Chen (2007) proposed a distance based method to identify insider malicious sensors while assuming neighbour nodes are monitoring the same attributes. Each sensor monitors its one hop neighbours and measures the Mahalanobis distance between the calculated and actual values received in multivariate instances to detect anomalies. They discovered that it is not practical in medical WBAN applications to exploit promiscuous mode and increase network node redundancy which monitor the same parameters.

Authors in Yim and Choi (2010) propose a voting based approach to detect abnormal network events. In Miao, Liu, He, Liu, and Papadias (2011), the authors propose a failure detection approach for WSNs which exploits metric correlations to detect abnormal sensors and to uncover failed nodes. A simple prediction and fault detection method for WSNs was proposed in Yao, Sharma, Golubchik, and Govindan (2010) and has been evaluated on short, long, and constant fault classes. The proposed algorithm is based on the detection of deviations between reference and the collected measurements. The reference time series is built using the linear Segmented Sequence Analysis (SSA) and when the remainder between the reference and measured values is greater than a threshold, an alarm is triggered.

Rule-based, estimation-based, time series analysis and learning-based methods are four methods for fault detection discussed in Sharma, Golubchik, and Govindan (2010). They conduct experiments which investigate various fixed and dynamic thresholds for linear least squares estimation, Auto Regressive Integrated Moving Average (ARIMA), Hidden Markov Model (HMM), etc. No superior class of detection methods was found to be suitable for every type of anomalous event as the accuracy is dependent on both the size and quality of the data. Rule-based methods require precise calibration and tuning threshold parameters, learning methods require training phases, estimation methods are unable to classify faults, and time series analysis has the highest rate of false positives.

Healthcare applications for patient monitoring require strict reliability on gathered data. Usually, many physiological attributes are monitored in the same time, such as heart rate, blood pressure, respirations, pulse and oxygenation. Alarms set for each attribute are triggered whenever the associated value falls outside a predefined interval. There are however correlations which exist between physiological parameters and the spatio-temporal correlations amongst monitored physiological attributes which may be exploited to detect anomalies and distinguish between faulty sensor measurements and medical emergencies. Faulty sensor readings tend to show irregular, random values unrelated to other attributes in the instance. Once detected, the instances containing the irregularities may be discarded to reduce false alarms, clean the data, and increase the reliability and the accuracy of the monitoring system.

In this paper, we seek to enhance fault detection for current medical WBAN systems. We use SVM and linear regression algorithms to detect abnormal records and to pinpoint abnormal sensors readings in the LPU. SVM is utilized to reduce the temporal complexity and for binary record classification into either normal or abnormal. If a record is classified as abnormal, the linear regression is used to predict values for the current attributes which may also uncover irregular attributes. Our system can detect anomalies in the data of a patient and prior to triggering an alarm, will uniquely distinguish between human physiological abnormalities and sensor node failure utilizing both the spatial and temporal parameters.

3. BACKGROUND

In Figure 1, we consider a patient wearing N medical WBAN sensor nodes $(S_1, S_2, ..., S_N)$ to observe specific physiological parameters where the nodes collect and transmit these observations to a smartphone or LPU. The data is gathered by the smartphone where it analysed in real time and is able to send prompt alert notifications to healthcare providers. Further authenticated local and remote data storage may be enabled through and transmitted by the LPU or smartphone. Due to greater resources on board modern smart devices, the LPU analyses and mines the data for irregularities using lightweight machine learning algorithms. It also maintains high accuracy when distinguishing between sensor errors and patient health irregularities and generating the appropriate alarm.

Physiological parameter measurements are collected which we declare as the data matrix $X=(X_{ij})$ where i represents the temporal growth and j represents a sensor metric. All gathered values for all parameters are stored as a single record incrementally at time instant k we represent with $X_k = \left(x_{k1}, x_{k2}, ..., x_{kn} \right)$. X_k is the line k in the data matrix X given in Equation (1). We also denote by $A = \left(A_1, A_2, ..., A_n \right)$ the set of monitored attributes, where A_i is the column i in the matrix X:

Figure 1. WSN for collecting vital signs and alerting caregivers

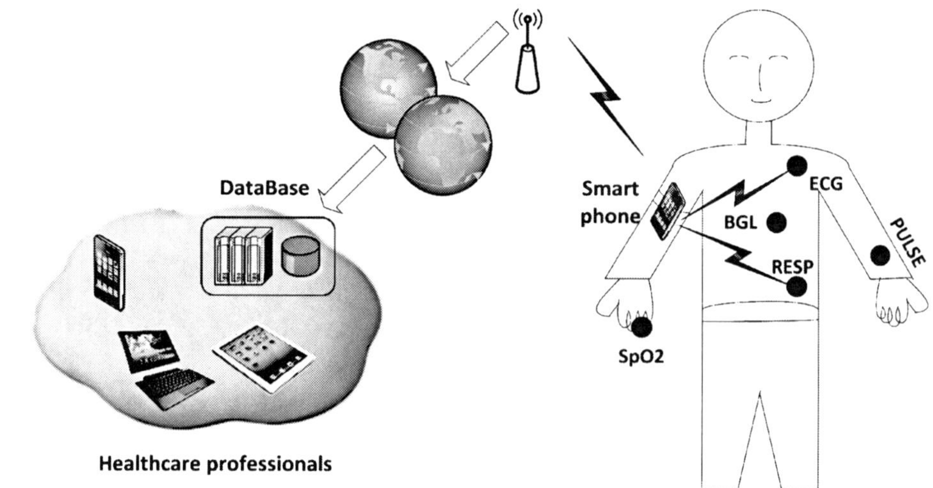

$$X = \begin{array}{c} \\ X_1 \\ X_2 \\ \vdots \\ X_m \end{array} \begin{matrix} A_1 & A_2 & A_3 & \cdots & A_n \\ \begin{bmatrix} x_{11} & x_{12} & x_{13} & \cdots & x_{1n} \\ x_{21} & x_{22} & x_{23} & \cdots & x_{2n} \\ \vdots & \vdots & \vdots & \ddots & \vdots \\ x_{m1} & x_{m2} & x_{m3} & \cdots & x_{mn} \end{bmatrix} \end{matrix} \quad (1)$$

To provide instantaneous online anomaly recognition we process in real time, the collected data on the smart device. These measurements are likely to be of low quality and unreliable due to the sensor hardware constraints and resources as well as the physiological condition of the individual (i.e. bodily sweat, sensor detachment) and the environmental conditions (i.e. sensor damage, fading, disrupted communication). The WBAN monitor is reliant on the received data to maintain its accuracy and robustness, where erroneous instances are identified and it may trigger false alarm notifications when necessary to alert authorized medical personnel. To boost the analysis accuracy and reduce false alarms or misdiagnosis, abnormal instances must be found, analysed, and isolated.

To detect abnormal values, we use Support Vector Machine (SVM) to detect outliers and classify each instance (received attributes at time t) as normal or abnormal. Upon finding an anomaly, we apply a linear regression model to predict values for each attribute in the abnormal instance. When the variance exceeds a predefined threshold, between the predicted and actual value, we analyse data correlations to differentiate faulty sensors from irregular or degrading patient health. We discuss briefly the algorithms used in our approach, SVM and linear regression, in the remaining paragraphs of this section. For more in depth information about the algorithms, please refer to Witten, Frank, and Hall (2011).

3.1. Support Vector Machine

Support Vector Machine (SVM) (Bishop, 2006) is a widely used supervised machine learning method for binary classification which uses the training data to build a model for classification. The SVM then uses this model to classify, using attribute data, each instance in the test set.

The main concept behind linear SVMs is to maximize the distance between two parallel boundaries or hyperplanes which are defined by support vectors:

$$w^T X_i + w_0 = 1 \text{ and } w^T X_i + w_0 = -1 \quad (2)$$

The objective is to construct a separating hyperplane which achieves maximum separation between the 2 classes:

$$w^T X_i + w_0 = 0 \tag{3}$$

When generating the model for classification, SVM looks for the maximum margin hyperplane which divides the training data into two categories. Given the training data set $X = (X_1, X_2, ..., X_T)$, with their associated class $y_i \in \{-1,1\}$ (-1 for abnormal & 1 for normal or healthy patient), for $i \in (1...T)$, the hyperplane is the solution of the optimization problem:

$$
\begin{aligned}
&\underset{w,w_0}{\text{Minimize}} && \frac{1}{2}\|w\|^2 + C\sum_{i=1}^{m}\xi_i \\
&\text{Subject to} && w^T X_i + w_0 \geq 1 - \xi_i && \text{if } X_i \in y_1 \\
& && w^T X_i + w_0 \leq -1 + \xi_i && \text{if } X_i \in y_2 \\
& && \xi \geq 0
\end{aligned}
\tag{4}
$$

The margin width (or distance) is equal to $2/\|w\|$ as shown in Figure 2. The margin errors, ξ_i, are used to prevent over fitting problems, and are positive for points inside the margin, or outside the margin on the wrong side of the classifier, and 0 for points in the correct side of the classifier. C is a user-defined constant. SVM uses the coordinates of the nearest training data points in both classes in order to create the largest possible separation between border values in each class. Those specific data points are called the support vectors and they have to satisfy:

$$y_i(w^T \cdot X_i + w_0) = 1 \tag{5}$$

where w is the normal vector to the hyperplane, and w_0 is the bias of the hyperplane function. The normal vector w is calculated using the values in the training data set:

Figure 2. Linear SVM and data separation

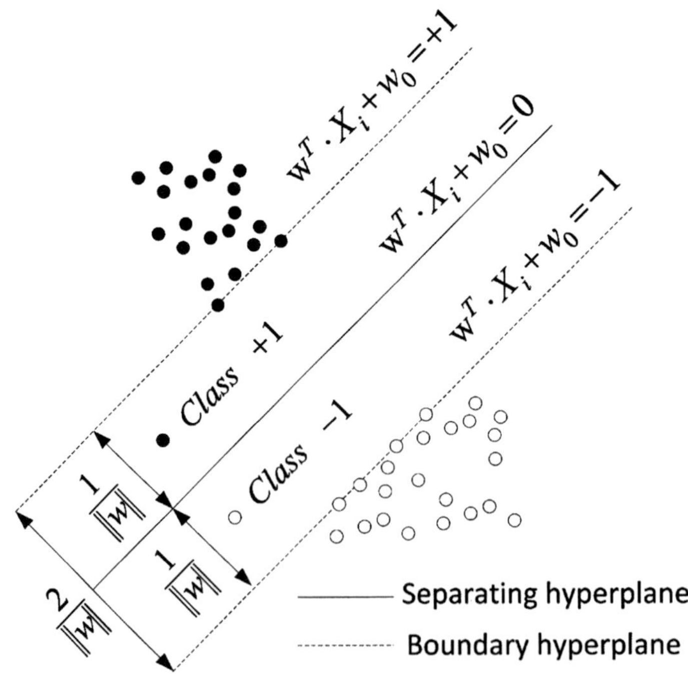

$$w = \sum_{i=1}^{n} \alpha_i y_i X_i \tag{6}$$

where α_i are the Lagrange multipliers of the optimization task, and they are different than zero only for points outside the margin and inside the correct side of the classifier. The classification of X_i is based on the sign of $h(X_i)$:

$$\begin{aligned} y_i &= sign\left(h(X_i)\right) \\ &= sign\left(w^T \cdot X_i + w_0\right) \end{aligned} \tag{7}$$

3.2. Linear Regression

The linear regression (Bishop, 2006; Witten, Frank, & Hall, 2011) is a statistical modeling method used to predict the current value of monitored attribute. For a given attribute A_j, it exploits spatial correlation to predict the current value $(\hat{x}_{ij})$, as linear combination of measured values for other attributes $x_{ik|k \neq j}$. The model of the predicted attribute value is given by:

$$\begin{aligned} \hat{x}_{ij} &= a_0 + a_1 x_{i1} \\ &\quad + a_2 x_{i2} + \cdots + a_n x_{in} \end{aligned} \tag{8}$$

where a_k are the coefficients of the regressors (weights). These coefficients are obtained during the training phase as the result of division of the covariance of A_i and A_j attributes, on the variance of A_j:

$$a_k = \frac{Cov(A_i, A_j)}{Var(A_i)} = \frac{\sum_k \left(x_{ki} - \overline{A}_i\right)\left(x_{kj} - \overline{A}_j\right)}{\sum_k (x_{ki} - \overline{A}_i)} \tag{9}$$

Once the model is computed from training data, it is used to predict the value of each attribute $(\hat{x}_{ij})$ at instance i. Afterward, we compare the predicted value $(\hat{x}_{ij})$ with the actual value (x_{ij}) to find if it fits within a small margin error and to classify p_i as normal or abnormal.

4. PROPOSED APPROACH

We consider a general scenario for remote patient monitoring, as shown in Figure 1, where many wireless motes with restricted resources are used to collect data, and a portable collection device (e.g. smart phone) with higher resources and higher transmission capabilities than motes, is used to analyze collected data, and to raise alarms for emergency team when abnormal patterns are detected. We seek to detect abnormal values in order to reduce false alarms resulted from faulty measurements, while differentiating faults from patient health degradation.

The proposed approach is based on decision tree and linear regression. It builds a decision tree and looks for linear coefficients from normal vital signs that fall inside restricted interval range of monitored attributes. In the rest of this paper, we focus only on the following vital signs:

$BP \in [60\text{-}110]$
$HR \in [60\text{-}100]$
$pulse \in [60\text{-}100]$
$respiration\ rate \in [12\text{-}30]$
$SpO2 \in [90\text{-}100]$

Attributes values that fall outside these (restricted) normal intervals are considered abnormal. HR and pulse reflect the same attribute from different sensors, where pulse is obtained from the pulse oximeter and HR is measured as the number of interbeat intervals (R-R) in ECG signal.

The proposed approach is based on two phases: training and detection. In the training phase, we build the classification models for SVM and linear regression methods, and in the testing phase, inputs are classified as abnormal if they deviate from established model. The linear SVM is used in our approach to classify each received record as normal or abnormal. The SVM is used due to its accuracy and low complexity, where the classification requires only the sign of $h(X_i)$ in Equation (7).

Abnormal instances detected by SVM will only activate the forecasting procedure using the linear regression, where we recursively assume that an attribute (x_{ik}) is missing, and the coefficients of linear regression are used to estimate the current value for this attribute $(\hat{x}_{ik})$ with respect to the others $(x_{ij|j \neq k})$ as given in Equation (10) for heart rate estimation:

$$\widehat{HR}_i = C_0 + C_1 Pulse_i + C_2 RESP_i + \cdots + C_5 BP_i \tag{10}$$

If the Euclidean distance between current (HR_i) and estimated $\left(\widehat{HR}_i\right)$ values is larger than the predefined threshold (10% of estimated value) for only one attribute, the measurement is considered faulty and replaced by estimated value with linear regression. Equation (11) shows the residual threshold used to detect abnormal measurement:

$$e_i = \left| x_{ik} - \hat{x}_{ik} \right| \geq 0.1 * \hat{x}_{ik} \tag{11}$$

However, if at least k readings are higher than the threshold, we trigger a medical alarm for response caregiver emergency team to react, e.g. heavy changes in the HR and reduced rate of SpO2 are symptoms of patient health degradation and requires immediate medical intervention. We assume that the probability of many attributes ($k=2$ in our experiments) being faulty is very low. The pseudo-code for our proposed algorithm is given in Algorithm 1.

The SVM is used to reduce the computation complexity, and to prevent the estimation of each attribute for each instance on the base station. SVM is based on sign comparison for classification, and the combination of both approach for fault detection and classification is used. Sliding window is not used in our experiments to reduce the complexity. When the model is specified with the training data, updating or rebuilding the model requires additional complexity (temporal & spatial) and reduce the accuracy of the classification model. Most of the time, the gathered measurements are normal, and updating the classification model using skewed data (normal data only for training) leads to erroneous classification.

5. EXPERIMENTAL RESULTS

In this section, we present the performance analysis results of the proposed approach for anomaly detection in medical WSN. Afterward, we conduct analysis to study the impact of decision threshold on true positive and false alarm ratio. We used real medical data set from the Physionet database (Physionet, 2013), which contains 7 attributes (ABPmean, ABPsys, ABPdias, HR, PULSE, RESP and SpO2). We only focus on 5 attributes in each record: ABPmean, HR, PULSE, RESP and SpO2.

The variations of Heart Rate (in beats per minute – bpm) are shown in Figure 3. We take notice of 4 abnormal measurements (spikes) where 2 between them falling down to zero. Other variations associated with a clinical change of the monitored patient can be clearly distinguished in Figure 3.

Algorithm 1. Detection algorithm

```
1:for each received record Xᵢ during T do
2:Classify Xᵢ using SVM
3:if Class(Xᵢ)=="ABNORMAL" then
4:for each xᵢₖ do
5: x̂ᵢₖ = Σⱼ₌₁,ⱼ≠ₖⁿ aⱼ.xᵢⱼ
6:ctr+ = ((|xᵢₖ − x̂ᵢₖ|) ≥ 0.1 × x̂ᵢₖ)?1 : 0
7:end for
8:if (ctr≥k) then
9:Raise alarm for healthcare
10:end if
11:end if
12:end for
```

The variation of Blood Pressure (in millimeters of mercury – mmHg), Pulse (in bpm), respiration rate (in respirations per minutes – rpm), and oxygenation ratio (in percentage) are presented in Figures 4, 5, 6 and 7 respectively.

In fact, HR and Pulse measure the same physiological parameter using two different devices, and usually they must present the same variations. However, when comparing Figures 3 and 5, they exhibit some differences especially for spikes at different time instant. The difference results from abnormal values reported by the sensor.

To prove the correlation between monitored attributes, we show the variation curves of the 5 parameters in Figure 8, where we can notice that clinical emergency induces changes in many parameters at the same time instant. However, there is no spatial correlation among monitored attributes for faulty measurements. It is important to note that some curves in Figure 8 are shifted to clarify the shape of their variations. We can visually distinguish zones of clinical change, where many attributes change at the same time instant.

As physiological parameters vary by individual and they are dependent on many physical characteristics (sex, age, weight, activity, etc.), the use of a static interval for anomaly detection is heavily reliant on additional dynamic parameters

Figure 3. Heart rate

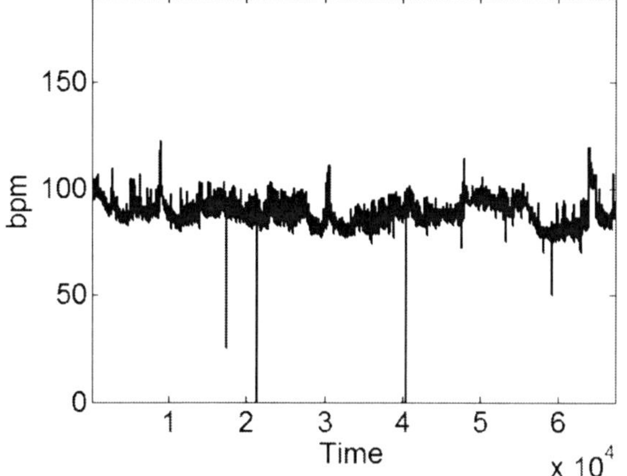

Figure 5. PULSE

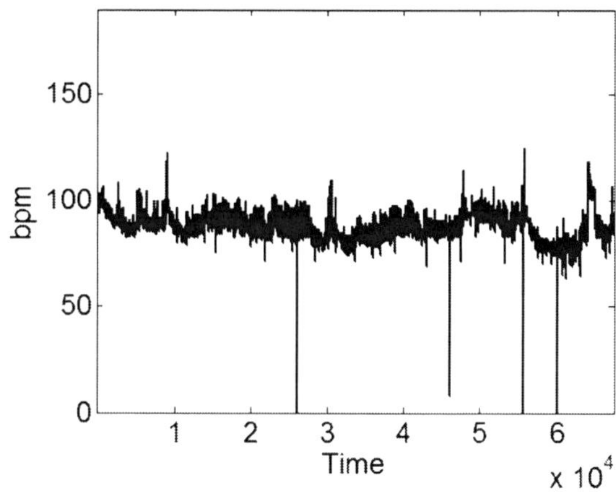

Figure 4. Blood pressure

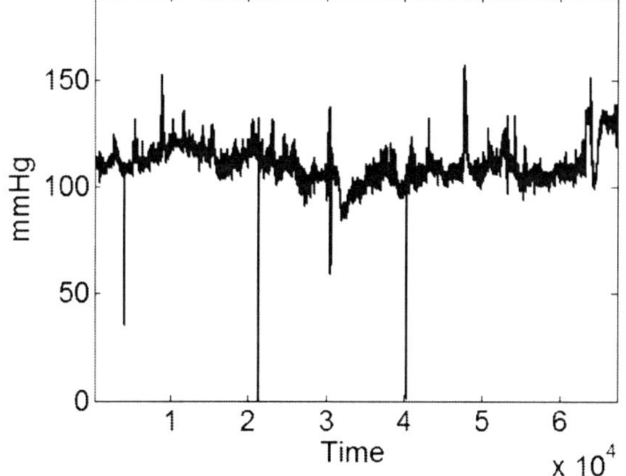

Figure 6. Respiration rate

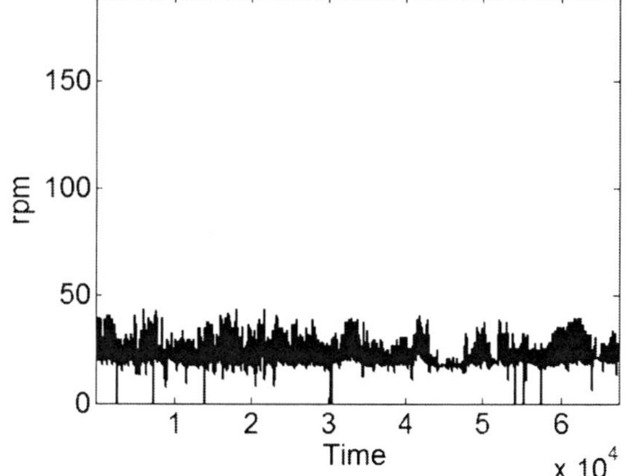

Figure 7. Oxygenation ratio

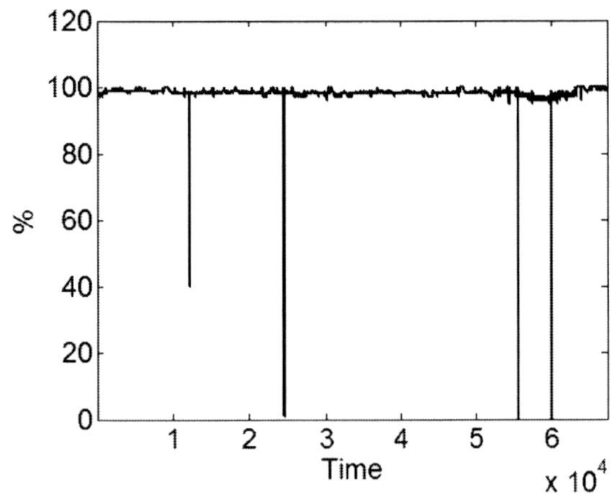

Figure 8. Variations of the 5 parameters

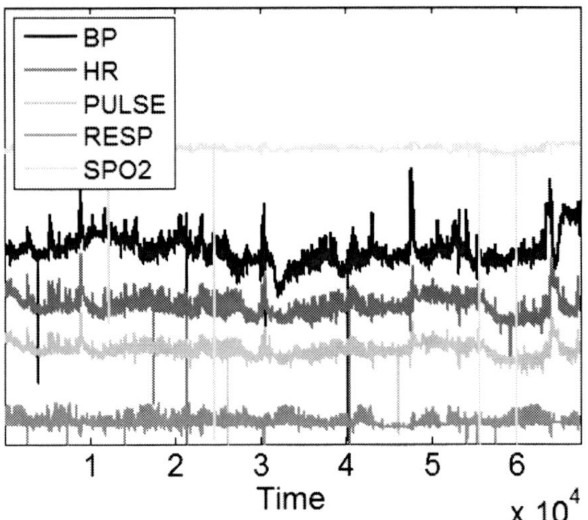

(environmental, ages, activities, etc.) which are difficult to set dynamically.

Figures 9 and 10 respectively show the predicted and error values for HR using linear regression. The measured values of HR (actual) are presented in Figure 3. The error represents the difference between actual and predicted values of HR. To test the efficiency of the used algorithms, we compare the results (predicted and error) with different classifiers using the WEKA (Hall, et al., 2009; WEKA, 2013) toolkit: Decision Stump, Decision Table, Additive Regression and K-NN for $K=1$.

Figures 11 and 12 show similar results (predicted and error respectively) using additive regression tree, where the prediction error is higher than linear regression. Figures 13 and 14 show the results of the decision stump classifier. Figures 15 and 16 show the results of the decision stump classifier. The results using KNN, which has a slower runtime due to the greater computational complexity, are shown in Figures 17 and 18 to have a lower error rate in comparison to additive regression, decision stump and decision table.

Figure 9. Predicted heart rate using linear regression

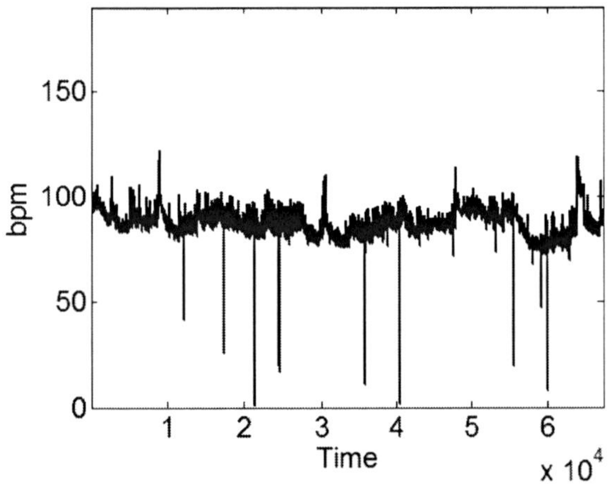

Figure 10. Prediction error using linear regression

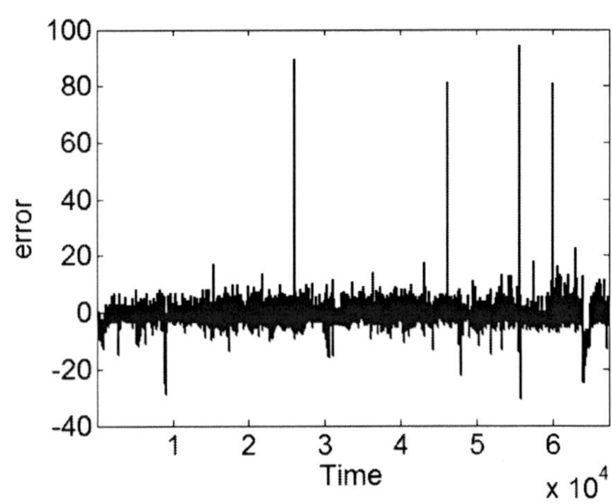

Figure 11. Predicted heart rate using additive regression

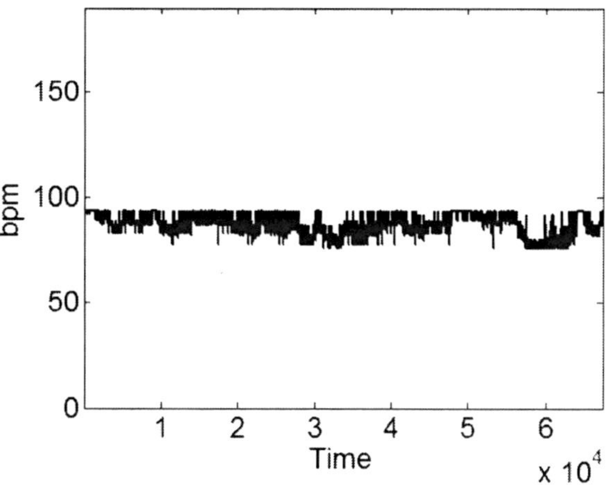

Figure 12. Prediction error using additive regression

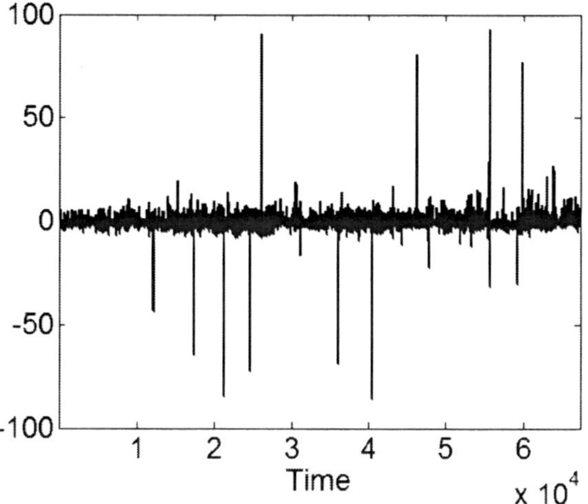

Figure 13. Predicted heart rate using decision stump

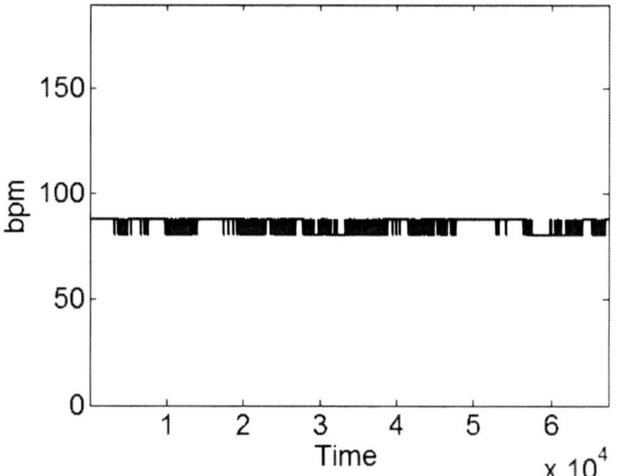

Figure 14. Prediction error using decision stump

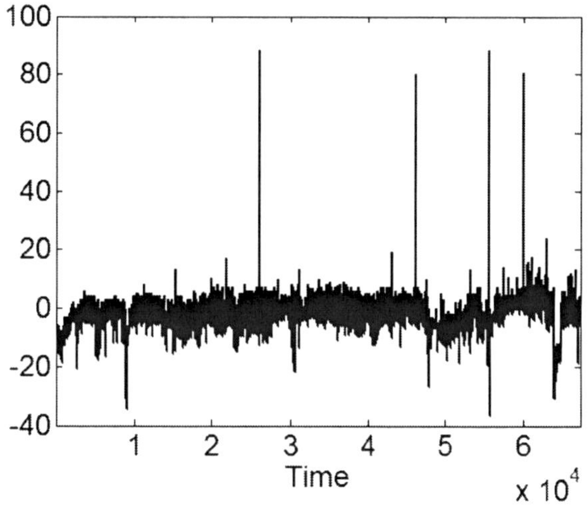

Figure 23 shows the mean absolute error for each of these classifiers, where decision table achieves the prediction with the highest mean error rate, followed in descending order by decision stump, additive regression, K-NN and linear Regression. A slight difference, in terms of the mean prediction error, between K-NN and additive regression is presented in Figure 23. During the experiment, we discover that the result of additive regression sometimes is better than K-NN when using other data set. That is to say, the accuracy of the prediction algorithm depends also on the data

in training phase. Linear regression had the lowest error percentage and the best overall performance out of the four classifiers, which is also why we use this classifier in the rest of this paper.

Figure 19 shows the raised alarms by the application using SVM. In our previous work (Salem, Guerassimov, Mehaoua, Marcus, & Furht, 2013), our approach applied J48 on real patient data. To compare the performance of both classifiers, the alarms triggered by J48 are shown in Figure 20. These results confirm that SVM slightly outper-

Figure 15. Predicted heart rate using decision table

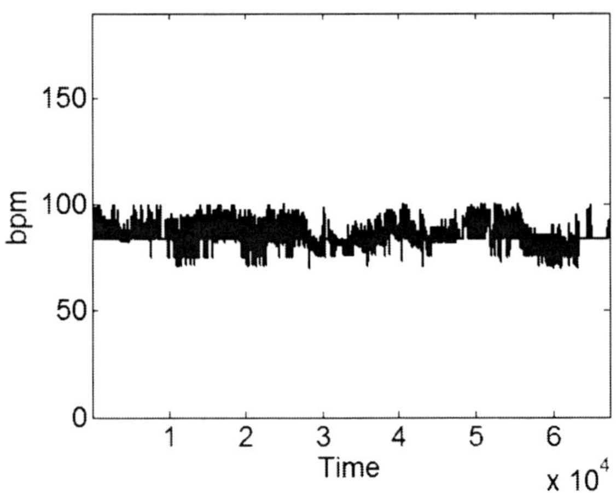

Figure 16. Prediction error using decision table

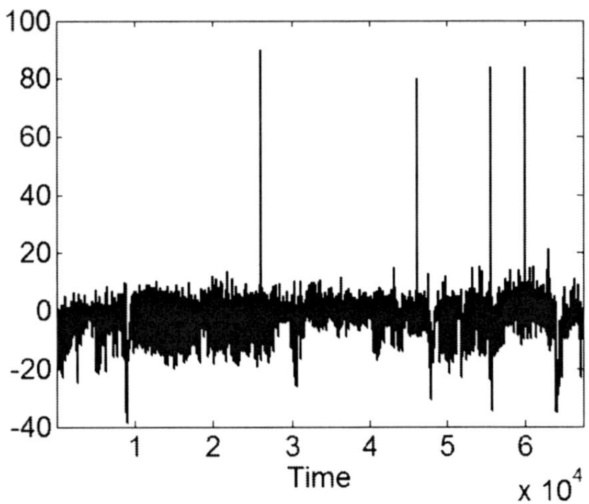

Figure 17. Predicted heart rate using K-NN

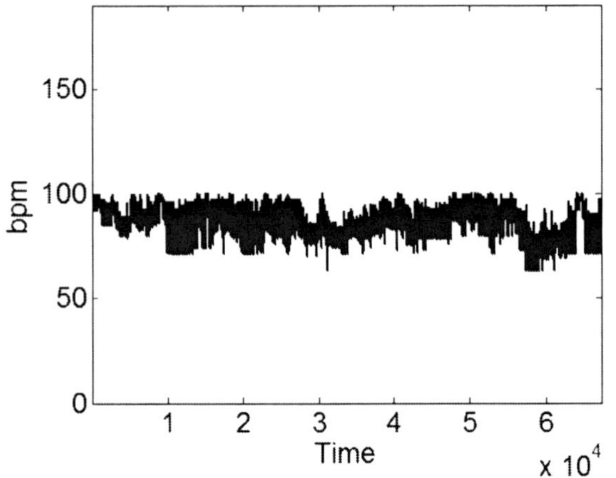

Figure 18. Prediction error using K-NN

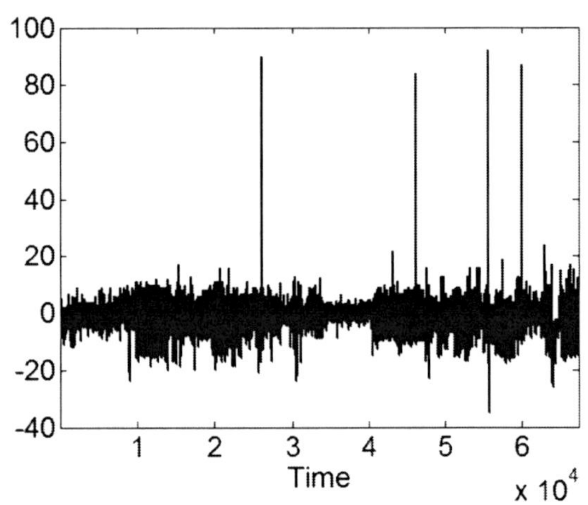

Figure 19. Raised alarms by SVM

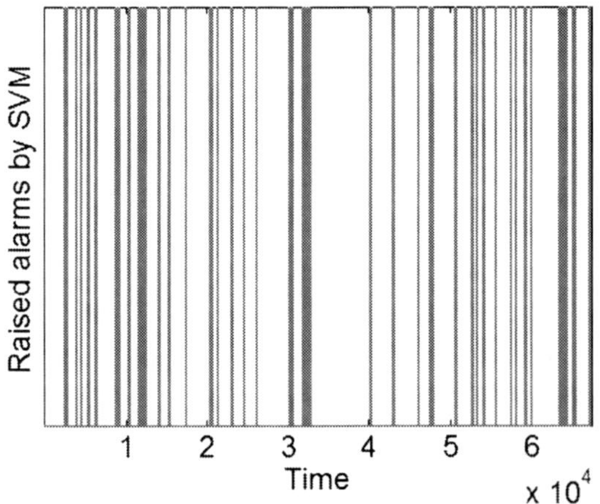

Figure 20. Raised alarms by J48

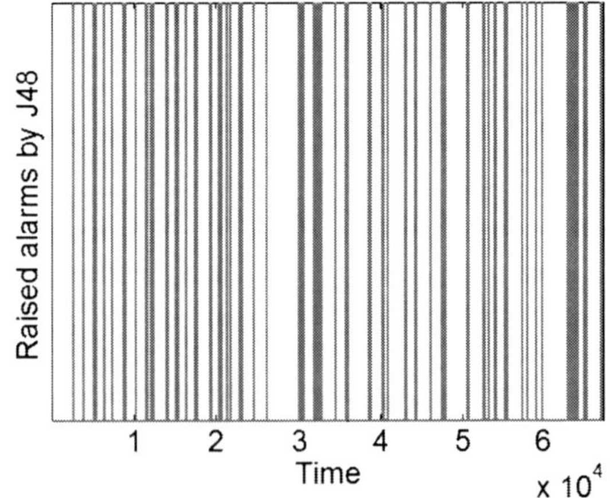

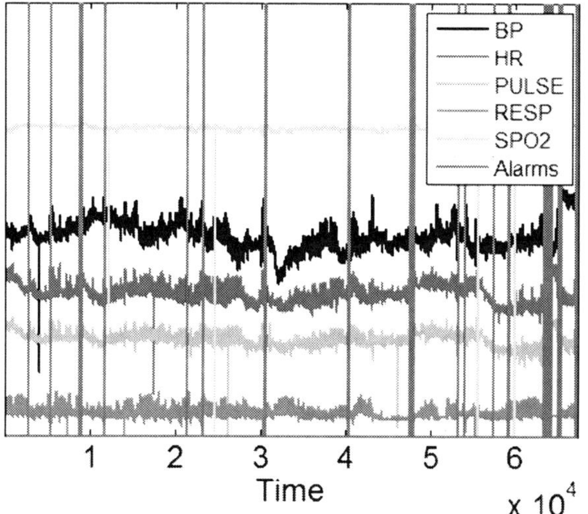

Figure 21. Raised medical alarms by SVM and linear regression

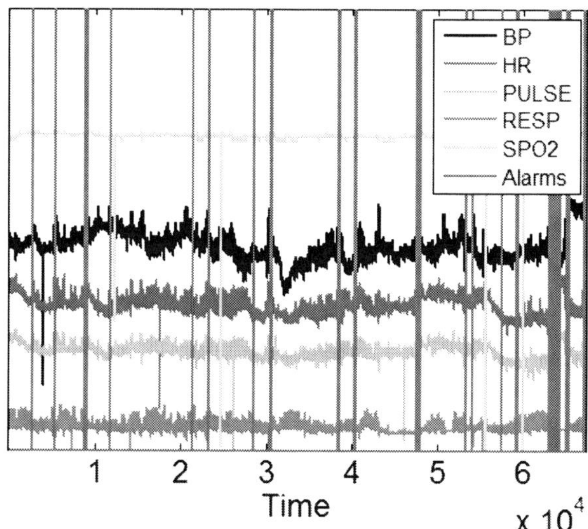

Figure 22. Raised medical alarms by J48 and linear regression

forms J48 in terms of detection accuracy, but J48 builds the classification model (decision tree) faster than SVM.

We used the Receiver Operating Characteristic (ROC) in the performance evaluation of the proposed approach to show the relationship between the true positive rate (Equation (12)) and the false positive rate (Equation (13)).

$$TPR = \frac{TP}{TP + FN} \qquad (12)$$

where TP represents the number of true positives, and FP is the number of false positives. The false positive rate (FPR) is defined as:

$$FPR = \frac{FP}{FP + TN} \qquad (13)$$

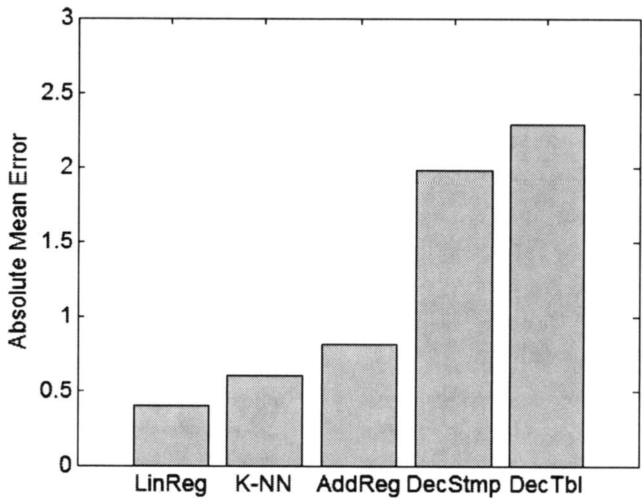

Figure 23. Mean error rate with different classifiers

Figure 24. Receiver Operating Characteristic (ROC)

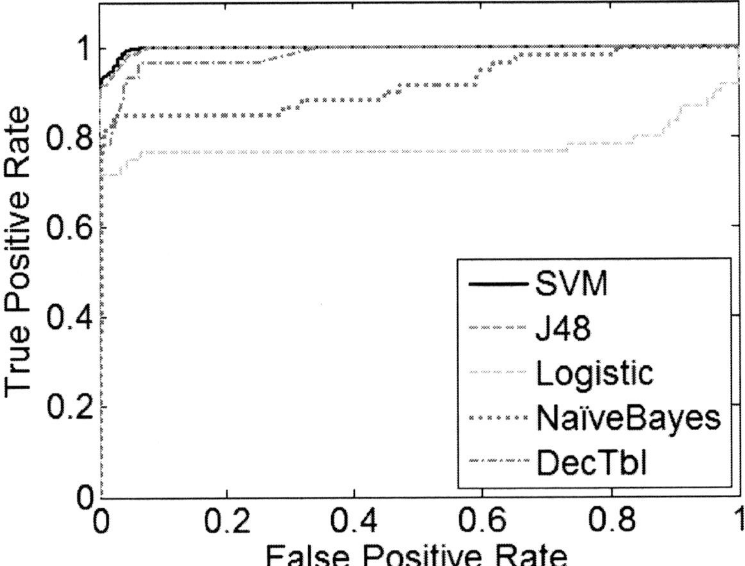

ROC curves are used for accuracy analysis where it represents, graphically, the true positive rate versus the false positive rate when varying the value of the decision threshold. In general, a good detection algorithm must achieve a high detection ratio with the lowest false alarm rate.

Figure 21 shows the raised medical alarms by the proposed approach. The raised alarms are triggered by heavy changes in at least k attributes. We can clearly notice in Figure 21 that faulty measurements (spikes), without correlated changes between physiological parameters (BP, HR, Pulse, SpO2 and RESP), don't trigger medical alarms. Figure 22 shows the raised alarms while replacing SVM by J48 in the proposed approach. The results are similar, and the raised alarms occur at the same time instants. We can notice some differences between Figures 21 and 22, where we get two additional alarms by J48 in Figure 22 (before 3.10^4 and 4.10^4 respectively).

Figure 24 shows the ROC for the proposed approach where the first nominal classifier is SVM, followed by J48, Logistic regression, Naïve Bayes and Decision Table respectively. SVM and J48 classifiers were the two most accurate

algorithms which achieved the best performances with TPR=100% for both, FPR=6.5% for SVM and FPR=7.4% for J48 respectively. The ROC for SVM and J48 is very similar having only minor difference. However, they achieve better performance compared to the other classifiers. The ROC validates that our claim that the proposed approach achieves high accuracy for detecting mote anomalies.

6. CONCLUSION AND PERSPECTIVES

Medical WBAN is a new emerging technology in the field of healthcare, providing vital care and access to patients, elderly, and infants. It allows continuously monitoring patients without restrictions in the movements and keeping the healthcare professional informed of any evolution of patients' condition.

These types of monitoring systems are tasked with providing humanity an outstanding instrument for patient observation and autonomous diagnostic, alarm, and emergency services. They also provide simple, remote patient data management and allow greater freedom for healthcare professionals which may, as a result, better serve clients from practically any location where network connectivity exists.

We described our architecture conceptually and detailed the results from preliminary experimentation conducted with our applications' analysis of real patient data. Furthermore, we discussed the issues and justified the need for medical WBANs for ubiquitous patient monitoring and authenticated remote patient data access for healthcare professionals.

The application, after mining the incoming data incrementally, applies machine learning algorithms to generated models based on algorithmically located correlations in the data. It is also able to distinguish between irregular patient attributes and faulty sensor data to maintain robustness and high accuracy. Considering the limitations associated with WSN technology and the spontaneity of our environment, we have constructed a reliable application for real time global patient monitoring from modern smart devices. The experimental results confirm the applications' high detection accuracy, low false alarm ratio and its' ability to quickly identify and differentiate between sensor faults and irregularities in a patient's health.

In the future, knowing that most collected sensor measurements are normal, we look to reduce the amount of exchanged data between the wireless sensors and the sink node, by transmitting only abnormal values on the sensor motes to reduce energy consumption by wireless transmissions.

ACKNOWLEDGMENT

This research was supported by Korea Science and Engineering Foundation, under the World Class University (WCU) program with additional support from NSF grants CCF-0545488 and OISE-0730065.

REFERENCES

Abduvaliyev, A., Pathan, A.-S. K., Zhou, J., Roman, R., & Wong, W.-C. (2013). On the vital areas of intrusion detection systems in wireless sensor networks. *IEEE Communications Surveys & Tutorials*, *99*, 1–15.

Alemdar, H., & Ersoy, C. (2010). Wireless sensor networks for healthcare: A survey. *Computer Networks*, *54*(15), 2688–2710. doi:10.1016/j.comnet.2010.05.003

Banerjee, T., Xie, B., & Agrawal, D. P. (2008). Fault tolerant multiple event detection in a wireless sensor network. *Journal of Parallel and Distributed Computing*, *68*(9), 1222–1234. doi:10.1016/j.jpdc.2008.04.009

Bishop, C. (2006). *Pattern recognition and machine learning (Information science and statistics)*. Springer-Verlag New York, Inc.

Chen, Y.-C., & Juang, J.-C. (2012). Outlier-detection-based indoor localization system for wireless sensor networks. *International Journal of Navigation and Observation*, 2012.

Cheng, X., Xu, J., Pei, J., & Liu, J. (2010). Hierarchical distributed data classification in wireless sensor networks. *Computer Communications*, *33*(12), 1404–1413. doi:10.1016/j.comcom.2010.01.027

Chipara, O., Lu, C., Bailey, T. C., & Roman, G.-C. (2010). Reliable clinical monitoring using wireless sensor networks: Experiences in a step-down hospital unit. In *Proceedings of the 8th ACM Conference on Embedded Networked Sensor Systems (SenSys'10)* (pp. 155-168).

Choi, J., Ahmed, B., & Gutierrez-Osuna, R. (2012). Developpement and evaluation of an ambulatory stress monitor based on wearable sensors. *IEEE Transactions on Information Technology in Biomedicine*, *16*(2), 279–286. doi:10.1109/TITB.2011.2169804 PMID:21965215

Cunha, J. P., Cunha, B., Pereira, A. S., Xavier, W., Ferreira, N., & Meireles, L. (2010). Vital-Jacket®: A wearable wireless vital signs monitor for patients' mobility in cardiology and sport. In *Proceedings of the International Conference on Pervasive Computing Technologies for Healthcare, PervasiveHealth.*

Curiac, D.-I., & Volosencu, C. (2012). Ensemble based sensing anomaly detection in wireless sensor networks. *Expert Systems with Applications, 39*(10), 9087–9096. doi:10.1016/j.eswa.2012.02.036

Farruggia, A., Giuseppe, L. R., & Ortolani, M. (2011). Probabilistic anomaly detection for wireless sensor networks. In *Proceedings of the 12th International Conference on Artificial Intelligence Around Man and Beyond* (pp. 438-444).

Grgic, K., Žagar, D., & Križanovic, V. (2012). Medical applications of wireless sensor networks – current status and future directions. *Medicinski Glasnik, 9*(1), 23–31. PMID:22634904

Hall, M., Frank, E., Holmes, G., Pfahringer, B., Reutemann, P., & Witten, I. H. (2009). The WEKA data mining software: An update. *SIGKDD Explorations, 11*(1). doi:10.1145/1656274.1656278

Havard Sensor Networks Lab. (2013). *CodeBlue: Wireless sensors for medical care.* Retrieved from http://fiji.eecs.harvard.edu/CodeBlue

Huang, F., Jiang, Z., Zhang, S., & Gao, S. (2010). Reliability evaluation of wireless sensor networks using logistic regression. In *Proceedings of the 2010 International Conference on Communications and Mobile Computing (CMC'10)* (pp. 334-338).

Jurdak, R., Wang, X. R., Obst, O., & Valencia, P. (2011). Wireless sensor network anomalies: Diagnosis and detection strategies. In D. A. Tolk & L. C. Jain (Eds.), *Intelligence-based systems engineering* (pp. 309–325). Springer. doi:10.1007/978-3-642-17931-0_12

Ko, J., Lim, J., Chen, Y., Musvaloiu-E, R., Terzis, A., & Masson, G. et al. (2010). MEDiSN: Medical emergency detection in sensor networks. [TECS]. *ACM Transactions on Embedded Computing Systems, 10*(1), 1–29. doi:10.1145/1814539.1814550

Kumar, P., & Lee, H.-J. (2012). Security issues in healthcare applications using wireless medical sensor networks: A survey. *Sensors (Basel, Switzerland), 12*(1), 55–91. PMID:22368458

Li, Y. (2010). *Anomaly detection in unknown environments using wireless sensor networks.* University of Tennessee.

Liu, F., Cheng, X., & Chen, D. (2007). Insider attacker detection in wireless sensor networks. *Proceedings - IEEE INFOCOM, 07*, 1937–1945. doi:10.1109/INFCOM.2007.225

Malan, D., Fulford-jones, T., Welsh, M., & Moulton, S. (2004). CodeBlue: An ad hoc sensor network infrastructure for emergency medical care. In *Proceedings of International Workshop on Wearable and Implantable Body Sensor Networks.*

Miao, X., Liu, K., He, Y., Liu, Y., & Papadias, D. (2011). Agnostic diagnosis: discovering silent failures in wireless sensor networks. *Proceedings - IEEE INFOCOM, 11*, 1548–1556.

Montgomery, K., Mundt, C., Thonier, G., Thonier, A., Udoh, U., Barker, V., et al. (2004). Lifeguard – A personal physiological monitor for extreme environments. In *Proceedings of the IEEE 26th Annual International Conference on Engineering in Medicine and Biology Society* (pp. 2192-2195).

Navarro, K. F., Lawrence, E., & Lim, B. (2009). Medical MoteCare: A distributed personal healthcare monitoring system. In *Proceedings of the International Conference on eHealth, Telemedicine, and Social Medicine (eTELEMED'09)* (pp. 25-30).

Otto, C., Milenkovi, A., Sanders, C., & Jovanov, E. (2005). System architecture of a wireless body area sensor network for ubiquitous health monitoring. *Journal of Mobile Multimedia, 1*(4), 307–326.

Physionet. (2013). Retrieved from http://www.physionet.org/cgi-bin/atm/ATM

Rajasegarar, S., Leckie, C., Bezdek, J. C., & Palaniswami, M. (2010). Centered hyperspherical and hyperellipsoidal one-class support vector machines for anomaly detection in sensor networks. *IEEE Transactions on Information Forensics and Security, 5*(3), 518–533. doi:10.1109/TIFS.2010.2051543

Sahoo, P. (2012). Efficient security mechanisms for mHealth applications using wireless body sensor networks. *Sensors (Basel, Switzerland), 12*(9), 12606–12633. doi:10.3390/s120912606 PMID:23112734

Salem, O., Guerassimov, A., Mehaoua, A., Marcus, A. M., & Furht, B. (2013). Sensor fault and patient anomaly detection and classification in medical wireless sensor networks. In *Proceedings of the IEEE ICC 2013 (ICC'13)* (pp. 4338-4343).

Sharma, A. B., Golubchik, L., & Govindan, R. (2010). Sensor faults: Detection methods and prevalence in real-world datasets. *ACM Transactions on Sensor Networks, 6*(3), 1–39. doi:10.1145/1754414.1754419

Siripanadorn, S., Hattagam, W., & Teaumroong, N. (2010). Anomaly detection in wireless sensor networks using self-organizing map and wavelets. *International Journal of Communication, 4*(3), 74–83.

Theodoridis, S., Pikrakis, A., Koutroumbas, K., & Cavouras, D. (2010). *Introduction to pattern recognition: A Matlab approach.* Academic Press.

Wang, H., Fang, H., Xing, L., & Chen, M. (2011). An integrated biometric-based security framework using wavelet-domain HMM in wireless body area networks (WBAN). In *Proceedings of the IEEE International Conference on Communications (ICC'11)* (pp. 1-5).

WEKA. (2013). The university of Waikato. *WEKA data mining tool.* Retrieved from http://www.cs.waikato.ac.nz/~ml/weka/

Witten, I. H., Frank, E., & Hall, M. A. (2011). *Data mining: Practical machine learning tools and techniques* (3rd ed.). Morgan Kaufmann Publishers Inc.

Wood, A., Virone, G., Doan, T., Cao, Q., Selavo, L., Wu, Y., & Stankovic, J. (2006). *ALARM-NET: Wireless sensor networks for assisted-living and residential monitoring.* University of Virginia.

Xiaozhen, Y., Hong, X., & Tong, W. (2011). A multiple linear regression data predicting method using correlation analysis for wireless sensor networks. In *Proceedings of the Cross Strait Quad-Regional Radio Science and Wireless Technology Conference* (pp. 960-963).

Xie, M., Hu, J., Han, S., & Chen, H.-H. (2012). Scalable hyper-grid k-NN-based online anomaly detection in wireless sensor networks. *IEEE Transactions on Parallel and Distributed Systems, 99*, 1–11.

Xu, S., Hu, C., Wang, L., & Zhang, G. (2012). Support vector machines based on K nearest neighbor algorithm for outlier detection in WSNs. In *Proceedings of the 8th International Conference on Wireless Communications, Networking and Mobile Computing (WiCOM'12)* (pp. 1-4).

Yang, X., Dinh, A., & Chen, L. (2010). Implementation of a wearerable real-time system for physical activity recognition based on naïve Bayes classifier. In *Proceedings of the International Conference on Bioinformatics and Biomedical Technology (ICBBT'10)* (pp. 101-105).

Yao, Y., Sharma, A., Golubchik, L., & Govindan, R. (2010). Online anomaly detection for sensor systems: A simple and efficient approach. *Performance Evaluation, 67*(11), 1059–1075. doi:10.1016/j.peva.2010.08.018

Yim, S.-J., & Choi, Y.-H. (2010). An adaptive fault-tolerant event detection scheme for wireless sensor networks. *Sensors (Basel, Switzerland)*, *10*(3), 2332–2347. doi:10.3390/s100302332 PMID:22294929

Ying-xin, X., Xiang-guang, C., & Jun, Z. (2011). Data fault detection for wireless sensor networks using multi-scale PCA method. In *Proc. of International Conference on Artificial Intelligence, Management Science and Electronic Commerce (AIMSEC'11)* (pp. 7035-7038).

Zhang, Y., Chao, H.-C., Chen, M., Shu, L., Park, C.-h., & Park, M.-S. (2010). Outlier detection and countermeasure for hierarchical wireless sensor networks. *IET Information Security*, *4*(4), 361–373. doi:10.1049/iet-ifs.2009.0192

Zhang, Y., Hamm, N., Meratnia, N., Stein, A., Van de Voort, M., & Havinga, P. (2012). Statistics-based outlier detection for wireless sensor networks. *26*(8), 1373-1392.

Zhang, Y., Meratnia, N., & Havinga, P. (2009). Adaptive and online one-class support vector machine-based outlier detection techniques for wireless sensor networks. In *Proceedings of the International Conference on Advanced Information Networking and Applications Workshops* (pp. 990-995).

Zhang, Y., Meratnia, N., & Havinga, P. J. (2010). Outlier detection techniques for wireless sensor networks: A survey. *IEEE Communications Surveys and Tutorials*, *12*(2), 159–170. doi:10.1109/SURV.2010.021510.00088

Chapter 25
Securing XML with Role-Based Access Control:
Case Study in Health Care

Alberto De la Rosa Algarín
University of Connecticut, USA

Timoteus B. Ziminski
University of Connecticut, USA

Steven A. Demurjian
University of Connecticut, USA

Yaira K. Rivera Sánchez
University of Connecticut, USA

Robert Kuykendall
Texas State University, USA

ABSTRACT

Today's applications are often constructed by bringing together functionality from multiple systems that utilize varied technologies (e.g. application programming interfaces, Web services, cloud computing, data mining) and alternative standards (e.g. XML, RDF, OWL, JSON, etc.) for communication. Most such applications achieve interoperability via the eXtensible Markup Language (XML), the de facto document standard for information exchange in domains such as library repositories, collaborative software development, health informatics, etc. The use of a common data format facilitates exchange and interoperability across heterogeneous systems, but challenges in the aspect of security arise (e.g. sharing policies, ownership, permissions, etc.). In such situations, one key security challenge is to integrate the local security (existing systems) into a global solution for the application being constructed and deployed. In this chapter, the authors present a Role-Based Access Control (RBAC) security framework for XML, which utilizes extensions to the Unified Modeling Language (UML) to generate eXtensible Access Control Markup Language (XACML) policies that target XML schemas and instances for any application, and provides both the separation and reconciliation of local and global security policies across systems. To demonstrate the framework, they provide a case study in health care, using the XML standards Health Level Seven's (HL7) Clinical Document Architecture (CDA) and the Continuity of Care Record (CCR). These standards are utilized for the transportation of private and identifiable information between stakeholders (e.g. a hospital with an electronic health record, a clinic's electronic health record, a pharmacy system, etc.), requiring not only a high level of security but also compliance to legal

DOI: 10.4018/978-1-4666-8756-1.ch025

entities. For this reason, it is not only necessary to secure private information, but for its application to be flexible enough so that updating security policies that affect millions of documents does not incur a large monetary or computational cost; such privacy could similarly involve large banks and credit card companies that have similar information to protect to deter identity theft. The authors demonstrate the security framework with two in-house developed applications: a mobile medication management application and a medication reconciliation application. They also detail future trends that present even more challenges in providing security at global and local levels for platforms such as Microsoft HealthVault, Harvard SMART, Open mHealth, and open electronic health record systems. These platforms utilize XML, equivalent information exchange document standards (e.g., JSON), or semantically augmented structures (e.g., RDF and OWL). Even though the primary use of these platforms is in healthcare, they present a clear picture of how diverse the information exchange process can be. As a result, they represent challenges that are domain independent, thus becoming concrete examples of future trends and issues that require a robust approach towards security.

1. INTRODUCTION

Today's world is dominated by systems with a wide range of technological approaches (e.g. application programming interfaces, Web services, cloud computing, data mining, etc.), where one major objective is to support information sharing and exchange as applications are constructed as meta-systems (systems of systems), with new applications interfacing with multiple technologies, comprised of many interacting components. In such an environment, the one major challenge is to ensure that local security policies (of constituent systems) are satisfied not only when the application accesses a single system, but also when considered from a higher-level perspective. That is, an application's security is the combination of the security that must be attained within each constituent system that is accessed. What happens when security privileges of individual systems are in conflict with one another? How do we reconcile these local security policies? Is it possible to define a global encompassing security process or framework that provides a level of guarantee to the local security policies from an enforcement perspective? As today's applications continue to become more and more complex, interacting with many other systems (or applications) using varied technological paradigms, there will be a need to

provide some degree of assurance that security for the application (global) satisfies the sum of the parts (local security of constituent systems). Information exchange has increased exponentially, due to the development of generic data standards (e.g., XML, JSON, RDF, OWL, etc.) and the ease of interconnection across systems, in domains such as biomedical, health informatics, library repositories, collaborative software development, etc. All of these domains present security challenges that, though not unique, have yet to be sufficiently addressed; often neither in the specific format or system (local security), and definitely not across multiple formats and meta-systems (global security).

In this effort to facilitate the intercommunication between heterogeneous systems, the *eXtensible Markup Language (XML)*[1] has become the de facto document standard for information exchange. In health care, which will serve as the case study for this chapter, XML is used for standards such as: the Health Level Seven's (HL7) Clinical Document Architecture (CDA) (Dolin, 2006) that underlies many Health Information Exchange (HIE) approaches; and, the Continuity of Care Record[2] (CCR), used for storage of administrative, patient demographics, and clinical data. In Health Information Technology (HIT), the clinical document architecture and the continuity of care record come together in systems such as Electronic Health Records (EHR) and Personal Health Records (PHR) (e.g., Microsoft HealthVault[3]). The clinical document architecture is used to support health information exchange among hospitals, clinics, physician practices, laboratories, etc., with the continuity of care record providing the means to model the data that needs to be exchanged. As documents derived from standards such as these are circulated among various systems and made available to particular users with specific needs, we must expand security from each individual system to a focus that is more expansive in controlling the document and its content, particularly for health information exchange. Current approaches to security only do so from the system's perspective, in which the security policies that govern it are the final authority, and no consideration is given to the policies that govern the data repositories or constituent systems. This level of security is inadequate to scenarios such as information exchange in which the data utilized could not be owned by any particular user, but by an external party. Added to this is the rapidly emerging mobile applications domain where, in the case of health care, patients manage personal health information for chronic diseases, and a need to securely access information and authorize its exchange with medical providers via mobile applications, electronic health records, secure emails, or other means is a key concern. A solution that achieves this will require document-level access control of XML schemas to allow XML instances to appear differently to authorized users at specific times based on criteria that include, but are not limited to, a user's role, time and value constraints on data usage, collaboration for sharing data, delegation of authority as privileges are passed among authorized users, etc.

The challenge of attaining customized XML security enforcement necessitates the addressing of legal and adaptability requirements. In health care, the Health Insurance Portability and Accountability Act[4] (HIPAA) provides a set of security guidelines in the usage, transmission, and sharing of Protected Health Information (PHI); in e-commerce, there would be a need to protect Personally Identifiable Information (PII) including names, addresses, accounts, credit card numbers, etc. Protected health information and personally identifiable information must be strictly adhered to in many applications and settings. From an adaptability perspective, XML security policies must be defined at the XML schema level to support the definitions of users grouped in different roles, each with possible different sets of permissions that act on the specific parts of the information (an XML instance), across millions of records (XML instances). For the purposes of this chapter, we focus on the attainment of the National Institute for Standards and Technology's[5] (NIST) standard Role-Based Access Control (RBAC) (Ferraiolo, 1995, 2001) for XML, which would support the definition of security policies at the XML schema level (for example, the continuity of care record document (patient data) at the schema) that can then be used to specify (allow or deny) different permissions on certain portions of an XML instance (for example, a continuity of care record's instance), allowing the same instance to appear differently to specific users (patients and medical providers) acting in a chosen role at different times. To accomplish this, we leverage a secure software engineering process that promotes the consideration of security at an early stage and throughout the process. The usage of an XML schema via a new Unified Modeling Language (UML) schema diagrams requires a security framework for XML that allows the design, implementation, and deployment of enforceable security policies to allow access to XML instances to be precisely controlled by role. The definition of security at the XML schema level via an external security policy separates the security from the XML instances, which avoids the overhead required when updating security policies that are otherwise embedded in instances and target a large amount of these.

In this chapter, we present our security framework for XML (De la Rosa Algarín, 2012) defined at the schema level and realized at the instance level through the creation and generation of eXtensible Access Control Markup Language (XACML)[6] policies, and demonstrate the work (design, mapping of policy and enforcement) via a case study of an in-house health care scenario composed of a set of health information technology applications. As shown in Figure 1, this generalized framework achieves granular security by taking the XML schemas and instances for any application (right hand side of Figure 1) and using them to define UML[7] diagrams for the respective XML schemas and the associated roles in order to create an enforcement XACML security policy that will be able to generate role-restricted (RR) instances that limit the information in the original instances based on the defined security (left hand side of Figure 1). Our approach provides separation of security concerns to tackle the challenge of changing security policies that can apply to millions of XML instances. In support of this framework, we leverage our prior work on secure software engineering using UML (Pavlich-Mariscal, 2008) and have created new UML diagrams: an XML Schema Class Diagram that captures the structure of the applications XML schemas; and an XML Role Slice Diagram that allows privileges on an XML schema's entities and attributes to be allowed/denied to different users by role at different times, thereby creating a role-restricted instance that is customized for that user. We note that Figure 1 is referring to any XML schemas, instances, and security definitions regardless of domain. In this chapter, after briefly reviewing our security framework for XML schemas and documents, we apply it to a case study of health care, consisting of the continuity of care record standard, utilized as the information exchange document, coupled with two in-house developed applications: the Personal Health Assistant (PHA), which consists of two mobile applications that support the exchange of information stored in a personal health record

(Microsoft HealthVault) between patients and providers; and, SMARTSync (Ziminski, 2012), a medication reconciliation application, built as a meta-system utilizing Microsoft HealthVault and the Harvard SMART Platform[8], that generates a list of potential overmedication, adverse interactions, and adverse reactions for the patient and provider. All of these applications require that the XML that is delivered be restricted by role (a filtering of the content of the instance) in order to insure that only the authorized information is provided to the user. Our in-house mobile and Web apps both share the same server, with the Web app accessing another server, using well accepted Web standards (XML, RDF, JSON) for information modeling and exchange; thus our work is applicable to any such architecture. The use of these in-house applications supports our ability to apply and experiment with our XML security solutions with actual working systems that, while health care based, are just mobile/Web apps and servers.

The remainder of this chapter has five sections. In Section 2, background is provided on the NIST RBAC standard, XML, and the continuity of care record for the reader's benefit and understanding of the examples used throughout the chapter. In Section 3, we briefly describe our existing security framework for XML (De la Rosa Algarín, 2012) with a review of the new UML diagrams (XML Schema Class Diagram and XML Role Slice Diagram in Figure 1) for XML schemas and security definition, the generation of enforcement XACML policy schemas from these new diagrams, and relevant related work. Section 4 presents our case study in health care using two in-house developed applications, Personal Health Assistant (PHA) and SMARTSync, by detailing: the overall architecture and associated technologies (Android[9], JSON[10], Microsoft HealthVault, and Harvard's SMART Platform), the Personal Health Assistant and SMARTSync applications, and the attainment of security for these applications using our security framework from Section 3. Note that while we

Figure 1. Security framework and enforcement process for XML

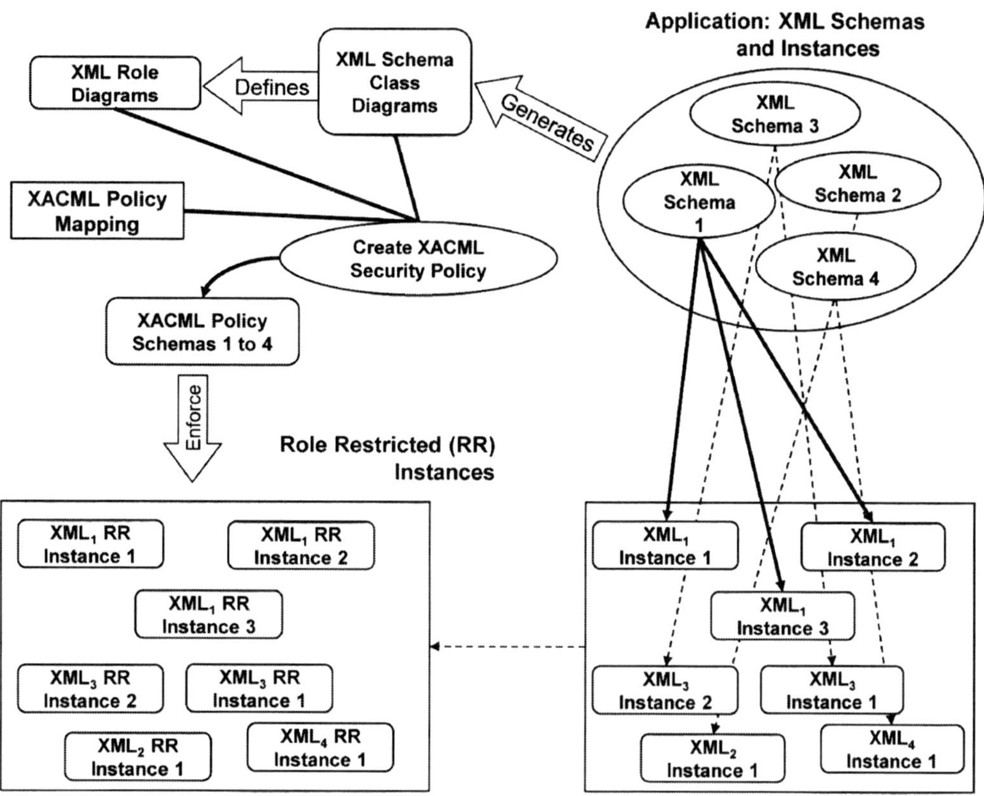

utilize the health care domain as the case study for our demonstration, this security framework can be applied in any domain where the document structure to be secured is XML and an XML schema that validates the instances is available. Following our case study of the health care domain, Section 5 presents future trends by detailing a large scale view of health information technology systems and applications, with an emphasis on the interplay of health information exchange among the various systems; and the role of security at global and local levels across such a complex architecture. As part of this discussion, accessible health information technology platforms are explored, including: Microsoft HealthVault personal health record; Open *m*Health[11], which promotes mobile health via an open architecture; and, the Harvard SMART platform for substitutable medical applications that promote reuse, are explored. The wide range of open electronic health records,

the myriad of XML standards, and the way that applications like Personal Health Assistant and SMARTSync interact to gather data effectively are also explored. These platforms, their role in the health information exchange process, and the large amount of data formats, standards and usage of data present concrete examples of research problems not unique to the health care domain, but present in domains that utilize information exchange, meta-systems or traditional system interoperability, as part of their daily workflow, requiring the intercommunication of information stored in different repositories with different formats and security policies. The end result is the recognition of a greater need for a comprehensive approach to security operating under information exchange. Towards this end, in Section 5, we also include a number of recommendations for the health care discipline and health information technology for improvements towards a more cohesive and shared future that promotes patient's health via electronic means. These recommendations, though directed to the health care domain as part of the case study, are presented in a general way so that the underlying, common application construction and interoperations issues are evident, and the proposed recommendation can be likewise achieved in this setting. We finish the chapter by offering concluding remarks in Section 6.

2. BACKGROUND

In support of this chapter, we provide background in three key areas: the National Institute for Standards and Technology (NIST) Role-Based Access Control (RBAC) model (Ferraiolo, 1995, 2001) which is intended to allow a user to be assigned permissions (read, write, etc.) to access objects (or portions of objects) based on his/her responsibilities as defined by a role; the eXtensible Markup Language (XML) a well-established standard for data representation that facilitates ease of exchange among users and systems; and, the health standard Continuity of Care Record (CCR) the represents data on patients (demographic, medications, allergies, medical history, etc.) using XML. Collectively, all three of these background areas establish the concepts and terms that are utilized throughout the paper. Health care is also an easy-to-understand domain, since most readers have experience with the stakeholders (medical providers) and their venues (offices, clinics, hospital, labs, etc.).

Role-based access control has long been utilized in the industry to represent permissions to an application based on a user's responsibilities. A role (e.g., Physician or Nurse) represents a category of permissions against objects (e.g., the way the role can access the data in a patient medical record), and by assigning permissions to roles, we can authorize users to roles against specific objects (e.g., Dr. Smith with Physician role can access objects of Patient Jones). When a role needs to change, we can change its permissions without impacting its authorization. The NIST RBAC (Ferraiolo, 1995, 2001) model organizes roles into different levels. First, $RBAC_0$ defines permissions on a role and authorizes a role to a user. Second, $RBAC_1$ allows for role hierarchies where permissions defined at the parent role can pass down to the child roles, e.g., the Nurse is a parent role with Staff_RN a role for taking care of patients, Discharge_RN a role for handling patient's upon leaving a hospital, Education_RN would teach patients about managing their chronic disease, etc. Third, $RBAC_2$ supports constraints, such as separation of duty and mutual exclusion, e.g., the roles Staff_RN and Physician are not allowed to assigned to the same individual (user); this prevents a user assigned a Staff_RN being assigned a Physician role in the future. Finally, from an authorization perspective, a user can be assigned multiple roles, but is only allowed to play a single role at any given time, which corresponds to the concept of sessions in $RBAC_3$, which provide the enforcement of permissions on specific objects authorized to a user playing a role at runtime. For example, Dr. Smith may have a Primary_MD role when treating patients in his practice while have an Attending_MD role when treating patients at a hospital.

XML is intended as a unifying means for data in terms of its representation to allow for it to be collected, transmitted, displayed, and exchanged among users and systems with ease. XML is a modeling language with the ability to define an *XML Schema* for the structure of the data being modeled (akin to a class in a UML diagram) which can then be instantiated to create *XML Instances* that are also referred to as XML documents. Collectively, a given application (like an electronic medical record) can have a set of XML schemas that describe the application and all of its instances. In this context, each XML schema serves as both the blueprint and validation agent for instances seeking to comply and be used for information representation and exchange. XML schemas support the definition of information to be hierarchically structured and tagged, and the tags themselves can be exploited to capture and represent the semantics of the information. The main modeling capability of XML schemas is the XML Schema Definition and associated XML Schema language. As an example, an XML schema can be composed of multiple xs:simpleType, xs:sequence, xs:element, etc, and these can be combined and nested in any way to form a more encompassing xs:complexType, a characteristic shared with classes in UML.

A continuity of care record document includes both protected health information and personally identifiable information such as demographics, social security number, insurance policy details, and health related information (such as medications, procedures, psychological notes, etc.). The continuity of care record schema defines all of the structure and interdependencies of information, but in practice, not all of the information at the schema level is available to all users based neither on role, nor at the instance level available to be written by some users based on role. For example, a Secretary role at a private practice performing financial operations might only need to see the patient's demographics and insurance policy details (personally identifiable information), whereas the Primary_MD role may to access the entire patient's information, but not the social security number. Select protected health information, such as psychiatric notes may not be available to the Primary_MD role, but be more constrained. Thus, when given information modeled using XML schemas (like the continuity of care record) and the associated instances (data for actual patients), the intent of the work presented in this chapter is to allow for the continuity of care record instances to be authorized to a user by role which will allow the instances appear differently at particular times and will also limit if the user (by the permissions of the role) will be able to read and/or write the authorized portions of an instance.

3. SECURITY FRAMEWORK FOR XML

Our security framework for XML schemas and instances (see Figure 1 again) separates the security policies from the schema by utilizing extended UML diagrams and a mapping algorithm that places the XACML policies at the same layer of the UML diagrams. These two diagrams, the XML Schema Class Diagram (XSCD) and the XML Role Slice Diagram (XRSD), are XML representative artifacts in the UML model, as we detail in Section 3.1, to address XML security from a software engineering perspective. Tackling the problem this way allows for the change of policies affecting large numbers of XML instances without the inherent cost of updating each instance. With our framework, designers can follow both a secure software engineering approach (Pavlich-Mariscal, 2008), and a secure information engineering approach for a more complete and secure solution. As a result, from the XSCD and XRSD artifacts, we generate a XACML policy that can enforce the defined security at the schema level, as we present in Section 3.2. To complete the discussion, Section 3.3 reviews related research. Note that we again stress that the security approach that is being demonstrated focuses on XML schemas and instances, and the generation of XACML policies; health care is simply an explanation vehicle.

3.1. XML Schema Class and Role Slice Diagrams in UML

UML provides multiple diagrams to visually model applications, but there is a lack of integrating security. Our prior work has defined new UML security diagrams for supporting RBAC (Pavlich-Mariscal, 2008) via the UML meta-model. Using this as a basis, we have extended this work to define two new UML artifacts (De la Rosa Algarín, 2012): the XML Schema Class Diagram (XSCD) in Figure 2a that contains architecture, structure characteristics, and constraints of an XML schema; and, the XML Role Slice Diagram (XRSD) in Figure 2b which has the ability to add permissions to the various elements of the XSCD, i.e. read/write, read/nowrite, noread/write, noread/nowrite. The set of all XML schemas for a given application are converted into a corresponding set of XSCDs. As a result, we provide secure software engineering to the XML design process where the creation of an XML schema is placed into the UML context alongside other diagrams. XSCD, in Figure 2a, presents the way that the XSCD for the continuity of care record's schema xs:complexType 'StructuredProductType' would be represented in an UML-like XSCD diagram. The XSCD allows for customized access control policies to be generated for the respective concepts of the XML schema. The XRSD in Figure 2b is capable of applying access control policies or

permissions on the attributes of the XSCD based on role, thereby achieving fine-grained control. Permissions on XML documents are read, no read, write, and no write permissions with respective stereotypes, <<read/write>>, <<read/nowrite>>, <<noread/write>>, and <<noread/nowrite>>. Figure 2b defines Physician and Nurse XRSDs with permissions against the XSCD in Figure 2a. Note that in Figure 2b, the continuity of care record's complexType 'StructuredProductType' element Product allows a Physician role all of the information on a drug and be able to create new instances following the continuity of care record schema, with the Nurse role limited to read the drug details and cannot create new records. Note that the XSCD (Figure 2a) and the XRSD (Figure 2b) do not cover the whole continuity of care record schema representation due to space limitations.

Figure 2. XSCD of a continuity of care record schema segment (a) and XRSD of the XSCD in a health care scenario (b)

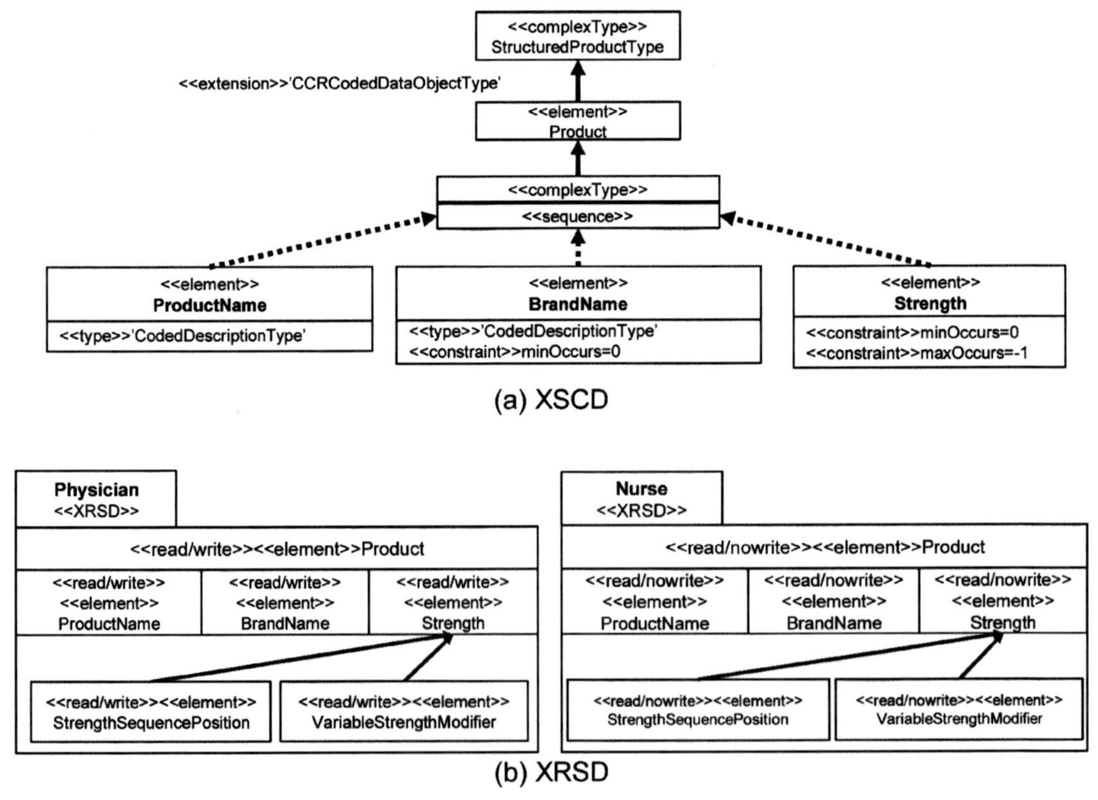

3.2. Generating XACML Policies from XSCD and XRSD

As given in Figure 2b, XRSDs act as the blueprint of the access-control policy for reading and writing permissions for a specific element or component of an XML schema for any given role, and are used to represent the portions of the application's XSCD (Figure 2a) that are to be allowed (or denied) access at an instance level to create role restricted instances (Figure 1), which can then be used to generate an XACML policy using the XACML Policy Mapping process in Figure 3. The architecture has a number of components: Policy Enforcement Point (PEP) allows a request to be made on a resource (a user playing a Physician role to access an continuity of care record instance); Policy Decision Point (PDP), which evaluates the request and provides a response according to the policies in place (evaluate if a Physician role can access (read and/or write) a portion of a continuity of care record schema); the Policy Administration Point (PAP) is utilized to write and manage policies (a realization of the XRSD against the continuity of care record schema and its associated instances); and, the Policy Information Point (PIP) to arbitrate very fine grained security issues (control access to psychiatric data). To map the XRSD in Figure 2b into an XACML policy, we utilize an XACML PolicySet to make the authorization decision via a set of rules in order to allow for access control decisions that may contain multiple Policies, and each Policy contains the access control rules. Note that multiple XACML Polices may be generated, resulting in a PolicySet for a specific set of XML schemas that comprise a given application. Our prior work (De la Rosa Algarín, 2012) has all of the details for this mapping process to generate XACML policies; and while we omit this discussion due to length considerations, in Listing 1 we present the generated XACML policy for the Physician XRCD in Figure 2b.

Briefly, we explain the generated XACML. First, the Policy's PolicyId attribute value is the Physician XRSD is concatenated to 'AccessControlPolicy'; the Rule's RuleId attribute value is the Physician XRSD value concatenated to the XRSD's higher order element (in Listing 1 it would be Product as defined in the XSCD in Figure 2b) and concatenated to 'ProductRule'; the Rule's Description value is the Physician XRSD is concatenated to 'Access Control Policy Rule'; and, the XACML Policy and Rules target and match the role (*Subject*, e.g., *Physician* in Figure 2b and Listing 1), the schema elements (*Resources*, e.g., ProductName, BrandName and Strength in Figure 2a, 2b and Listing 1), and the permissions (*Actions*, e.g., read and write in Figure 2b and Listing 1). Second the XACML *Subject* Physician is identified as an attribute. Third, the resources are identified; namely, the *AttributeValue's* value is the Physician XRSD's element names from the XSCD (e.g., ProductName, BrandName and Strength in Figure 2a, 2b and Listing 1). Finally, the XACML *Actions* as operations and values (read and write in Figure 2b and Listing 1) are defined.

Figure 3. XACML mapping from XRSD's and enforcement architecture

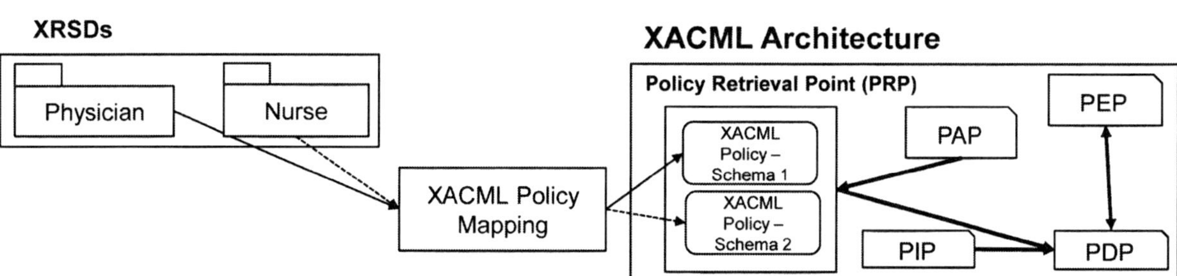

The end result in Listing 1 is an XACML policy that when applied to a continuity of care record instance for the Physician role will generated a role restricted XML instance that limits the visibility and usage of the continuity of care record instance for a particular patient.

3.3. Related Work

In this section, we present related work in a number of areas. First in, XML security frameworks, one effort on enterprise resource planning consists of an integrated packaged software that serves as a single solution for database and communication utilizing XML (Chandrakumar, 2012) by focusing on the XML Signature specification (Ardagna, 2007), and another effort (Ammari, 2010) presents an architecture capable of handling the receiving of XML messages from heterogeneous systems. Second, in embedded XML security, the work of (Damiani, 2000) presents an access control system that embeds the definition and enforcement of the security policies in the structure of the XML documents in order to provide customizable security using document type definitions (outmoded XML) that incurs high overhead since security changes impact all instances, while the work of (Damiani, 2008.) details a model that combines the embedding of policies and rewriting of access queries to provide security to XML datasets.

Third, in XML and access control, one effort (Bertino, 2002; Bertino, 2004) presents Author-X, a Java-based system for discretionary access control in XML documents (using document type definitions) that provides customizable protection to the documents with positive and negative authorizations. A second effort (Leonardi, 2010) considers the scenario of a federated access control model, in which the data provider and policy enforcement are handled by different organizations, while a third effort (Kuper, 2005) presents a model consisting of access control policies over a document type definition with XPath expressions in order to achieve XML security. Last, the work of (Müldner, 2009) uses an approach of supporting RBAC to handle the special case of role proliferation, which is an administrative issue that happens in RBAC when roles are changed, added, and evolve over time, making security of an organization difficult to manage. Finally, in encryption-based XML security, the XML Security Working Group[12] (SWG) works on three different security aspects: XML signatures, XML encryption, and XML Security Maintenance, a second effort (Bertino, 2002) encrypts different sections of an XML document with different encryption keys which are distributed to the specific users based on the access control policies in place, and a third effort (Rahaman, 2008) presents a distributed access control model for collaborative environments where XML documents are used.

4. CASE STUDY OF HEALTHCARE APPLICATIONS

In this section, we present a case study of attaining security in XML for two in-house developed health applications, demonstrating the generation and enforcement of XACML policies on XML instances based on an a subset of the continuity of care record schema. The first, a mobile health application, the Personal Health Assistant (PHA), consists of two perspectives for medication management. One perspective allows a patient to keep track of their medications, nutritional supplements, allergies, etc., and also authorize that protected health information (continuity of care record information), which is stored in Microsoft HealthVault, to his/her specific medical providers at different times. The second perspective allows a provider to select and view the authorized protected health information on a patient-by-patient basis as determined by his/her assigned role. The second application, SMARTSync for medication reconciliation (Ziminski, 2012), takes patient

Listing 1. Mapped XACML policy from physician XRSD

```xml
<?xml version="1.0" encoding="UTF-8"?>
  <Policy xmlns="urn:oasis:names:tc:xacml:2.0:policy:schema:os"
  xmlns:xsi="http://www.w3.org/2001/XMLSchema-instance"
  xsi:schemaLocation="urn:oasis:names:tc:xacml:2.0:policy:schema:os
  http://docs.oasis-open.org/xacml/access_control-xacml-2.0-policy-schema-os.xsd"
  xmlns:md="http:www.med.example.com/schemas/record.xsd"
  PolicyId="urn:oasis:names:tc:xacml:2.0:example:policyid:PhysicianAccessControlPol
icy"
  RuleCombiningAlgId="urn:oasis:names:tc:xacml:1.0:rule-combining-algorithm:deny-
overrides">
  <Target/>
   <Rule RuleId="urn:oasis:names:tc:xacml:2.0:example:ruleid:PhysicianProductRule"
       Effect="Permit">
    <Description>Physician Access Control Policy Rule</Description>
    <Target>
      <Subjects>
        <Subject>
        <SubjectMatch MatchId="urn:oasis:names:tc:xacml:1.0:function:string-equal">
          <AttributeValue DataType="http://www.w3.org/2001/XMLSchema#string">
            Physician
          </AttributeValue>
        <SubjectAttributeDesignator
          AttributeId="urn:oasis:names:tc:xacml:2.0:example:attribute:role"
          DataType="http://www.w3.org/2001/XMLSchema#string"/>
        </SubjectMatch>
      </Subject>
    </Subjects>
    <Resources>
    <Resource>
      <ResourceMatch MatchId="urn:oasis:names:tc:xacml:1.0:function:string-equal">
        <AttributeValue DataType="http://www.w3.org/2001/XMLSchema#string">
          ccr:schema:product:productname
        </AttributeValue>
      <ResourceAttributeDesignator
        AttributeId="urn:oasis:names:tc:xacml:1.0:resource:target-namespace"
        DataType="http://www.w3.org/2001/XMLSchema#string"/>
      </ResourceMatch>
      </Resource>
      <Resource>
      <ResourceMatch MatchId="urn:oasis:names:tc:xacml:1.0:function:string-equal">
          <AttributeValue DataType="http://www.w3.org/2001/XMLSchema#string">
          ccr:schema:product:brandname
```

continued on following page

Listing 1. Continued

```
        </AttributeValue>
      <ResourceAttributeDesignator
        AttributeId="urn:oasis:names:tc:xacml:1.0:resource:target-namespace"
        DataType="http://www.w3.org/2001/XMLSchema#string"/>
      </ResourceMatch>
      </Resource>
      <Resource>
      <ResourceMatch MatchId="urn:oasis:names:tc:xacml:1.0:function:string-equal">
        <AttributeValue DataType="http://www.w3.org/2001/XMLSchema#string">
            ccr:schema:product:strength
        </AttributeValue>
      <ResourceAttributeDesignator
        AttributeId="urn:oasis:names:tc:xacml:1.0:resource:target-namespace"
        DataType="http://www.w3.org/2001/XMLSchema#string"/>
      </ResourceMatch>
      </Resource>
   </Resources>
  <Actions>
   <Action>
     <ActionMatch MatchId="urn:oasis:names:tc:xacml:1.0:function:string-equal">
        <AttributeValue DataType="http://www.w3.org/2001/XMLSchema#string">
            read
        </AttributeValue>
      <ActionAttributeDesignator
        AttributeId="urn:oasis:names:tc:xacml:1.0:action:action-read"
        DataType="http://www.w3.org/2001/XMLSchema#string"/>
      </ActionMatch>
   </Action>
     <Action>
      <ActionMatch MatchId="urn:oasis:names:tc:xacml:1.0:function:string-equal">
         <AttributeValue DataType="http://www.w3.org/2001/XMLSchema#string">
             write
         </AttributeValue>
      <ActionAttributeDesignator
        AttributeId="urn:oasis:names:tc:xacml:1.0:action:action-write"
        DataType="http://www.w3.org/2001/XMLSchema#string"/>
      </ActionMatch>
    </Action>
   </Actions>
  </Target>
 </Rule>
</Policy>
```

medications from HealthVault and the Harvard SMART Platform Reference Electronic Health Record and from this information is able to generate a summary list of medications/supplements added by patients (in HealthVault) with those prescribed by a patient's medical provider. The intent is to generate a color-coded list of potential overmedication, adverse interactions, and adverse reactions for the patient and provider. Both applications have been coded by undergraduate, masters, and doctoral students as part of research related to biomedical and health informatics and its security and interoperability issues. The remainder of this section begins the case study by presenting the overall architecture of Personal Health Assistant and SMARTSync in Section 4.1. Then, Personal Health Assistant and SMARTSync are described in Sections 4.2 and 4.3, respectively, with a focus on their functional capabilities and user interfaces. Finally, in Section 4.4, we explore the way that XACML based security is achieved in the Personal Health Assistant application (where the documents to secure are XML instances) and in SMART-Sync (where information is represented in RDF/XML and JSON-DL that must then be converted to XML in order to allow the information to be appropriately secured). Note, from a generalized perspective, we have a mobile app (PHA) and Web-based app that both interact with a server (MSHV) using JSON with XML conversion occurring to retrieve data entered by the end-user (patient), with the Web app (SMARTSync) also interacting with another external system (SMART EHR) which is effectively a database controlled by a third party (physician's office with patient data). If you reread the prior sentence without the parenthetical remarks, you have a mobile app and Web app interacting with one server, and the Web app interacting with another, all with information flowing with standard formats (XML, JSON, RDF); clearly the architecture is generalizable in this way to many other business and industrial domains.

4.1. Overall Architecture

The overall architecture of the two healthcare applications is given in Figure 4, where the bottom of the figure indicates Personal Health Assistant and SMARTSync. Microsoft HealthVault acts as the data source (server) for both applications, and stores information in a proprietary format which to be exported via a.NET API which can then be used to generate a continuity of care record compliant document in XML. The HealthVault Middle-Layer Server (center of Figure 4) acts as the contained solution of policy access, information, decision, and enforcement points (see right hand side of Figure 3). The XACML policies created and stored in the account of each respective user limits access to HealthVault through the HealthVault Middle-Layer Server, which handles the requests (where data is sent as JSON) of both applications. To store the relations between the authorized list of providers and their respective patients, the Middle-Layer Server uses MySQL[13]. JSON is utilized for the communication of the two applications and the Middle-Layer Server, allowing us to insure a uniform communication with any application (not only with Personal Health Assistant) that can be created for users. The communication between the Personal Health Assistant (patient version) and the Middle-Layer Server is done with unmodified JSON objects, while the communication between the Personal Health Assistant - (provider) version and SMARTSync and the Middle-Layer Server is a combination of unmodified (for the initial request of patients) and filtered (for the resulting data allowed by the policies enforced) JSON. From HealthVault, XML role restricted instances are generated. Requests done by the provider application determine the format of the data. If a provider is requesting information in the patient's continuity of care record document, then data from HealthVault is exported as a continuity of care record schema compliant XML document with policy enforce-

Figure 4. Medication management and reconciliation applications

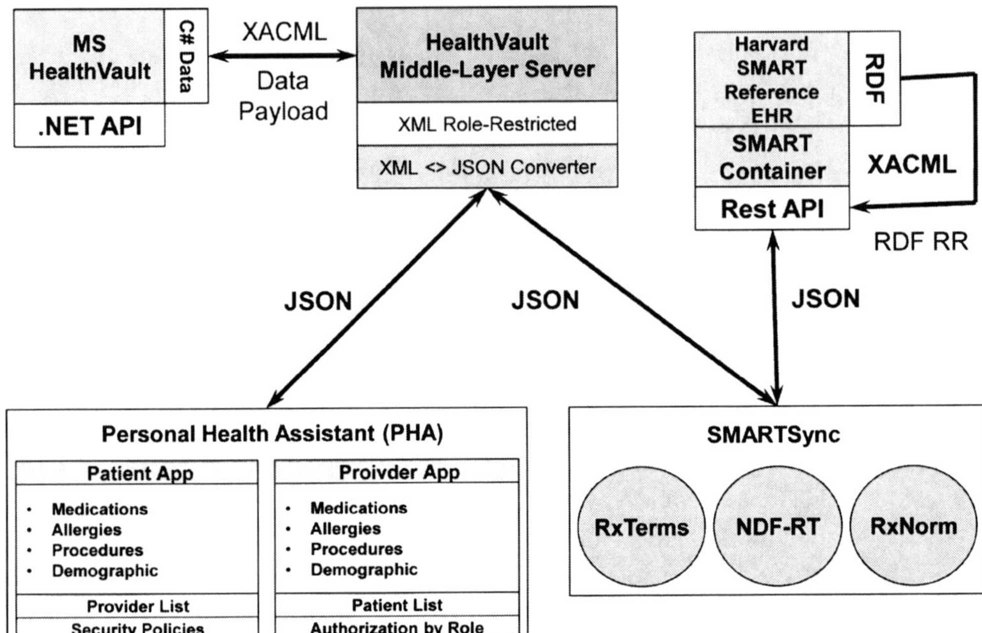

ment performed, whereas any input from the provider to HealthVault is first received as a JSON payload, converted to an XML document based on the continuity of care record schema, enforced with policies (Section 4.3), and once authorized, translated to HealthVault objects for write back. A similar process occurs on the SMARTSync side to merge and save the data from HealthVault and SMART Reference Electronic Health Record (another server) back into HealthVault.

4.2. Personal Health Assistant (PHA)

Personal Health Assistant (PHA) is an in-house developed mobile (not publicly available), test-bed Android application for medication management that allows: patients to view and update their personal health record stored in their HealthVault account and authorize medical providers to access certain portion of protected health information; and, for providers to obtain the permitted information from their respective patients that they have been authorized to view. The patient version of

Personal Health Assistant allows users to perform a set of actions regarding their health information. Users can view and edit their medication list, allergies, observations of daily living, and set security policies for read/write permissions on their medical providers by role per the discussion in Section 3. Security settings can be set at a fine granular level, and each provider gets view/update authorizations to the different information components available in Personal Health Assistant. The provider version of Personal Health Assistant allows the users (health professionals or medical providers) to view and edit the medical information of their patients as long as they are permitted to do so as dictated by the security set by the user (patient).

4.3. SMARTSync Application

SMARTSync is an in-house developed (not publicly available), Web-based test-bed medication reconciliation application used to create and preserve a patient's medication list through transfers among locations of care, preventing immediate interactions, and avoiding dosage errors in situations where brand and generic drugs are received or multi-component drugs are used (Barnsteiner, 2005; Poon, 2006). Significant risks include (Huang, 2004): *overmedication* when a provider prescribes a new medication (or one from the same class) or when an interacting medication is prescribed; *adverse interactions*, the result of conflicts between medications, which can change effect strength or serum concentration; and *adverse reactions*, allergic/other effects, experienced by patients which can result in a patient being wrongly labeled as allergic to a medication, unnecessarily excluding it as a treatment option in the future. To accomplish this, we gather data form HealthVault and SMART Reference Electronic Health Record as shown in Figure 4. Any medical data source (e.g., an electronic medical record, a personal health record, etc.) can be turned into a SMART container by exposing the SMART REST API, the SMART Connect API, and the related RDF/XML based data model[14].

In the SMART framework, applications are grouped on the SMART dashboard, which offers authentication and a set of basic services based on RDF/SPARQL for accessing the underlying medical data source in the SMART container. SMARTSync is also operated through this user interface component. In addition, SMARTSync communicates with HealthVault and takes advantage of the RxNorm, RxTerms, and the National Drug File – Reference Terminology[15] nomenclature/terminologies for semantic navigation of clinical drugs. The graphical user interface for SMARTSync is designed provide the alert information to the user in a quick and easily recognizable fashion, geared towards simplicity in order to serve a wide range of patients and to be easily portable to mobile devices. The main application screen is currently divided in two tabs, visualizing the personal health record (HealthVault) and the SMART Reference Electronic Health Record. Patients can switch between the tabs to see the list of medications stored in each record. The *Reconcile Medications* and the *Find Medication Interactions* buttons perform on-demand reconciliation and interaction searches. In the HealthVault tab, the user is presented with the reconciled list of medications. If any of the entries interact, the severity of interaction is indicated by a yellow (significant interaction) or red (critical interaction) background. Entries for which no interactions are found are displayed with a neutral background color. There are up to three buttons located next to each of the medications, over the counters, and natural supplements on either tab: *View Interactions*, *Details*, and *Remove*. Since a patient cannot modify the information located in the provider's EMR, the only button visible in this tab is *Details*. *View Interactions* presents the user with a listing of cross-interactions between the specified medication (over the counter/natural supplement) and any other reconciled entry. *Details* presents information of the medication ingredients, generic names, and the dates when the user started and stopped taking the medication. *Remove*, only available in the personal health record tab, allows the user to permanently delete the medication from their personal health record.

4.4. Achieving Security in Personal Health Assistant and SMARTSync

Securing the protected health information in Personal Health Assistant and SMARTSync is accomplished by utilizing the new UML-like XSCD and XRSD diagrams that define the security (see Section 3.1) in order to generate the XACML security policies (see Section 3.2). While Personal Health Assistant strictly uses HealthVault to store and retrieve information, SMARTSync (by the nature and objective of the SMART Platform) is capable of obtaining information from heterogeneous data sources that do not share the same XML standard. These two cases present the diversity of formats and standards (sometimes equivalent, often non-equivalent) on which not only the health care domain operates, and must be considered in order to effectively secure information that is being exchanged in different formats among a range of health information technology systems. This approach of using XML to exchange and share information is occurring using a mobile app, a Web app, and multiple servers; this is a very typical model for any application domain. In the remainder of this section, we describe the way that the XACML policy is enforced when handling reading and writing requests on XML instances whose schema has been secured in Personal Health Assistant, as well as the realization of the security framework in SMARTSync which requires additional steps to deal with additional data formats.

Providing security on the continuity of care record utilized by Personal Health Assistant is achieved by the enforcement in the HealthVault Middle-Layer server (see Figure 4). The read and write operations to be enforced are initialized by the provider perspective of Personal Health Assistant, handled by the HealthVault Middle-Layer server, and realized in the generated XACML (see Listing 1 in Section 3.2). When a request is initiated from a provider to read the protected health information of a patient, the Middle-Layer Server retrieves the patient's information exported as a continuity of care record along with the targeting XACML policy. After this step, enforcement is performed and those elements with read permissions denied for the provider are filtered out and deleted from the continuity of care record using the XACML policy (Listing 1). Once this has occurred, the filtered instance of the patient's continuity of care record is then converted into an equivalent JSON object for Personal Health Assistant utilization; JSON is utilized to provide a common abstraction layer in data model for any other developed application that wishes to utilize HealthVault data. Consider an example scenario where a user with a role of Nurse is requesting information on a patient's personal health record. The permission of read for the Nurse role has been

allowed for medications and allergies, and denied for medical procedures. The permission of write has been disallowed for all data elements. When a nurse utilizes the provider's Personal Health Assistant, s/he selects the patient named Jane Doe. As explained, the Middle-Layer Server retrieves the Jane Doe continuity of care record along with the XACML policy, and enforces security by filtering the continuity of care record as directed by the XACML policy. The filtered continuity of care record is then converted into a JSON object so that the Personal Health Assistant application can present the information to the user.

The steps to enforce security on writing operations done by a provider are similar. Starting with a write-back request with the JSON payload of new information, the Middle-Layer Server utilizes the XACML (see Listing 1) to evaluate which elements the provider is allowed to update. Only these elements are then updated in the continuity of care record, which goes through a validation process with the continuity of care record schema (for consistency in structure and integrity), and then written back to HealthVault in their respective objects. If the user requesting a write operation has a role with a permission that allows it to occur, the continuity of care record instance is updated with the sent data, and validated with the continuity of care record schema before the write-back to HealthVault. If validation against the schema is successful, then the write-back occurs, and the update performed by the provider is saved in the patient's HealthVault record. If the requester has a role that is not allowed to perform writing operations on the desired element, the Middle-Layer Server drops the request. Our approach provides a means for updating XML documents (in this case continuity of care record instances) that is controlled via an XACML security policy with the assistance of the Middle-Layer Server.

While HealthVault provides the information in continuity of care record, the SMART Platform's data model is capable of providing information in RDF/XML[16], N-TRIPLES[17], TURTLE[18] and

JSON-LD[19]. RDF[20], which is a semantically augmented extension to XML, shares similar design, structure and hierarchical characteristics. The RDF/XML format provides XML syntax for RDF. This syntax is defined with respect to the XML namespaces, information set, and base. By using N-TRIPLES, the formal grammar for RDF/XML is annotated from the RDF graph. N-TRIPLES is an RDF graph-serializing format that enables the precise recording of the RDF graph mapping to machine-readable form. TURTLE allows the writing of RDF graphs in textual form, consisting of directives and triple-generating statements. Finally, JSON-LD is a linked data format utilized to provide context to data. Based on JSON, JSON-LD is capable of augmenting RESTful[21] services into providing data to the semantic-Web (Lanthaler, 2012). To secure the information obtained from the SMART Platform that is utilized by SMARTSync, we make use of the JSON-LD format. While an RDF/XML instance is at its core an XML instance annotated with RDF, it lacks a unique serialization from which an XML schema can be abstracted. That is, multiple XML schemas exist that validate against the different RDF/XML serializations. This presents a scalability problem in our approach, as we only consider a unique and valid XML schema to secure. The use of JSON-LD provides a unique JSON representation from which an equivalent XML instance can be generated using a variety of tools that are available for this purpose. To properly apply our security framework to JSON-LD, we first apply an XML transformation to the JSON-LD instance. Since JSON-LD is extended JSON, any JSON to XML transformation tool will do the conversion and create an equivalent XML document, from which an XML schema can then be generated. To demonstrate, the Listing 2a has JSON-LD for the medication AMITRIPTYLINE (for depression), while the right hand side has the resulting XML instance. Since the generated XML instance only has one serialization, the one obtained from the transformation operation, abstracting a unique

XML schema that can validate is possible using an XML schema generator or tool, e.g., Microsoft's Visual Studio[22], Stylus Studio[23], Eclipse's Oxygen XML Plugin[24], Trang[25], etc. This XML Schema abstracted from AMITRIPTYLINE instance is shown in Listing 3a.

To complete the process, we again leverage the XSCD and XRSD's from Section 3.1 to generate XACML Policies (using the process in Section 3.2). In Listing 3, the XML Schema for the medication (Listing 3a) is then enforced using an XACML policy (Listing 3b). The XACML Policy only changes, with respect to the continuity of care record targeting policy, in the resources and their references. Note that we utilize the same color-coding scheme from Section 3.2 to illustrate the different aspects of the XACML with respect to the shading for policy, and blue and red lettering for read and write, respectively. While the SMART Platform does not currently support writing data back to the data sources, we still provide the mechanism to enforce security on write operations. That is, the Action elements in the XACML policy are still defined for read and write operations (and evaluated to Deny or Permit based on the credentials deduced from the XRSD). The SMARTSync example clearly illustrates that it is possible for our XACML security framework to work in many different settings, as long as there are tools available to allow the data translation to occur and the appropriate XML schema to be generated.

5. FUTURE TRENDS AND RESEARCH DIRECTIONS

Future trends and research directions in security are related to taking a high-level view of the information data exchange process, in general, and its application to the healthcare domain, in particular. Our focus in this section, with respect to health care as shown in Figure 5, considers all of the different health information technology systems

Listing 2. SMART JSON-LD for medication (a) and transformed XML instance (b)

(a) JSON-LD

```
{
    "@context": ".../contexts/smart_context.jsonld",
    "@graph": [
      {
          "@type": "Medication",
          "belongsTo": {
              "@id": "http://sandbox-api.smartplatforms.org/records/2169591"
      },
      "drugName": {
        "@type": "CodedValue",
        "code": {
          "@id": "http://purl.bioontology.org/ontology/RXNORM/856845"
        },
        "dcterms__title": "AMITRIPTYLINE HCL 50 MG TAB"
    },
    "endDate": "2007-08-14",
    "frequency": {
      "@type": "ValueAndUnit",
      "unit": "/d",
      "value": "2"
    },
    "instructions": "Take two tablets twice daily as needed for pain",
    "quantity": {
      "@type": "ValueAndUnit",
      "unit": "{tablet}",
      "value": "2"
    },
    "startDate": "2007-03-14"
    },
    {
    "@id": "http://purl.bioontology.org/ontology/RXNORM/856845",
    "@type": [
      "spcode__RxNorm_Semantic",
      "Code"
    ],
    "dcterms__identifier": "856845",
    "dcterms__title": "AMITRIPTYLINE HCL 50 MG TAB",
    "system": "http://purl.bioontology.org/ontology/RXNORM/"
    }
  ]
}
```

continued on following page

Listing 2. Continued

(b) Transformed XML

```
<?xml version="1.0" encoding="UTF-8" ?>
      <@context>
               …/contexts/smart_context.jsonld
      </@context>
      <@graph>
            <@type>Medication</@type>
            <belongsTo>
                    <@id>http://sandbox-api.smartplatforms.org/records/2169591</@
id>
            </belongsTo>
            <drugName>
                    <@type>CodedValue</@type>
                    <code>
                          <@id>http://purl.bioontology.org/ontology/RX-
NORM/856845</@id>
                    </code>
                    <dcterms__title>AMITRIPTYLINE HCL 50 MG TAB</dcterms__title>
            </drugName>
            <endDate>2007-08-14</endDate>
            <frequency>
                    <@type>ValueAndUnit</@type>
                    <unit>/d</unit>
                    <value>2</value>
            </frequency>
            <instructions>Take two tablets twice daily as needed for pain</in-
structions>
            <quantity>
                    <@type>ValueAndUnit</@type>
                    <unit>{tablet}</unit>
                    <value>2</value>
            </quantity>
            <startDate>2007-03-14</startDate>
      </@graph>
      <@graph>
            <@id>http://purl.bioontology.org/ontology/RXNORM/856845</@id>
            <@type>spcode__RxNorm_Semantic</@type>
            <@type>Code</@type>
            <dcterms__identifier>856845</dcterms__identifier>
            <dcterms__title>AMITRIPTYLINE HCL 50 MG TAB</dcterms__title>
             <system>http://purl.bioontology.org/ontology/RXNORM/</system>
      </@graph>
```

Listing 3. Segment of XML schema (a) and a segment of the targeting XACML policy (b)

```
(a) Segment of XML Schema
<?xml version="1.0" encoding="UTF-8"?>
<xs:schema xmlns:xs="http://www.w3.org/2001/XMLSchema"
elementFormDefault="qualified">
  <xs:element name="graph">
    <xs:complexType>
      <xs:sequence>
        <xs:element ref="type"/>
        <xs:element ref="belongsTo"/>
        <xs:element ref="drugName"/>
        <xs:element ref="endDate"/>
        <xs:element ref="frequency"/>
        <xs:element ref="instructions"/>
        <xs:element ref="quantity"/>
        <xs:element ref="startDate"/>
      </xs:sequence>
    </xs:complexType>
  </xs:element>
<xs:element name="belongsTo" type="id"/>
  <xs:element name="drugName">
    <xs:complexType>
      <xs:sequence>
        <xs:element ref="type"/>
        <xs:element ref="code"/>
        <xs:element ref="dctermstitle"/>
      </xs:sequence>
    </xs:complexType>
  </xs:element>
<xs:element name="code" type="id"/>
<xs:element name="dctermstitle" type="xs:string"/>
<xs:element name="endDate" type="xs:NMTOKEN"/>
  <xs:element name="frequency">
    <xs:complexType>
      <xs:sequence>
        <xs:element ref="type"/>
        <xs:element ref="unit"/>
        <xs:element ref="value"/>
      </xs:sequence>
    </xs:complexType>
  </xs:element>
<xs:element name="instructions" type="xs:string"/>
  <xs:element name="quantity">
```

continued on following page

Listing 3. Continued

```
  <xs:complexType>
    <xs:sequence>
      <xs:element ref="type"/>
      <xs:element ref="unit"/>
      <xs:element ref="value"/>
    </xs:sequence>
  </xs:complexType>
</xs:element>
<xs:element name="startDate" type="xs:NMTOKEN"/>
<xs:element name="type" type="xs:NCName"/>
<xs:complexType name="id">
```

(b) Segment of Targeting XACML Security Policy

```
<?xml version="1.0" encoding="UTF-8"?>
  <Policy xmlns="urn:oasis:names:tc:xacml:2.0:policy:schema:os"
   xmlns:xsi="http://www.w3.org/2001/XMLSchema-instance"
   xsi:schemaLocation="urn:oasis:names:tc:xacml:2.0:policy:schema:os
   http://docs.oasis-open.org/xacml/access_control-xacml-2.0-policy-schema-os.
xsd"
   xmlns:md="http:www.med.example.com/schemas/record.xsd"
   PolicyId="urn:oasis:names:tc:xacml:2.0:example:policyid:PhysicianAccessCont
rolPolicy"
   RuleCombiningAlgId="urn:oasis:names:tc:xacml:1.0:rule-combining-
algorithm:deny-overrides">
    <Target/>
      <Rule RuleId="urn:oasis:names:tc:xacml:2.0:example:ruleid:PhysicianProdu
ctRule"
                Effect="Permit">
     <Description>Physician Access Control Policy Rule</Description>
     <Target>
       <Subjects>
         <Subject>
         <SubjectMatch MatchId="urn:oasis:names:tc:xacml:1.0:function:stri
ng-equal">
         <AttributeValue DataType="http://www.w3.org/2001/XMLSchema#string">
             Physician
         </AttributeValue>
         <SubjectAttributeDesignator
             AttributeId="urn:oasis:names:tc:xacml:2.0:example:attribute:ro
le"
           DataType="http://www.w3.org/2001/XMLSchema#string"/>
         </SubjectMatch>
         </Subject>
```

continued on following page

Listing 3. Continued

```
        </Subjects>
        <Resources>
          <Resource>
          <ResourceMatch MatchId="urn:oasis:names:tc:xacml:1.0:function:stri
ng-equal">
              <AttributeValue DataType="http://www.w3.org/2001/
XMLSchema#string">
                    generated:schema:graph:type
              </AttributeValue>
              <ResourceAttributeDesignator
                AttributeId="urn:oasis:names:tc:xacml:1.0:resource:target-
namespace"
                DataType="http://www.w3.org/2001/XMLSchema#string"/>
              </ResourceMatch>
          </Resource>
          <Resource>
          <ResourceMatch MatchId="urn:oasis:names:tc:xacml:1.0:function:str
ing-equal">
              <AttributeValue DataType="http://www.w3.org/2001/
XMLSchema#string">
                    generated:schema:graph:belongsTo
              </AttributeValue>
              <ResourceAttributeDesignator
                AttributeId="urn:oasis:names:tc:xacml:1.0:resource:target-
namespace"
                DataType="http://www.w3.org/2001/XMLSchema#string"/>
              </ResourceMatch>
          </Resource>
          <Resource>
          <ResourceMatch MatchId="urn:oasis:names:tc:xacml:1.0:function:s
tring-equal">
              <AttributeValue DataType="http://www.w3.org/2001/
XMLSchema#string">
                    generated:schema:graph:drugName
              </AttributeValue>
              <ResourceAttributeDesignator
```

and relevant standards that are utilized in the care and treatment of patients, with an emphasis on the interplay of health information exchange among various health information technology systems with security at global and local levels across such a complex architecture. Content wise, the lower left of Figure 5 contains open electronic health record systems (openEHR[26], PatientOS[27], VistA[28]) that all share an ability to export patient data in XML formats (XML, continuity of care record, and clinical document architecture); this is in contrast to commercial electronic health records (GE Centricity) which often have proprietary formats that hinder health information exchange. The upper left of Figure 5 contains various emerging platforms: Open *m*Health to promote mobile health via an open architecture, the Harvard SMART platform for substitutable medical applications that promote reuse), and Microsoft HealthVault, a personal health record. Open *m*Health and SMART have JSON and JSON-LD, respectively, to model patient data, which must be converted (XML-C diamond) before it can be secured. HealthVault has .NET classes that can export to XML instances. The bottom right contains the medical applications that must be securely managed, Personal Health Assistant and SMARTSync, as reviewed in Section 4. The upper right contains the various standards and services involving medications (RxTerms[29] and RxNorm[30]), medical codes (SNOMED[31]), medical nomenclature (UMLS[32] and MeSH[33]), and laboratory codes (LOINC[34]) that are used by all of the systems and applications. Again, we note that the architecture shown in Figure 5 has many servers (left side), access to standards (upper right), and end user applications (lower right); this can logically be mapped to another domain that has a similar architecture.

The two complementary aspects to allow all of the interactions to occur across the diagram is overlaid in Figure 5 via: health information exchange (pentagon) that uses dotted lines to indicate the need to share information among health information technology systems and applications;

and, the Global Security Policy and Control (octagon) that provides a centralized location from which secure interactions can locally occur within the framework. The end result and major challenge, represented in Figure 5 for the health care domain, is the recognition of a greater need for a comprehensive approach to security at global and local levels operating within an environment that is driven to share data through health information exchange. This need for a global approach towards security, addressed at the document-level, is not unique to healthcare, as other domains (such as e-commerce, etc.) also make use of data found in distributed repositories, each with their own local and global security policies to enforce. Note that Figure 5 does not contain all of the possible scenarios and possibilities that can arise from the interplay of information exchange in healthcare or another domain with a similar architecture. First, other security threats (intrusion detection, name server attacks, etc.) can take place. These vulnerabilities and the effects they have in the information exchange process must be protected proactively. We have realized that, in current security approaches, these types of attacks are found retroactively (e.g., when audits of systems are performed). The impact of these attacks can create a disparity between system trust and sharing policies (local and global security). For example, as shown in the lower left of Figure 5, electronic health record systems that share information typically do so via the use of a Health Information Exchange (HIE) server that contains data from the production counterpart offloaded at regular intervals. In the event of a security compromise, only the information deemed sharable would be breached. This layer of defense allows the systems to only share the data they seem comfortable with in case of a security threat such as intrusion or server attacks.

Second, another major component in health information exchange is the data analytics and mining across the entire interoperating systems to allow clinicians and clinical researchers to query

Figure 5. The interplay of health information exchange and security

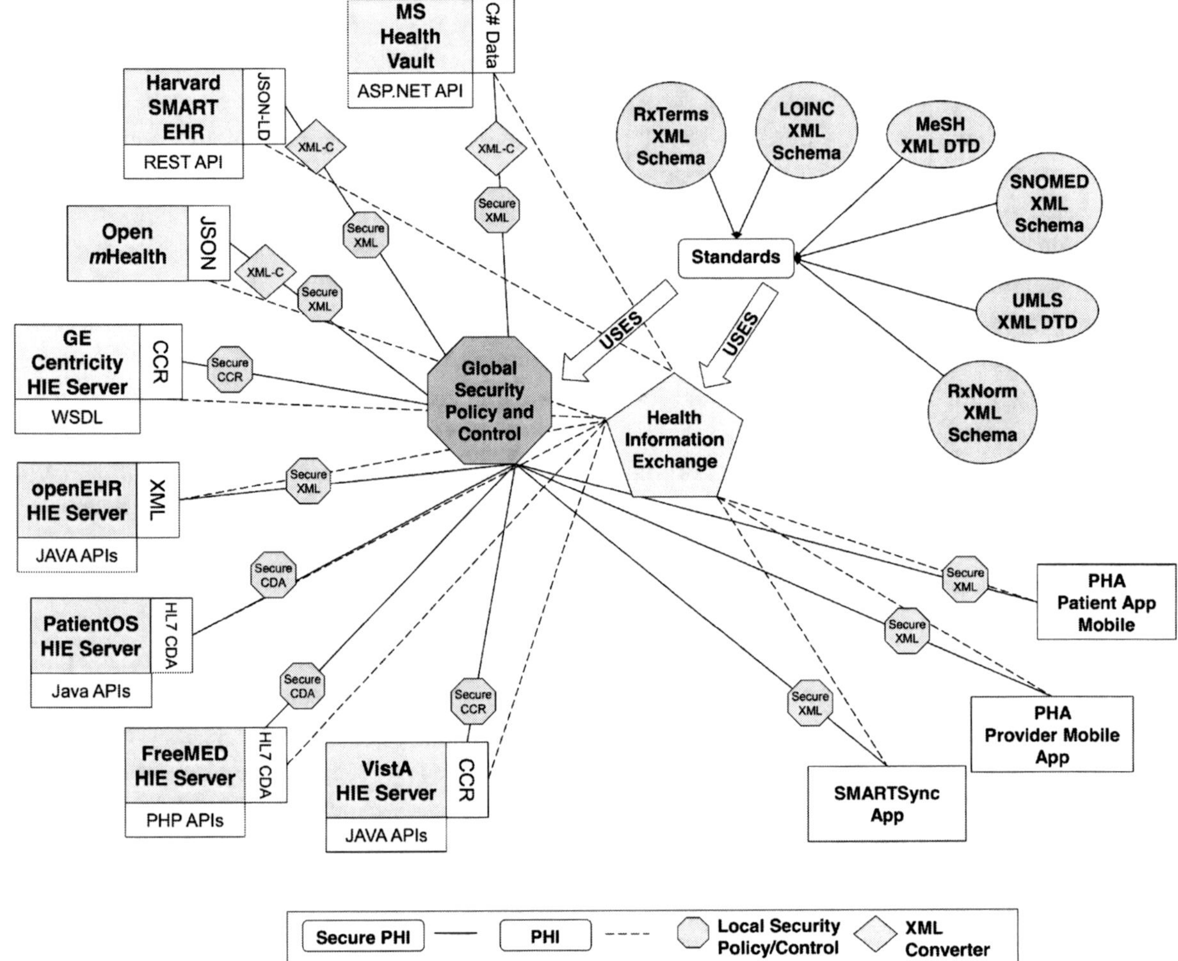

the data in support of analyzing health data towards improving medical care. Institutions and individuals who are placed under this component typically use data dispersed throughout repositories under a set of terms of conditions and agreement of fair usage. The case of such data analytics and mining presents a challenge in terms of security since the users of the data are not usually the owners, and therefore must abide by the security policies set in each individual system. In the case of health care, privacy of protected health information and personal identifiable information is controlled by an array of policy enforcement or computational methods, some which prove sufficient for a set of cases, but not all. For example, there exist generic data publishing methods (e.g., k-anonymity and (α, k)-anonymity) that are not useful for cases with demographic data and the specific needs of electronic health records. An example of this is that, if age is not to be disclosed, removing the age from the shared dataset might not be enough since health codes (e.g., International Classification of Diseases – 9[35] codes) can reveal a person's age. Towards the goal of providing proper security while maintaining data usefulness, several machine learning techniques have been developed not only as mechanisms of verification for privacy enforcement, but also as mechanisms for feedback on the quality and completeness of the desired security policies.

Third, a scenario, which is not typically discussed, is what happens in the event where information providers decide to enter and/or leave the information exchange architecture. In these situations, global and local security is impacted in not only the constituent systems of the information exchange process, but also in those meta-systems already deployed that make use of resources found on information providers that left; in this case, both outdated resources and information from new systems can skew data analysis. Such events require the constant need of updating the security policies on those systems that share and utilize share data. Currently, when such an event happens, each information provider still part of the architecture must scramble to update their sharing and security policies to the new architecture's components.

In Section 4, we reviewed security for XML as attained with Personal Health Assistant and SMARTSync. Our intent in this section is to provide a look at future trends in regards to the attainment of security for XML data exchange in health care from two perspectives. First, in Section 5.1, we explore the accessible technology platforms in the health care domain, more specifically we focus on Open *m*Health, Harvard SMART, and Microsoft HealthVault, that are all intended for widespread use by different users and in different contexts, to provide a means for various stakeholders (patients, clinicians, medical researchers, medical vendors, health information technology companies, etc.) to more easily interact with one another in different ways. These are concrete examples of the variety of platforms that can be found in an information exchange process, and while we focus on the healthcare counterpart as part of our case study, the content can be generalized to other domains with respect to the different platforms available to them. Next, in Section 5.2, we examine the open and free data repositories in the form of open electronic

health records, namely, openEHR, PatientOS, and VistA. These repositories are intended to promote an environment of open access and sharing via a community approach, as viable alternatives to commercial products that are difficult to install and maintain, particularly for medical providers that lack information technology staff. In the same manner as Section 5.1, these electronic health records serve as concrete examples of the diversity and distributed nature of repositories in the information exchange process found across domains. Collectively, both perspectives demonstrate the significant level of complexity needed in regards to information exchange, and the diverse scenarios under which a security policy and control approach with both global and local components must effectively operate. Finally, Section 5.3 takes a concerted look at the information exchange and security issues from the health care perspective, their underlying computational issues, and makes recommendations that stakeholders in any domain would need to pursue in order to utilize information exchange process to insure that information can be successfully shared, exchanged, and secured. Again, many applications will have accessible platforms (open), proprietary systems (commercial), require the use of standards (in XML, RDF, OWL), and interact with Web-based and mobile apps via different protocols (JSON, SOAP, Web services, etc.); our work is generalizable.

5.1. Accessible Technology Platforms

In terms of accessible health information technology platforms, we focus on Microsoft HealthVault, Open *m*Health, and Havard SMART, all of which offer different capabilities to specific stakeholders for particular purposes. HealthVault, launched in 2007, is a personal health record intended to allow patients to manage their own medical information including demographic data, personal data (height, weight), medications, allergies, etc. The larger scale intent is to provide a means for this to be stored securely (protected health information and HIPAA compliant) while simultaneously facilitating interactions with health care providers, medical device companies, health information technology applications, etc. For example, there are a wide range of applications and devices[36] for managing medical conditions such as diabetes meters, blood pressure monitors, etc. that can connect to HealthVault. Also, major pharmacies (CVS and Walgreens) allow patients to be able to link their prescription records into HealthVault. Such a capability would greatly improve our Personal Health Assistant Patient and Provider applications, and the accuracy of medication reconciliation in SMARTSync. Other HealthVault partners include the American Cancer Society, American Diabetes Association, and the American Heart Association. The reach of HealthVault from a patient centered personal health record to one that can reach out into application, devices, and the medical provider community at large is an important future trend.

Harvard University's SMART (Sustainable Medical Applications, Reusable Technologies) is one of the projects funded by The Office of the National Coordinator for Health Information Technology through the Strategic Health IT Advanced Research Projects[37] (SHARP) program. The goal of the SMART project is to provide a uniform, well-defined, reusable infrastructure for applications to interact with medical-record data. The creators of SMART motivate their work with the argument that environments which are constantly changing and evolving such as the health care system have the inherit need for information technology infrastructures that are of general purpose nature rather than monolithic and pre-designed (Mandl, 2009). SMART has a diverse range of partners, including Microsoft, CVS/Caremark, Athena Health, the Massachusetts Department of Public Health, etc.; all share the objective of improving the delivery of health care to patients via technology. However, SMART's focus differs from HealthVault since it is emphasizing the promotion of the platform for research endeavors with the recent launch of

a SMART app at Boston Children's hospital. The future trend to promote the exchange and sharing of information to positively impact patient care is a laudable objective.

Lastly, the Open *m*Health organization has defined an open source architecture with mix and match components for mobile health applications to be constructed from reusable units; the intent is to use the architecture to make data an information more meaningful to patients and clinicians via personal evidence that is provided by patients and analyzing by clinicians. To support this, Open *m*Health provides *Data Processing Units (DPU)* and *Data Visualization Units (DVU)* (Estrin, 2012). A data processing unit is a Web service that defines a set of data inputs and outputs (via an application programming interface) and provides an underlying algorithmic capability to extract, infer, and analyze a data set from one or more sources. For example, a data processing unit may take as input a set of glucose readings and insulin dosages with date time stamps, along with patient time (weight, age, etc.) and be able to output an analysis to determine the trends in terms of diabetes care (e.g., low glucose levels too often, etc.). A data visualization unit provides the means via a returned browser component to display information from a data processing unit in a form that is conducive to the recipient (patient, provider, researcher, etc.). Open *m*Health, via its data processing and visualization units, will provide access to a myriad of information including sensors from mobile devices, sensor data collected from the cloud (via glucose meters that update values to cloud repository), data from public sources (Food and Drug Administration DailyMed[38], nutrition), data from electronic health records, etc. One of their major initiatives is the Post Traumatic Stress Disorder collaboration with the Department of Veteran Affairs, having a mobile post-traumatic stress disorder Coach to help veterans cope with post-traumatic stress disorder. This future trend has the features of HealthVault (putting care under a patient's control) with a simultaneous eye to providers and researchers interested in treating patients or analyzing data sets.

These three platforms present the diversity of purpose and orientation (user-oriented for HealthVault, developer oriented for Open *m*Health, developer and user-oriented for SMART) in platforms that are constituents of the information exchange process, yet must act in harmony in order to provide the best and/or intended functionality and results for their end users. They also demonstrate the differences in the use of technologies and standards that can be found across platforms, from completely proprietary products (HealthVault) to community driven efforts (SMART) to semi-private/collaborative approaches (Open *m*Health). These differences result in different policies for usage and data sharing, and in turn result in conflicts of which policy should be enforced completely, partially, or not at all.

5.2. Open and Free Data Repositories

The adoption of electronic health records has increased in the previous years because of the benefits they provide and enacted laws, such as the Affordable Care Act of 2010[39]. The shift from paperwork to electronic data has pushed vendors to seize the opportunity and create their own respective versions of electronic health records for consumer adoption. We focus on those alternatives that are open source and free to implement: openEHR, PatientOS and VistA. openEHR[40] serves as a framework and standard to describe the administration and storage of patient data for electronic clinic history. This electronic clinic history acts as the repository of patient information, and is independent of the technology utilized for its access. The openEHR specifications are maintained by the openEHR foundation. These specifications, which arise from research done throughout a decade, include information and data models for the electronic clinic history, demographic information, clinical procedures, etc., and are implemented to provide a base for

health information exchange. With the ongoing binding of Systematized Nomenclature of Medicine – Clinical Terms to openEHR, as well as the addition of a virtual electronic health record for the user interface, openEHR serves as an open source, complete solution framework for users and institutions to implement their own EHRs capable of complying with information exchange standards and data storage. This important future trend sets the standard for all electronic health records to target.

The objective of PatientOS[41] is to make the user's (medical provider) workflow a rapid one. To achieve this, PatientOS provides detailed observations on which values should be default in which forms, an almost never-changing user interface (as the tool is updated), automated functions and using the least amounts of clicks necessary to complete a task. PatientOS permits the user workflow to be customized based on the user, his/her role, and the institution in which the user works. While other software solutions are plagued by a scarce maintenance and update schedule, PatientOS has been designed to be scalable and easily maintained. These two factors reduce the bar on updating the electronic health record to a newer version by assuring users that the backend does not change. For developers, PatientOS offers a Java application programming interface that permits the development of plugins, customized forms, and user interface themes. By partnering with businesses such as MResult Healthcare, new alternatives to reducing the cost of implementation of electronic health records are possible. As a future trend, PatientOS targets the ease of both deploying and integrating health information technology into medical practices for usage by providers, a vital problem that hinders adoption of electronic health records.

Lastly, VistA[42] (Veterans Health Information Systems and Technology Architecture) is an open source information system built around an electronic health record. Developed by the United States Department of Veterans Affairs (VA), VistA consists of hundreds of clinical, financial, infrastructure and patient-Web functions. Clinical functions range from Admission Discharge Transfer, clinical procedures, pharmaceutical, laboratories, and mental health. Financial and administrative functions include an automated information collection system, incident reporting, fugitive felon program, and others. The infrastructure functions cover the maintenance of the backend, as well as communication standards, e.g., capacity management tools, Health Level 7 (messaging), broker, an SQL interface, and a network health exchange. The last sets of functions, the patient-Web functions, provide clinical information decision support, health record keeping, and a personal finance system. With the Veterans Health Administration utilizing VistA, the electronic health record is considered the largest medical system in the United States, spanning the largest health information exchange system and covering over 8 million patients. This widespread use also translates to physician usage: 60% of United States trained physicians rotate through the Veterans Health Administration, making VistA the most familiar and widely used electronic health record in the country. The widespread use of VistA has spanned different iterations, including Austronaut VistA[43], WorldVistA[44], OpenVistA[45], and vxVistA[46]. As a future trend, VistA is often cited as the "trend setting" and model for electronic health records and their adoption across the world.

VistA, openEHR and PatientOS demonstrate the way that data formats utilized for export and import functionalities, as well as internal operations, can differ between solutions intended for the same domain. These differences in data structures and formats utilized by repositories is not unique to the health care domain, and demonstrate a need to present an encompassing approach that handles all of the possibilities in term of document standards and secure information exchange. Added to this are the proprietary solutions that are widespread (for example, in the health care domain

GE Centricity[47]) that could only support one of the many available standards due to development and economic reasons.

5.3. Recommendations for Success

The computing profession operates in the world where standards are the norm rather than the exception. After a tumultuous period in the late 1980s/early 1990s, where there were many different incompatible versions of C++, the profession has striven to an emphasis and strong reliance on the standards definition and approval process. In the early years of UML, every vendor's tool was incompatible; today, the UML via OMG has a standard of not just the language but the structure of the diagrams, allowing XMI to be exported for importing into any other UML tool. The same is true for database systems, which easily allow the porting of relational schemas and databases of all sizes via XML and XMI, allowing data to easily move from MySQL to Oracle or to SQL Server. In the process, the standards community in computing has provided the tools, and all of the vendors have accepted the responsibility to allow for designs, information, and data of all formats to be easily and effectively exchanged.

One troubling trend in widespread information exchange, especially in health care, is the lack of such a commitment by vendors and a promotion of data exchange. Clearly, as shown in Figure 5 for health care, there are many standards that have been adopted and are in use, ranging from JSON to RDF to XML to the continuity of care record and clinical document architecture standards; but those standards and the modeling of data have not been unified. Further, when one attempts to share information across commercial vendors (for example, between the electronic health records such as GE Centricity, AllScripts[48], etc.), it ends up requiring n^2 custom mappings of data between n different systems, as vendors are more concerned with proprietary protection of information as opposed to facilitating sharing; one major issue is competition as hospitals in a region see sharing information leading to the potential of losing patients. In health care this is clearly evident, as vendors do not want to provide the ability to export to a common XML format for medical data, since then it would allow the medical provider to potentially change vendors (akin to changing from Oracle to SQL Server in order to save licensing costs).

Another troubling trend is the inability to access information in repositories (for example, electronic health records) in a manner that would be able to present information that cuts across multiple instances of common information (patient's record); patient's visit multiple providers, labs, health facilities, etc., and if each has their own repository, the ability to get a complete collection of all of the information has not been achievable to date. Following the theme of health care, consider than an electronic health record is set up to manage individual patients and their medical records electronically including medications, allergies, immunizations, etc. However, suppose a medication is recalled, as Vioxx[49] was back in 2004, then every medical provider would need to contact his/her patients to switch their medication. But, electronic health records don't provide the ability to easily do this. In fact, for it to occur, one would need to have enough technical expertise to understand and access the underlying relational schema and database to write an ad-hoc query. There is a further hindrance in regards to supporting analysis of a medical provider's practice from a data and treatment perspective. For example, if you are a medical provider who wants to check on all of the diabetes patients in your practice taking a specific medication and determine commonalities related to other diseases (say congestive heart failure) or conditions (obesity), there is no way for you to make such an investigation without sophisticated ad-hoc queries.

Another issue to consider is the legal implications involved in data sharing and exchange, especially data that is confidential or otherwise protected by legal statues. For example, the Ethical, legal and social implications (ELSI) of human genomics are tied to the Genetic Information Nondiscrimination Act (GINA) of 2008[50] and the Health Insurance Portability and Accountability Act of 1996 (HIPAA). GINA protects a patient's genetic information against discrimination in health insurance and employment; this includes: genetic test of patient, his/her family members, fetus of individual or family member, family medical history, and request/receipt of genetic services that may including clinical research trials. HIPAA's Privacy Rule insures that protected health information is securely maintained by entries with patients retaining rights to access that information while still allowing entities to disclose the information under certain situations. HIPAA's Security Rule defines the "series of administrative, physical, and technical safeguards for covered entities to use to assure the confidentiality, integrity, and availability of electronic protected health information". For ELSI, protection of information must be reconciled across HIPAA and GINA to securely deliver the appropriate combination of clinical, genomic, and phenotypic information to all of the involved stakeholders (medical, researchers, clinical providers, support personnel, insurers, and patients).

Based on these issues and their underlying computational, political and acceptance limitations, we propose three major recommendations to facilitate information exchange in domains clouded by different standards, platforms, purposes and orientations. *First*, we note that there is a need for a *formal and unifying standards process* for data to allow the easy exporting and importing of data across information technology systems. This does not only mean to achieve a common format, but also one that uses the most up-to-date technologies. For example, in the health care scenario (see Figure 5), there are not just XML schemas used in current standards, but outdated and outmoded standards such as the document type definitions

(XML DTD). One unifying standard or a set of standards with the most up-to-date features is a must to successfully achieve information exchange. We know this works well, since the UML community with its standard allows the easy exchange of UML designs between different tools and the database community provides export in XML to allow ease of porting a database across vendor products.

Second, open source and commercial data repositories need to be more conducive towards *cross platform access*, providing the potential for more effective tools and applications that improve the functionality, analysis or usage of information to improve end-user experience. In the case of health care, this involves open and commercial electronic health record vendors to provide *cross patient access* in order to provide better tools for medical providers so patient care and treatment improves. The computing community has been a leader in this regard, and these successful approaches need to be applied.

Third, involving the combination of legal statutes on domains that utilize and exchange data that is protected (for example, in health care with GINA and HIPAA for ELSI), will require careful consideration of the *policy, cost, usage, and exchange of information in a secure manner* across a wider range of data (for example, clinical, genomic, and phenotypic) than has normally been required. HIPAA gets involved in many non-medical settings, as does the need to manage personal identifiable information for many domains.

6. CONCLUSION

This chapter has presented a security framework for XML (see Section 1 and Figure 1) that is intended to allow security to be defined at the XML schema level to be enforced on XML instances using NIST Role-Based Access Control (RBAC) in Section 2. In the process, the XML instances delivered to users (by role) are customized to insure

that a user is only able to see and/or modify what has been authorized, effectively yielding role restricted XML instances. To achieve the security, we leverage XACML to define policies against XML schemas that can then be enforced on all XML instances; our approach separates the security privileges from both the XML schema and their instances, allowing changes as security policies evolve to have no impact on schemas and existing instances. Our approach has been demonstrated on a healthcare domain case study with an emphasis on medical or clinical patient data as represented by the continuity of care record standard (see Section 2 and Figure 2), and we have briefly reviewed our earlier work (De la Rosa Algarín, 2012) that has created UML diagrams: an XML Schema Class Diagram (XSCD) to graphically represent an XML schema, and XML role slice diagram (XRSD) to define roles and their privileges (read, write, etc.) against XML schema elements (see Section 3.1). Using this as a basis, we described the generation of an XACML security policy for enforcement purposes, as detailed in Section 3.2, and illustrated in Listing 2. Collectively, the work in Section 3 was applied to in Section 4 to two applications: the Personal Health Assistant (PHA) in Section 4.2 hooked to Microsoft HealthVault for a patient to track of medications, nutritional supplements, allergies, etc., and also authorize that protected health information to his/her specific medical providers who can use their own app to select and view the authorized protected health information on a patient-by-patient basis as determined by his/he assigned role; and SMARTSync, an application for medication reconciliation in Section 4.3 hooked to Microsoft HealthVault and Harvard SMART's Reference Electronic Health Record to gather information from multiple sources. For each application, we demonstrated the generation of XACML policies in different ways from an eventual XML representation (Section 4.4). While we demonstrated the work in a health care domain, our architecture is simply servers, mobile, and Web apps, interacting with one another using many different mans (XML, JSON, SOAP, Web services, etc.). The XML security approach that we have presented is intended to target the wide array of apps on the World Wide Web.

Our future trends in Section 5 has taken a larger scale view of the security process for XML in regards to secure data sharing and exchange; while the work in this chapter (Section 3) is applicable to any domain, Section 5 focuses on the health care domain and the unique challenges of security at global and local levels that must interact with health information exchange across a myriad of health information technology systems and applications that have differing data formats that must be reconciled. The emerging trends in Sections 5.1 and 5.2 include accessible information technology platforms: the HealthVault system that allow patients to manage their health information with increasing linkages to applications, medical devices, pharmaceutical records, etc.; the Harvard SMART platform promoting a reusable infrastructure for health care data sharing and exchange, with diverse partners and roll out of research tools at a major medical center; the Open *m*Health platform trending to both satisfy patient, provider, and research requirements through an innovative and open means to collect and visualize information; and, a set of open and free data repositories, more specifically the electronic health records openEHR, PatientOS, and VistA, all striving to promote open access and sharing via a community approach, as viable alternatives to commercial products that are difficult to install and maintain. These platforms and systems served as concrete examples to pinpoint the major issues currently present to attain information exchange, and in Section 5.3 we presented a number of recommendations, some controversial, chastising the adoption of standards and free exchange of information by commercial information technology vendors, and hindering the attempt to utilize and exchange information in information technology systems for more effective usability, such as patient care in health care. Many of these recommendations are

accepted practice in computing and information technology, and there needs to be a migration of these successes by applying those approaches to health care and other domains.

REFERENCES

Ammari, F., & Lu, J. (2010). Advanced XML security: Framework for building secure XML management system (SXMS). In *Proceedings of the 2010 Seventh International Conference on Information Technology: New Generations (ITNG)* (pp. 120-125). ITNG.

Ardagna, C., Damiani, E., Capitani di Vimercati, S., & Samarati, P. (2007). XML security. In *Proceedings of Security, Privacy, and Trust in Modern Data Management* (pp. 71-86). Springer. doi:10.1007/978-3-540-69861-6_6

Barnsteiner, J. (2005). Medication reconciliation: Transfer of medication information across settings-keeping it free from error. *The American Journal of Nursing*, *105*(3), 31. doi:10.1097/00000446-200503001-00007 PMID:15802996

Bertino, E., Carminati, B., & Ferrari, E. (2004). Access control for XML documents and data. *Information Security Technical Report*, (9): 19–34. doi:10.1016/S1363-4127(04)00029-9

Bertino, E., Castano, S., Ferrari, E., & Mesiti, M. (2002). Protection and administration of XML data sources. *Data & Knowledge Engineering*, (43): 237–260. doi:10.1016/S0169-023X(02)00127-1

Bertino, F., & Ferrari, E. (2002). Secure and selective dissemination of XML documents. *ACM Transactions on Information and System Security*, (5): 290–331. doi:10.1145/545186.545190

Chandrakumar, T., & Parthasarathy, S. (2012). Enhancing data security in ERP projects using XML. *International Journal of Enterprise Information Systems*, (8): 51–65. doi:10.4018/jeis.2012010104

Damiani, E., De Capitani di Vimercati, S., Paraboschi, S., & Samarati, P. (2000). Design and implementation of an access control processor for XML documents. *Computer Networks, 33*(1), 59–75. doi:10.1016/S1389-1286(00)00053-0

Damiani, E., Fansi, M., Gabillon, A., & Marrara, S. (2008). A general approach to securely querying XML. *Computer Standards & Interfaces, 30*(6), 379–389. doi:10.1016/j.csi.2008.03.006

De la Rosa Algarín, A., Demurjian, S. A., Berhe, S., & Pavlich-Mariscal, J. (2012). A security framework for XML schemas and documents for healthcare. In *Proceedings of 2012 International Workshop on Biomedical and Health Informatics (BHI 2012)*, (pp. 782-789). BHI.

Dolin, R. H., Alschuler, L., Boyer, S., Beebe, C., Behlen, F. M., Biron, P. V., & Shvo, A. S. (2006). HL7 clinical document architecture, release 2. *Journal of the American Medical Informatics Association, 13*(1), 30–39. doi:10.1197/jamia. M1888 PMID:16221939

Estrin, D., & Sim, I. (2010). Open mHealth architecture: An engine for health care innovation. *Science, 330*(6005), 759–760. doi:10.1126/science.1196187 PMID:21051617

Ferraiolo, D., Cugini, J., & Kuhn, D. R. (1995). Role-based access control (RBAC): Features and motivations. In *Proceedings of 11th Annual Computer Security Application Conference* (pp. 241-248). CSAC.

Ferraiolo, D. F., Sandhu, R., Gavrila, S., Kuhn, D. R., & Chandramouli, R. (2001). Proposed NIST standard for role-based access control. *ACM Transactions on Information and System Security, 4*(3), 224–274. doi:10.1145/501978.501980

Huang, S., & Lesko, L. (2004). Drug-drug, drug-dietary supplement, and drug-citrus fruit and other food interactions: What have we learned? *Journal of Clinical Pharmacology, 44*(6), 559. doi:10.1177/0091270004265367 PMID:15145962

Kuper, G., Massacci, F., & Rassadko, N. (2005). Generalized XML security views. In *Proceedings of the 10th ACM Symposium on Access Control Models and Technologies* (pp. 77-84). ACM.

Lanthaler, M., & Gütl, C. (2012). On using JSON-LD to create evolvable RESTful services. In *Proceedings of the 3rd International Workshop on RESTful Design (WS-REST 2012) at WWW2012* (pp. 25-32). Lyon, France: ACM Press.

Leonardi, E., Bhowmick, S., & Iwaihara, M. (2010). Efficient database-driven evaluation of security clearance for federated access control of dynamic XML documents. In *Database Systems for Advanced Applications* (pp. 299–306). Academic Press. doi:10.1007/978-3-642-12026-8_24

Mandl, K., & Kohane, I. (2009). No small change for the health information economy. *The New England Journal of Medicine, 360*(13), 1278–1281. doi:10.1056/NEJMp0900411 PMID:19321867

Müldner, T., Leighton, G., & Miziołek, J. (2009). Parameterized role-based access control policies for XML documents. Information Security Journal: A Global Perspective, Taylor & Francis, (18), 282-296.

Pavlich-Mariscal, J., Demurjian, S., & Michel, L. (2008). A framework of composable access control definition, enforcement and assurance. In *Proceedings of the SCCC'08. International Conference of the IEEE* (pp. 13–22). IEEE.

Poon, E., Blumenfeld, B., & Hamann, C. et al. (2006). Design and implementation of an application and associated services to support interdisciplinary medication reconciliation efforts at an integrated healthcare delivery network. *Journal of the American Medical Informatics Association*, *13*(6), 581–592. doi:10.1197/jamia.M2142 PMID:17114640

Rahaman, M., Roudier, Y., & Schaad, A. (2008). Distributed access control for XML document centric collaborations. In *Proceedings of the EDOC'08. 12th International IEEE* (pp. 267-276). IEEE.

Ziminski, T. B., De la Rosa Algarín, A., Saripalle, R., Demurjian, S. A., & Jackson, E. (2012). SMARTSync: Towards patient-driven medication reconciliation using the SMART framework. In *Proceedings of 2012 International Workshop on Biomedical and Health Informatics (BHI 2012)*, (pp. 806-813). BHI.

ADDITIONAL READING

Baumer, D., Earp, J., & Payton, F. (2000). Privacy of medical records: IT implications of HIPAA. *ACM SIGCAS Computers and Society*, *30*(4), 40–47. doi:10.1145/572260.572261

Berhe, S., Demurjian, S., & Agresta, T. (2009). Emerging trends in health care delivery: Towards collaborative security for NIST RBAC. In *Proceedings of Research Directions in Data and Applications Security LNCS* (Vol. 5645, pp. 283–290). Berlin: Springer. doi:10.1007/978-3-642-03007-9_19

Berhe, S., Demurjian, S., Gokhale, S., Pavlich-Mariscal, J., & Saripalle, R. (2011). Leveraging UML for security engineering and enforcement in a collaboration on duty and adaptive workflow model that extends NIST RBAC. [LNCS]. *Proceedings of Research Directions in Data and Applications Security*, *6818*, 293–300.

Berhe, S., Demurjian, S., Saripalle, R., Agresta, T., Liu, J., & Cusano, A. … Gedarovich, J. (2010). Secure, obligated and coordinated collaboration in health care for the patient-centered medical home. In *Proceedings of the AMIA Annual Symposium* (p. 36). AMIA.

Bernauer, M., Kappel, G., & Kramler, G. (2003). *Representing XML schema in UML - An UML profile for XML schema (Tech. Rep.)*. Citeseer.

Bernauer, M., Kappel, G., & Kramler, G. (2004). Representing XML schema in UML – A comparison of approaches. In *Proceedings of Web Engineering* (pp. 767–769). Web Engineering. doi:10.1007/978-3-540-27834-4_54

Blechner, M., Sariapalle, R., & Demurjian, S. (2012). A proposed star schema and extraction process to enhance the collection of contextual and semantic information for clinical research data warehouses. In *Proceedings of 2012 International Workshop on Biomedical and Health Informatics (BHI 2012)*. BHI.

Demurjian, S., Ren, H., Berhe, S., Devineni, M., Vegad, S., & Polineni, K. (2010). Improving the information security of collaborative web portals via fine-grained role-based access control. In S. Murugesan (Ed.), *Handbook of Research on Web 2.0, 3.0 and X.0: Technologies, Business and Social Applications* (pp. 430–448). Hershey, PA: IGI Global.

Demurjian, S., Saripalle, R., & Berhe, S. (2009). An integrated ontology framework for health information exchange. In *Proceedings of 21st International Conference on Software Engineering and Knowledge Engineering (SEKE09)* (pp. 575–580). SEKE.

Doan, T., Demurjian, S., Ting, T. C., & Phillips, C. (2004). RBAC/MAC security for UML. *Research Directions in Data and Applications Security*, *144*, 189–204. doi:10.1007/1-4020-8128-6_13

Klyne, G., Carroll, J. J., & McBride, B. (2004). *Resource description framework (RDF), concepts and abstract syntax*. W3C Recommendation, 10.

Mandl, K., Mandel, J., & Murphy, S. et al. (2012). The SMART platform: Early experience enabling substitutable applications for electronic health records. *Journal of the American Medical Informatics Association*, 19(4), 597. doi:10.1136/amiajnl-2011-000622 PMID:22427539

Montelius, E., Astrand, B., Hovstadius, B., & Petersson, G. (2008). Individuals appreciate having their medication record on the web: A survey of attitudes to a national pharmacy register. *Journal of Medical Internet Research*, 10(4). doi:10.2196/jmir.1022 PMID:19000978

Pavlich-Mariscal, J., Demurjian, S., & Michel, L. (2010). A framework for security assurance of access control enforcement code. *Computer & Security Journal*, 29(7), 770–784. doi:10.1016/j.cose.2010.03.004

Pavlich-Mariscal, J., Demurjian, S., & Michel, L. (n.d.). A framework of composable security features: Preserving separation of security concerns from models to code. *Computer & Security Journal*, 29(3), 350-379.

Pavlich-Mariscal, J., Doan, T., Michel, L., Demurjian, S., & Ting, T. C. (2005). *Role slices: A notation for RBAC permission assignment and enforcement. Research Directions in Data and Applications Security (LNCS)* (Vol. 3654, pp. 40–53). Berlin: Springer.

Phillips, C., Demurjian, S., & Bessette, K. (2005). A service-based approach for RBAC and MAC security. In Z. Stojanovic & A. Dahanayake (Eds.), *Service-Oriented Software System Engineering: Challenges and Practices* (pp. 317–339). Hershey, PA: IGI Global.

Routledge, N., Bird, L., & Goodchild, A. (2002). UML and XML schema. *Australian Computer Science Communications*, 24(2), 157–166.

Saripalle, R. Knath, Demrjian, S., & Berhe, S. (2011). Towards a software design process for ontologies. In *Proceedings of 2011 International Conference on Software and Intelligent Information (ICSII 2011)*. ICSII.

Skogan, D. (1999). UML as a schema language for XML based data interchange. In *Proceedings of the 2nd International Conference on the Unified Modeling Language (UML'99)*. UML.

KEY TERMS AND DEFINITIONS

Continuity of Care Record (CCR): A document standard for health information typically used for Personal Health Records (PHR) with the intended purpose of information exchange. It provides a universal structure to the patient's information that can be utilized by different personal health records, applications and systems.

Electronic Health Record (EHR): An electronic version of the patient's medical record. An electronic health record contains all related health information, from medications to procedures, and is managed by the institution in which it is stored (e.g. hospital, private practice, clinic, etc).

eXtensible Access Control Markup Language (XACML): A security policy language designed from XML. Its specifications allow for a uniform policy language that can be enforced in heterogeneous systems. XACML policies can be enforced at a systems level, software level, or information level, depending on the policies' targets and rules.

eXtensible Markup Language (XML): A structured language utilized for information exchange, standards and information validation via the use of schemas. Its extensibility allows developers and experts to design and implement common standards for the use across systems and domains.

Health Information Exchange (HIE): The ability to share information among health information technology systems by linking information for the same patient across multiple repositories to provide a complete health care view.

Health Information Technology (HIT): Information technologies (e.g. mobile applications, computer programs, decision support systems, etc.) whose use is intended for the healthcare domain.

Meta-System: A system or platform built from many constituent systems that makes use of functionality or data distributed among its components or external data repositories.

Personal Health Record (PHR): An electronic version of a medical record that is managed by the patient. PHRs typically provide the means to manage medication lists, allergies, procedures, emergency contacts, and other clinical data.

Personal Identifiable Information (PII): Information that contains attributes and values that can help determine a person's identity.

Protected Health Information (PHI): Clinical and other health related information regarding a patient that is protected under laws, or must be protected as dictated by laws.

Role-Based Access Control (RBAC): An access control model where permissions are assigned directly to roles, which are assigned to users.

Role-Restricted (RR): A filtered version of a document. Its filtering depends on the role of the user requesting the information, and the security policies in place.

Substitutable Medical Apps, Reusable Technologies (SMART): A platform that permits the development and reusability of applications by targeting a common abstraction layer, removing the need to target specific data repositories.

XML Role-Slice Diagram (XRSD): The XRSD is a diagram containing the role's credentials and the elements of the XML schema on which these credentials act.

XML Schema Class Diagram (XSCD): The XSCD is an UML artifact that serves as an equivalent representation of an XML schema in a UML diagram.

ENDNOTES

[1] eXtensible Markup Language, http://www.w3.org.com/XML/

[2] Continuity of Care Record (CCR), http://www.astm.org/Standards/E2369.htm

[3] Microsoft HealthVault, http://www.microsoft.com/en-us/healthvault/

[4] Health Insurance Portability and Accountability Act of 1996 (HIPAA), http://www.hhs.gov/ocr/privacy/

[5] National Institute of Standards and Technology, http://www.nist.gov/index.html

[6] OASIS XACML, https://www.oasis-open.org/committees/xacml/

[7] Unified Modeling Language, http://www.uml.org/

[8] SMART Platforms, http://www.smartplatforms.org/

[9] Android, http://www.android.com/

[10] JavaScript Object Notation, http://www.json.org/

[11] Open *m*Health, http://openmhealth.org/

[12] XML Security Working Group (SWG), http://www.w3.org/2008/xmlsec/

[13] MySQL, http://www.mysql.com/

[14] SMART RDF/XML Data Model, http://dev.smartplatforms.org/reference/data_model/

[15] NDF-RT, http://www.pbm.va.gov/NationalFormulary.aspx

[16] RDF/XML, http://www.w3.org/TR/REC-rdf-syntax/

[17] N-TRIPLES, http://www.w3.org/2001/sw/RDFCore/ntriples/

[18] Terse RDF Triple Language (TURTLE), http://www.w3.org/TeamSubmission/turtle/

[19] JSON for Linking Data (JSON-LD), http://json-ld.org/

[20] Resource Description Framework (RDF), http://www.w3.org/RDF/

[21] RESTful Services, http://www.ibm.com/developerworks/Webservices/library/ws-restful/

22   MS VisualStudio XML Schema Definition Tool, http://msdn.microsoft.com/en-us/library/x6c1kb0s(v=vs.80).aspx

23   StylusStudio, http://www.stylusstudio.com/

24   Eclipse's Oxygen XML Plugin, http://oxygenxml.com/eclipse_plugin.html

25   Trang, http://www.thaiopensource.com/relaxng/trang.html

26   openEHR, http://www.openehr.org/home.html

27   PatientOS, http://www.patientos.org/

28   VistA, http://worldvista.org/AboutVistA

29   RxTerms, http://wwwcf.nlm.nih.gov/umlslicense/rxtermApp/rxTerm.cfm

30   RxNorm, http://www.nlm.nih.gov/research/umls/rxnorm/

31   SNOMED, http://www.ihtsdo.org/snomed-ct/

32   UMLS, http://www.nlm.nih.gov/research/umls/

33   MeSH, http://www.ncbi.nlm.nih.gov/mesh

34   LOINC, http://loinc.org/

35   ICD-9 codes, http://www.icd9data.com/

36   HealthVault App Directory, https://account.healthvault.com/Directory

37   Strategic Health IT Advanced Research Projects, http://goo.gl/62K5d

38   FDA DailyMed, http://dailymed.nlm.nih.gov/dailymed/about.cfm

39   Affordable Care Act of 2010, http://www.healthcare.gov/law/full/

40   openEHR, http://www.openehr.org/home.html

41   PatientOS, http://www.patientos.org/index.html

42   VistA, http://worldvista.org/AboutVistA

43   Austronaut VistA, http://astronautvista.com/

44   WorldVistA, http://www.worldvista.org/

45   OpenVistA, http://www.medsphere.com/solutions/openvista-for-the-enterprise

46   vxVista, https://www.vxvista.org/display/vx4h/Welcome

47   GE Centricity, http://goo.gl/LCvU7

48   AllScripts, http://www.allscripts.com/

49   Vioxx, http://www.merck.com/newsroom/vioxx/

50   Genetic Information Nondiscrimination Act of 2008, http://www.genome.gov/24519851/

Chapter 26
Design Principles in Health Information Technology:
An Alternative to UML Use Case Methodology

Sabah Al-Fedaghi
Kuwait University, Kuwait

ABSTRACT

Electronic health record (EHR) systems are said to be the cornerstone of a modernized health service. They improve health care, allow for integrated information, and help prevent lost and duplicated records as well as occurrence of administrative errors. Studies have consistently shown, however, that introducing EHR systems is a complex task, with difficulties stemming from technical designs that fit poorly with the details of clinical work practices. Given the evolving role of EHRs and the importance of information design, the need exists for further exploration of EHRs with the purpose of advancing innovations in health IT with the potential for significant positive effects on clinical practice. This paper focuses on a subfield of EHR studies that is working to establish a foundation for applying information design principles to implementation of health information technology in primary care settings. Without loss of generality, the paper examines a specific attempt that includes documenting patterns of clinician information use and developing "use cases" and tools for evaluating EHR implementation. The paper proposes an alternative approach based on a new flow-based specification methodology. It is shown that the method can be applied uniformly at the conceptual requirements level and simultaneously at the user interface level. The new method seems to be a viable technique for expressing situations arising in clinical work practices.

DOI: 10.4018/978-1-4666-8756-1.ch026

CONCEPTUAL FOUNDATION FOR ELECTRONIC HEALTH RECORD SYSTEMS

An electronic health record (EHR) system involves methodological collection and organization of health information in electronic format that is theoretically capable of being shared across different health care settings (Gunter, 2005). EHRs include several types of health information, including medical history, medications and allergies, laboratory test results, radiology images, age and weight, and billing data, generated and maintained within a healthcare institution to give patients, physicians, and care providers access to medical records.

EHRs are said to be the cornerstone of a modernized health service (Greenhalgh et al., 2009). They improve health care, allow for integrated information, and help prevent administrative errors and lost and duplicated records (Department of Health, 2008; Institute of Medicine, 2009). An EHR system can improve efficiency in workflow, effectiveness of healthcare services, and synthesis of patient data with medical evidence to support the decision-making process (Kupersmith et al., 2007; Stead & Lin, 2009).

In such systems, "the key challenge was seen as getting the design right, implementing the technology, and ensuring that clinicians used it" (Greenhalgh et al., 2009). Some researchers have reservations about such a holistic approach to organizing electronic health information (Avison et al., 2007; Kreps & Richardson, 2007), however, and failures in this context have been reported recently (Røed, 2011).

Nevertheless, despite apparently negative conclusions, research in this area is still quite extensive for several reasons, including the fact that

There is considerable scope for more flexible and technologically sophisticated forms ... (e.g., mobile devices) to overcome current limitations. But for this to happen, technology [re]design must occur in intimate proximity to the work process and actively involve users and potential users ... (Greenhalgh et al., 2009, referencing Hartswood et al., 2003; Oudshoorn & Pinch, 2005).

Also, according to Armijo et al. (2009),

Given the evolving role of EHRs in clinical practice and the importance of information design and display to meaningful use, further exploration of EHR usability ... [is] an opportunity for innovation in health IT with the potential for significant impact on clinical practice.

Problem and Proposed Solution

Studies have consistently shown that introducing EHR systems is a complex task in which difficulties arise because "technical designers typically missed these subtleties and produced artefacts that fitted poorly with the situated nature of knowledge and the micro-detail of clinical work practices" (Greenhalgh et al., 2009). Currently, efforts have been insufficient to evaluate EHR systems in terms of identifying best practices in information design. Recognition of usability as a critical issue is inconsistent, and objective evidence is insufficient for design considerations. Hence, the need exists for standards for the design of user interfaces to guarantee efficiency and quality (Armijo et al., 2009a). Greenhalgh et al. (2009) identified a number of "tensions" in relation to users, organizational context, clinical work, the process of change, implementation success, and complexity and scale.

Many approaches and solutions have been proposed related to the establishment and development of EHR systems. An extensive (600-page) review in this area can be found in Car et al. (2008). The present paper focuses on a narrow subfield of EHR systems concerned with establishing a foundation for the application of information design principles to the use of health information technology in primary care settings. Without loss of generality regarding the methodology, the paper examines a specific attempt by Armijo et al. (2009a) to build a framework for "the usability of these systems and their ability to effectively integrate with clinical decision making and workflow." These aspects of EHR systems have "not been adequately explored to date," while financial and technical issues have received much attention (Gans et al., 2005).

Information design, the art and science of preparing information so that it can be used by human beings efficiently and effectively, is central to system usability and implementation success. As such, the further exploration of EHR information design ...[is]... an opportunity for innovation in health IT that will improve the safe, efficient, effective, patient-centered, equitable, and timely delivery of care... Only through a full understanding of workflow, practice patterns, and physician information needs will it be possible to develop technologies that truly integrate with and enhance the practice of medicine. (Armijo et al., 2009b)

Accordingly, Armijo et al. (2009b) recommended documentation of patterns of clinician information use, and development of "use cases" and tools for evaluating usability and best practices in EHR implementations. They utilized representative use cases as initial approaches to information design principles tailored to EHR considerations. "Use cases" implemented by Unified Modeling Language (UML) graphic notation techniques are applied to categorize and describe scenarios and to show how computer interactions are carried out. These use cases and design principles provide a starting point for evaluating EHR adherence to information design principles (Armijo et al., 2009a).

In this context this paper proposes an alternative to the UML methodology of use cases. This methodology is contrasted with Armijo et al.'s (2009a) use case–based approach, but it can serve as a systematic base for a broader philosophy of system design.

Use Case

A use case is a description of a system's behavior as it responds to stimulus and serves both in defining *conceptual requirements* of a system and in evaluating compliance with user requirements (Armijo et al., 2009a). In view of that, Armijo et al. (2009a) develop the following use cases:

- Acute Care Use Case
- Chronic Care Use Case
- Preventative and Health Promotion Use Case
- Undifferentiated Symptoms Use Case

These serve as a common framework for an EHR design incorporating other aspects for the most effective use of information technology in clinical practice (Walsh, 2004).

The present paper claims that

Conceptual requirements of a system can be specified in a new methodology of high-level description, called the Flowthing Model (FM) that presents a viable alternative to methods based on use cases.

To substantiate this claim, the first use case in Armijo et al.'s list, Acute Care, will be recast in FM, with the aim of showing the advantages and disadvantages of each method. To lay the foundation for such a task, the next section reviews FM from previous publications in various application areas (Al-Fedaghi, 2009–2013).

Flowthing Model

The Flowthing Model (FM) was inspired by the many types of flows that exist in diverse fields, such as, for example, supply chain flow, money flow, and data flow in communication models. This model is a diagrammatic schema that uses flowthings to represent a range of items, including data, information, and signals. An FM representation is a depiction of the structure of a scheme resembling a road map of components and conceptual flows. A component comprises *spheres* (e.g., those of a hospital, a laboratory, a physician, a pharmacy) that enclose or intersect with other spheres (e.g., the sphere of a hospital contains departments and wards, which in turn include rooms). A sphere embeds flows (called *flowsystems*). Things that flow in a flowsystem are referred to as *flowthings*. The life cycle of a flowthing is defined in terms of six mutually exclusive *stages*: creation, process (may change the form, but no new flowthing is generated), arrival, acceptance, release, and transfer (See Figure 1).

The six stages in FM can be described as follows:

1. **Arrival:** A flowthing reaches a new flowsystem (e.g., a patient arrives at the reception desk in a hospital, where his/her arrival is registered)
2. **Accepted:** A flowthing is permitted to enter the system (e.g., medical treatment can begin when the patient's insurance is confirmed); if *arriving* flowthings are also always *accepted*, Arrive and Accept can be combined as a *Received* stage.
3. **Processed (Changed):** The flowthing passes through some kind of transformation that changes its form but not its identity (e.g.,

the form of medication in a prescription is changed from pills to liquid).

4. **Released:** A flowthing is marked as ready to be transferred (e.g., an officially discharged patient still waiting in a hospital room for transportation).
5. **Created:** A new flowthing is created in the system (e.g., a baby is born in the hospital, hence the appearance of a new patient record).
6. **Transferred:** The flowthing is transported within or outside the flowsystem (e.g., an outpatient progresses from laboratory services to the radiology department for various tests).

These stages are mutually exclusive, i.e., a flowthing in the *Process* stage cannot be in the *Created* stage or the *Released* stage at the same time. An additional stage of *Storage* can also be added to any FM model to represent the storage of flowthings; however, storage is not a generic stage, because there can be stored processed flowthings, stored created flowthings, etc.

Basic notions of FM can be further explained as follows.

- **Spheres and Subspheres**: These are the environments of the flowthing. A sphere can have multiple flowsystems in its construction if needed, and it can be an entity.

Figure 1. Flowsystem, assuming that no released flowthing is returned. The dark dots denote flowthings at different stages of the flowsystem. The figure may be considered like net marking (instantaneous location of all tokens in the net; Petri net terminology).

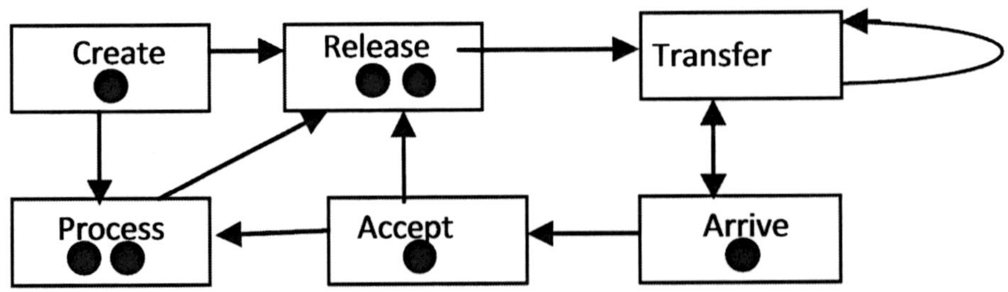

A flowsystem is a subsphere that embodies the flow; it itself has no subsphere. Control of the movement of flowthings is assumed to be embedded in the stages; e.g., in the **Process** stage: *if flowthing (e.g., patient) is finished processing (e.g., being tested) then it flows (moves) to **Release** (is allowed to exit laboratory)*. In principle, no difficulties should exist in conceptualizing such a control on the edges, in the manner of Petri nets (Diaz, 2010).

- **Triggering**: Triggering is an activation (denoted in FM diagrams by a dashed arrow) of one flow by another. It is dependent on flows and parts of flows. A flow is said to be triggered if it is created or activated by another flow, e.g., a flow of electricity triggers a flow of heat (See Figure 2A), or if it is activated when a condition in the flow is satisfied, e.g., *processing* of logical formulas x and y triggers the *creation* of z (x AND y => z) in the flowsystem of true formulas (See Figure 2B).

A flowsystem may not need to include all the stages; for example, an archiving system might use only the stages Arrive, Accept, and Release. Multiple systems captured by FM can interact with each other by triggering events related to one another in their spheres and stages.

In addition to the fundamental characteristics of flow in FM, the following types of possible operations exist in different stages:

1. **Copying:** Copy is an operation such that *flowthing* f => f. That is, it is possible to copy f to produce another flowthing f in a system S. In this case, S is said to be S *with copying* feature, or, for short, *Copy S*. For example, any informational flowsystem can be copy S, while physical flowsystems are non-copying S. Notice that in copy S, stored f may have its copy in a non-stored state. It is possible that copying is allowed in certain stages and not in others.

2. **Erasure:** Erasure is an operation such that *flowthing* f => e, where e denotes the *empty flowthing*. That is, it is possible to erase a flowthing in S. In this case, S is said to be S *with erasure* feature, or, for short, *erasure S*. Erasure can be used for a single instance, all instances in a stage, or all instances in S.

3. **Canceling:** *Anti-flowthing* f^- (f with superscript $-$) is a flowthing such that $(f^- + f)$ => e, where e denotes the empty flowthing, and + denotes the presence of f^- and f.

It is possible that the anti-flowthing f^- is declared in a stage or a flowsystem. If flowthing f triggers the flow of flowthing g, then anti-flowthing f^- triggers anti-flowthing g^-.

An example of the use of these FM features is erasure of a flow, as in the case of a customer who orders a product, then cancels the order, an action that might require cancellation of several flows in different spheres triggered by the original order.

Figure 2. Samples of triggering

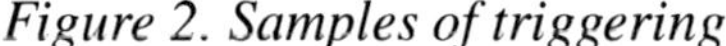

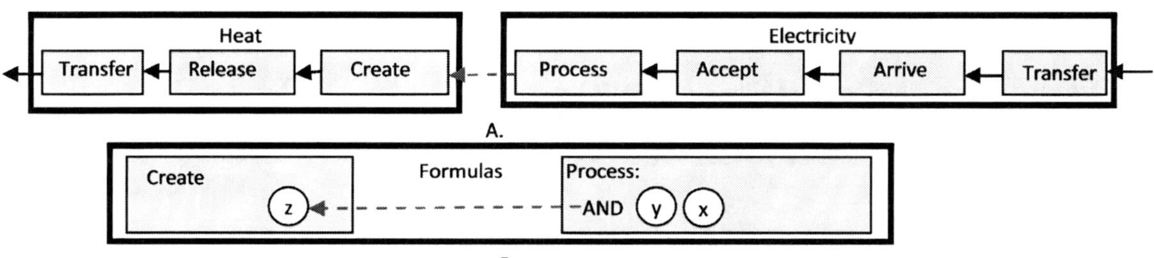

Formally, FM can be specified as FM = $\{S_i$ ($\{F_j\}$, T_i), $\{(F_{ij}, F_{ij})\}$, $1 \leq i \leq n$, $1 \leq j \leq m$, $1 \leq l \leq t\}$

That is, FM is a set of spheres $S_1,...S_n$, each with its own flowsystems $F_{ij}... F_{im}$. T is a type of flowthing $T_1,..., T_t$. Also, F is a graph with vertices V that is a (possibly proper) subset {Arrive*, Accept*, Process*, Create*, Release*, Transfer*}, where the asterisks indicate secondary stages. For example, {Copy, Store, and Destroy} can represent these secondary stages.

Example: In many scenarios that adopt UML diagrams, the requirements specification contains a conceptually fragmented collection of these diagrams. As a sample, consider a model of nursing receptionists registering basic information about patients, given by Juan et al. (2005) and shown in Figure 3. The corresponding FM representation is depicted in Figure 4. It includes two flows: information and repeat/not-repeat messages and three

spheres: Patient (circle 1 in Figure 4), Receptionist (2), and (information) System (3). Starting at circle 4, information (Social Security number) is created by the patient and flows to the receptionist (5), who inputs it into the system (6). The system processes the information (7) by comparing it with its database (8). This processing triggers (9) creation (10) of a message asking whether the data is already in the system. This message flows to the receptionist (11), who processes it (12); if the patient's data is not in the system (13), a request is triggered (14) for additional information from the patient (create; 4).

Use Case: Acute Care

"An acute episode is defined by the period of time when injury or illness is at its worst, usually right after the injury or flare-up has occurred" (Armijo et al., 2009a), and it often requires speed and ac-

Figure 3. Use case diagram for adding visitor (left – partial) and Activity diagram for adding visitor (right)

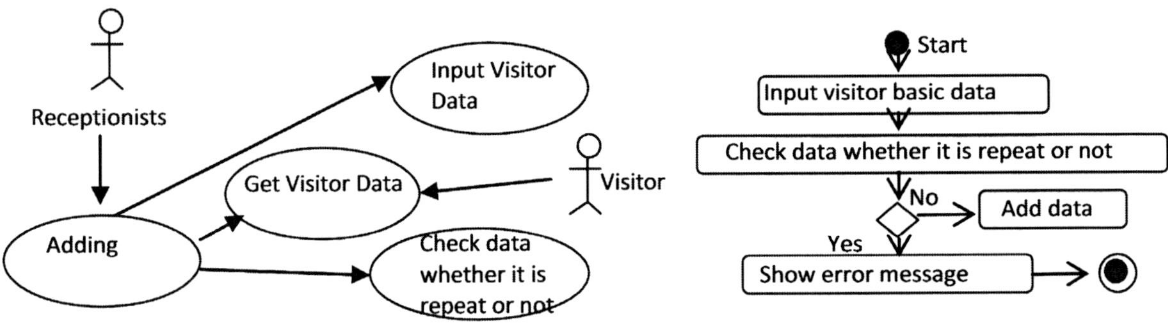

Figure 4. FM representation corresponding to Figure 3

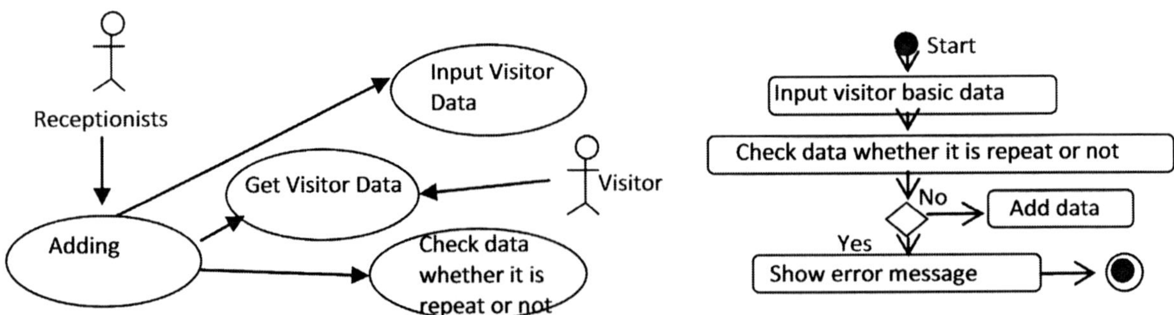

Figure 5. Acute care display use case

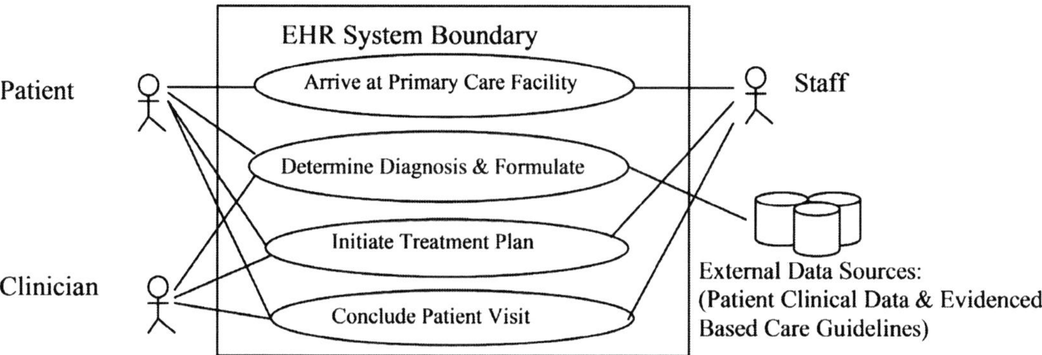

curacy in delivery of care. Its corresponding use case (See Figure 5) highlights design principles relevant to judging patient history while incorporating knowledge necessary to develop diagnoses and treatment plans.

Stakeholder roles include the following (Armijo et al., 2009a):

- **Clinicians**. Enter and review information, conduct a physical examination to determine a diagnosis, formulate a treatment plan, instruct staff, …
- **Staff**. Collect patient data, document results, enter vital signs,...
- **Patients**. Review information for accuracy, describe symptoms…

Once a patient presents, clinicians require the ability to enter current vital information into the EHR and electronically conduct real-time eligibility and prior-authorization activities. Information required to support these capabilities are *Patient and clinician identification* and *Patient administrative data*. Design characteristics that enhance this function include ease of data entry and effective use of default information.

The use case is designed to include all events related to care delivery from the point the patient presents, to the determination of a diagnosis, the formulation of a treatment plan, execution of the treatment plan and the implementation of any follow-up care after the acute episode has ended. Each of these major events has specific requirements for display of data to support care of the whole patient. (Armijo et al., 2009a)

Acute Care FM Specification

Flows in the acute care system involve streams of patients, information, treatments, clinicians and other staff, and instructions, as illustrated in Figure 6 (Armijo et al., 2009a). Some of these elements are represented in Figure 7, showing an FM representation of the acute care use case depicted in Figure 5. The FM description is based on identification of spheres and flows. Four spheres are involved: Patient (circle 1 in Figure 5), Staff (2), Clinician (3), and System (4).

Use of the figure to identify flows is analogous to using a city map to describe traffic flow. It is a conceptual depiction that can be shared by diverse stakeholders. The related scenario depicted in Figure 7 proceeds as follows.

The patient checks in (circle 1 in Figure 5) to be processed (examined). This processing triggers (dashed arrows) the activation of *Patient and clinician identification* (5) and *Patient administrative data* (6) in the context of staff. The staff can create data by examining the patient, or they can download data gathered at previous visits from the system database (7 and 8). The staff's handling of

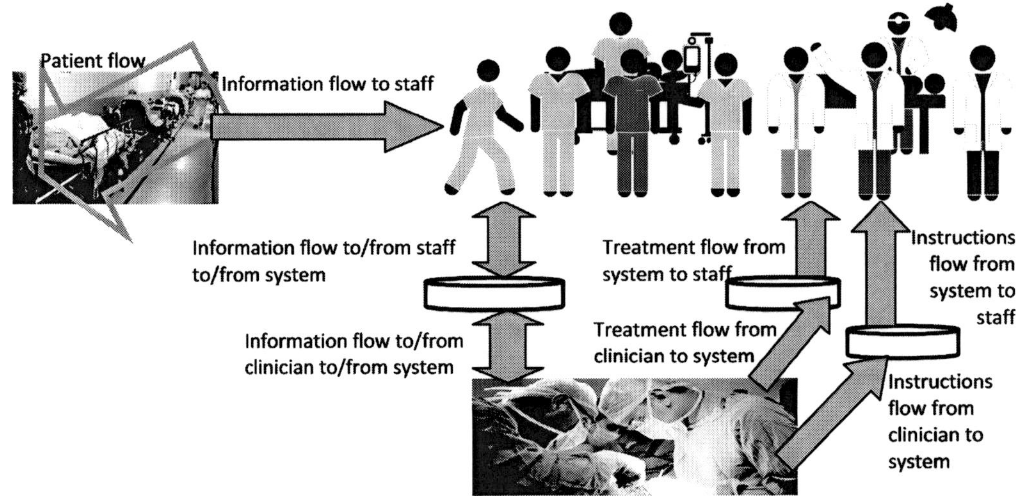

Figure 6. Flows in the acute care situation

Figure 7. FM representation of the acute care situation

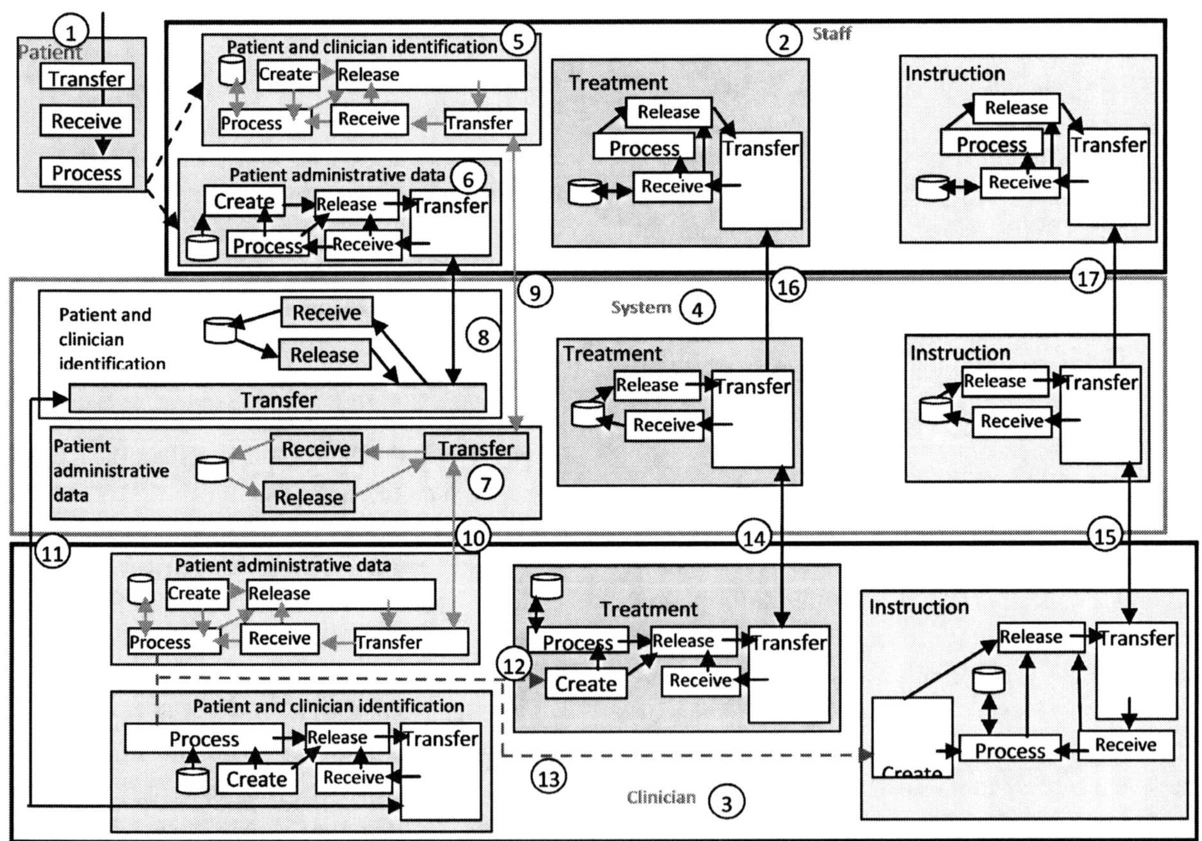

information might also involve processing (e.g., summarizing, diagramming, printing, etc.).

When clinicians take over from staff, they find all related information in the system database (10 and 11). They can create new data about treatments (12) and instructions (13) to be stored by the system (14 and 15). Treatments and instructions can be downloaded by staff (16 and 17) from the database.

Contrasting the FM representation with the use case representation shows that the FM depiction reflects a complete and uniform specification of the event, including the types of operations applied by each stakeholder. It can serve as a foundation for other notions such as constraints, synchronization, logical operations (AND, OR), and rules that can be superimposed over the streams of flows and stages. It is a conceptual description in the sense that it is not oriented toward any specific domain (e.g., computer specialists, physicians, managers, …), thus it can assist in communication and understanding among stakeholders. In comparison, the use case appears sketchy and vague, a heterogeneous collection of entities and relationships.

Usability

One of the important requirements emphasized by Armijo et al. (2009a) and others regarding EHR systems is "adherence to *usability* principles":

This concept is critically important in promoting both the widespread adoption and "meaningful use" of EHRs… Developing an understanding of, and ways to measure the impact of usability and information design on ergonomic and cognitive workload, data comprehension, usability, patient safety, clinician decision making, and clinical outcomes. (Armijo et al., 2009a)

According to Linder et al. (2006), usability is a major factor in the acceptance of EHRs in the clinical setting.

EHRs are used by physicians, nurses, and other staff to input, display, and share medical information. The presentation of such information has a great influence on their work (Marchionini et al., 2007). Designing intuitive and agreed-on displays can improve system usability with trivial cognitive effort (Tufte, 2001). In FM, the design elements and principles for EHR interfaces can be built utilizing the same flow-based foundation. That is, FM can be applied uniformly to the conceptual requirements level and simultaneously at the user interface level.

Consider building an interface for staff in the form of Web pages, as shown in Figure 8.

If staff members participate in developing the conceptual requirements as FM streams of flow, their interfaces will use the same model to interact with the system. Suppose a staff member logs in when receiving a patient; a screen appears (See Figure 8A) asking the staff member to choose among Patient and clinician identification, Patient administrative data, Treatment, or Instruction.

Notice the correlation between the subspheres specified in the FM representation and these selections. Assume the staff member selects to work on *Patient and clinician identification*; screen B in Figure 8 appears, allowing selection in *Process* of entering data manually or downloading data from the system's database. Suppose the person selects processing data manually; screen C appears. The screens reflect the flowsystem shown in the FM representation with different stages included. The user can handle data at any stage and move such data among them. Suppose he or she selects to create data (input); screen D appears, where the staff member can input data in a form like that shown on the screen.

Suppose that on screen C, the staff member selects *Arrival*; screen E appears, showing all notes sent specifically to the staff member handling a particular patient, e.g., data sent from an ambulance attendant. Suppose that, instead, the staff member selects *Transfer* on C; screen F then appears, where he or she can send the data to the printer or database.

Figure 8. Illustration of staff interface and its mapping to the underlying FM description

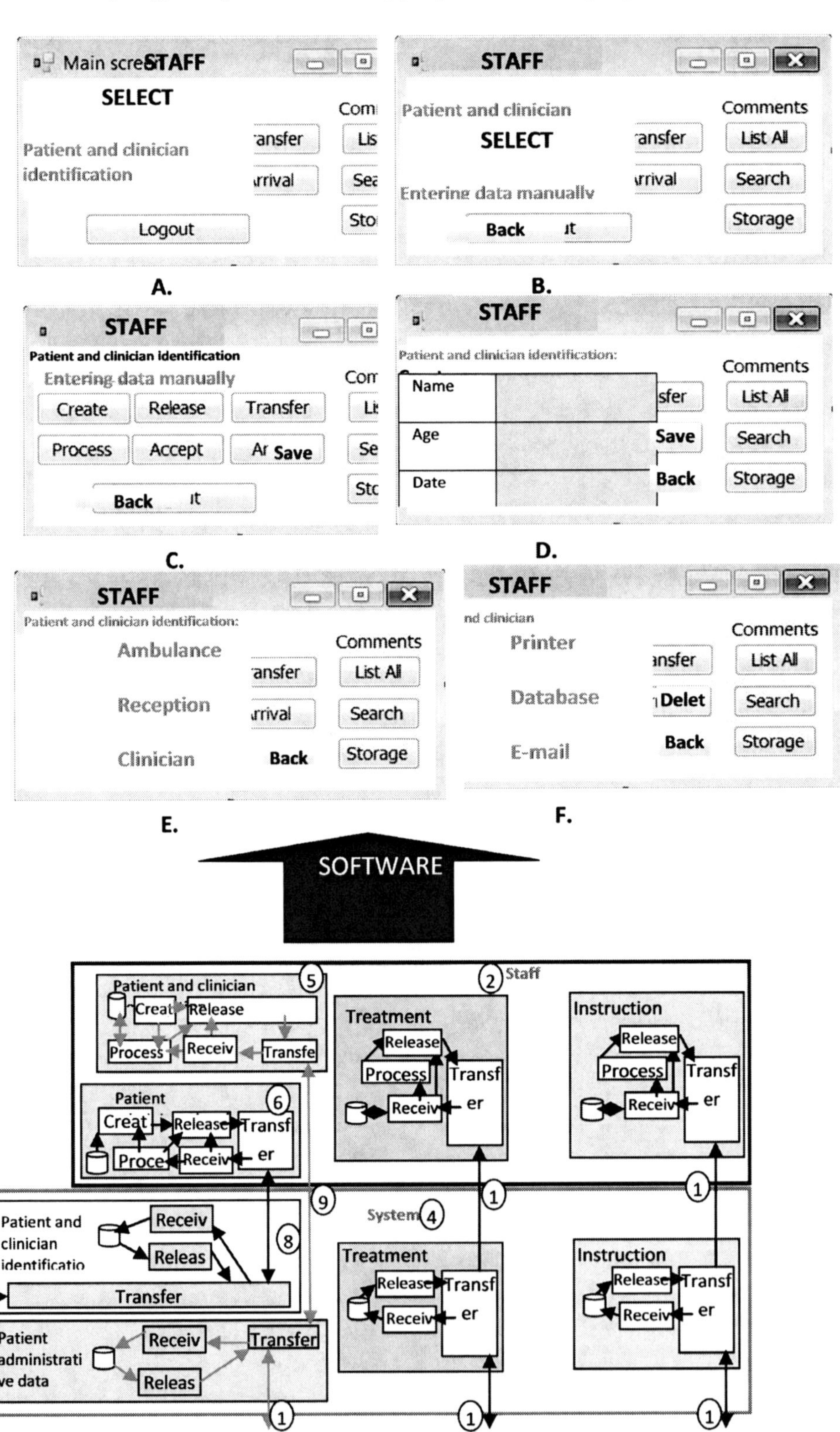

Modifications and Additional Events

In their Acute Care use case, Armijo et al. (2009a) include other events related to this situation, such as "some of the information needs when determining a diagnosis and formulating a treatment plan for an acute episode [including]: Medical resources–Diagnosis and treatment plan formulation may require the support of external sources of clinical information and guidance." The FM representation can easily be modified to include such cases. Figure 9 shows the clinician sphere, where the *Patient administrative data* flowsystem is omitted, based on the assumption that clinicians do not need such data.

Additionally, flowsystems of *Request for clinical information and guidance* and *Response for clinical information and guidance* are added (circles 1 and 2 in Figure 9). Treatment can be triggered by this response (circle 3) or by entry of data into *Patient and clinician identification*.

The interfaces to this request/response can be developed as in Figure 10. In the request, the clinician can select the type of request. It is possible to develop a page where he or she can create, release, process, and transfer requests. Such a page is beneficial in case a clinician creates several requests for different patients, where a request can be released but still not transferred (waiting to confirm final content). Later, the clinician could modify the request by moving it to Process, then releasing and transferring it.

Figure 9. Modified clinician sphere of the acute care situation

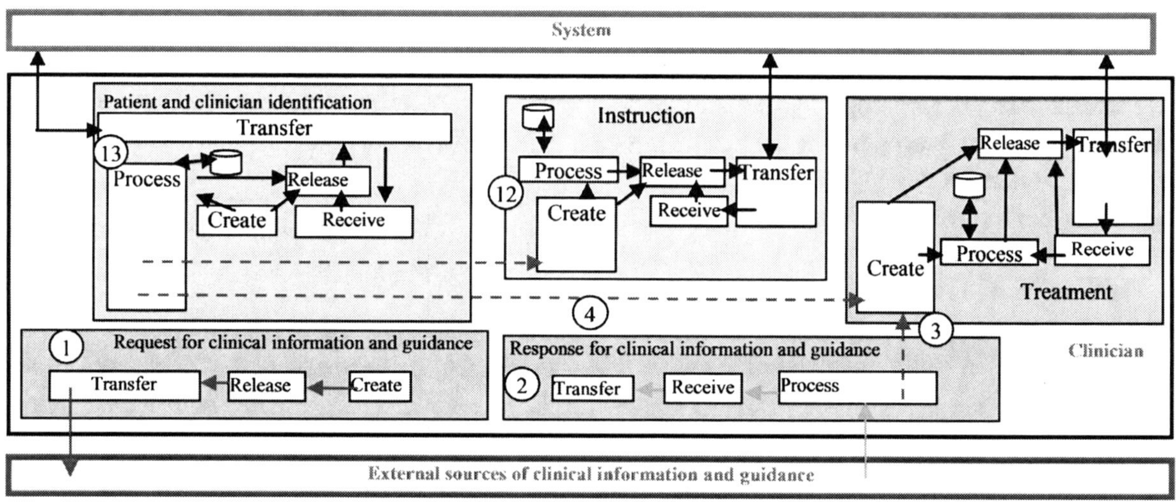

Figure 10. Possible interface for requesting clinical information and guidance

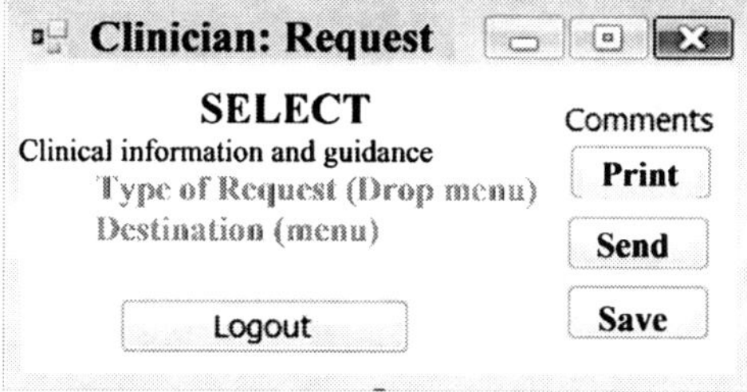

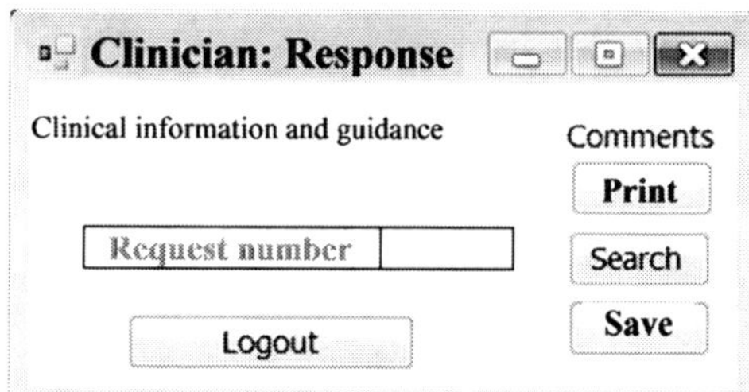

CONCLUSION

This paper proposes establishing a foundation for the application of information design principles to the use of health information technology in primary care settings. This proposal imitates a specific attempt in this direction (Armijo et al., 2009a) that includes documenting patterns of clinician information use and developing "use cases" and tools for evaluating EHR implementation. The paper introduces an alternative approach based on a new flow-based specification methodology. It is shown through examples that the method can uniformly specify health information operations in various phases and across roles. It also provides a more exact description in which "things" (e.g., information, treatments, instructions, and patients) are separated into different streams of flow with six generic internal operations: create, release, transfer, arrive, accept, and process. The method can be applied uniformly to the conceptual requirements level and, simultaneously, at the user interface level. The proposal seems to be a viable technique for expressing situations arising in clinical work practices and as an alternative to "use cases" for the purpose of standardizing EHR implementation.

Current work in this area involves further exploration of the potential and features of FM-based modeling in building of theoretical and actual systems.

REFERENCES

Al-Fedaghi, S. (2009). States and conceptual modeling of software systems. [IRECOS]. *International Review on Computers and Software*, *4*(6), 718–727.

Al-Fedaghi, S. (2010). System-based approach to software vulnerability. In *Proceedings of the IEEE Symposium on Privacy and Security Applications (PSA-10)*, Minneapolis, MN.

Al-Fedaghi, S. (2011). A conceptual foundation for data loss prevention. *International Journal of Digital Content Technology and its Applications*, *5*(3), 293–303.

Al-Fedaghi, S. (2012). Information management and valuation. *International Journal of Engineering Business Management*, *4*(47), 1–11.

Al-Fedaghi, S. (2013, April 15-17). Alternative representation of aspects. In Proceedings of the *HCI International 2013, 10th International Conference on Information Technology: New Generations, (IEEE ITNG 2013)*, Las Vegas, NV.

Armijo, D., McDonnell, C., & Werner, K. (2009a). *Electronic health record usability: Evaluation and use case framework. AHRQ Publication No. 09(10)-0091-1-EF*. Rockville, MD: Agency for Healthcare Research and Quality.

Armijo, D., McDonnell, C., & Werner, K. (2009b). *Electronic health record usability: Interface design considerations. AHRQ Publication No. 09(10)-0091-1-EF*. Rockville, MD: Agency for Healthcare Research and Quality. October.

Avison, D., & Young, T. (2007). Time to rethink healthcare and ICT? *Communications of the ACM*, *50*(6), 69–74. doi:10.1145/1247001.1247008

Car, J., Black, A., Anandan, C., Cresswell, K., Pagliari, C., McKinstry, B., … Sheikh, A. (2008). *The impact of eHealth on the quality and safety of healthcare: A systematic overview and synthesis of the literature, Report for the NHS Connecting for Health Evaluation Programme*.

Department of Health. (2008). *The NHS Informatics review report*. London, UK: The Stationery Office.

Diaz, M. (2010). *Petri nets: Fundamental models, verification and applications*. John Wiley & Sons.

Gans, D., Kralewski, J., Hammons, T., & Dowd, B. (2005). Medical school groups' adoption of electronic health records and information systems. *Health Affairs (Project Hope)*, *24*(5), 1323–1333. doi:10.1377/hlthaff.24.5.1323 PMID:16162580

Greenhalgh, T., Potts, H. W. W., Wong, G., Bark, P., & Swinglehurst, D. (2009). Tensions and paradoxes in electronic patient record research: A systematic literature review using the meta-narrative method. *The Milbank Quarterly*, *87*(4), 729–788. doi:10.1111/j.1468-0009.2009.00578.x PMID:20021585

Gunter, T. D., & Terry, N. P. (2005). The emergence of national electronic health record architectures in the United States and Australia: Models, costs, and questions. *Journal of Medical Internet Research*, *7*(1). doi:10.2196/jmir.7.1.e3 PMID:15829475

Hartswood, M., Procter, R., Rouncefield, M., & Slack, R. (2003). Making a case in medical work: Implications for the electronic medical record. *Computer Supported Cooperative Work*, *12*(3), 241–266. doi:10.1023/A:1025055829026

Institute of Medicine. (2009). *Health and human sciences in the 21st century: Charting a new course for a healthier America*. New York, NY: National Academies Press.

Juan, Y. C., Ma, C. M., & Chen, H. M. (2005). Applying UML to the development of medical care process management system for nursing home residents. *International Journal of Electronic Business Management*, *3*(4), 322–330.

Kreps, D., & Richardson, H. (2007). IT success and failure: The problem of scale. *The Political Quarterly*, *78*(3), 439–446. doi:10.1111/j.1467-923X.2007.00871.x

Kupersmith, J., Francis, J., Kerr, E., Krein, S., Pogach, L., Kolodner, R. M., & Perlin, J. B. (2007). Advancing evidence-based care for diabetes: Lessons from the Veterans Health Administration. *Health Affairs*, *26*(2), w156–w168. doi:10.1377/hlthaff.26.2.w156 PMID:17259199

Linder, J. A., Schnipper, J. L., Tsurikova, R., Melnikas, A. J., Volk, L. A., & Middleton, B. (2006). Barriers to electronic health record use during patient visits. *AMIA 2006 Symposium Proceedings*, 499-503.

Marchionini, G., Rimer, B. K., & Wildemuth, B. (2007). *Evidence base for personal health record usability: Final report to the National Cancer Institute*. University of North Carolina at Chapel Hill, School of Information and Library Science.

Oudshoorn, N., & Pinch, T. E. (2005). *How users matter: The co-construction of users and technology*. Cambridge, MA: The MIT Press.

Røed, K. (2011). *Socio-technical integration in health care: A case study from a hospital-based laboratory context*. Ph.D. dissertation, Faculty of Health Sciences, Department of Clinical Medicine, University of Tromso, Norway.

Stead, W. W., & Lin, H. S. (Eds.). (2009). *Computational technology for effective health care: Immediate steps and strategic directions*. Washington, DC: National Academies Press.

Tufte, E. (2001). *The visual display of quantitative information* (2nd ed.). Graphics Press.

Walsh, S. H. (2004). The clinician's perspective on electronic health records and how they can affect patient care. *BMJ (Clinical Research Ed.)*, *328*(7449), 1184–1187. doi:10.1136/bmj.328.7449.1184 PMID:15142929

This work was previously published in the International Journal of Healthcare Information Systems and Informatics (IJHISI), 9(1); edited by Joseph Tan, pages 30-41 copyright year 2014 by IGI Publishing (an imprint of IGI Global).

Tools and Technologies

This section presents an extensive coverage of various tools and technologies available in the field of E-Health and Telemedicine that practitioners and academicians alike can utilize to develop different techniques. These chapters enlighten readers about fundamental research on the many tools facilitating the burgeoning field of E-Health and Telemedicine. It is through these rigorously researched chapters that the reader is provided with countless examples of the up-and-coming tools and technologies emerging from the field of E-Health and Telemedicine. With 21 chapters, this section offers a broad treatment of some of the many tools and technologies within the E-Health and Telemedicine field.

Chapter 27
Healthinfo Engineering:
Technology Perspectives from Evidence-Based mHealth Study in WE-CARE Project

Anpeng Huang
Peking University, China

Linzhen Xie
Peking University, China

ABSTRACT

Driven by the commission to proliferate information and communication technologies to health services globally, a new multidisciplinary direction is born, which can be named as Health Information (termed as a new word, Healthinfo) Engineering. To highlight the significances of Healthinfo Engineering, the evidence-based mHealth study in the WE-CARE project demonstrates technology perspectives. In this project, the authors built up a WE-CARE system, which integrate various necessary information and communication technologies to fulfill online healthcare services, even including advances from related math/modelling, physics sciences, etc. Without any doubt, such a system is a promising tool to change healthcare delivery. But this project also reveals there are many explicit and implicit factors left when using system-level integration in order to perform healthinfo applications. In general, in contrast to an explicit factor, an implicit factor is hidden from practical applications, which is the critical risk that may break down a healthinfo system. This phenomenon motivates us to investigate what's real bottlenecks in healthinfo systems. Based on the motivation, this paper summarizes healthinfo challenges from evidence study in the WE-CARE project, for instance, scheduling strategy, system light-loading, virtual clinical perception, privacy protection, etc. This technology summary shows that more extensive attention should be needed for healthinfo study not only in mobile and medical areas, and also in computer science, maths, physics, even including ethic, law, etc. In return, the new interdisciplinary cutting-edge science, Healthinfo Engineering, can make contributions to offer a practical life-cycle health management for all human being, including cancer supportive care.

DOI: 10.4018/978-1-4666-8756-1.ch027

INTRODUCTION

According to the reports from WHO (World Health Organization) (WHO and ITU Joint Report, 2014; WHO and ITU Joint Report, 2013), healthcare cost is becoming the unaffordable socio-economic problem in the world. Let us take cardiovascular disease (CVD) as an example. Only cardiovascular disease has contributed counting up to 29% of the total global deaths (Huang, 2014). Official statistics in (Huang, 2014) show that 230 million people in China - 1/5 of Chinese adults - suffer from cardiovascular diseases. On average, one patient dies from CVD every 10 seconds in China. In return, if the mortality rate from CVD could be reduced by 1% in next 3 decades, the reduction in total social cost would be about 10.7 trillion US dollars (68% of the 2010 Chinese fiscal year GDP). The cost of CVD has attracted attention from academic and industry communities in order to develop an early warning system for CVD monitoring (Global Survey Report, 2011; Estrin, 2010; Collins, 2012; Silva, 2013). The main causes of fatal cardiovascular disease include serious myocardial ischemia (acute myocardial infarction), heart failure, and malignant arrhythmia. As shown in (Bacquer, 1998; Falchuk, 2010; Usher, 2013), most of these symptoms can be predicted by observing certain specific manifestations of electrocardiogram (ECG) signals. If a system can detect such manifestations at an early phase, it can save valuable time for taking precautions against the cardiovascular disease (Caldeira, 2012; Zhang, 2012; Caldeira, 2013; Xie, 2014). To satisfy the requirement above, health conditions of CVD affected people must be collected and delivered to a professional healthcare center online, without unexpected disruption and distortion. Recent advances in information and communication technologies and engineering have provided an opportunity to accomplish this objective. Correspondingly, technology and engineering are becoming the indispensable ingredients for health information services today and future. Driven by this new trend, a new multidisciplinary area, Healthinfo Engineering, is born, which is changing health-care delivery today and at the core of responsive health systems in the future.

The rest of the paper is organized as follows: Section II introduces related works and presents a common architecture for Healthinfo Engineering. In Section III, we discuss real challenges to Healthinfo Engineering, which are revealed from an implementation of WE-CARE project. Finally, we discuss system tests and clinical trials of WE-CARE in Section IV.

A COMMON ARCHITECTURE FOR HEALTHINFO SYSTEMS

As well known, healthcare cost is becoming the huge socio-economic problem. Only in terms of falling-related injuries, the annual direct and indirect cost is expected to reach $67.7 billion by 2020 (the dollar value in the 2012 fiscal year) (CDC Report, 2014). To handle this challenge, there is a new trend to proliferate information and communication technologies for offering healthcare services over cyber-infrastructures, called Health Information (Healthinfo) Engineering. So far, there are already a number of Healthinfo systems that can be classified into three types below.

The first type focuses on signal sensing and acquisition (Woojae, 2010; Peng, 2010; Paglinawan, 2009; Chen, 2007). The reference (Woojae, 2010) proposed an enhancement of CMRR (Common Mode Rejection Ratio) for higher amplifier gain and lower noises when extracting physiological signals. In the literature (Peng, 2010), an acquisition function of multi-physiological parameters was embedded into a healthinfo system. In the literature (Paglinawan, 2009; Chen, 2007), the authors discussed the sensor power consumption issue with CMOS (Complementary Metal Oxide Semiconductor) and RF (Radio Frequency) circuit techniques. In the literature (Xie, 2014), the developed WE-CARE system can offer a 7-lead

ECG real-time monitoring service over mobile networks, which is objective to collect adequate clinical ECG information while considering user mobility needed.

The second type aims at signal transmission (Zhang, 2013; Mulyadi, 2009; Yu, 2008). In (Zhang, 2013), the authors proposed a BCD (Best-fit Carrier Dial-up) algorithm to guarantee medical image and video transmission in mobile networks. In (Mulyadi, 2009), the authors tested ZigBee and Bluetooth technologies for local robust wireless connection. In (Yu, 2008), wireless communication technology is applied for a distributed monitor system.

The third type is to interpret the acquired medical signals in Healthinfo applications (Lee, 2011; Chang, 2009). In (Lee, 2011), a decision-support system is conceived for a specific disease of diabetes. In (Chang, 2009), the Bayesian theorem and decision trees are used to construct a web-based decision-support system.

In all kinds of these systems above, we found there are a number of major common enabling technologies. This phenomenon is very useful while devising a common framework for Healthinfo systems. As shown in Fig. 1, a common framework is suggested, which consists of three layers: sensing layer, network layer, and application layer.

In Healthinfo systems, the sensing layer is served as the frontier, in which biological electrode sensors and biosensors are used to detect, monitor and control physiological signals, such as temperature, blood pressure, blood oxygen saturation, pulse rate, respiration, ECG (Electrocardiogram), EEG (Electroencephalogram). Besides these biosensors, there are some new approaches for information acquisition. For example, RFID (Radio Frequency Identification) is broadly used in hospitals for patient tracking, ownership identification, drug control, baby location services, etc. Typically, the sensing layer collects and displays physiological signal/data, and performs signal and data processing if necessary. For the state-of-the-art constraints of silicon-based chip performance

and computing complexities at sensing terminals, local processing should be simplified as much as possible. This is also the reason that main data processing functions are carried out in the application layer.

To make the best use of collected digital data, they should be available upon an authorized request on demand. Therefore, the sensing data are carried and transmitted over networks at a required reliability. In the network layer, there are wired and wireless transmission technologies in terms of access media, e.g., fiber, cable, radio, infrared, etc. Of course, a wireless technology is integrated as the natural component of Healthinfo systems, because it can offer services without time and location limitations (Xie, 2014; Zhang, 2013). On the other hand, wireless radio channels are badly suffering from interference, fading, path loss, shadow and other many negative effects. As a consequence, the QoS (Quality of Service) of Healthinfo applications are greatly depending on unreliable radio channels. Moreover, when mobile networks are evolving into the full-IP (Internet Protocol) switching pattern, for example, Long-Term Evolution (LTE)-Advanced mobile networks (Sesia, 2009), the existing 'Best Effort' service pattern is absolutely unsuitable for Healthinfo applications. To solve the concern above, a scheduling strategy plays a special role in the mobile networks (Sesia, 2009). Additionally, other related topics in this layer include authentication, authorization, accounting, etc. In a Healthinfo architecture, the network layer serves information transmission with required reliability and survivability.

Ultimately, the collected data are used for current or future healthcare applications, e.g., homecare, disease control and prevention, emergency rescue, allergy test, genetic disease tracking, privacy-sensitive treatment of sexually communicable diseases, cancer supportive care, and so on. In the application layer, enabling technologies essentially include application infrastructure and middleware, information processing, application

Figure 1. A basic common framework for Healthinfo systems.

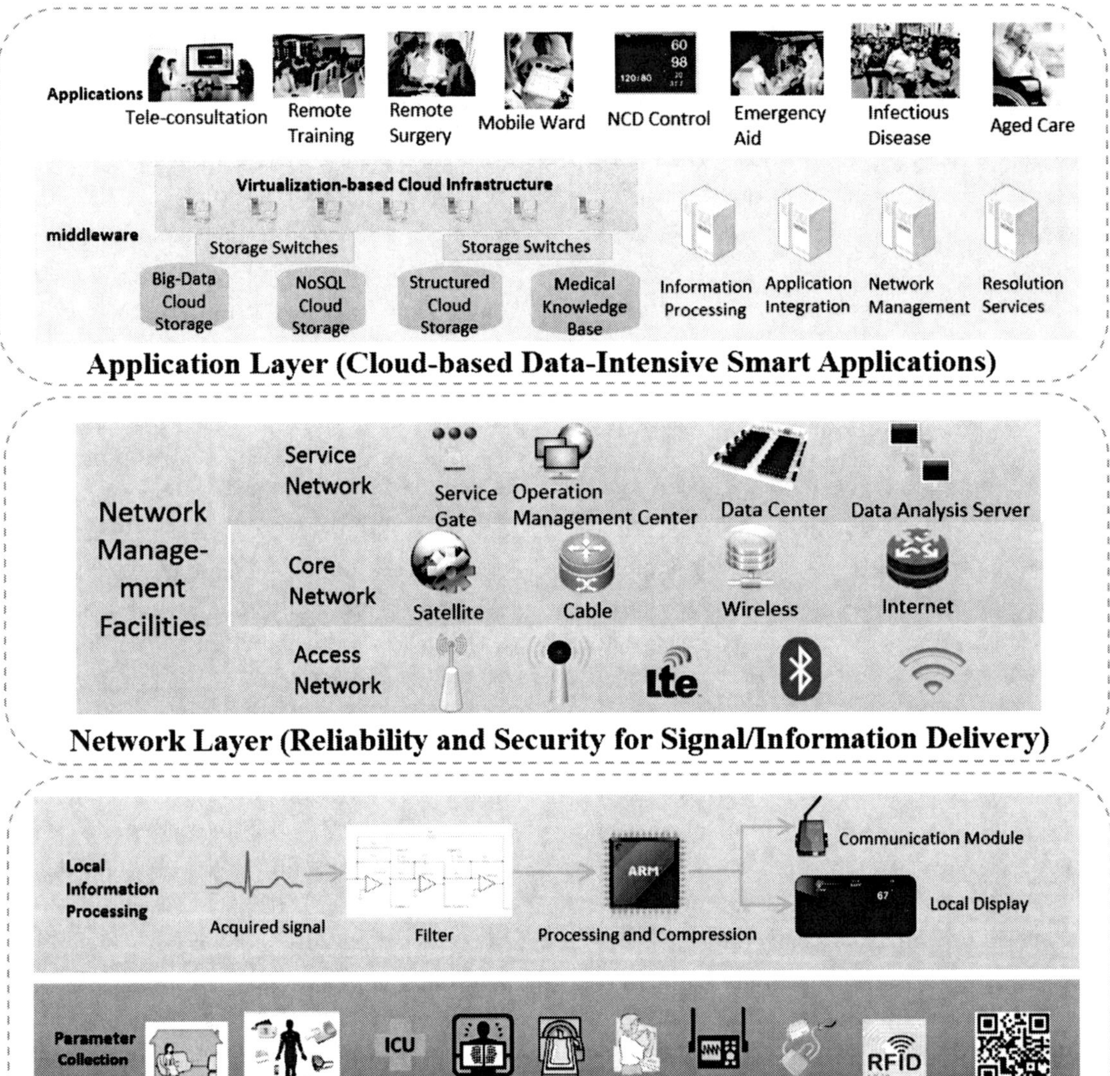

integration, and service management. With healthcare applications emerging, the collected data are explosively increasing. To effectively analyze and structurally archive the digital data that are accumulated with time passing, cloud computing is a powerful tool. It can provide dynamic deployment and smooth the expansion of computing, storage, communications, and other resource requirements at an effective and efficient way.

As explained above, the devised common Healthinfo framework can cover existing system technologies, and is also open to incorporate any advanced or future technologies, e.g., decision-support system, life-cycle health management, nano-chip sensor, quantum communications, math/statistic models. To take advantages from Healthinfo systems, people can access online professional healthcare services, which helps health-conditioned persons living in a normal lifestyle (this is more closely related with the more recent topic of AAL (Ambient Assisted Living) (AAL, 2004)).

Science and Technology Challenges to Healthinfo Engineering

Driven by this successful future of Healthinfo Engineering, we developed and tested WE-CARE (Wearable Efficient teleCARdiology systEm), which generates real-time disease risk alerts without sacrificing user mobility or losing important clinical information, please see the usage style in Fig. 2 (Huang, 2014). In the WE-CARE system, several key enabling technologies are developed and tested upon requests emerging in our system experiments and clinical trials, e.g., de-noising technology for clean signal capture, power-saving wearable mobile user device, ECG signal frame design and data compression over IP/TCP in mobile networks for reliable transmission, privacy-sensitive data center architecture, and clinical decision-support system for data mining. Even though each individual technology of them works properly in tests, the real-time alert function is still broken downs quite often in clinical trials. Obviously, there are some challenges that are still tacit knowledge, which may be the real bottleneck to online healthcare applications. Below, we highlight these tacit knowledge.

Scheduling Strategies to Offer 'Better Than Best Effort (Bbe)' Services

Let us start with a typical example first. If a Healthinfo user needs health information to be 'accurate' and 'real-time' in LTE (Long-Term Evolution) Advanced mobile networks, how to realize this requirement? In order to support different Quality of Service (QoS) requirements for different applications, QCI (QoS Class Identifier) levels are standardized by the 3rd Generation Partnership Project (3GPP)), please see

Table I (3GPP, 2014). Each QCI is characterized by priority, acceptable packet delay budget and packet loss rate, in which these regulated budgets consider the compositive effect contributed from both user and control planes in LTE-A mobile networks. The packet delay budget and the acceptable packet loss rate from the QCI level determine how the evolved Node Base Station (eNB) scheduler handles packets sent over wireless radio resources. For instance, a packet with a higher priority can be expected to be scheduled before a packet with a lower priority across the radio interface.

As observed in Table I, QCI No. 5 is ranked as the top priority because it can take account of both packet delay budget and packet loss rate requirements. In fact, there is the tradeoff between delay budget and packet loss rate. This is because these two metrics often interact in a contradictory fashion. This fact has forced the 3GPP organization accepts compromises when legislating industrial standards. This is also why the packet delay budget in QCI No. 5 set at 100 ms with the smallest packet loss rate, rather than targeting the smallest 50 ms that LTE-advanced mobile networks can offer. In the most advanced mobile network today, QCI No. 5 is the available top-priority service. Nevertheless, the top-priority

Figure 2. The PKU WE-CARE system for monitoring real-time miocardial infarction in mobile networks (the first licensed mHealth clinical-support system in the world).

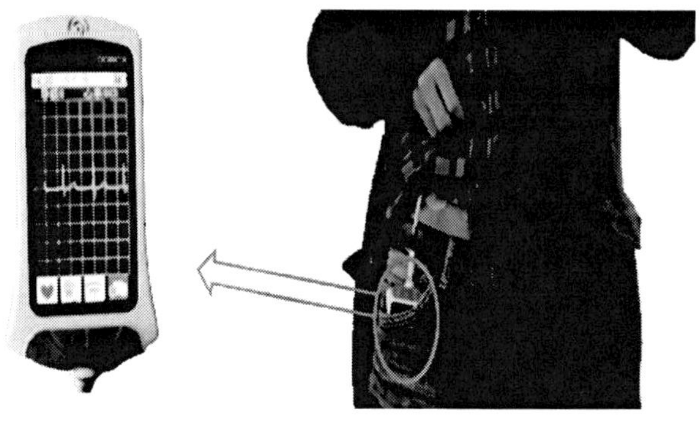

Table 1. Standardized QCIs for Healthinfo in LTE-A networks (3GPP, 2014).

QCI Index	Priority Level	Packet Delay	Error Rate	Typical Examples from mHealth Applications
1	2	100 ms	10^{-2}	Emergency VoIP Call
2	4	150 ms	10^{-3}	Consultation Video Call
3	5	300 ms	10^{-6}	Daily Health Monitoring
4	3	50 ms	10^{-3}	Online Consultation Video Meeting
5	1	100 ms	10^{-6}	Real-time Operation Video
6	7	100 ms	10^{-3}	Medical and Healthcare Education
7	6	300 ms	10^{-6}	Medical Data Transmission w/ TCP
8	8	300 ms	10^{-6}	Daily Health Condition Notices
9	9	300 ms	10^{-6}	Medical Image Download, etc.

service of QCI No. 5 is obtained at the cost of reduced resource utility (i.e., occupying more wireless bandwidth). However, radio resources are always limited, which explains why the QCI No. 5 service is only dedicated to control-level information for guaranteeing system signaling delivery in LTE-A mobile networks right now. In terms of QoS requirements from Healthinfo applications, the most critical mission, for example, the real-time operation video (e.g., robot-assisted surgical system), should be served the top-priority, namely, QCI No. 5. For other kinds of Healthinfo services, each of them should be mapped with a corresponding QCI level, please refer to the examples listed in Table I. Back to the history, the QCI issue is originated from computer IP networking. Thanks to simple and open interconnection protocols deployed, computer IP networking is predominating over most of infrastructures. As mobile networks carry original IP traffic in an all-packet-switching manner, the original 'best effort' in IP networking definitely conflicts with the native requirements in Healthinfo applications. Furthermore, a Healthinfo user is more sensitive to QoS performance because a radio channel is full of uncertainties in comparison to a wired channel (e.g., cable, fiber). Thus, it is significant to study how to offer the "Better than Best Effort (BBE)" services for Healthinfo and other emerging

mobile internet applications, without jeopardizing resource efficiency in mobile networks.

To achieve "Better than Best Effort" services for Healthinfo applications in different scenarios, a scheduling strategy should be robust and agile to handle variations and uncertainties over unreliable radio channels in relation to the service quality requirements in Table I. Unfortunately, most scheduling strategies in OFDM-based mobile networks are depending on the Channel Quality Indicator (CQI)-based scheduling metric. For the CQI-based scheduling, its goal is to maximize 'system throughput' by fully utilizing CQI information, e.g., in the Max C/I (Carrier-to-Interference Ratio) scheduling algorithm (Wang, 2004). For a user in the LTE-advanced mobile network, wideband and sub-band CQI information are dynamically reported to the eNB scheduler in order to respond properly to variations in wireless radio channels. Then CQI information is incorporated into the scheduling process of a CQI-based scheduling algorithm (Awal, 2011). In addition, CQI-based scheduling creates a fairness issue to co-existing users because it allows higher-priority users to preempt resources. To handle the issue of fairness, proportional fair scheduling and opportunistic fair scheduling in (Kong, 2009) were proposed, which consider historical scheduling information (e.g., average throughput). There also exist studies on how to improve CQI measurements for better scheduling performance, see (Mokari, 2010; Wang, 2008) for investigation of CQI-related interference and power control issues. In fact, CQI-based scheduling mainly focuses on how a telecommunication system can utilize its own resources optimally, without considering whether its utilization pattern matches with its users' requirements or not. To deal with this concern, some cross-layer solutions were proposed with QoS (Quality of Service) considerations in (Kong, 2007; Koutsopoulos, 2006). In these CQI-based cross-layer scheduling algorithms, a higher QoS requirement can be served by allocating more radio resources statistically, e.g. a higher QoS user consumes larger bandwidth. Since the wireless resources are limited, enabling a larger number of higher QoS users may force other users to share smaller bandwidth. Thus, the problem of fairness for co-existing users with different QoS requirements arises in this scenario (Bohge, 2007). As a result, these CQI-based scheduling algorithms face a common challenge on how to appropriately use radio resources to provide 'Better than Best Effort' services for Healthinfo applications. Furthermore, if a Healthinfo user needs the top-priority service in both packet loss rate and packet delay budget, what does this mean to coexisting users? Thus, scheduling design is also a multiuser optimization problem over a volatile radio channel in mobile networks, where the intent is to prevent wireless capacity from immediate exhaustion when the number of Healthinfo users increases.

Based on these observations, it is significant to exploit potentials in various self-adaptive mechanisms (e.g., AMC (Adaptive Modulation and Coding), HARQ (Hybrid ARQ), ARQ (Automatic Repeat-reQuest)) to handle uncertainties and various factors (for example, interference, pathloss, fading, and other mobility effects), and incorporate them into a scheduling strategy for providing QoS-benchmarked stable services for Healthinfo users (Yang, 2014; Chang, 2013), in which QCI and CQI factors could be considered

together without a bias. Furthermore, computational complexity of the designed scheduling should be kept low for the time-sensitive concern in Healthinfo applications.

Light-Loading Technology to Maintain Stable System Operation

Besides the scheduling problem, system overload is also the implicitly critical challenge when a Healthinfo system is applied for 24/7 daily health monitoring. In our WECARE clinical trials, we experienced a serious conflict between the necessary clinical information amount and the system stable operation. Furthermore, professionals may be lost in the cumulating digital data. Specifically, in the WE-CARE system (Xie, 2014), the ECG sampling rate must be above 500Hz to guarantee necessary details in acquired ECG data. On the other hand, the amount of 7-lead ECG data in WE-CARE is more than 28 Kbps, while its embedded GPRS (General Packet Radio Service) wireless transmission capacity is limited to 20 Kbps or even less (only a few Kbps in some real deployments due to interference, fading, etc.). In return, this phenomenon causes more congestion, delay, distortion, and collapse into the system operation. If the newly developed LTE-Advanced wireless access technologies are deployed for Healthinfo systems, similar problems also occurred when carrying high definition medical consultation video (Zhang, 2013). This challenge reveals a secret that a Healthinfo system should be lightly loaded. Otherwise, a Healthinfo system may lose stable operation in practice. In addition, user connectivity is also disrupted by power consumption on terminal devices because of over local computing and communications. To lighten the load in a Healthinfo system, the acquired raw data should be filtered to eliminate redundancy. This filtering, however, must maintain data fidelity in order to avoid misdiagnosis. Conventionally, a compression approach could be used to process raw data at a required data fidelity. Generally, compression approaches can be classified into three categories: direct methods, parameter extraction methods and transform methods (Huang, 2014). To keep fidelity at a required level, the compression ratio is still relatively low. This situation leaves a large amount of raw data to be transmitted in a Healthinfo system, which is a concrete obstacle in real-time applications. Moreover, the reverse process, decompression, is needed as well, which is a precondition of biosignal analysis at a datacenter. For considering these constraints, conventional compression approaches are unsuitable for Healthinfo systems, specially, for real-time applications. If clinical features in raw biosignal data can be abstracted and preserved at a high-fidelity level, it is ideal for daily health-risk monitoring applications. In the literature (Huang, 2014), a feature-purification algorithm is studied to reduce redundancy by mapping high-dimensional raw data into a low-dimensional space, in which manifold learning theory is applied into the manifold nature of ECG raw data, without loss of original clinical information. This reference (Xie, 2014) showed that its method can reduce the size of transmitted raw data while preserving its effectiveness on the system level, and decrease power consumption in daily online monitoring. In terms of the light-loading issue, an anomaly discrimination approach can play a vital role. For example, in 24/7 homecare applications, it causes too much system load if converting all ingress digital raw data into the medical conventional pattern (please see next subsection for the conventional pattern). In such a case, it is desired to only turn abnormal data into medical conventional forms while keeping normal data in the digital archive center. Accordingly, professional workload can be reduced since only abnormal signals get inspection attention. Thus, an anomaly detection algorithm has the function of transmission load reduction. In a Healthinfo system, the anomaly detection may be only used to differentiate abnormal signals from normal data, without involving the specific abnormal analysis online (which is left for professional diagnoses).

When an anomaly discrimination method is used for traffic reduction, its complexity should be minimized so that it can be embedded into a Healthinfo system. If physiological signals have numerical characters (such as heat rate, blood pressure, body temperature), then a numerical threshold can be applied in the anomaly discrimination. For example, the heart rate of healthy adults is 60 to 100 times/min. Then a heart rate value out of this range belongs to an anomaly. Of course, the numerical threshold needs to be customized for every one because of individual differences and time-varying health conditions. No doubt, this threshold type is best-fit for numeric physiological signals. How about complex physiological signals, such as ECG signal? To only differentiate anomalies from the multiplexed signals without involving quantitative analysis of abnormal formation, the widely cited SVM (Support Vector Machine) method (Vapnik, 1999) may be useful for its unique role of the binary classification problem in machine learning field. In (Zheng, 2013), a SVM (Support Vector Machine)-based anomaly discrimination algorithm is proposed for this function. Of course, there are more works left for further study on this topic, which is also beneficial for the real-time risk alert, life-cycle health management, system stable operation, etc.

Augmented Reality to Enable Online Professional Healthcare

When the real-time alert is activated in the WE-CARE with the light-loading technology, there are still some critical challenges from purpose-directed applications. In terms of healthcare applications, clinical diagnosis is still a semi-empirical science due to the 3I (Incomplete, Indeterminate and Individual) features of biosignals. To be worse, the 3I features themselves are also of the time-varying nature. For instance, the 3I-featured data of a patient in this evening may be quite different from those captured in the tomorrow morning. In reality, doctors make clinical decisions by the combination of their medical professional knowledge and skillful experiences. In other words, to see a doctor means the doctor has to sense a disease in his/her patient in person. As a result, "clinical perception" is the decisional step for any medical diagnosis and treatment. In medical science, "clinical perception" is defined as the ability to observe, to recognize, to discriminate and to interpret clinical evidence (Cox, 2009; Shaw, 2003). Medical professionals obtain cumulating sensory and perceptual experience when they investigate the clinical phenomena themselves. Because creative activity is involved, the clinical perception is an integration of clinical features and underlying medical symptoms. Please note, the clinical perception is an active process, not a passive reception of observational data. Thus, the semi-empirical "clinical perception" is of 'making sense and judgement' of directly experiencing 'a disease in a patient' rather than 'diseases in data.' In a Healthinfo system, digital data turned from electrophysiological signals are captured and delivered for healthcare purpose, in which any kinds of biosignals if necessary must also be converted into digital data for digital transmission (Zhang, 2012). Without any doubt, it loses the real and essential "clinical perception" process, because a patient is detached from the 'direct sense and judgement' of a professional although they are connected online. As a consequence, it is expected to restore the delivered digital information into the conventional medical pattern for approaching the virtual reality of "clinical perception" in a Healthinfo system. In essence, the challenge is greatly amplified due to the natural and time-varying 3I features in clinical perception that are totally inherited by the Healthinfo system. To deal with this challenge, a promising technology option is about how to realize effective virtual "clinical perception" for online healthcare users who is tied to a Healthinfo system. In (Zhang, 2012), the designed 3R (Retiming, Regeneration, and Reshaping) dataflow engine is dedicated for this objective, which can restore digital bit

streams into the medical conventional patterns for facilitating professional examinations, please see Fig. 3. In fact, the augmented reality of virtual clinical perception is the reverse process of digital data collection and transmission in a Healthinfo system, namely, which is similar to the conversion from digital to analogy in a digital communication system.

Furthermore, to support online professional healthcare, the other major concern is privacy protection. To address the privacy problem, a biometric-based encryption algorithm can prevent any illegal access or hacker invasion, and keep the medical data safely. When a biometric-based encryption algorithm is used for the online healthcare purpose, it should be effective and simple. In an encryption algorithm, the key generation is the core of information security process. Currently, biological natures are broadly used for biometric identification (Jain, 2002; Bringer, 2010). Usually, biodata captured from a person are individual, unique and time-varying, which is qualified to be an encryption key. In the developed WE-CARE system, the RR-interval[1] nature abstracted from ECG signals is chosen as the initial value of key generation. Same as other challenges above, there are more open problems for further study about virtual clinical perception and privacy protection.

TEST RESULTS AND DISCUSSION

In this paper, we mainly focus on the real challenges to Healthinfo Engineering, which are demonstrated from the developed WE-CARE (a Wearable Efficient tele-CARdiologysystEm) (Xie, 2014). In system tests and clinical trials, two connection modes are implemented in deployment scenarios. One of them is a socket connection for real-time monitoring applications. For example, in a point-of-care field, all captured data should be delivered to doctors for professional examination in real-time, and archived in the cloud datacenter concurrently. The other connection is Hyper-

Figure 3. A basic architecture of the designed 3R dataflow engine in WE-CARE project.

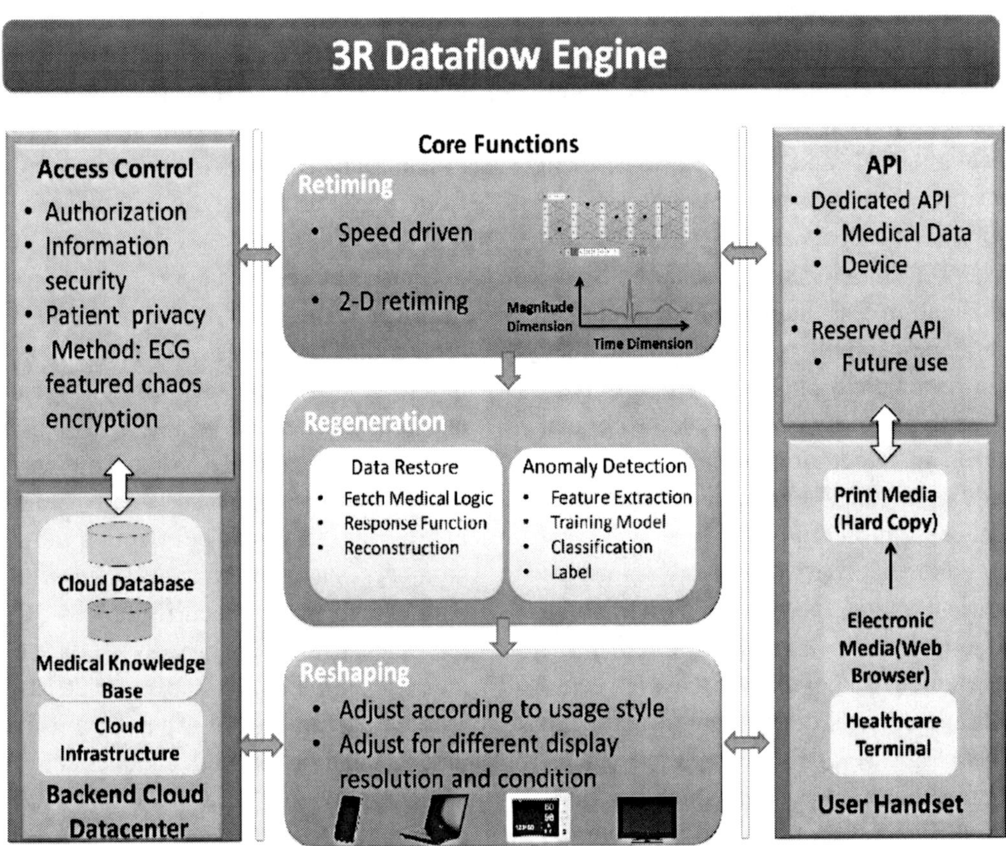

text Transport Protocol (HTTP) mode, which is typically for general purposes, e.g., offline backtracking historical anomalies, periodical data collection of 24/7 homecare services, postoperative healthcare, etc. (Liao, 2012). When an urgent request or health risk alert happens, the HTTP mode can be automatically switched to the socket communication for real-time monitoring. In both socket and HTTP connections, users employ digital signatures to enhance access authentication, so as to prevent any illegal access or hacker invasion. Additionally, all requests are recorded in an audit log in the health datacenter. If an authorized connection is set up, data-flow transmission between the user and its professional (or the datacenter) is activated. While physiological signals are sent to doctors, the data presentation needs to match with different application requirements, which

is performed by the Application Programming Interfaces (APIs). An API can adjust data delivery modes according to specific healthcare requirements. In the WE-CARE, the standard ECG waveform has a default 10 mm/mV sensitivity and 25 mm/s chart driving speed. For matching with different conditions, sensitivity of 5 mm/mV or 2.5 mm/mV, and chart driving speed of 12.5 mm/s and 6.25 mm/s may be requested through APIs. In Fig. 4, we observe that a detection rate of 99.4% for R wave detection and that of 97.7% for T wave detection in WE-CARE clinical trials, while applying a SVM-based anomaly detection into 300-second long data sets from the European ST-T Database (ESD) (Zheng, 2013). If readers are interesting to learn more test results about WE-CARE, please refer to (Huang, 2014; Zhang, 2013; Zheng, 2013; Zhang, 2012) for details.

Figure 4. Evaluation of R Wave and T Wave detection in WE-CARE system.

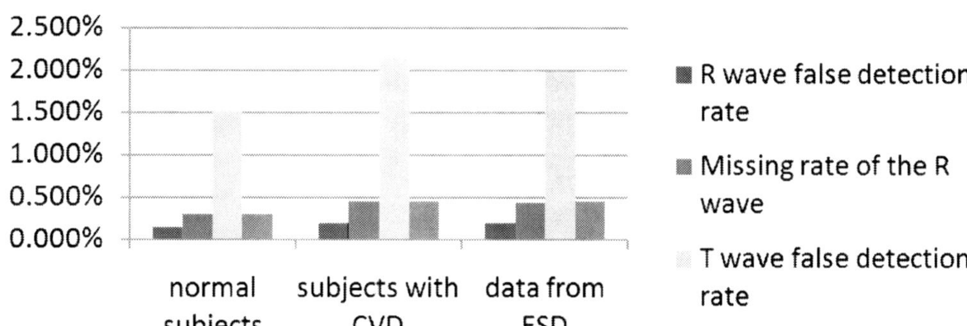

To the end, the emerging concepts, e.g., eHealth, Mobile Health (mHealth), AAL, Digital Hospital, telemedicine, cloud health, pervasive health, ubiquitous health, etc., all of them might be constructive elements of Healthinfo Engineering, in which the interdisciplinary cutting-edge study is not limited to mobile and medical scopes, and also extended to computer sciences, maths, chemistry, physics, even including ethic, law, etc. With solving science challenges from Healthinfo Engineering, various Healthinfo systems are hopefully becoming powerful medical tools in the health delivery. Since we focus on the tacit knowledge from the WE-CARE system tests, there are more challenge problems open for future study in Healthinfo Engineering, for example, lower power-consumption sensor chip in the sensing layer, reliability of control information in the network layer, data mining for clinical decision-support system and life-cycle health management in the application layer, etc. All these efforts in Healthinfo Engineering can make online healthcare services truly available for the public in the promising future.

ACKNOWLEDGMENT

This work was supported in part by the National Science and Technology Major Projects in Wireless Mobile Healthcare Projects under Contract 2012ZX03005013 and Contract 2013ZX03005008, in part by the National Key Technologies R&D Program under Contract 2013BAI05B07, and in part by the Seeding Grant for Medicine and Information Sciences of Peking University (2014-MI-02). This paper was presented in part at the IEEE BSN 2012, IEEE Healthcom 2012, and IEEE ICC 2013. Authors thank to contribution from PKU mHealth lab graduated students Miss Yingrui Zhang, Mr. Chao Chen, Mr. Zhinan Li, Mr. Min Chen, Miss Qian Zheng, Mr. Hongqiao Gao, Mr. Chao Meng, Miss Shiming Liang, and our co-workers and friends Dr. Wenyao Xu, Prof. Jason Cong, Prof. Bingli Jiao, Prof. Xiaohui Duan, Prof. Majid Sarrafzadeh, Dr. Kaigui Bian, Prof. Xiaoming Li, and Prof. Yuanting Zhang.

REFERENCES

Awal, M. A. and Boukhatem, Lila (2011). Dynamic CQI Resource Allocation for OFDMA Systems. *IEEE Wireless Communication and Networking Conference (WCNC2011)* (pp. 19–24). Quintana-Roo, Mexico. doi:10.1109/WCNC.2011.5779132

Bacquer, D. D. et al.. (1998). Prognostic Value of Ecg Findings for Total, Cardiovascular Disease, and Coronary Heart Disease Death in Men and Women. *Heart (British Cardiac Society), 80*(6), 570–577. doi:10.1136/hrt.80.6.570 PMID:10065025

Bohge, M., Gross, J., Wolisz, A., & Meyer, M. (2007). Dynamic Resource Allocation in OFDM Systems: An Overview of Cross-Layer Optimization Principles and Techniques. *IEEE Network*, *21*(1), 53–59. doi:10.1109/MNET.2007.314539

Bringer, J., Chabanne, H., & Kindarji, B. (2010). Identification with Encrypted Biometric Data. *Security and Communication Networks*, *4*(5), 548–562. doi:10.1002/sec.206

Caldeira, J. M. L. P., Rodrigues, J., & Lorenz, P. (2012). Towards Ubiquitous Mobility Solutions for Body Sensor Networks on HealthCare. *IEEE Communications Magazine*, *50*(5), 108–115. doi:10.1109/MCOM.2012.6194390

Caldeira, J. M. L. P., Rodrigues, J. J. P. C., & Lorenz, P. (2013). Intra-Mobility Support Solutions for Healthcare Wireless Sensor Networks – Handover Issues. *IEEE Sensors Journal*, *13*(11), 4339–4348. doi:10.1109/JSEN.2013.2267729

Chang, C. C., & Lu, H. M. (2009). Integration of Heterogeneous Medical Decision Support Systems Based on Web Services. *The 9th IEEE International Conference on Bioinformatics and BioEngineering (BIBE '09)* (pp. 415-422). Taichung, China.

Chang, T. et al.. (2013). A Self-Adaptive Scheduling (SAS) Solution for Enhancing VoIP Service Quality in OFDM-based Mobile Networks. *IEEE International Conference on Communications 2013 (ICC 2013)* (pp. 1084-1088). Budapest, Hungary. doi:10.1109/ICC.2013.6654907

Chen, C. A. et al.. (2007). Low-Power 2.4-GHz Transceiver in Wireless Sensor Network for Biomedical Applications. *2007 IEEE Conference in Biomedical Circuits and Systems (BIOCAS 2007)* (pp. 239-242). Montreal, Canada. doi:10.1109/BIOCAS.2007.4463353

Collins, F. (2012). The Real Promise of Mobile Health Apps: Mobile Devices Have the Potential to Become Powerful Medical Tools. Scientific American, http://www.scientificamerican.com/article.cfm?id=real-promise-mobile-health-apps

Cox, K. (2009). Teaching and Learning Clinical Perception. *Medical Education*, *30*(2), 90–96. doi:10.1111/j.1365-2923.1996.tb00725.x PMID:8736243

Estrin, D., & Sim, I. (2010). Open mHealth Architecture: An Engine for Health Care Innovation. *Science*, *330*(6005), 759–760. doi:10.1126/science.1196187 PMID:21051617

Falchuk, B. et al.. (2010). The mHealth Stack: Technology Enablers for Patient-Centric Mobile Healthcare. [IJEHMC]. *IGI-Global International Journal of E-Health and Medical Communications*, *1*(1), 1–17.

Global Survey Report. (2011). mHealth: New Horizons for Health through Mobile Technologies, www.who.int/goe/publications/goe mhealth web.pdf, World Health Organization.

GPP TS 23.203. (2014). Policy and Charging Control Architecture. http://www.3gpp.org/specifications

Huang, A., Xu, W., Li, Z., Xie, L., Sarrafzadeh, M., Li, X., & Cong, J. (2014). System Light-Loading Technology for mHealth: Manifold-Learning-Based Medical Data Cleansing and Clinical Trials in WE-CARE Project. *IEEE Journal of Biomedical and Health Informatics*, *18*(5), 1581–1589. doi:10.1109/JBHI.2013.2292576 PMID:25192569

Jain, A. K. et al.. (2002). *Biometrics: Personal Identification in Networked Society* (pp. 1–41). Kluwer Academic Publishers.

Kong, Z. et al.. (2007). A New Cross Layer Approach to QoS-Aware Proportional Fairness Packet Scheduling in the Downlink of OFDM Wireless Systems. *2007 IEEE International Conference on Communications (ICC)* (pp. 5695–5700). Glasgow, UK. doi:10.1109/ICC.2007.944

Kong, Z. et al.. (2009). A Low-Complexity QoS-Aware Proportional Fair Multicarrier Scheduling Algorithm for OFDM Systems. *IEEE Transactions on Vehicular Technology, 58*(5), 2225–2235. doi:10.1109/TVT.2008.2009874

Koutsopoulos, I., & Tassiulas, L. (2006). Cross-Layer Adaptive Techniques for Throughput Enhancement in Wireless OFDM-based Networks. *IEEE/ACM Transactions on Networking, 14*(5), 1056–1066. doi:10.1109/TNET.2006.882842

Lee, C. S., & Wang, M. H. (2011). A Fuzzy Expert System for Diabetes Decision Support Application. *IEEE Transactions on Systems, Man, and Cybernetics. Part B, Cybernetics, 41*(1), 139–153. doi:10.1109/TSMCB.2010.2048899 PMID:20501347

Liao, L., Chen, M., Rodrigues, J. J. P. C., Lai, X., & Vuong, S. (2012). A Novel Web-enabled Healthcare Solution on HealthVault System. [JOMS]. *Springer Journal of Medical Systems, 36*(3), 1095–1105. doi:10.1007/s10916-010-9572-2 PMID:20703631

Mokari, N., Javan, M. R., & Navaie, K. (2010). Cross-Layer Resource Allocation in OFDMA Systems for Heterogeneous Traffic with Imperfect CSI. *IEEE Transactions on Vehicular Technology, 59*(2), 101–1017. doi:10.1109/TVT.2009.2035131

Mulyadi, I. H. et al.. (2009). Wireless Medical Interface Using ZigBee and Bluetooth Technology. *Third Asia International Conference on Modelling & Simulation (AMS '09)* (pp. 276-281). Bali, Indonesia. doi:10.1109/AMS.2009.134

Paglinawan, A. C., Wang, Y.-H., Cheng, S.-C., Chuang, C.-C., & Chung, W.-Y. (2009). CMOS Temperature Sensor with Constant Power Consumption Multi-level Comparator for Implantable Bio-medical Devices. *Electronics Letters, 45*(25), 1291–1292. doi:10.1049/el.2009.2115

Peng, Y., & Le, S. (2010). Embedded Multi-Physiological Parameter Collecting and Displaying System Based on Windows CE. *2010 International Conference on Computational Intelligence and Software Engineering (CiSE)* (pp. 1-4). Hubei, China.

Report, C. D. C. (2014). Costs of Falls Among Older Adults, http://www.cdc.gov/homeandrecreationalsafety/falls/fallcost.html

Sesia, S. et al.. (2009). *LTE – The UMTS Long Term Evolution: From Theory to Practice.* Wiley. doi:10.1002/9780470742891

Shaw, A., Latimer, J., Atkinson, P., & Featherstone, K. (2003). Clinical Perception and Clinical Judgment in the Construction of a Genetic Diagnosis. *New Genetics & Society, 22*(1), 3–19. doi:10.1080/1463677032000069682

Silva, B. M. C., Rodrigues, J. J. P. C., Lopes, I. M. C., Machado, T. M. F., & Zhou, L. (2013). A Novel Cooperation Strategy for Mobile Health Applications. *IEEE Journal on Selected Areas in Communications, 31*(9), 28–36. doi:10.1109/JSAC.2013.SUP.0513003

The Ambient Assisted Living (AAL) Joint Programme. (2004). Retrieved November 15, 2009, from http://www.aal-europe.eu/

Usher, W. et al.. (2013). The Connective Matric of Emerging Health Technologies: E-Health Solutions for People with Chronic Disease. [IJEHMC]. *IGI-Global International Journal of E-Health and Medical Communications, 4*(3), 94–114. doi:10.4018/jehmc.2013070107

Vapnik, V. N. (1999). An Overview of Statistical Learning Theory. *IEEE Transactions on Neural Networks, 10*(5), 988–999. doi:10.1109/72.788640 PMID:18252602

Wang, L. C., & Lin, W. J. (2004). Throughput and Fairness Enhancement for OFDMA Broadband Wireless Access Systems Using the Maximum C/I Scheduling. *2004 IEEE 60th Vehicular Technology Conference, VTC2004-Fall., vol. 7* (pp. 4696–4700). Los Angeles, U.S.A.

Wang, R., & Lau, V. K. N. (2008). Robust Optimal Cross-Layer Designs for TDD-OFDMA Systems with Imperfect CSIT and Unknown Interference: State-Space Approach Based on 1-bit ACK/NACK Feedbacks. *IEEE Transactions on Communications, 56*(5), 754–761. doi:10.1109/TCOMM.2008.060100

WHO and ITU Joint Report. (2013). Be Health, Be Mobile: mHealth 2013 Progress.

WHO and ITU Joint Report. (2014). mHealth for Noncommunicable Diseases (NCDs) Initiative.

Woojae, L.,.... (2010). CMRR Enhancement Technique for IA using Three IAs for Bio-medical Sensor Applications. *2010 IEEE Asia Pacific Conference on Circuits and Systems (APCCAS)* (pp. 248-251). Kuala, Lumpur.

Xie, L. et al.. (2014). WE-CARE: An Intelligent Mobile Telecardiology System to Enable mHealth Applications. *IEEE Journal of Biomedical and Health Informatics, 18*(2), 693–702. doi:10.1109/JBHI.2013.2279136 PMID:24608067

Yang, H., Huang, A., Gao, R., Chang, T., & Xie, L. (2014). Interference Self-Coordination: A Proposal to Enhance Reliability of System-level Information in OFDM-based Mobile Networks via PCI Planning. *IEEE Transactions on Wireless Communications, 13*(4), 1874–1887. doi:10.1109/TWC.2014.030514.130447

Yu, C., & Xi, W. (2008). Design of Distributed Intelligent Physiological Parameter Monitor System Based on Wireless Communication Technology. *International Seminar on Future BioMedical Information Engineering, 2008 (FBIE '08)* (pp. 403-406). Hubei, China.

Zhang, Y.,.... (2012). A 3R Dataflow Engine for Restoring Electrophysiological Signals in Telemedicine Cloud Platforms. *Prodeedings of 2012 IEEE 14th International Conference on e-Health Networking, Applications and Services (Healthcom 2012) (the best student paper award)* (pp. 486-489). Beijing, China.

Zhang, Y.,.... (2013). To Enable Stable Medical Image and Video Transmission in Mobile Healthcare Services: A Best-fit Carrier Dial-up (BCD) Algorithm for GBR-Oriented Applications in LTE-A Networks. *IEEE International Conference on Communications 2013 (ICC 2013)* (pp. 2961-2965). Budapest, Hungary.

Zheng, Q. et al.. (2013). A Novel Multi-Resolution SVM (MR-SVM) Algorithm to Detect ECG Signal Anomaly in WECARE Project. *Proceeding of 4th IEEE Biosignals and Biorobotics conference 2013(BRC2013)* (pp. 1-6). Rio de Janeiro, Brazil.

ENDNOTES

[1] RR-interval: R wave to R wave interval, or R wave length connecting two QRS complex. It represents the time required from a ventricular depolarization to the next ventricular depolarization.

This work was previously published in the International Journal of E-Health and Medical Communications (IJEHMC), 6(1); edited by Joel J.P.C. Rodrigues, pages 22-35 copyright year 2015 by IGI Publishing (an imprint of IGI Global).

Chapter 28
Cloud–Based Monitoring for Patients with Dementia

Philip Moore
Lanzhou University, China

Fatos Xhafa
Universitat Politécnica de Catalunya, Spain

Mak Sharma
Birmingham City University, UK

ABSTRACT

Demographic changes are resulting in a rapidly growing elderly population with healthcare implications which importantly include dementia, which is a condition that requires long-term support and care to manage the negative behavioural symptoms. In order to optimise the management of healthcare professionals and provide an enhanced quality of life for patients and carers alike, Remote Electronic Health Monitoring forms a crucial role. This requires myriad functions and components to achieve patient monitoring while accommodating the technological, medical, legal, regulatory, ethical, and privacy considerations. The chapter considers the relevant components and functions of the current state-of-the-art to the provision of effective Remote Electronic Health Monitoring. The authors present the background and related research, and then they focus on the technological aspects of Remote Electronic Health Monitoring to which Cloud-Based Systems and the closely related Cloud Service Modules are central. A number of scenarios to illustrate the concepts are discussed in the chapter.

INTRODUCTION

There is a demographic challenge, which has potentially serious social geopolitical and financial consequences for individuals, families, and the wider society globally driven by the growing elderly population. A significant aspect of this issue is the prevalence of Alzheimer Type Disease (ATD) (a leading cause of dementia) (Rosenblatt, 2005). Effective management of dementia demands both medical treatment and patient management; both approaches include long term care to manage the negative behavioural symptoms which are primarily exhibited in terms of agitation and aggression.

DOI: 10.4018/978-1-4666-8756-1.ch028

Caring for patients with Alzheimer's disease and related disorders (ADRD) is conservatively estimated to cost 80 to 100 billion dollars annually (Rosenblatt, 2005). The scale of the challenge for all stakeholders is clear.

In considering the prevalence of dementia, there is a direct correlation between the demographic changes alluded to and the incidence of dementia (Finkel *al.,* 1996). The results of the *Behavioral Symptoms of Dememtia* (BPSD) are manifested in suffering, premature institutionalisation, increased costs of care, and significant loss of quality-of-life for the patient and family and carers (Finkel *al.,* 1996). This chapter identifies the scale of the problem and the issues around *Alzheimer's Disease and Related Disorders* (ADRD) and dementia and demonstrates the correlation between an ageing population and dementia. To address the issues and challenges identified and provide for an increase in the Quality of Life (QoL) for patients and carers, while mitigating the burgeoning costs in managing patients with dementia and ADRD related conditions.

Dating from the early 1990's pervasive computing and its corollary, the use of context to enable Personalised Service Provision (PSP) (Moore *al.,* 2010) to individuals and entities (Dey & Abowd, 1999) has been the subject of a large body of research and application development. In recent years Cloud-Based Systems (CBS) (Moore & Sharma, 2013) have moved from the domain of computer research to the mainstream and have gained significant traction; the interest in and uptake of CBS applies to individuals, industry, commerce, academia, and importantly the healthcare sector to enable Electronic Patient Records (EPR) and Electronic Staff Records (ESR). In practice the use of EPR has been extensively discussed in the literature however ESR is a topic that received far less discussion and analysis.

The interest in CBS is motivated by many factors including the need to effectively utilise computing resources in an era when there is a general requirement to provide scalable data storage and processing to accommodate the exponential growth in the volume of data. Context and context-awareness have been the subject of much research in a computing laboratory environment however as with Translational Research (Ashford al., 2010) in the medical field there is a need to provide an effective approach to enable non-technical [from a computational perspective] users [who have domain knowledge and expertise] to build context-aware systems in a diverse range of domains and systems. To this end we propose a new CBS service model: Context-as-a-Service (CaaS) which is conceived as a framework designed to provide the components required to build context-aware systems (Moore *al.,* 2014).

This Chapter considers the issues and challenges with the technological developments, which may provide a solution to (or at least mitigate) the challenges faced in the healthcare sector. Patient monitoring with electronic health records is introduced and the relative merits and de-merits of patient monitoring for patients with dementia are discussed. As we have alluded to the use of Internet including the Internet-of-Things (IoT) in CBS. It is postulated that technology enhanced patient management based on situational awareness in intelligent context-aware systems has the capability to improve the patient experience and improve the QoL for both patients with dementia and carers along with improvements in resource utilization.

The chapter is structured as follows: dementia related research is discussed followed by consideration of Remote Electronic Health Monitoring (REHM). Data processing and temporal considerations are discussed with issues and challenges related to patient data monitoring. Internet technologies and health monitoring with the IoT and the Cloud-of-Things (CoT) are introduced along with consideration of CBS and the closely related Cloud Service Models (CSM) including the novel CaaS. Developments in sensor technologies are introduced with IoT based patient monitoring and patient monitoring using IoT and Cloud Based

Solutions. We present illustrative Scenarios demonstrating how electronic health monitoring may function is real world situations; we show patient monitoring in a hospital Setting and using REHM we consider monitoring in a smart domestic setting. Conclusions drawn, lessons learned, and research challenges are presented; the Chapter closes with a discussion, challenges, and future work.

SECTION 1: DEMENTIA RELATED RESEARCH

Dementia is a degenerative condition (Pugh *al.,* 2007) and is a progressive cognitive disabling disease which effects around 5% of people over 65 and in excess of 40% of people aged over 90. Dementia is one of the main causes of disability later in life, ahead of cancer, cardiovascular disease and stroke. Typical symptoms include:

1. Memory loss,
2. Speech impediments,
3. Deteriorating thought processes, and
4. Impaired perception and reasoning (Lauriks *al.,* 2007).

Additionally, there are changes in personality, behaviour, and mood, which include depressive symptoms, apathy, agitation, and aggression.

Alzheimer's disease (AD) is a leading cause of dementia and characterised by progressive cognitive impairment with neuropsychiatric symptoms such as anomalous motor behaviour, depression (Peng *al.,* 2011), anxiety, weight loss, irritability and agitation. The stages of dementia have been modelled by Vickland & Brodaty (Vickland & Brodaty, 2008) based on the BPSD (Finkel *al.,* 1996). The BPSD has gained acceptance from health care practitioners and in computer science research; seminal work being conducted by, for example, Cohen-Mansfield *et al* (Cohen-Mansfield *et al.,* 1989).

A seven tiered conceptual model (Vickland & Brodaty, 2008) sets out a graphical representation of BPSD in which patients with dementia are classified according to the severity of symptoms and their need for different levels of health care services, the seven tiered model is constructed as follows. The prevalence % are estimates; for tier 7 prevalence is the estimated percentage of people with dementia who fall into this category and for tiers 5 and 6 estimates are based on clinical observations in, for example Burgio (1996).

Tier 1: No dementia. Management: universal prevention, although specific strategies to prevent dementia remain unproven.

Tier 2: Dementia with no BPSD. Prevalence 40%. Management: by selective prevention, though preventive or delaying interventions (not widely researched).

Tier 3: Dementia with mild BPSD – e.g., night time disturbance, wandering, mild depression, apathy, repetitive questioning, shadowing. Prevalence 30%. Management: by primary care workers.

Tier 4: Dementia with moderate BPSD – e.g., major depression, verbal aggression, psychoses, sexual inhibition, wandering. Prevalence 20%. Management: by specialist consultant in primary care.

Tier 5: Dementia with severe BPS – e.g., severe depression, psychoses, screaming, severe agitation. Prevalence 10%Management: in dementia specific nursing homes or by case management under a specialist team.

Tier 6: Dementia with very severe BPSD – e.g., physical aggression, severe depression, suicidal tendencies. Prevalence <1%. Management: in psychogeriatric or neurobehavioral units.

Tier 7: Dementia with extreme BPSD – e.g., physical violence. Prevalence rare. Management: in intensive specialist care unit.

In considering Tier 1, this can be managed by regular consultations with healthcare professionals where diagnosis and management can implemented however while management of the condition can be achieved through universal prevention, specific strategies to prevent dementia remain unclear (Vickland & Brodaty, 2008).

Tiers 6 and 7 require institutionalisation and retention of a domestic living arrangement is impractical and potentially dangerous for both patients and carers. Tier 5 is more problematic as management [of the patient] may be in: "dementia specific nursing homes or by case management under a specialist team. Thus, for Tier 5 patients the spectrum of BPSD severity varies; as such there may be patients within Tier 5 who display symptoms and behaviours closely related to Tier 4 behaviours who may be capable of remaining in a domestic environment while monitored. For a patient classified as Tier 5 IAL is patient specific and whilst there may be a case made for retention of IAL arrangement the likelihood is that institutional care is the sensible option. In considering Tiers 2, 3, and 4 the status(s) classified under these tiers offer the optimal scope for retention of IAL supported by 24/7 remote monitoring using sensor technologies with mobile technologies.

Based on this analysis retention of IAL for domestic settings can be restricted to Tiers 2, 3, and 4 with possible Tier 5 patients displaying behaviours closely related to tier 4 patients as set out in the 7 tier model. This conclusion is supported by the observations in (Vickland & Brodaty, 2008); from a dementia management perspective the estimated prevalence of BPSD in dementia patients in specific tiers is: 40% for Tier 2, 30% for Tier 3, 20% for Tier 4, 10% for Tier 5, and 1% for Tier 6. The incidence in Tier 7 is noted as 'rare' (Vickland & Brodaty, 2008).

In practice the clear demarcation between the tiers is not realistic as the boundaries are fuzzy however the conclusions drawn from the analysis remain valid. From this analysis it can be seen that the manageable tiers from an IAL perspective

(tiers 2, 3, and 4) represent 90% of the population of patients with dementia and retention of IAL for these cases present opportunities to improve the QoL for patients and carers while realising significant financial savings for all stakeholders in the management of ADRD and dementia.

There is a large body of documented research addressing Alzheimer type conditions in general and dementia in particular (Pugh *al.*, 2007; Lauriks *al.*, 2007; Vickland & Brodaty, 2008); the literature reviewed has focused on agitation and aggression as these behaviours relate to dementia. Agitated behaviour is one of the most frequent reasons that patients with dementia are placed in long-term care settings. These behaviours are indicators of distress and are associated with increased risk of injury to the patients and their caregivers (Bankole *al.*, 2011). Biswas *et al* (2006) have noted that Agitated behaviours are common in patients with dementia and represent a challenge for all stakeholders in dementia management.

There is a direct correlation between the demographic changes alluded to and the incidence of dementia. A number of studies have investigated the prevalence of BPSD in nursing home populations and have found that the [BPSD] symptoms occur in up to 90% of patients. The prevalence of BPSD (Finkel *al.*, 1996, 1998) is shown in Table 1 which shows the prevalence of dementia as it relates to the age range of the total population. The tabulated results clearly demonstrate the correlation between age range and the prevalence of dementia in the population. A commonly accepted measure of the impact of dementia [on both patients with dementia and possibly more importantly the carers] is the Behavioural and Psychological Symptoms of Dementia (BPSD) (Finkel and Burns, 2000). The results of are BPSD are manifested in suffering, premature institutionalization, increased costs of care, and significant loss of Quality-of-Life (QoL) for the patient and h/her family and carers (Finkel *al.*, 1996). The impact of BPSD can:

Table 1. The relationship between age and the prevalence of dementia

Total Population (Age Range)	Prevalence (%)
60-64	0.6
65-69	1.6
70-74	3.5
75-79	7.4
80-84	15.7
85-89	26.2
90-94	41.0
>95	46.3

(Source: Finkel *al.*, 1996).

1. Interrupt patient care and frustrate caregivers (Rosenblatt, 2005), and
2. Lead to premature institutionalisation in residential care with reduced QoL for both patients and carers.

The issues around ADRD and dementia demonstrate the correlation between an ageing population and dementia. To address the issues and challenges identified and provide for an increase in the QoL for patients and carers, while mitigating the burgeoning costs in managing patients with dementia and ADRD related conditions, this paper considers Independent Assisted Living (IAL) implemented using e-Health monitoring to manage the BPSD using intelligent context-aware systems incorporating decision-support (Moore *al.*, 2013).

Qiu *et al* (2007) have observed that if agitation is not detected or addressed (the failure to address the early signs of BPSD) or there is a "poor reaction" to a patient demonstrating "agitated dementia" can result in "a catastrophic reaction" Research dating back to the 1960's by Cutler & Sramek (1966) has observed that a catastrophic reaction as: "as "any strenuously difficult reaction to an overwhelming situation". The development of a catastrophic reaction by a patient not only results in trauma to the individual with reduced

activity living but also increased stress for carers, and in increased costs for all stakeholders in dementia management.

SECTION 2: REMOTE ELECTRONIC HEALTH MONITORING (REHM)

Traditionally, patient monitoring has been a labour intensive activity with the related manuscript patient records and while computerisation with database technologies has improved the availability of patient data the collection and processing of the collected patient data remains a labour intensive operation.

Additionally, we have introduced the concept of IAL (Moore *al.*, 2013) for patients with dementia. Consider the potentially huge benefits to be realised for patients and carers in terms of quality of life if effective IAL implemented using REHM. There are efficiency benefits [to be derived from implementing IAL using Intelligent Context-Aware Decision Support (ICADS) systems for healthcare professionals and the wider society where reductions in premature institutionalization offer the potential for huge financial savings on a global scale (Moore *et al.* 2013a).

However IAL with patient management and treatment is very restricted and remains a labour intensive operation provided by care assistants, healthcare professionals, and clinicians [who visit the patient's home] in the domestic setting. Effective IAL however requires REHM implemented in "Smart Spaces" as discussed in Thomas *et al.* (2013). Effective REHM has the potential to enable improvements in the quality of patient care combined with efficient utilisation of healthcare staff and resources (Parks *al.*, 2011).

While the focus of this Chapter lies in dementia there are clear correlations with the monitoring of other conditions including: post-operative care, depression, mental illness, Parkinson's disease (Thomas *et al.* 2013) and related cognitive degenerative conditions on the Alzheimer spectrum where there is a general imperative to institute premature institutionalisation (Moore al., 2013a). As we have alluded to in this Chapter IAL with REHM and ICADS has positive and beneficial implications in both financial and quality-of-life for all stakeholders involved in patient care, management, and planning.

There are however ethical considerations (including informed consent) and technical challenges implicit in the implementation of IAL with REHM and ICADS. In the subsequent sections these considerations and challenges with related potential solutions envisaged in our research are discussed.

Data Processing and Temporal Considerations

The processing of the captured data into useful information can be viewed under two headings:

1. In 'real-time' data processing in e-health monitoring, and
2. The processing of data in 'big-data' solutions in which data is mining is applied to realise long-term prognoses.

The goal of 'real-time' data processing in a health-monitoring scenario is to measure a patient's current state at time t0 and the changed state a time t1 (the time intervals between t0 and {t1 … tn} will be defined by the clinician and will be patient and condition dependent). The developments in Smartphone technologies offer the prospect of implementing local data processing with decision support thus enabling full remote health monitoring. Health monitoring clearly involved a very large volume of data. The requirement in 'real-time' health monitoring is for health monitoring applications which can run on low-powered devices (such as high-end mobile phones) and can process the sensor derived data to reach instant decisions relating to a patients dynamic state at times {t0 … tn}. Ideally, health-

monitoring systems will only communicate current patients state if there is an issue or problem (see the brief illustrative scenario later in this article).

Clearly there is a requirement for any number of reasons for the patient monitoring information to be sent at periodic intervals for logging and possibly further analysis. The time interval at which such uploading of the collected data is made is again a clinical decision. The analysis of the data from multiple patients can be viewed as a big-data challenge.

Issues and Challenges with Patient Data Monitoring

Unlike traditional patient records, which tend to be standardized ways of collecting and storing data into relational database systems, the patient data monitoring presents several challenges and issues. Indeed, to start with, the amount of data produced is an endless data stream, due to continuous patient monitoring. This leads to the need of using Big Data technologies. Big-Data science (Dobre & Xhafa, 2014) relates to a scenario in which very large volumes of data are gathered and processed to identify (in the case of health monitoring systems) trends in the data and potential prognoses based on the data collected and results obtained from multiple patients. Clearly, big-data solutions require massive data storage and computing power (as opposed to the 'real-time' data processing). Recent research studies have shown that relational databases cannot cope with such amount of data, giving rise to solutions based on 'NoSQL' technologies.

Additionally, patient data monitoring requires addressing issues of data cleansing, data provenance and governance. Indeed, it is needed to clean the data, detect potential missing data and errors and bring it to a format for later analysis and processing. There is therefore a data cycle identified from data capturing to final data persistence and analysis. This serves also as a basis for regulatory issues (regarding access and use of data) and building national archives, with access to data by all actors involves (doctors, nurses, carers and stakeholders).

SECTION 3: INTERNET TECHNOLOGIES AND HEALTH MONITORING

This section provides a discussion related to sensor technologies with examples to illustrate how sensor networks can be used to capture and potentially pre-process data into useful information. We consider approaches to intelligent processing of e-health monitoring data in effective decision-support systems. In this section we will discuss the IoT and the developing CoT with a new concept in CSM which is CaaS which is designed to provide a platform and framework to enable the creation of context-aware systems.

We have considered the motivation and background for health monitoring generally and REHM to enable IAL using ICADS decision-support systems. We now turn to the focus of this Chapter, which is the use and implementation of CBS and the related CSM available within a CBS environment. We will initially introduce and discuss the (arguably related) concepts of the Internet-of-Things (IoT) and the Cloud-of-Things (CoT). These concepts are very important in the realisation of REHM where communications and the realisation of effective data capture, collection, storage, and processing forms a critical element in the cocktail of functional requirements that is REHM and the essential EPR and ESR.

The Internet-of-Things and Cloud-of-Things

Recent developments in CBS have resulted in what has been termed: the IoT which in a medical context has been referred to as: the *Internet-of-Health* (IoH) (Thomas *al.,* 2013a). There is a close affinity between the IoT and CBS; in actuality in

a modern context the IoT may be more correctly referred to as the CoT (Thomas *al.,* 2013a).

There is a large body of research around cloud-based systems and the health sector has an abundance of services that could be serviced by the cloud; there is however a great deal of scrutiny as to the suitability of cloud services for use in the health sector. In actuality the term "Cloud" has no clear and commonly agreed definition; there is a large body of documented research in which a definition for the term: "Cloud" has been considered and it has been suggested by Wyld (2009) that the term "Cloud be viewed as an acronym standing for: "Common, Location-Independent, Online, Utility that is available on Demand".

If we dissect this acronym, it is relevant to the offering today, there are Common services, i.e. shared with individuals and companies; we do not generally know where these services are unless we ask suppliers for the location, so services can geographically dispersed and user generally do not care, i.e., Location independent; these services are generally web based and so Online; finally the demand is elastic and we can use as little or as much dependent on requirements and Service Level Agreements (SLA), therefore available on-Demand. As with utility services, Cloud solutions are usually auto configuration and reconfiguration on the fly, based on agreed SLA, with properties such as auto monitoring, fault recovery and healing, to provide high resilience and minimum outage times (Thomas *al.,* 2013a).

These definitions are exactly the kinds of services that are required for enhanced patient management. We need the common data, presentation and equipment available to all health care professionals. A similar visualization is required for all the users, consumers, and practitioners and in limited capacity the patient (subject to access rights, permissions, and protocols) as the geospatial location of staff will not be generally known to the system. The services need to be available on any device, *anytime and anywhere* by the various health care professionals, dependent on requirements as one day it may be an emergency and on another day it may be an outpatient, i.e. the system must enable Situational Awareness (SA) (ref) to deliver the service. Finally when there is an unpredictable event or major crisis, these services may be needed a lot more than normal hence are required to be available on demand, just like more electricity and gas is used in cold weather. This is one of the reasons that cloud services are referred to as a Utility (Sotomayor *al.,* 2009; Wyld, 2009).

Cloud Based Systems

Cloud-Based Systems (CBS) generally fall into three distinct types:

1. Public Clouds,
2. Private Clouds, and
3. Hybrid Clouds.

Figure 1 graphically models the [three] CBS and the relationships that exist between a private and public cloud when used in concert to create a hybrid cloud.

There is generally an element of confusion around the concept of the 'Cloud'; there being no generally agreed definition of the term. In asking: "What is Cloud computing?" Hartig

Figure 1. Cloud-based systems and their conceptual relationships

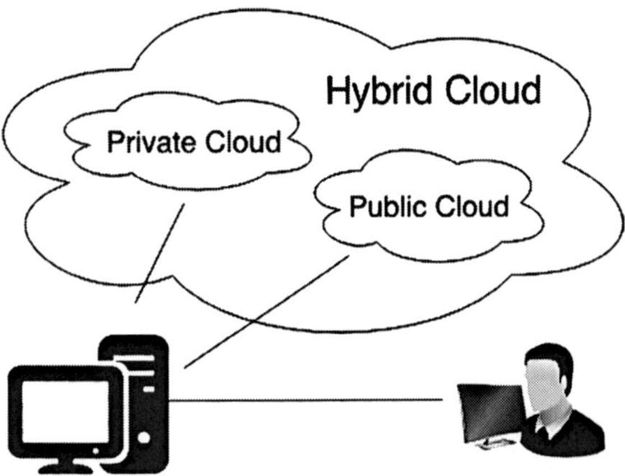

(2008) observes: "the Cloud is a virtualisation of resources that maintains itself". This definition, while adequate in a general sense fails to capture the complexities that characterise Cloud-based solutions. In relation to the medical context an interesting discussion on: "ubiquitous access to cloud emergency services" can be found in Koufi *et al* (2012). Ubiquitous access on-demand and anytime-anywhere (within the provisions of location and access rights and permissions) is an essential requirement in the health domain and Cloud-based solutions offer this service.

As we have discussed context and SA encompasses much more than location; this aspect of SA however remains a pivotal component in context-aware patient management Morton *et al* (2012) address this in respect of "location and activity tracking in the cloud". The IoT and sensing of entities is, as we have discussed, central to enhancing patient management; Rao et al (2012) consider these elements in a paper entitled: 'Cloud Computing for the Internet of Things & Sensing-Based Applications'. While the work of Rao is not patient management focused their work has a clear relationship to patient management and the sensing of entities (as we have discussed) in a hospital setting.

Mazhelis *et al* (2012 investigate the: "Impact of Storage Acquisition Intervals on the Cost-Efficiency of the Private vs. Public Storage"; this forms a strategic decision both in the option to use a Cloud-based solution (as opposed to a traditional in-house approach) and also in the cloud system to be adopted.

In general usage Public Clouds are generally open for public use. While from a technical perspective there are no significant differences between public and private cloud architectures when considering privacy and security there are important differences in services [including: applications, storage, and other resources] provided. The security and privacy limitations inherent in public clouds are driven by the availability of CBS using public open non-trusted networks (see: Table 1).

Public Clouds

A Public cloud refers to offsite, multi-shared occupancy of services that provide the potential to optimise service efficiencies. However, as we have alluded to (see: Table 1) a public cloud may suffer from security issues in domains of interest (e.g., health monitoring) where data security is a primary consideration. Security issues are driven by the limited set of control measures that can be applied when using a public cloud. A Public cloud is best suited for multiple users and the deployment of standard software. While public cloud solutions provide a number of potential benefits including: scalability (to meet demand variability) and efficiencies in hardware usage [3], there are contractual, legal, regulatory, and security issues which must be addressed including:

1. The requirements to develop, test, and validate application code,
2. The implementation of a security strategy, and
3. Support for collaborative working.

A cloud is called a 'Public cloud' when the services are rendered over a network that is open for public use. Technically there is no difference between public and private cloud architecture, however, security consideration may be substantially different for services (applications, storage, and other resources) that are made available by a service provider for a public audience and when communication is effected over a non-trusted network. Generally, public cloud service providers such as Amazon (Amazon, 2014), Google (Google, 2014), and Microsoft *Azure* (Microsoft, 2014). These prominent examples of public clouds own and operate the infrastructure with access offered only via Internet.

A Public cloud refers to offsite, multi-shared occupancy of hardware services, hence providing optimum efficiency of use. Because of the shared nature of the services, these they are more susceptible to issues than Private cloud as there are a limited set of control measures that can be applied. A Public cloud is best suited for large number of users for the deployment of standard issue software or Software as a Service application with a well implemented security strategy (Sotomayor *al.,* 2009). This is as there may be a large number of users requiring the same application, data and interface. This will help provide a good service that can be expanded and contracted as needed and will be welcomed by IT departments.

A Public cloud pushes the responsibilities to a third party and there is a perceived lack of control and this is why HCP are concerned with the security aspects around patient data. A Public cloud also provides other opportunities that not relevant to this paper, for a detailed exposition see (Rao *et al.,* 2012) however in summary there are contractual, legal, regulatory, and security issues which must be addressed including:

- The requirements to develop, test, and validate application code.
- The Software-as-a-service (SaaS) provider must implement a robust and reliable security strategy.
- The service must be incrementally scalable to meet peak demand (in a hospital setting this is generally uncertain both in time and scale).
- There must be the capability to support collaborative projects and activities.

In addition to these items the support for ad-hoc software development project using a Platform as a Service (PaaS) offering cloud. In the PaaS model, cloud providers deliver a computing platform, typically including operating system, programming language execution environment, database, and web server.

Application developers can develop and run their software solutions on a cloud platform without the cost and complexity of buying and managing the underlying hardware and software layers.

With some PaaS offers, the underlying computer and storage resources scale automatically to match application demand so that the cloud user does not have to allocate resources manually.

We consider the types of Cloud in detail in subsequent section however in summary of potential interest from a healthcare perspective is the Hybrid Cloud which, as we discuss below, may address the privacy and security concerns while leveraging the power of cloud-based solutions where, for example, Software-as-a-Service may provide for efficiencies in technology and system management.

Private Clouds

A private cloud employs a service infrastructure operated solely by, and for, a specific organization (generally for sole use), whether managed internally or by a third-party and hosted internally or externally. A significant benefit of a private cloud lies in increased security and privacy however a private cloud requires a significant investment, effort, and day-to-day engagement to virtualize the business environment. Thus from an organisational perspective a private cloud requires significant re-evaluation of decisions relating to service provision and the implementation of existing resources.

When considering private clouds users remain responsible for the infrastructure costs along with building and maintenance; thus the efficiencies of the public cloud model are lost. However, when correctly implemented (notwithstanding the additional organisational, maintenance costs) security and privacy considerations can be significantly improved. However, realising the additional security demands a significant degree of in-house design capability to prevent serious vulnerabilities.

A Private cloud refers to a company's investment into capital, revenue and staffing, with local staff providing all aspects of support. Therefore rendering this solution is generally more secure as there is direct control over all facets of the operation. This is an expensive option primarily due to

the CAPEX, on-going replacement of equipment and the larger revenue costs of staff (OPEX). It is generally recognised that private IT provision is not efficiently used however a Private Cloud is possibly the best option as it is best suited for meeting legislative benchmarks or data protection regulation. Health informatics is characterized by "mission-critical" functionality and a Private Cloud can be the best choice when data is the critical component of the system. This seems the ideal choice for the patient management systems discussed in this paper as HCP are focused on patient records. If the health service can afford this option, it could meet the legislative needs and met regulatory body approval.

Private cloud is cloud infrastructure operated solely for a single organization, whether managed internally or by a third-party and hosted internally or externally. Undertaking a private cloud project requires a significant level and degree of engagement to virtualise the business environment, and requires the organization to re-evaluate decisions about existing resources. When done right, it can improve business, but every step in the project raises security issues that must be addressed to prevent serious vulnerabilities. They have attracted criticism because users "still have to buy, build, and manage them" and thus do not benefit from less hands-on management, essentially "[lacking] the economic model that makes cloud computing such an intriguing concept".

Hybrid Clouds

A Hybrid Cloud is a composite created using a combination of Public Clouds and Private Clouds (Sotomayor *al.*, 2009). While the constituent Clouds remain unique entities they are bound together in a hybrid structure. A Hybrid Cloud provides a basis upon which multiple deployment models can be implemented thus expanding deployment options for Cloud-Based services and systems. The Hybrid Cloud option allows organisations [such as in the healthcare domain] to use Public Clouds and Private Clouds to meet specific and defined implementation demands and systemic security requirements.

Hybrid Cloud architectures enable degrees of fault tolerance combined with locally immediate usability without a dependency upon Internet connectivity (for Private Cloud functionality). However Hybrid Cloud architectures require both on-site resources and off-site (remote) server-based Cloud infrastructure. Additionally, a Hybrid Cloud architecture enables an expansion of deployment options for cloud services, allowing IT organizations to use public cloud computing resources to meet temporary needs. This capability enables Hybrid Clouds to employ 'cloud bursting' with scaling across Clouds. Cloud bursting is an application deployment model in which an application runs in a Private Cloud [or alternatively in a data centre] and when the demand for computing capacity increases utilises Public Cloud capacity.

A primary advantage of cloud bursting and the Hybrid Cloud model is that an organization only pays for extra computing resources when they are required. Cloud bursting enables data centers to create an in-house IT infrastructure that supports average workloads, and use cloud resources from Public Clouds and/or Private Clouds during 'spikes' in processing demands. Hybrid clouds may lack the security and certainty of Private Clouds however the corollary is that a Hybrid Cloud provides flexibility and increased fault tolerance with the scalability enabled by the use of Public Clouds with enhanced control over security, which is a characteristic Private Clouds implemented using in-house applications and systems.

A Comparative Analysis

It has often been observed that: 'every cloud has a silver lining'; it has also been noted by sceptics that: 'every silver lining has a cloud'. In considering the Cloud solutions, a comparison between Public and Private Clouds demonstrates that each has positive and negative aspects; a summary is presented in Table 2. The tabular comparison identifies the differing functional properties that characterise Public and Private clouds. It is however incorrect to refer to positive and negative characteristics; the correct interpretation must be related to the domain of interest. For example in a health domain security of patient data is critical, thus a public cloud is not a practical solution however a public cloud would provide the scalability to address non-critical functions. In such a case a hybrid cloud may be the optimal approach. A brief overview of each characteristic is as discussed below.

While the initial cost comparison is clear this may not be the overriding factor in the selection of a cloud solution type. The other factors identified arguably have greater prominence. As with the initial cost, the Running Cost is domain specific and will be influenced by the capabilities realised based on the remaining factors.

Customisation is central to a user requirements specification. Where customisation forms a central plank in the requirements (as in the case of the healthcare domain) a Public Cloud alone is arguably not an optimal option. A Private Cloud would offer the facility to tailor the service to suit the domain specific requirements of a healthcare domain. As for Customisation, a Public Cloud fails where Privacy is concerned; this is pivotal

Table 2. Cloud types: a comparative analysis

Characteristics	Public Cloud	Private Cloud
Initial Cost	Low	High
Running Cost	Variable	Variable
Customization	No	Yes
Privacy	No	Yes
Security	Problematic	Manageable
Regulation	Problematic	Manageable
Single Sign On	No	Yes
Scalability	Simple	Difficult

where security, privacy, legal, and regulatory requirements are concerned. A Private Cloud may offer the facility (in a hospital setting) to implement the security requirements with clearly defined access rights and permissions based on defined roles (e.g., clinicians, nursing, auxiliary and management staff).

Compliance with regulatory regimes including: data protection statutes [which are clearly vital in healthcare systems] and implementing security [principally data security] while problematic for a public cloud is manageable for private clouds. The capability to implement a Single Sign On is, as for other characteristics, domain specific and may be a useful function or alternatively a security risk. Scalability is crucial in a hospital domain where the dynamic nature of the environment demands scalability both in the immediate demands but also over time. In a public Cloud solution scaling up is relatively easy while within defined limits however in a private Cloud solution scaling up is more laborious and may entail significant infrastructure investment in terms of hardware, software, and human cost; the scope to scale up is however potentially limitless.

Each option has its advantages and negative characteristics and while the Private Cloud meets the privacy, data security, and access conditions it may fail in terms of scalability to meet spikes in computing demands. A Public Cloud however, while scalable, fails to meet the privacy, data security, and access conditions A primary function in a hospital setting is the sharing of patient records between clinicians and outside organizations within the NHS; in this area a Public Cloud offers many advantages however the security and privacy issues probably outweigh these advantages. In summary it is clear that neither cloud type alone fulfils the demands of health informatics in REHM and EPR.

Figure 2 illustrates the principal CSM. Readers will have noted the additional CSM, the Context-as-a-Service (CaaS). This brief overview of CBS identifies the relative benefits attributable to each Cloud classification. In the following Section we consider the Cloud-Service-Models (CSM) and CaaS.

Cloud Service Models

We have considered the problem this paper considers and introduced CBS. An integral part of CBS is Cloud-Service-Models (CSM) (Moore al., 2013b). There are a number of mainstream Cloud Service Models:

1. Software-as-a-Service (SaaS),
2. Platform-as-a-Service (PaaS), and
3. Infrastructure-as-a-Service (IaaS).

In addition to the 3 service models identified there is also a service model termed Network-as-a- Service (NaaS); an overview of this service model is set out below. Access, control and management of CSM is generally achieved using Cloud Clients (CC).

Figure 2 graphically models the relationship between the CSM and the CC. We have provided

Figure 2. The topology of cloud service models

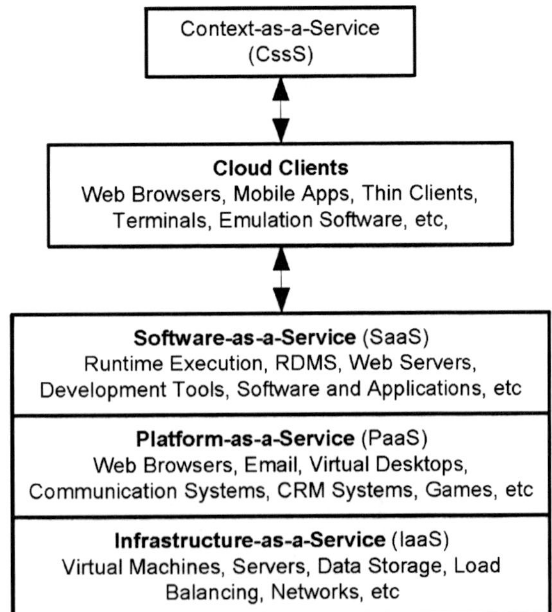

an overview of CBS and CSM including: CC, SaaS, PaaS, IaaS, and NaaS; shown in Figure 3 is the novel Context-as-a-Service (CaaS) CSM architecture which we have proposed in (Moore *al.,* 2014). In operation the CC's, when taken with the appropriate CSM, form the essential components that combine to create the CaaS framework. Section 9 presents a discussion around the CaaS CSM.

Cloud Clients

The Cloud Service Models are accessed using a range of device and interface specific cloud clients designed to address the range and diversity of the potential devices. Clearly, there is a need to personalise the presentation of information in a suitable visualisation. For example, in a hospital setting there is a need to provide appropriate visualisations to suit individual roles such as: clinicians, nursing staff, auxiliary staff, management functions, technical staff, and patients; this can be realised using CC.

Software-as-a-Service

SaaS is typically accessed using a thin client or a web browser. SaaS has become a relatively ubiquitous delivery model for many business applications and may be viewed in terms of a 'utility' as provision may be accessed 'anytime and anywhere' and 'on-demand'. The SaaS CSM is generally implemented on a 'pay-per-use' basis and as such can be viewed as a 'utility'. Additionally, SaaS provides users with a central hosting model in which updates can be released automatically on a scheduled basis without the need for users to manage updates or install new software.

Platform-as-a-Service

The PaaS model cloud providers deliver a computing platform which typically includes:

1.   The operating system software,

Figure 3. A conceptual model of the CaaS architecture

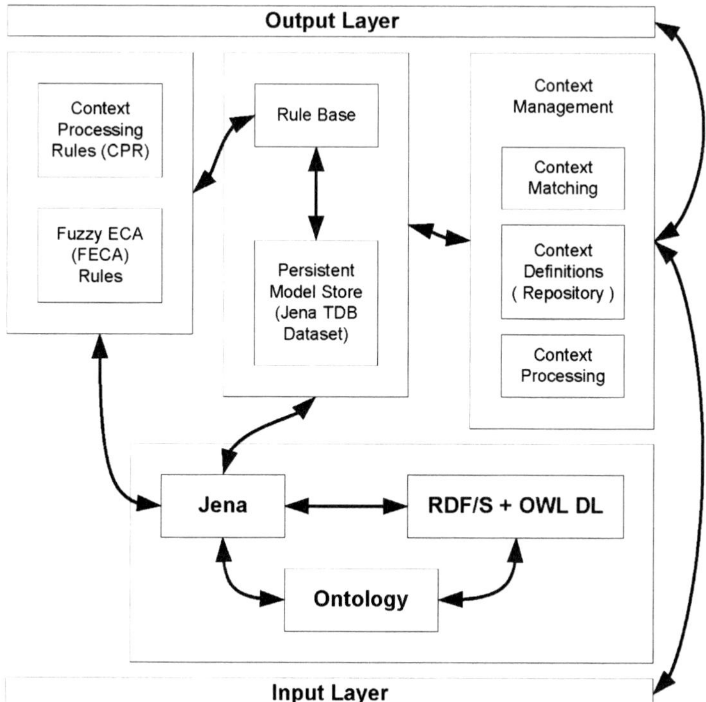

2. The programming language execution environment,
3. A data structure and database, and
4. A web server application.

Developers are able to build and operate software solutions in a cloud environment without the expense (technical, financial and time) and complexity of purchasing and managing the underlying hardware and software layers. A PaaS model may additionally offer the potential for the underlying computer and storage resources to scale automatically to meet the demands of application(s), thus manual resource allocation and the resultant time and expense incurred can be avoided.

Infrastructure-as-a-Service

Possibly the most basic CSM is IaaS. This model generally encompasses provision of computing facilities based on two general approaches:

1. Physical hardware, and
2. Virtual machines.

Pools of hypervisors [within the cloud operational support systems] can support large numbers of virtual machines and the ability to scale services to suit the dynamic user requirements over time. Service provision is generally on-demand from data centres. Connectivity is realised using the Internet or 'carrier clouds' (dedicated virtual private networks) (ref). Cloud providers typically charge for IaaS services on a utility computing basis with cost reflecting the amount of resources allocated and consumed.

Network-as-a-Service

As noted above there is a fourth service model: NaaS. This cloud service model is a category of cloud services where the capability provided to the user is the use of network/transport connectivity services and/or inter-cloud network connectivity services.

NaaS involves the optimization of resource allocation by considering network and computing resources using a holistic approach. Traditional NaaS services include flexible and extended VPN, and bandwidth on demand. NaaS concept materialization may also include the provision of a virtual network service by the owners of the network infrastructure to a third party.

Context-as-a-Service (CaaS)

We have provided an overview of CBS and CSM including: CC, SaaS, PaaS, IaaS, and NaaS. In operation the CC's, when taken with the appropriate CSM, form the essential components that combine to create the CaaS framework. In this section we introduce the concept of Context-as-a-Service (CaaS); the CaaS model architecture is graphically modelled in Figure 3.

The CaaS system architecture essentially consists of 3 modules: the data structure, the context management module, and the rule-base (Moore *al.*, 2013).

- **The Data Structure Module:** This provides a basis upon which persistent and in-memory data representation and storage can be realised. While the data structure shown in Figure 3 employs Semantic Web technologies (Semantic Web, 2014) implemented using the Java based Jena (Jena, 2014) API the proposed CaaS framework may employ an alternative approach to suit the domain specific requirements.
- **The Context Management Module:** provides for the Context-Management and Context-Processing function. The *Rule-Base*: this provides the rule repository. The rules include:
  - Context-Processing Rules (CPR), and
  - Fuzzy Context-Processing Rules (FCPR). The CPR will implement control and constraints [e.g., in a healthcare domain: access rights, permissions, and

visualisations] while the FCPR are designed to realise effective context processing. A detailed discussion around context processing and the rule-based approach implemented to achieve intelligent context processing may be found in (Moore *al.,* 2013); a discussion on fuzzy rule-based systems may be found in Berkan, & Trubatch (1997).

In summary, the posited approach employs an event driven rule-based approach, which uses an Event-Condition-Action (ECA) approach with an IF-THEN logic structure. Figure 3 shows an Input Layer (to enable the creation and accessing of the CaaS application) and an Output Layer (to provide the result in an appropriate visualisation. The Input and Output layers will be designed to incorporate appropriate visualisation capabilities to suit:

1. The role of the individual accessing the application, and
2. The devices used to access the CaaS system.

The CaaS system architecture is a conceptual view of the principal components that combine to enable the creation and accessing of a context-aware system.

The CaaS system is currently conceived as a real-time approach however the data structure using Ontology-Based Context-Modelling (OBCM) may be accessed by other applications. For example, we envisage a Data-as-a-Service (DaaS) (Xhafa *et al.* 2014a, 2014b; Terzo *al.,* 2013) CSM, which may provide sophisticated data analytics and data mining in 'big-data' solutions.

SECTION 4: DEVELOPMENTS IN SENSOR TECHNOLOGIES

With any monitoring system it is essential that sensors be fit for purpose and value for money. Due to the volumes required it is particularly important in

healthcare. Advances in sensor technologies have resulted in the formulation of specific of standards and simpler protocols such as IEEE 802.1.5.4 for low power, low data rate application's in sensors and other similar devices. Specifically Zigbee sensors utilise small foot print operating systems e.g. *TinyOS* (Khazraee *al.,* 2013).

These sensors need some local data storage and processing before transmission to the main data warehouse to be used in the decision-making. Typically Body Areas Networks (BAN) (Khazraee al., 2013) comprise multiple sensors in mesh networks that work together as a group or independently around body to transmit health data. As an example, sensors can be sewn into clothing to have direct body monitoring of vital signs. These will have some use however; it is more effective to have contactless sensors where possible. For example it is possible measure weight and body movement fairly easily using pressure sensors attached to mattresses and pillows. Using the correct sensors it is possible to determine respiration and cardiac beat as well. Similarly, body temperature can be measured using thermistors these have been deployed effectively as show in (Motoi *et al.,* 2009).

As with dementia patients, weight and gait is of interest these can be measured, but the sensors will be more costly. To measure weight, is possible install a load cell bearing platform and weigh in motion for example moving from lounge to kitchen. However an example in (Motoi *et al.,* 2009) the platform is placed around the toilet, here there is less movement and more accurate. In the example of gait analysis has been carried out with low cost pressure transducers in show, however these are problematic as sensors deform easily and the wireless module is prohibitively large.

The latest technology that could be employed is MEMS Micro Electro Mechanical Systems or MOTES typically these are the size of 2AA batteries, such as that they Google IO device, which monitors environmental conditions (Hewlett Packard, 2014). These motes are the largest of the current batch of intelligent sensors and we could use these to monitor the surroundings and correlate the results to the health conditions of patients. Hewlett Packard (HP) (Hewlett Packard, 2014b) are also currently working on a project termed: 'Central Nervous System for the Earth (CeNSE), consisting of a trillion nanoscale sensors and actuators'. "We would propose to leverage this work and us these smart dust sensors around the body, bed, chair, toilet bath, shower and kitchen" (Hewlett Packard, 2014b). Typically these sensors are approx. 5cm square with functionality for movement, light, temperature, barometric pressure, airflow and humidity [(Hewlett Packard, 2014a).

The Wireless Identification and Sensing Platform (WISP) architecture (OpenWISP, 2014) has been used to create miniature sensors that harvest UHF energy from the reader to power the device, sense, process, store and transmit the sensor data. Although more expensive than self-adhesive RF tags, these sensors are effectively intelligent RFID tags containing miniature computers. Generally these are best used for short usage or very long term sensing applications that are ultralow power (Buettner *al.,* 2008). Buettner *et al* have demonstrated the use of this device in a home environment, however, in our application we could use, for example use the Intel WISP device to monitor patient temperature and movement (acceleration). The sensors could be activated when the patient passes the RF readers in the door way or even placed around the room. The HP devices are small and lightweight to be sewn into clothing or built into standard every day object such jewellery and watches where skin contact is needed.

There are many examples with the latest consumer products such as fitbit (fitbit, 2014). This range of cost effective products includes a nylon-rubber bracelet that monitors activity, food, weight and sleep; and wirelessly creates a history log on a smart phone, it is possible to combine this with other sensors to describe the patient's life style and health condition. These may be used in DSS to create an intervention plan for a

healthier lifestyle. Similarly Jawbone functions the same way, the Nike+ Fuel Band is a simpler to use version of the others on the market. The Nike+ Watch provides additional functionality and can be used for example for the rehabilitation of patients with limb injuries by measuring their activity with GPS their location. All these devices can connect wirelessly to computers or smart phones to show the parameters measured in a simple graphical format.

These devices all use similar sensing technologies based on the smart dust. Our proposal is to use these devices to provide a range of conditions on which decisions can be made. For the proof of concept, the software developed will use the data provided and where possible the application will use the APIs provided by the sensor devices. However, for production purposes eventually the OEM version of the sensors will be used with specifically designed hardware and bespoke application software.

This software will also have APIs to allow other applications to be developed and the data structure will be published. If these devices have GPS, it is possible to have context aware, intelligent devices; therefore it is possible to determine if the patient is driving walking, cycle sleeping and then relating the health of the patients to these patterns. Indeed this intelligence is now in a majority of smart phones, so maybe we could, with the addition of few external sensors, using them as patient health monitors. The evolving sensor technologies are shown in Figure 5 (Source: Gartner 2012).

Lloyds pharmacy are collaborating with Proteus (Proteus, 2014) in a trial an indigestible electronic chip (see Figure 4). The chip is ingested by mouth and functions on the potato battery technique (Proteus, 2014) to power the electronics. The chip transmits physical health data, the data to a to a receiver worn by the user. As with the majority of the sensor-based devices considered the receiver may conceivably be a Smartphone as we have discussed in this Chapter. Such an approach has the potential to enable

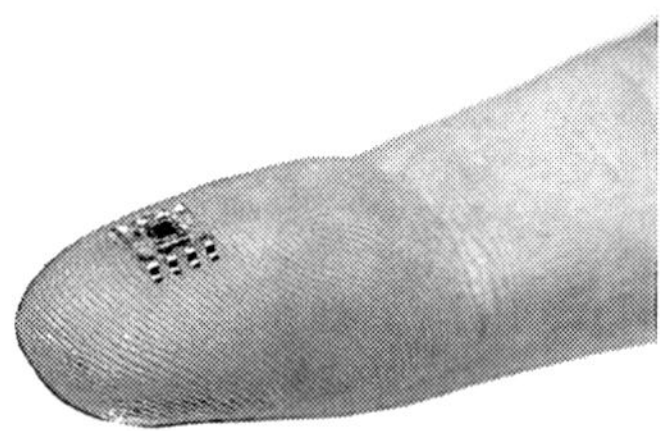

Figure 4. An example of an ingestible sensor

data processing with data sent to clinical services where appropriate intervention(s) using intelligent contest-aware systems.

Patient Monitoring using Cloud Based Solutions

A central function in effective patient monitoring and management is the personalization of service provision (the care pathway) based on their current prevailing state. The IoT [in a medical context] in capturing sensor-derived data and processing it into information useful to clinicians and healthcare professionals provides a basis upon which effective personalised healthcare can be provided while optimising the use of hospital resources and facilities.

Patient Monitoring using the Internet-of-Things

The revolution in smart-phone technologies along with their ubiquity has provided opportunities to inform behaviour and prompt interventions where required at an appropriate level. In the case of the iPhone, it has even been used for microscopy and spectral-analysis of blood and tissue samples using very simple adaptors.

Similarly, GPS is widely used in the health sector, such as locating emergency vehicles and personnel, and has potential for locating patient's

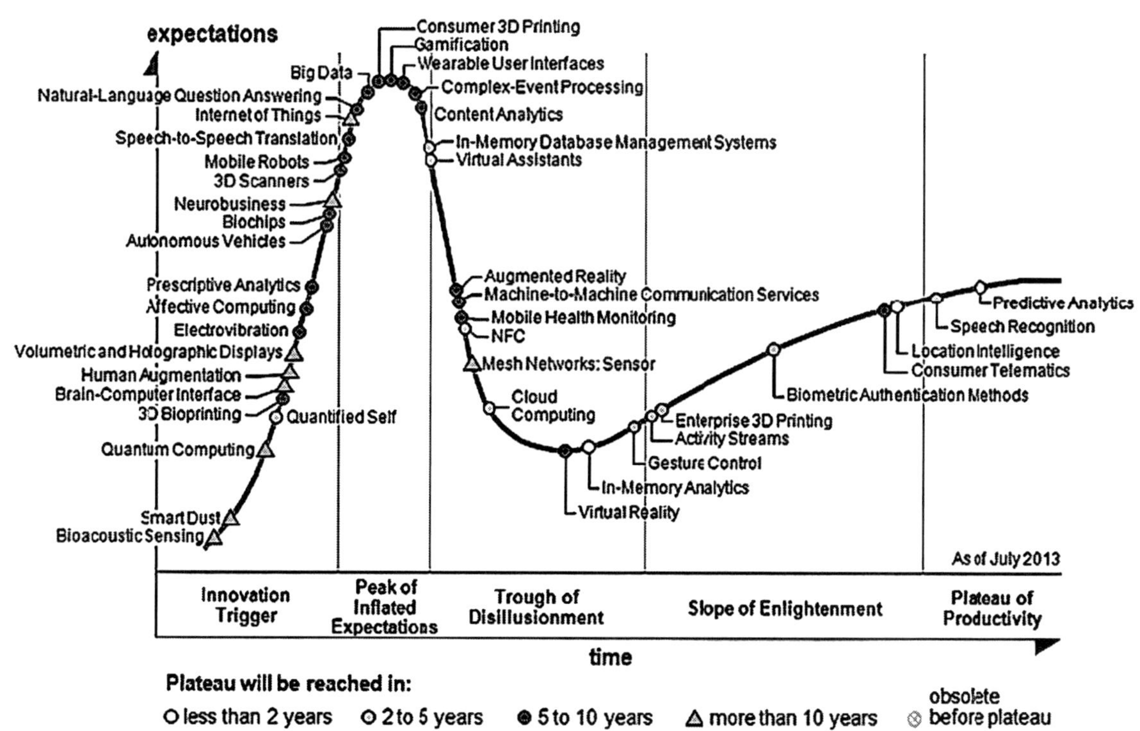

Figure 5. Hype cycle for emerging technologies, 2012 (Source: Gartner).

en-route to hospital, for advance scheduling, via their phones. Accelerometers and gyroscopic sensors are a particularly exciting aspect of mobile devices, allowing simple testing to aid diagnosis, especially when combined with knowledge bases about conditions and symptoms. Mobile phones and tablets are also able to interface with medical equipment over wired (e.g. USB and RS232) and wireless (e.g. Bluetooth and Wi-Fi) connections, including through the cloud. Therefore, they have the potential for revolutionising access to medical data, sensor data and expert systems, greatly augmenting the abilities of clinicians and carers. For patients and clinicians alike, they also have the potential for quick and simple scheduling input, and communication of needs and even emotions.

Additionally, the integration of the CoT with smart-phone technologies opens up many interesting areas related to the sensing of behaviour(s). Figure 6 shows some commonly used sensors.

The applicability of such RFID technologies has a clear application in a hospital setting where a range of uses can be envisaged including: smart clothing (for staff and patients), equipment, facilities, wheelchairs, and trolleys etc. Many other technologies also exist for inclusion in an Internet-of-Health (IoH).

A discussion on the IoH is beyond the scope of this paper however wireless patient and healthcare professional location (simply achieved through received-signal strength data in, for example, Bluetooth and Wi-Fi, and for more localised use via ZigBee enabled sensor (Zigbee, 2014) should be noted. Also, devices such as the Microsoft Kinect have shown themselves capable of useful 3D positioning over short distances and also have applications within interactive recuperation software.

Patient Monitoring using Cloud Based Solutions

As discussed earlier the continuous patient monitoring leads to the need of Big Data technologies and Cloud-based solutions. Different from traditional patient data record, in patient data monitoring requires access efficient access to huge volumes of data. To this end, Terzo et al (2013) developed a Data-as-a-Service (DaaS) approach. DaaS is based on data virtualization to overcome limitations of state-of-the-art approaches in data technologies, according to which data is stored and accessed from repositories whose location is known and is relevant for sharing and processing. Besides limitations for the data sharing, current

Figure 6. Commonly used sensors

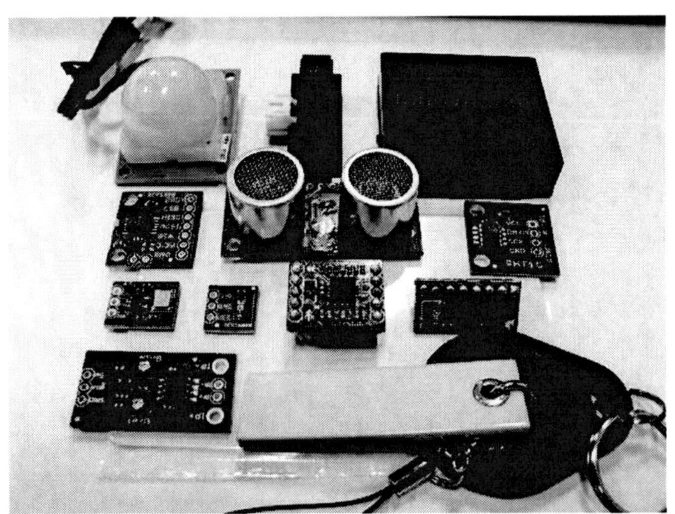

approaches also do not achieve to fully separate/decouple software services from data and thus impose limitations in inter-operability. Additionally, DaaS can support large communities of users that need to share, access, and process the data for collectively building knowledge from data. It also address the needs of accessing the same data from different actors (doctors, nurses, carers and stakeholders) and achieving thus different data views according to access rights.

While DaaS provides a solution to data sharing and access, the security of patient data monitoring is dealt with by recent approaches as well. Xhafa *et al.* (2014a), consider security of patient record data at Cloud using fuzzy keyword search to ensure fine-grained access control. Additionally, in Xhafa *et al.* (2014b) attribute-based encryption techniques are used to design cloud-based electronic health record system with attribute-based encryption, which guarantees security and privacy of medical data stored in the cloud.

Illustrative Scenarios

We have introduced CBS and CSM and presented an overview of the proposed CaaS. To illustrate the implementation of the CaaS this section will present two illustrative scenarios based on e-health monitoring and healthcare systems in domestic and hospital settings. Figure 7 shows a conceptual model of an e-health monitoring system in a hospital setting; a similar conceptual model applies to e-health monitoring in a 'smart' domestic setting.

Hospital Setting

Under this heading we consider two typical potential scenarios:

1. A procedure-scheduling scenario, and
2. A scenario related to routine patient observations.

Figure 7. A smart space patient monitoring model

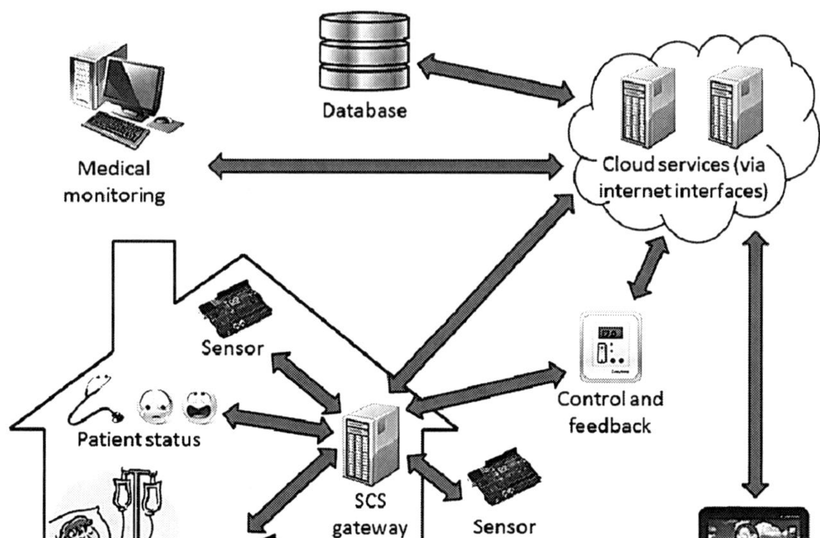

Procedure Scheduling

A typical scenario relates to a patient in a hospital setting who requires an elective or pre-planned procedure (say: an X-Ray examination). Given that a hospital setting is characterised by dynamic uncertainty the need to dynamically change treatment pathways to prioritise urgent or emergency procedures is a regular and potentially frequent occurrence.

A patient has a pre-planned X-Ray examination requiring transport to and from the ward to the X-Ray department. Prior to the planned procedure an emergency admission of a number of patients [in say: a road traffic accident] demands a number of emergency X-Ray examinations. This clearly requires prioritisation over the pre-planned X-Ray examination; therefore the scheduling of the X-Ray workload is required with concomitant revisions in the facility, staffing and transport scheduling. In such a case to maximise the effectiveness of patient treatment pathways Intelligent Context-Aware Decision Support (ICADS) systems provide an effective basis for the re-scheduling of the essential services that combine to provide the treatment pathway. Additionally, there is a need to maximise the effectiveness of staff (at all functional levels) and facilities (e.g., the X-Ray department) with the provision of transport (e.g., wheelchairs, trolleys, etc).

An ICADS system should be aware of the current and changing state (or context) of all entities (an entity has been defined by Dey & Abowd (1999) as a: "person, place, or physical or computational object"). Thus an ICADS must know the location and current context of all patients, staff, and facilities (e.g., X-Ray facilities) including the current and scheduled workload, availability. Additionally, an ICADS should know the state of patient(s) and their planned and emergency treatment requirements. Given this knowledge it is possible to dynamically re-schedule treatment options to provide improved quality of care for all patients with efficiencies in the utilisation of staff and facilities.

Patient Observations

In scenario (1) we briefly considered a dynamic situation, which is a characteristic of a hospital setting. In considering patient treatment pathways it must be recognised that patients resident in hospital (including emergency accident and emergency patients) are generally ill; patients will therefore require regular monitoring [the time intervals and the metrics recorded being condition specific] of vital physiological metrics such as: blood pressure, pulse, respiration, temperature, etc.

Historically patient observations and the recording of the results have generally been monitored manually; this may be by manuscript charts with a computerised database record being made later. Clearly this process is very time and labour intensive, which mitigates against the desired aim of nursing which is to maximise the time with patients. To improve the effectiveness of nursing staff and maximise nursing patient time consider how an ICADS system with autonomic patient observations and updating of patient records may provide not only improved nursing effectiveness but also with intelligent data processing in a ICADS system (with appropriate visualisation of data and results) but may also improve treatment options by highlighting changes in a patients state (or context) in real time; such change may of course be both in negative and positive states calling for appropriate action (or possibly no action) where required.

In action, patient monitoring using an ICADS system with autonomic data and record keeping may enable:

1. Patients treatment can be improved,
2. Change in patients state(s) can be more effectively monitored, and
3. Nursing effectiveness and time management with patients can be improved including the prioritisation of patients requiring urgent care.

Smart Domestic Setting

A very important potential use of context in an ICADS system lies in e-health monitoring in a 'smart' (i.e., sensor equipped) settings (Moore *al.,* 2014) (see Figure 7), which may include domestic settings. Consider, for example, cognitive degenerative conditions on the Alzheimer spectrum where there is a general imperative to institute premature institutionalisation. This course of action has implications in both financial and quality-of-life for all stakeholders involved in patient care, management, and planning.

A very important potential use of context in an ICADS system lies in e-health monitoring in a 'smart' (i.e., sensor equipped) settings, (see Figure 7) which include domestic settings. Consider, for example, cognitive degenerative conditions on the Alzheimer spectrum where there is a general imperative to institute premature institutionalisation. This course of action has implications in both financial and quality-of-life for all stakeholders involved in patient care, management, and planning.

An important aim is to provide an environment in which patients with dementia may be capable of Independent Assisted Living (IAL). Space restricts a discussion on this topic however a detailed exposition may be found in. We have the technologies to implement smart sensor enabled spaces, the challenges lie in effective data processing in ICADS systems as discussed in this paper.

Consider the potentially huge benefits to be realised for patients and carers in terms of quality of life if effective IAL can be implemented. Additionally, there are efficiency benefits [to be derived from implementing IAL using ICADS systems] for healthcare professionals and the wider society where reductions in premature institutionalization offer the potential for huge financial savings on a global scale.

SECTION 5: CONCLUSION, LESSONS LEARNED, AND RESEARCH CHALLENGES

The use-cases have introduced typical scenarios and have identified a number of important aspects relating to patient care and facilities / staff utilisation. Space restricts a detailed analysis however there are a number of conclusions to be drawn from the use-cases.

Hospital settings are characterised by dynamic uncertainty, which is reflected in time constraints, which may be (and frequently are) life threatening. Given that the central consideration of all healthcare systems must be the patient providing efficient, effective and informed patient care pathways is central to quality of care. ICADS systems provide an effective basis to accommodate the dynamic uncertainty inherent is a hospital setting while minimising the potential for changes in patients' treatment pathways.

It is essential for the implementation of ICADS systems that effective and unambiguous data collection and updating is realised. This demands a scalable, secure, reliable, robust, approach to data collection along with a suitable approach to context modelling in a data structure capable of storing patient data in a format that is readily accessible and updatable.

Accommodating different classes of user for a computerised patient records system is essential as doctors, nurses, auxiliary staff, management staff, and the public (patients) require differing levels of access to such a system with graduated rights and permissions. An ICADS system must provide differing visualisation of the data and results to accommodate differing classes of user and a range of devices (e.g., intelligent white boards, computer monitors, tablets, and wearable / mobile devices). The CaaS framework provides a basis for the creation of an ICADS system usable in a range of domains including the healthcare field. We have considered the growing use of CBS and the associated privacy and security imperatives that healthcare systems must address. As discussed in and in this paper the use of a hybrid cloud may provide the essential the scalability demanded in the dynamic setting while addressing the security considerations that are central to patient record keeping.

Discussion

In this chapter we have considered the challenges inherent in the creation of context-aware systems as they relate to context and its use by individuals and organisations. We have introduced CBS and CSM and have presented our new CaaS framework designed to provide the components required to enable individuals, organisations, or collaborating groups [e.g., healthcare and computing experts] can create an effective context-aware systems.

We have presented a number of illustrative scenarios to identify typical scenarios in which CaaS may be implemented. CaaS has been conceived to enable individuals and organisations that have the required domain knowledge but lack adequate computational skills to implement an ICADS system can utilise context and build a context-aware system. Similarly, computer literate individuals and organisations (who may lack domain knowledge) may use CaaS to create context-aware systems using domain knowledge incorporated in the CSM.

We have observed that context and context-aware systems are highly domain specific, thus, we view CaaS as being representative of specific domains. In this paper we have discussed e-healthcare systems in hospital and domestic settings however we view the CaaS framework [with appropriate domain knowledge] as a general framework applicable to a broad and diverse range of domains, systems and technologies. In actuality, even within a specific domain (e.g., healthcare) there will be sub-domains such as: dementia care, mental illness, post-operative care, and translational research, as such each sub-domain will require specific domain knowledge.

Challenges and Future Work

In this chapter we have presented the CaaS CSM, which is based on previously documented research into ICADS, ontological context modelling, and related data structures. While many issues have been explored there remain a number of open research questions including disambiguation of context properties and the related literal values with optimal data structure development.

While many of the hardware (sensor) challenges have been addressed in the literature, there are significant issues in implementing non-invasive data collection with associated privacy and informed consent issues. Addressing these issues and challenges forms the basis for future work however we prose the CaaS framework as a basis within which these issues and challenges can be accommodated.

REFERENCES

Abowd, G. D., Dey, A. K., Brown, P. J., Davies, N., Smith, M., & Steggles, P. (1999). Towards a better understanding of context and context-awareness. In *Proc. of the First International Symposium on Handheld and Ubiquitous Computing* (LNCS), (vol. 1707, pp. 304–307). Springer. doi:10.1007/3-540-48157-5_29

Amazon. (2014). *Amazon web services*. Retrieved July 2014 from http://aws.amazon.com

Ashford, R., Moore, P., Hu, B., Jackson, M., & Wan, J. (2010). Translational research and context in health monitoring systems. In *Proc. of the Fourth International Conference on Complex, Intelligent and Software Intensive Systems (CISIS 2010)* (pp. 81-86). Academic Press. doi:10.1109/CISIS.2010.44

Bankole, A., Anderson, M., Knight, A., Kyunghi, O., Smith-Jackson, T., & Hanson, M. A. ... Lach, J. (2011). Continuous, non-invasive assessment of agitation in dementia using inertial body sensors. In Proc. of Wireless Health 2011. Academic Press.

Berkan, C., & Trubatch, S. L. (1997). *Fuzzy systems design principles: Building fuzzy if-then rule bases*. Piscataway, NJ: IEEE Press.

Biswas, J., Jayachandran, M., Thang, P. V., Fook, V. F. S., Choo, T. S., Quiang, Q., & Lin Kiat, P. Y. et al. (2006). Agitation monitoring of persons with dementia based on acoustic sensors, pressure sensors and ultrasound sensors: A feasibility study. In W. C. Mann & A. Helal (Eds.), *Promoting independence for older persons with disabilities*. IOS Press.

Brodity, E. (1971). Excess disabilities of mentally impaired aged: Impact of individualized treatment. *The Gerontologist*, 25, 124–133.

Buettner, M., Prasad, R., Sample, A., Yeager, D., Greenstein, B., Smith, J. R., & Wetherall, D. (2008). RFID sensor networks with the Intel WISP. In *Proc. of the 6th ACM Conference on Embedded Network Sensor Systems* (pp. 393-394). ACM. doi:10.1145/1460412.1460468

Burgio, L. (1996). Direct observation of behavioral disturbances of dementia and their environmental context. *International Psychogeriatrics*, 8(S3), 343–346. doi:10.1017/S1041610297003591 PMID:9154586

Cohen-Mansfield, J., Marx, M., & Rosenthal, A. (1989). A description of agitation in a nursing home. *Journal of Gerontology*, 44(3), M77–M84. doi:10.1093/geronj/44.3.M77 PMID:2715584

Culter, N. R., & Sramek, J. J. (1966). *Understanding Alzheimer's disease: For general readers a guide to understanding a devastating illness that affects a significant segment of the elderly population*. Mississippi University Press.

Dobre, C., & Xhafa, F. (2013). Intelligent services for big data science. *Future Generation Computer Systems*. doi:10.1016/j.future.2013.07.014

Finkel, S., & Burns, A. (2000). Behavioural and psychological symptoms of dementia: A clinical and research update. *International Psychogeriatrics*, 12(1), 9–12. doi:10.1017/S1041610200006694 PMID:10798450

Finkel, S. I., Costa, E., Silva, J., Cohen, G. S. M., & Sartorius, N. (1996). Behavioural and psychological signs and symptoms of dementia. *International Psychogeriatrics*, 96(8suppl3), 497–500. PMID:9154615

Finkel, S. I., Costa e Silva, J., Cohen, G. D., Miller, S., & Sartorius, N. (1998). Behavioural and psychological symptoms of dementia: A consensus statement in current knowledge and implications for research and treatment. *The American Journal of Geriatric Psychiatry*, 6(2), 97–100.

Fitbit. (2014). *Fit health into every occasion*, Retrieved July 2014 from http://www.fitbit.com/uk

Google. (2014). *Google cloud platform: Tools for modern applications*. Retrieved July 2014 from https://cloud.google.com

Hartig, K. (2008). *What is cloud computing? The cloud is a virtualization of resources that maintains and manages itself*. SYS-CON Media.

Hewlett Packard. (2014a). Retrieved July 2014 from http://www.hpl.hp.com/news/2009/oct-dec/cense.html

Hewlett Packard. (2014b). Retrieved July 2014 from http://googlecloudplatform.blogspot.co.uk/2013/05/data-sensing-lab-at-google-io-2013.html

Jena. (2014). *Apache Jena*. Retrieved July 2014 from http://jena.apache.org/

Khazraee, M., Zamani, A., Hallajian, H., & Ehsani, S. P. Moghaddam, Parsafar, H. A., & Shabany, M. (2013). A novel hardware implementation for joint heart rate, respiration rate, and gait analysis applied to body area networks. Academic Press.

Koufi, V., Malamateniou, F., & Vassilacopoulos, G. (2010). Ubiquitous access to cloud emergency medical services. In *Proc. of the 10th IEEE International Conference on Information Technology and Applications in Biomedicine* (ITAB'10). IEEE. doi:10.1109/ITAB.2010.5687702

Lauriks, S., Reinersmann, A., van der Roest, H., Meiland, M., Davies, R. J., Moelaert, F., & Dröes, R. M. et al. (2007). Review of ICT-based services for identified unmet needs in people with dementia. *Ageing Research Reviews, 6*(3), 223–246. doi:10.1016/j.arr.2007.07.002 PMID:17869590

Mazhelis, O., Fazekas, G., & Tyrväinen, P. P. (2012). Impact of storage acquisition intervals on the cost-efficiency of the private vs. public storage. In *Proc. of the 5th IEEE International Conference on Cloud Computing* (CLOUD'12). IEEE. doi:10.1109/CLOUD.2012.101

Microsoft Azure. (2014). *The cloud for modern business*. Retrieved July 2014 from http://azure.microsoft.com/en-us/

Moore, P., Hai, V., & Pham, H. V. (2013). *Personalization and rule strategies in data intensive intelligent context-aware systems*. Cambridge University Press.

Moore, P., Hu, B., & Jackson, M. (2010). Fuzzy ECA rules for pervasive decision-centric personalized mobile learning. Studies in Computational Intelligence, 273. doi:10.1007/978-3-642-11224-9

Moore, P., Thomas, A., Tadros, G., Xhafa, F. & Barolli, L. (2013). Detection of the onset of agitation in patients with dementia: real time monitoring and the application of big–data solutions. *International Journal of Space-Based and Situated Computing*, (3), 136-154.

Moore, P., Xhafa, F., & Barolli, L. (2014). Context as a service for achieving personalisation in context-aware systems. In *Proc. of the Eighth International Conference on Complex, Intelligent, and Software Intensive Systems 2014* (CISIS-2014). Birmingham, UK: IEEE CPS.

Moore, P. T., & Sharma, M. (2103). Enhanced patient management in a hospital setting. *IT Convergence Practice, 1*(3), 1-21. Retrieved July 2014 from http://isyou.info/inpra/papers/inpra-v1n3-01.pdf

Morton, T., Weeks, A., House, S., Chiang, P., & Scaffidi, C. (2012). Location and activity tracking with the cloud. In T. Morton, A. Weeks, S. House, P. Chiang, & C. Scaffidi (Eds.), *Proc. of the 2012 Annual International Conference on IEEE Engineering in Medicine and Biology Society* (EMBC'12). San Diego, CA: IEEE. doi:10.1109/EMBC.2012.6347323

Motoi, K., Ogawa, M., & Ueno, H., Kuwae, Ikarashi, A., Yuji, H., … Yamaskoshi, K. (2009). A fully automated health-care monitoring at home without attachment of any biological sensors and its clinical evaluation. In *Proceedings of IEEE EMBS* (pp. 4323-4326). IEEE.

OpenWISP. (2014), *OpenWISP: Wireless everywhere*. Retrieved July 2014 from http://openwisp.org

Parks, R., Chu, C.-H., & Xu, H. (2011). Healthcare information privacy research: Issues, gaps and what next?. In *Proceedings of AMCIS 2011*. Retrieved July 2014 from http://aisel.aisnet.org/amcis2011_submissions/180

Peng, H., Hu, B., Liu, Q., Dong, Q., Zhao, Q., & Moore, P., P. (2011). User entered depression prevention: An EEG approach to pervasive healthcare. In *Proc. of the 5th International Conference on Pervasive Computing Technologies for Healthcare* (pp. 325-330). Academic Press.

Proteus. (2014). *Proteus digital health*. Retrieved July 2014 from http://www.proteus.com

Pugh, P. L., Richardson, J. C., Bate, S. T., Upton, N., & Sunter, S. (2007). Noncognitive behaviours in an APP/PS1 transgenic model of Alzheimer's disease. *Behavioural Brain Research*, *178*(1), 18–28. doi:10.1016/j.bbr.2006.11.044 PMID:17229472

Qiu, Q., Foo, S. F., Wai, A. A. P., Pham, T. P., Maniyeri, J., Biswas, J. J., & Yap, P. (2007). Multimodal information fusion for automated recognition of complex agitation behaviours of dementia patients. In *Proc. of the 10th International Conference on Information Fusion (Fusion 2007)*. Academic Press.

Rao, B. B. P., Saluja, P., Sharma, N., Mittal, A., & Sharma, S. V., S. V. (2012). Cloud computing for internet of things & sensing based applications. In *Proc. of the 6th International Conference on Sensing Technology* (ICST'12) (pp. 374–380). Academic Press. doi:10.1109/ICSensT.2012.6461705

Rosenblatt, A. (2005). The art of managing dementia in the elderly. *Cleveland Clinic Journal of Medicine*, *72*(3), S3–S12. doi:10.3949/ccjm.72.Suppl_3.S3 PMID:16265939

Sotomayor, B., Montero, R. S., Llorente, I. M., & Foster, I. (2009). Virtual infrastructure management in private and hybrid clouds. *IEEE Internet Computing*, *13*(5), 14–22. doi:10.1109/MIC.2009.119

Terzo, O., Ruiu, P., Bucci, E., & Xhafa, F. (2013). Data as a service (DaaS) for sharing and processing of large data collections in the cloud. In *Proc. of Seventh International Conference on Complex, Intelligent, and Software Intensive Systems* (CISIS 2013) (pp. 475-480). IEEE CPS. doi:10.1109/CISIS.2013.87

Thomas, A., Parkinson, J., Moore, P., Goodman, A., Xhafa, F., & Barolli, L. (2013a) Nudging through technology: Ethical choice architectures and the mobile information revolution. In *Proc. of The 8th International Conference on P2P, Parallel, Grid, Cloud and Internet Computing* (3PGCIC'13). IEEE CPS.

Thomas, A. M., Moore, P., Shah, H., Evans, C., Sharma, M., Xhafa, F., & Chima, P. et al. (2013). Smart care spaces: Needs for intelligent at-home care. *International Journal of Space-Based and Situated Computing*, *3*(1), 35–44. doi:10.1504/IJSSC.2013.051988

Vickland, V., & Brodaty, H., H. (2008). Visualisation of clinical and non-clinical characteristics of patients with behavioural and psychological symptoms of dementia. In *Proc. of the 5th International Conference BioMedical Visualization: Information Visualization in Medical and Biomedical Informatics* (pp. 23-28). Academic Press. doi:10.1109/MediVis.2008.20

W3C. (2014). *Semantic web activity*. Retrieved July 2014 from http://www.w3.org/2001/sw/

Wyld, D. C. (2009). The utility of cloud computing as a new pricing-and consumption-model for information technology. *International Journal of Database Management Systems*, *1*(1), 1–20.

Xhafa, F., Li, J., Zhao, G., Jin Li, J., Chen, X., Duncan, S., & Wong, S. D. (2014). Designing cloud-based electronic health record system with attribute-based encryption. *Multimedia Tools and Applications, Springer*. doi:10.1007/s11042-013-1829-6

Xhafa, F., Wang, J., Chen, X., & Joseph, K. (2014). An efficient PHR Service system supporting fuzzy keyword search and fine-grained access control. *Soft Computing*.

Zigbee. (2014). *Zigbee alliance*. Retrieved July 2014 from https://www.zigbee.org

Zorpette, G. G. (2014). Electronic tattoos for baby and you. *IEEE Spectrum*. Retrieved July 2014 from http://news.discovery.com/tech/biotechnology/electronic-tattoos-for-baby-and-you-140311.htm

KEY TERMS AND DEFINITIONS

Alzheimer's Disease and Related Disorders (ADRD): A term that describes Alzheimer's disease or related dementia where patients are susceptible to excess disability. This relates to a discrepancy that exists when a person's functional incapacity is greater than that warranted by the actual impairment (Brodity, 1971).

Behavioural and Psychological Symptoms in Dementia (BPSD): An umbrella term that embraces a heterogeneous group of non-cognitive symptoms and behaviours that occur in people with dementia.

Cloud-Based Systems (CBS): Refers to applications, services or resources made available to users on demand via the Internet from a cloud computing provider's servers. CBS is seen an important way to increase capacity, enhance functionality or add additional services on demand without having to execute potentially expensive infrastructure costs.

eHealth (Electronic Health): The use of computer systems and telecommunications networks to improve the processes involved in medicine, both for diagnosis and relationship between professionals and users.

Independent Assisted Living (IAL): A housing facility for people with disabilities, which provides supervision or assistance with activities of daily living (ADLs); coordination of services by outside health care providers; and monitoring of resident activities to help to ensure their health, safety, and well-being.

Infrastructure-as-a-Service (IaaS), Platform-as-a-Service (PaaS), Software-as-a-Service (SaaS), Data-as-a-Service (DaaS): Mainstreaming Cloud Service Models.

Intelligent Context-Aware Decision Support (ICADS): In health domain, systems that provide an effective basis for the re-scheduling of the essential services that combine to provide the treatment pathway.

MCI (Mild Cognitive Impairments): Sensorial or memory slight failures, usually associated to initial stages of dementia and mental or cognitive diseases.

Quality of Life (QoL): The general well-being of individuals and societies in a wide range of contexts, especially in the field of healthcare.

Remote Electronic Health Monitoring (REHM): A technology to enable monitoring of patients outside of conventional clinical settings (e.g. in the home), which may increase access to care and decrease healthcare delivery costs.

This work was previously published in Advanced Technological Solutions for E-Health and Dementia Patient Monitoring edited by Fatos Xhafa, Philip Moore, and George Tadros, pages 211-237 copyright year 2015 by Medical Information Science Reference (an imprint of IGI Global).

Chapter 29
An Android Mobile–Based Environmental Health Information Source for Malaysian Context

Lau Tiu Chung
Swinburne University of Technology – Sarawak, Malaysia

Lau Bee Theng
Swinburne University of Technology – Sarawak, Malaysia

H. Lee Seldon
Multimedia University, Malaysia

ABSTRACT

An anticipated research activity in healthcare is the involvement of populations and social media to identify health problems, including environmental ones. In this chapter, the authors propose an Android mobile-based system for collection and targeted distribution of the latest alerts and real-time environmental factors to the Malaysian population. This mobile system is designed to facilitate and encourage research into environmental health quality issues by providing a comprehensive tracking and monitoring tool correlated to social media networks. This system is embedded with Google Maps and Geocoding services to visualize the location and environmental health reports from the aggregated social media news feeds; the output is also shared across the social media networks.

INTRODUCTION

Social media networks help in creating big impact and public awareness toward environmental health tracking and monitoring. Tracking disease through online activity has been done before; Google found that search terms were good indicators of flu activity in 2008 and 2009 (Lowensohn, 2008; Google, 2012). Later Google introduced public estimation for flu activity through Google flu tracking system. Unlike basic internet searches from traditional search engines like Google or

DOI: 10.4018/978-1-4666-8756-1.ch029

Yahoo, social media networks seem to have introduced crowd-sharing and posting information across the given platforms. "Traditional" search requests are generally motivated only by a desire to learn more about given subject, such as infectious disease and healthcare topics, but social media networks seem to be motivated by the desire to gain more popularity by doing what one's friends do. For example, if haze is forming near one's living location, the person can easily make a short written post on Facebook or Twitter, so the short written post can ideally "go viral" and be exposed to others in the social media network. In other words, social media networks inherently explore more contexts to the individual's situation surrounding them. For someone who reads and writes a lot about the environment, Twitter and Facebook provide a great way to keep track of what others in the same field are working on.

Social media network is nowadays inseparable from Mobile. With smart phone usage projected to grow exponentially across the region, and with mobile data speeds increasing, and with the roll-out of wireless internet services and social media networks improving their mobile offering, social networking is becoming more mobile-oriented by nature (Firefly, 2012). There is no denying that the growth of social networking cannot be separated from increasing mobility, and will only be fuelled further by the advance of the smart phone in consumer's lives. So does the growth of the smart phone and increased mobility signify a new phase or dimension for social media? These situations imply and drive mobile users' behavior towards the way they receive environmental health information.

In this research, the establishment of an Android mobile-based environmental health information system associated with social media networks will play a key role in helping to provide the information needed to ideally improve public health. This paper presents several study areas such as environmental health tracking, the use of social media networks in tracking diseases, the social media network in RSS, and the use of mobile health technologies in Malaysia. Besides, it also includes the proposed solutions such as multi-tier architecture that used in developing Android mobile applications, word level n-gram approach used to match social media text inputs against a dictionary of known patterns, integrated environmental health ontological model in Malaysian context adopted in Android mobile-based environmental health information system, and the evaluation of system accuracy testing results.

BACKGROUND

In the past, many environmental health issues were not delivered to the public efficiently. The print and television press often did not headline environmental news. The mobile technologies revolution in the late 1990s mostly served the purpose of providing voice communication over the phone. People were passive consumers of news reports about environmental health hazards, seldom ones which could affect their own health.

In the early 2000s several studies of environmental health tracking tools were established with a main goal: to protect communities by providing federal, state, and local agencies with information they could use to plan, apply and evaluate environmental health actions (California Environmental Health Investigation Branch, 2012; Center for Disease Control and Prevention, 2010; European Environment Agency, 2011; Freifeld & Brownstein, 2007; Wisconsin Department of Health Services, 2011). While existing environmental health surveillance systems have been proven to serve as an effective mode for spreading health information to their respective users, the idea of "borderless" information dissemination should be also considered.

The Rise of Environmental Health Tracking

Environmental health tracking is the on-going, systematic collection, integration, analysis, interpretation, and dissemination of data from monitoring of environmental hazards and health effects (California Environmental Health Investigation Branch, 2012; Center for Disease Control and Prevention, 2012; HealthMap, 2012; New York Department of Health, 2009).The component parts of environmental health tracking are hazard identification and mapping, exposure assessment and quantification, development of biomonitoring, systematic review of health outcomes and disease surveillance, horizon scanning, and development of environment and health indicators (Health Protection Agency, 2012).

Environmental health tracking serves to protect the health of people by monitoring environmental contaminants and their related diseases, study the impact of these contaminants on human health, and inform the public about how to best protect their health from harmful pollutants (California Environmental Health Investigation Branch, 2012). It is interesting to know that checking the weather forecast every morning may help one with more than just deciding which clothes to wear; it may help one to prepare for how one feels that day, health wise. Weather forecasts may show a high level of humidity which may lead to headache or acne in certain people if they do not prepare themselves in advance. In this particular research context, environmental health tracking is a type of surveillance that endeavours to bring together specific health and environmental monitoring data in Malaysia from a number of different online media news.

The Use of Social Media Networks in Tracking Diseases

Social media has been widely used to predict some desirable results such as weekend box office takings for movies and elections (Taylor, 2013).

However, a social media network in tracking disease raised curiosity and attention in public and health officials. Many serious researchers are becoming more interested in the reliability of social media in delivering quality health messages to the public (Avnet, 2013). According to Schmidt (2012), traditional flu surveillance by the Center for Disease Control and prevention (CDC) relies on outpatient reporting and virological test results supplied by laboratories nationwide. However, the system confirms outbreaks within about two weeks after they begin, but social media can flag more immediate concerns and actions. Tweets with location information may allow officials to plot points on a map to detect a trend, then alert providers to gear up for a possible outbreak (Bautista, 2013). Besides, the use of Twitter to track levels of disease activity and public concern in the U.S. during the Influenza A H1N1 pandemic in 2009 by several researchers has demonstrated that Twitter traffic can be used not only descriptively, i.e. to track users' interests and concerns related to H1N1 influenza, but also to estimate disease activity in real time, i.e., one to two weeks faster than current practice allows. According to Taylor (2013), 250,000 social media users in U.S said they got the flu. To make use of Twitter as a source of collecting environmental health data can be very impressive due to volume and speed. One interesting statistic is that 87.9% of Malaysians has internet access via Facebook (Factbroser.com, 2012), Another fact is that Malaysia's mobile penetration is more than 100%, compared to 59% for internet and 41% for social media (Factbroser.com, 2012).

Social Media Network in RSS

Social media networks are becoming great tools for tapping into news and conversations about issues critical to the environment, both from public health and healthcare agencies (Chunara, Andrews, & Brownstein, 2012). Recently it has been suggested that the existing real-time platforms such as Facebook (Facebook, 2012)

Figure 1. Twitter user name

```
← → C  🔒 Twitter, Inc. [US] https://twitter.com/statuses/user_timeline/healthmap.rss                    ☆ O

<?xml version="1.0" encoding="UTF-8"?>
<rss xmlns:atom="http://www.w3.org/2005/Atom" xmlns:georss="http://www.georss.org/georss" xmlns:twitter="http://api.twitter.com" version="2.0">
  <channel>
    <title>Twitter / healthmap</title>
    <link>http://twitter.com/healthmap</link>
    <atom:link type="application/rss+xml" rel="self" href="https://twitter.com/statuses/user_timeline/healthmap.rss"/>
    <description>Twitter updates from HealthMap.org / healthmap.</description>
    <language>en-us</language>
    <ttl>40</ttl>
    <item>
      <title>healthmap: RT @WHOAFRO: Ministry of Health #Uganda has reported a cumulative number of 59 suspected cases of #Ebola including 16 deaths</title>
      <description>healthmap: RT @WHOAFRO: Ministry of Health #Uganda has reported a cumulative number of 59 suspected cases of #Ebola including 16 deaths</description>
      <pubDate>Mon, 06 Aug 2012 20:28:48 +0000</pubDate>
      <guid>http://twitter.com/healthmap/statuses/232573963321085952</guid>
      <link>http://twitter.com/healthmap/statuses/232573963321085952</link>
      <twitter:source>&lt;a href=&quot;http://twitter.com/download/iphone&quot; rel=&quot;nofollow&quot;&gt;Twitter for iPhone&lt;/a&gt;</twitter:source>
      <twitter:place/>
    </item>
    <item>
      <title>healthmap: #DiseaseDaily New Study Finds Rabies May Not Always Be Fatal http://t.co/XyRoOWmw #HealthMap</title>
      <description>healthmap: #DiseaseDaily New Study Finds Rabies May Not Always Be Fatal http://t.co/XyRoOWmw #HealthMap</description>
      <pubDate>Mon, 06 Aug 2012 18:59:09 +0000</pubDate>
      <guid>http://twitter.com/healthmap/statuses/232551401270689792</guid>
      <link>http://twitter.com/healthmap/statuses/232551401270689792</link>
      <twitter:source>&lt;a href=&quot;http://twitterfeed.com&quot; rel=&quot;nofollow&quot;&gt;twitterfeed&lt;/a&gt;</twitter:source>
      <twitter:place/>
    </item>
    <item>
      <title>healthmap: #DiseaseDaily Latest on Ebola, Aug. 6 2012, 12h: Two Suspected Cases in Tanzania, WHO Update for Uganda http://t.co/jOddjXW7 #HealthMap</title>
      <description>healthmap: #DiseaseDaily Latest on Ebola, Aug. 6 2012, 12h: Two Suspected Cases in Tanzania, WHO Update for Uganda http://t.co/jOddjXW7
#HealthMap</description>
```

and Twitter (Twitter, 2012) can be used as main sources to improve public health. Social media is a great choice of data input because of the simple structure of their reports – RSS feed. Every news feed may consist of the following details:

1. **The Title:** It describes the main topic of the news report.
2. **The Published Date:** It describes the date when the news is released.
3. **URL:** It describes where the online report is located on the web server.
4. **Description:** It describes the content of the news report.
5. **Address:** It describes either the news report published location or incident reported location.

RSS feed eases data collection as one can track down the user post through Twitter/Facebook user account timeline. There are two ways to access Twitter RSS feeds: through user id or user name. Both create the same outcome, in XML format. For example, a Twitter user name can be written in https://Twitter.com/statuses/user_timeline/healthmap.rssor while a Twitter user id can be written in https://Twitter.com/statuses/user_timeline/20149254.rss (Woodfin, 2011). Figure 1 shows an example of twitter user name while Figure 2 shows an example of twitter user ID.

Figure 1 and Figure 2 show twitter's information format that is encoded in plain view or can be described as XML document. XML contains markup symbols to describe the contents of a page that allow processing by RSS feed reader. Many application programming interfaces (APIs) such as Twitter and Facebook have been developed to aid RSS feed reader with processing XML data. The rise of "Web 2.0" technologies (O'Reilly, 2005) including the proliferation of Really Simple Syndication (RSS) (Cayzer, 2004) and Asynchronous JavaScript and XML (AJAX) (Garrett, 2005) make the process of data collection simple. All these RSS feeds, regardless from Twitter or Facebook, are structured in XML. With given the RSS feed, it allows many automated mechanisms such as RSS readers to retrieve the information from the given site URL.

The Use of Mobile Health Technologies in Malaysia

According to Vodafone (2012), cost-effective and easy-to-deploy mobile devices, with their ability to quickly capture and transmit data on disease

Figure 2. Twitter user ID

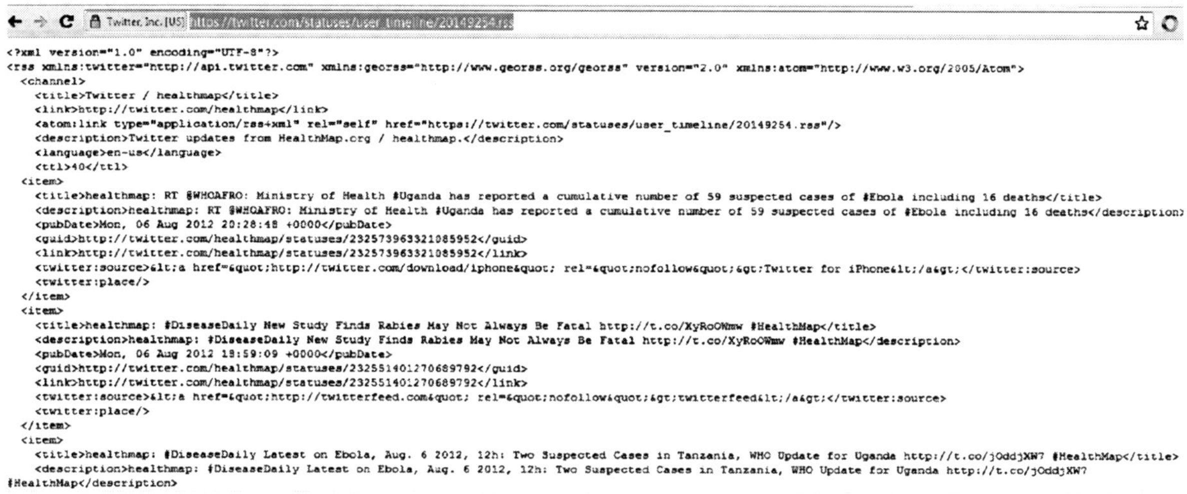

```
<?xml version="1.0" encoding="UTF-8"?>
<rss xmlns:twitter="http://api.twitter.com" xmlns:georss="http://www.georss.org/georss" version="2.0" xmlns:atom="http://www.w3.org/2005/Atom">
  <channel>
    <title>Twitter / healthmap</title>
    <link>http://twitter.com/healthmap</link>
    <atom:link type="application/rss+xml" rel="self" href="https://twitter.com/statuses/user_timeline/20149254.rss"/>
    <description>Twitter updates from HealthMap.org / healthmap.</description>
    <language>en-us</language>
    <ttl>40</ttl>
  <item>
    <title>healthmap: RT @WHOAFRO: Ministry of Health #Uganda has reported a cumulative number of 59 suspected cases of #Ebola including 16 deaths</title>
    <description>healthmap: RT @WHOAFRO: Ministry of Health #Uganda has reported a cumulative number of 59 suspected cases of #Ebola including 16 deaths</description>
    <pubDate>Mon, 06 Aug 2012 20:28:48 +0000</pubDate>
    <guid>http://twitter.com/healthmap/statuses/232573963321085952</guid>
    <link>http://twitter.com/healthmap/statuses/232573963321085952</link>
    <twitter:source>&lt;a href=&quot;http://twitter.com/download/iphone&quot; rel=&quot;nofollow&quot;&gt;Twitter for iPhone&lt;/a&gt;</twitter:source>
    <twitter:place/>
  </item>
  <item>
    <title>healthmap: #DiseaseDaily New Study Finds Rabies May Not Always Be Fatal http://t.co/XyRoOWmw #HealthMap</title>
    <description>healthmap: #DiseaseDaily New Study Finds Rabies May Not Always Be Fatal http://t.co/XyRoOWmw #HealthMap</description>
    <pubDate>Mon, 06 Aug 2012 18:59:09 +0000</pubDate>
    <guid>http://twitter.com/healthmap/statuses/232551401270689792</guid>
    <link>http://twitter.com/healthmap/statuses/232551401270689792</link>
    <twitter:source>&lt;a href=&quot;http://twitterfeed.com&quot; rel=&quot;nofollow&quot;&gt;twitterfeed&lt;/a&gt;</twitter:source>
    <twitter:place/>
  </item>
  <item>
    <title>healthmap: #DiseaseDaily Latest on Ebola, Aug. 6 2012, 12h: Two Suspected Cases in Tanzania, WHO Update for Uganda http://t.co/jOddjXW7 #HealthMap</title>
    <description>healthmap: #DiseaseDaily Latest on Ebola, Aug. 6 2012, 12h: Two Suspected Cases in Tanzania, WHO Update for Uganda http://t.co/jOddjXW7
#HealthMap</description>
```

incidence, can be decisive in the prevention and containment of outbreaks. With the right information and effective monitoring of both social media networks and environmental health issues, mobile health technologies are supporting effective environmental health tracking and enabling the identification of health trends. This literally allows governments and health authorities to allocate resources more effectively and, if required, adapt the programme and policies in place to manage emergency.

In Malaysia the internet digital divide limited the reach of computerized health behavior interventions for lower socioeconomic groups for years, if not decades. In contrast, mobile phone use has been rapidly and widely adopted among virtually all demographic groups. Malaysia has 34 million mobile subscribers and 17.5 million internet users (Factbrowser.com, 2012) in a population of about 27 million. Mobile health technologies are not unfamiliar in Malaysia as people begin to appreciate having health information at their fingertip. Malaysian Ministry of Health initiated myHealth application which provides information on Malaysia's healthcare system from health facilities, and the list of registered practitioners to registered medical products (Ministry of Health,

2013). Some other mobile applications such as Sime Darby Healthcare (Sime Darby Healthcare, 2013) provide free service to mobile users to book doctor appointments (at Sime Darby facilities). Malaysia telecommunication service providers such as Celcom (Celcom, 2013) and Maxis (Maxis, 2012) are also participating in innovative mobile healthcare solutions to dispense medical services more efficiently. Again, the question is: "Can environmental health surveillance systems be merged into mobile health technologies (in Malaysia)?"

RESEARCH PROBLEMS

There are some state-wide or regional health effect registries or surveillance systems that contain data of sufficient completeness, timeliness and quality to allow reporting of valid estimates of health effect prevalence, incidence, or mortality for a population, namely, CDC, HealthMap, Air pollutant index management system, Wisconsin Environmental Public Health Tracking, Air pollution monitoring system, California Environmental Health Tracking Program (Brownstein & Freifeld, 2007; California Environmental Health Investigation Branch, 2012; Center for Disease Control and Prevention, 2010; European Environment Agency, 2011; Wisconsin Department of Health Services, 2011;). Although real-time environmental health surveillance system is a promising area in improving public health, little attention has been paid to the use of the social media networks as sources of data input and real time collaboration. Besides, social media network is rife with real-time data that can help public users quickly anticipate demand for environmental health data, health services and prevention. Therefore, an environmental health information system was developed by embedding an integrated ontological model to serve as dictionary of pattern to attract data sources from social media networks and vice versa.

The environmental health data often comes in different data formats for different reasons by different environmental health tracking and monitoring systems (California Environmental Health Investigation branch, 2012). For example, some environmental health agencies such as healthcare providers are not required to report asthma-related office visits to the state. Hospital data are collected for the purpose of tracking health care quality, rather than for public health surveillance (California Environmental Health Investigation branch, 2012). Traditional environmental health surveillance systems do not collect data input from social media networks (Schmidt, 2012).

More than ever, people use social media networks to learn about what is happening in the world, and the traditional news outlets become increasingly less relevant to the digital generation (Laird, 2012). Some environmental health surveillance systems were not made accessible to the public, and the surveillance data are also not explicitly interpretable by public users, which can make it difficult for the public audiences to use. Most of the environmental health surveillance systems included only selected location in their systems to keep track on event location and this may become cumbersome without an ideal

channel to keep track the location (World Health Organization, 2008). In this research, it is proposed that with social media, it would be much easier to determine the true location of outbreaks.

Some of the surveillance systems have low adaptability to different electronic devices such mobile-based device (Robertson, et al, 2010). This reduces the accessibility of the public users to the environmental health surveillance systems for quick update and response. Some of the environmental health surveillance systems are not operated in real-time to deliver outbreak reports (Lemon, et al., 2007). Non-real-time reporting of environmental health is referred as batch reporting.

The data inputs are given by their own selected healthcare agencies, collaborative programs and partnerships, and it sometimes take weeks to process, filter, summarize and store them in the database before they can be released to the public. Despite a common interest in monitoring the impact of environmental health, due to the wide variety of environmental health issues existing everywhere in the world, researchers could only track a fraction of the environmental health issues (California Environmental Health Investigation branch, 2012), usually covering only the most emergent environmental health issues in their own countries – this is also referred to as categorical surveillance (Nsubuga, et al, 2006). Some systems do only "passive surveillance" (Center for Disease Control and Prevention 2011), i.e. only receive reports submitted from hospitals, clinics, public health units, or other sources (Nsubuga, et al., 2006).

With the supporting evidence, the research problems have been identified and we aim to develop a comprehensive Android mobile-based and real-time environmental health information source to achieve the goals and are committed to taking personal responsibility to manage and mitigate the impacts of their corporate, professional and daily living activities on the environment.

System Architecture and Methods

As social media is exploding, the networking activities do not end when one leaves the computer. Thus people can update it and get themselves updated by their mobile phones now. Various social media applications are available for all varieties of smart phones These make it easy to stay connected and share information with friends within minutes. However, accessing large portions of user's timeline data without proper filter and classification can be tedious. Android mobile-based application of environmental health information source is proposed in this research. The proposed solution involves several study areas:

- Multi-tier architecture (also known as N-tier approach) (Jain, Dahlin & Tewari, 2005) as a classifier to identify location and Environmental Health Data from social media networks,
- Word-level N-gram approach (BodHuin & Totorella, 2003; Caynar & Trenkle, 1994) to be used as matching inputs against a known patterns dictionary (Environmental health ontological model),
- Android mobile application has to be designed, developed and installed in Android mobile (Android, 2012),
- Selected social media networks such as Facebook and Twitter are being used as target sources of inputs and sharing of outputs,
- Integrated environmental health ontological model in Malaysian context by various existing environmental health surveillance systems/ontological models.

The main purpose of this research is to provide an Android application that allows public users to access the desired environmental health data. The benefit of social media networks is they provide RSS feed just like the services widgets given by the online media news. This RSS feed eases data collection as it can track down the user post through Twitter/Facebook user account timeline. In return, the RSS feed can be shared across other social media networks.

The development of real-time environmental health source emphasizes collecting and disseminating reliable environmental health events to public population whenever there is internet connectivity, computers and smartphones in order to display the data. Since the early 1990s, the Geographical Information System (GIS) has grown substantially, and it was later adopted in the public health sector (Richards et al, 1999), especially epidemiologic studies (Zhang et al., 2009). Environmental Wellness/Environmental Health model plays an essential role as an indicator and to develop a holistic ontological model in aggregating the data from Social Media networks.

Proposed Ontological Model

A proposed ontological model is an integrated environmental health model from existing diseases surveillance systems, environmental health surveillance systems and environmental health ontological models presented by various vendors and researchers. The integration process of proposed ontological model development involves three stages:

In stage 1, develop priority environmental health issues in Malaysian context through literature review and observation of Malaysian-based environmental health-related systems such Air Pollutant Index Management System (APIMS). The literature review indicated various types of environmental health issues and potential health effects covered in different countries. The uncountable types of environmental health issues made it hard to identify them in detail. The most efficient way is to rely on the reliable publications to determine the priority environment health issues in Malaysia. Then the information was used to develop the most appropriate direction and flexible ontological model for environmental health issues in Malaysia without making tricky and tedious work on the model's structure. Stage 1 aims to determine the primary scope of environmental health topics in Malaysia and later the keywords will be extracted and compared with other existing environmental health surveillance system and ontological models in stage 2. For example, many studies (CIA World Factbook, 2012; Department of Environment, 2009; Ministry of Health Malaysia, 2007; Mokhtar & Murad, 2010; WHO, 2005) mentioned "infectious diseases", "air pollution", and "water pollution" as the most critical environmental health issues, therefore these keywords will be collected in a new proposed ontological model in Malaysian context. Table 1 shows a proposed environmental health ontological model that covers major topics in Malaysia. Precisely, it is a summary of environmental health topics from several publications such as Malaysia environmental health country profile (WHO, 2005), Malaysia environmental quality report (Department of Environment, 2009), Issue and framework of environmental health in Malaysia (Mokhtar & Murad, 2010), CIA World Factbook (CIA World Factbook, 2012), and Communicable disease control information system (Ministry of Health Malaysia, 2007).

In Table 1, the left column indicates the major environmental health topics or dimensions while the right column indicates their attributes or properties. The attributes or properties refer to dimension's sub-indicator. For example, sulphur dioxide (SO_2) is part of air pollution topic. All these keywords are gathered and taken from the above mentioned publications (CIA World Factbook, 2012; Department of Environment, 2009; ; Ministry of Health Malaysia, 2007; Mokhtar & Murad, 2010; WHO, 2005;). It is essential to know that the stage 1 only illustrates the environmental health issues covered in Malaysia; however, it is the core work of the ontological model.

In stage 2, integrate with other six environmental health surveillance systems and two environmental health ontological models such as National Environmental Public Health Tracking Networks by CDC (Center for Disease Control and Prevention, 2012), Malaysia Air Pollutant Index Management System (Department of Environment, 2011), California Environmental Health Tracking Program (California Environmental Health Investigation Branch, 2012), Wisconsin Environmental Public Health Tracking (Wisconsin Department of Health Services, 2011), Environmental Health Monitoring System (European Environment Agency, 2011), HealthMap (2012), MedlinePlus Health (n.d), and CRISP Thesaurus (2006). This task aims to collect alternative keywords described in other existing surveillance systems and ontological models. The alternative keywords are also referred as indicators or information objects (Center for Disease Control and Prevention, 2012). The integration process removes duplicate keywords and adds new keywords from various existing environmental health surveillance systems and ontological models. For example, "air" can be also named as "air pollutant", "air quality" or "air pollution". Table 2 shows identified alternate keywords for two environmental health dimension (Air pollution and Water pollution) from various ontological models listed.

Table 2 shows the "air pollution" and "water pollution" are alternate main keywords in various ontological models/surveillance systems. The left column represents the alternate keywords used by other surveillance systems/ontological models while the right column indicates the vendors' names. In this research, it is assumed that the more alternative keywords collected from other surveillance systems and ontological models, the higher chances for the new proposed ontological model to meet the keyword expectation from social media. In this case, "air quality", "air" and "air pollutant" are discarded. The keyword "air quality" is likely to indicate measurement of air pollutant index, therefore it is more suitable to be used as supporting keywords. The keyword "air" is likely to be vague when the ontological needs narrow the definition. The keyword "air

Table 1. Proposed environmental health ontological model

Environmental Health Dimensions	Attributes or Properties
air pollution	Sulphur dioxide (SO2), Carbon Monoxide (CO), Nitrogen Dioxide (NO2), Lead (Pb), Particulate Matter (PM10 and PM2.5), Ozone (O3)/ Ozone depletion, Air Pollution Index (API)/ Air Quality Index (AQI), Open burning, Haze, General air pollution, Industrial waste, smog
Water pollution	Biochemical Oxygen Demand (BOD), sewerage, Daily waste, ammonia, River water pollution, Marine ecosystem issue, Chemical organic demand
Soil pollution	Pesticide
Environmental Radiation	Radioactive waste
Noise pollution	*None*
Climate Change	Carbon Monoxide Co2
Deforestation	Illegal logging
Infectious Diseases	Cancroids, Cholera, Dengue fever (DF) & Dengue Hemorrhagic Fever (DHF), Diphtheria, Dysenteries, Ebola, Food Poisoning, Gonoccocal Infection, Leprosy, Malaria, Measles, Myocarditis, Plague, Poliomyelitis, Rabies, Relapsing Fever, Syphilis, Tetanus, Tuberculosis, Typhus & Other Rickettsioses, Typhoid & Paratyphoid Fevers, Viral Encephalitis, Viral Hepatitis, Whooping Cough, Yellow Fever, Any other life Threatening Microbial Infection, HIV infection
Occupational Health	Coordination of occupation health agencies
Road Safety	*None*
Traffic crashes	*None*
Cross cutting issues	Health care waste
Solid waste	*None*
Toxic, Chemical and Hazardous wastes	*None*
Death and Effects of warmer temperatures	Airborne, food-borne, waterborne, Insect/mosquito-borne infections,
Biodiversity	Number of species, Diverse, Genetic, Organism, Community, Ecosystem level, Loss of Biodiversity
Afforestation	*None*
Bio-indicators	*None*
Biomass	*None*
Dichloro-diphenyl-trichloro-ethane (DDT)	*None*
Ecosystem	Complex communities of organism and their specific environments
Endangered Species	*None*
Inuit Circumpolar Conference (ICC)	Long-range transport of pollutants, Sustainable development, Climate change
Noxious substances	*None*
Overgrazing	*None*
Ozone Shield	*None*
Poaching	*None*
Ultraviolet radiation (UV)	*None*
Water-borne disease	*None*

Table 2. Identified alternate keywords for air and water from various ontological models

Alternate Keywords Used	Existing Ontological Models/Surveillance Systems
Air Quality	National Environmental Public Health Tracking Networks by CDC
	Malaysia Air Pollutant Index Management System
Air	California Environmental Health Tracking Program
Air Pollutant	Wisconsin Environmental Public Health Tracking
Air pollution	CRISP Thesaurus, 2006
	Environmental Health Monitoring System by European Environment Agency
Water Pollution	MedlinePlus Health
	CRISP Thesaurus, 2006
Community Water	National Environmental Public Health Tracking Networks by CDC
Well Water	National Environmental Public Health Tracking Networks by CDC
Drinking Water	California Environmental Health Tracking Program
	Wisconsin Environmental Public Health Tracking
Water	Environmental Health Monitoring System by European Environment Agency

pollution" and "air pollutant" show different vocabularies but the same context. However, social media networks are used to decide which keyword can attract more results by constructing a query in the search field. The keyword "air pollution" was chosen as an appropriate keyword in the proposed ontological model rather than the keyword "air pollutant" as it has a higher rank of results than others. Besides, the keywords "community water", "well water", "drinking water" and "water" would be discarded because these words lack strong context to represent the issue of water. However, they are rather suitable to be sorted in the category of supporting keywords. Fuzzy keywords may attract irrelevant news from social media networks. Lastly, the keyword "water pollution" was chosen as the appropriate keyword in the new proposed ontological model.

In stage 3, while integrating with other environmental health surveillance systems and two environmental health ontological models, the next task is define the level of indicators and continue to search for second level of alternative keywords and indicators. For example, under the main indicator – air pollution -- there are various sub-issues related to air pollution such "lead poisoning", "passive smoking" and "energy sector air pollution". Alternative keywords for "lead poisoning" are "heavy metal lead", "lead" or "lead emissions" in other surveillance systems and ontological models.

Table 3 shows the identification of attributes or properties of environmental health dimensions from various ontological models/surveillance systems were sorted in "Air pollution" and "Water pollution". In this case, the duplicated keywords would be appropriately removed while the new keywords would be added into the proposed ontological model. Apart from general water issues mentioned by MedlinePlus Health, CRIPS Thesaurus, and Environmental Health Monitoring system by European environment agency, other ontological models/surveillance systems included relevant keywords that may help to form an ontological model in Malaysian context.

After the development of the proposed ontological model in Malaysian context, this new environmental health ontological model will serve as a known pattern dictionary in matching the input from social media by using word-level N-gram approach (BodHuin & Totorella 2003; Caynar & Trenkle 1994). In this research, there are 24 main indicators and 412 secondary indicators. It is worth to take note that keywords discovery and integration from stage 1 to stage 3 aimed to develop a suitable ontological model in Malaysian context before accuracy testing in part 1 and part 2. And this will be discussed in a later section.

Table 3. Attributes identification of environmental health dimension

Environmental Health Dimensions	Environmental Hazards, Exposures and Health
Air Pollution	Ozone, Particulate Matter 2.5, Arsenic, Haloacetic Acid, Nitrates, Trihalomethane (*Source: Wisconsin Environmental Health Tracking Program*)
	Carbon Monoxide, Dust, Engine Exhaust, passive smoking (*Source: CRISP Thesaurus, 2006*)
	Annual PM 2.5 Level (Monitor + Modeled), Annual PM 2.5 Level (Monitor only), Ozone Days above regulatory standard (Monitor + Modeled), Ozone Days above regulatory standard (Monitor only), PM2.5 - Days above regulatory standard (Monitor + Modeled), PM2.5 - Days above regulatory standard (Monitor only) (*Source: National Environmental Public Health Tracking Networks*)
	Habuk Halus (PM10), Sulfur Dioksida (SO2), Nitrogen Dioksida (NO2), Ozon (O3), Karbon Monoksida (CO) (*Source: Malaysia Air Pollutant Index Management System (APIMS)*)
	exposure to PM2.5, exposure to PM10, exposure to ozone, exposure to traffic pollution (*Source: California Environmental Health Tracking Program*)
Water Pollution	Arsenic, Disinfection Byproducts, Public water use, Domestic well water use, Levels of Contaminants in Domestic (self-supplied) well water (*Source: National Environmental Public Health Tracking Networks by CDC* and *California Environmental Health Tracking Program*)
	Nitrate Levels in Drinking Water (*Source: California Environmental Health Tracking Program*)
	Arsenic, Haloacetic Acid, Nitrates, Trihalomethane (*Source: Wisconsin Environmental Public Health Tracking*)
	General Water issues
	(*Source: MedlinePlus Health, CRISP Thesaurus, 2006, Environmental Health Monitoring System by European Environment Agency*

Software Architecture

Figure 3 briefly illustrates the overview of the (Malaysian) Environmental Health Monitoring and tracking System, also named MyEHMS, that allows public access to monitor the trends, impacts, links, and effects in a national baseline tracking network for environmental health. This system is embedded with customized Google Maps in order to visualize the location and deliver the early warnings of critical environmental health threats. Public users (Social media users) would be able to join the responsive feedback discussion, search for particular environmental health events, share the events through social network, and submit any critical environmental health threat which is not located in the system.

In Process, this level is where it handles *user request from Web Frontend, data acquisition from news feed sources*, and *text classifications*. The request from user is received and converted into a database query. The database then returns the alarm reports that match these queries. The query results are displayed on Google Map with built-in markers.

Data acquisition allocates data from News Feed Source based on several criteria. In general, the system identifies and converts each source of news feed into a standard report format, containing five main fields: title, link, description, location, and date. The title is the report title, link is the URL, location is the specific position in physical place, date is the date of issue of the report, and description is a brief summary of the report. The parsing process involves extracting the elements from the documents that are useful. For instance, with Star Online News, the system extracts the parts according to the five main fields and removes the rest of the original publication. The Classification engine decides the primary locations and environmental data (exposure, hazard, and health) associated with each report acquired from web sources.

Figure 3. The architecture of proposed environmental health information system

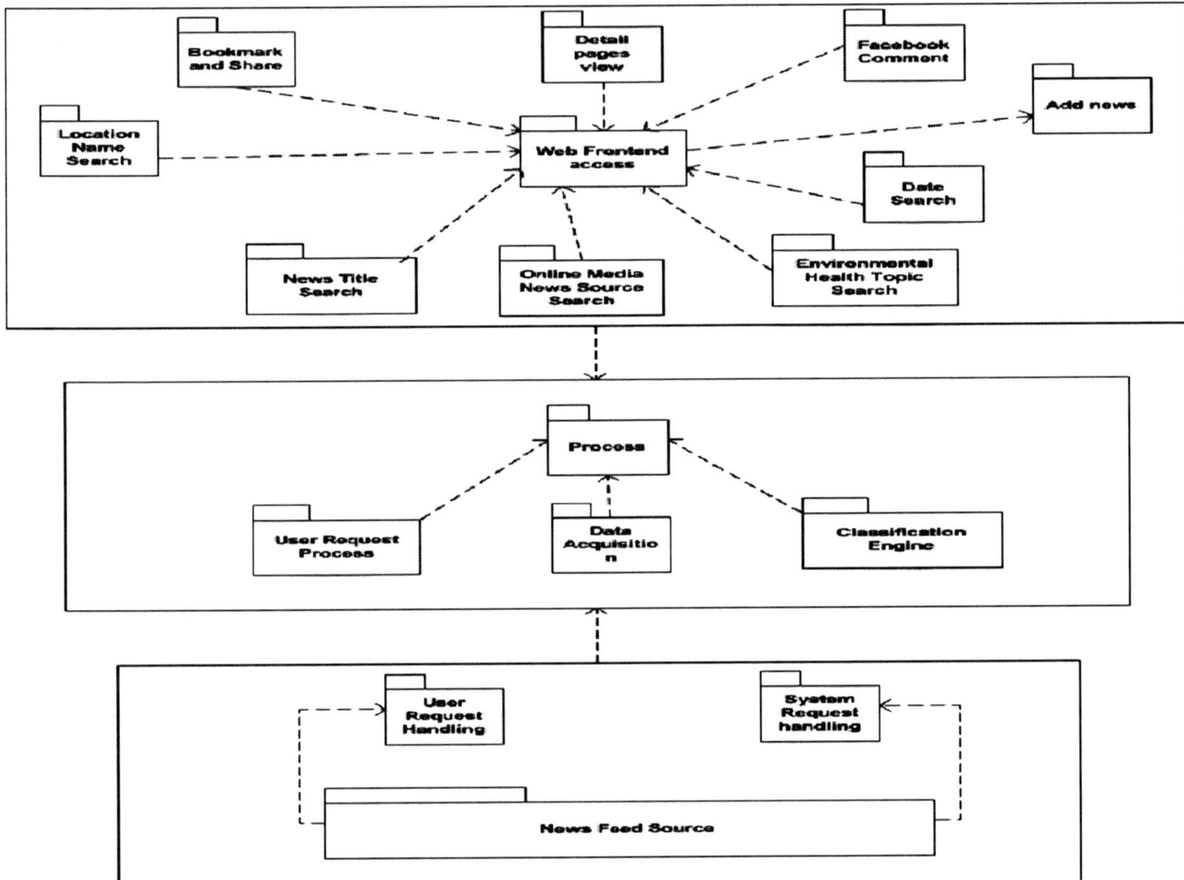

The classification engine has two modules that process the raw input and final output, which are the Reader module and Parser module. While the Reader module takes the raw input from the web source, segments it and prepares it for input to the parser, the Parser module takes segmented input and produces location and environmental data as output.

Reader module uses multi-tier architecture (also known as N-tier approach) (Jain, Dahlin & Tewari 2005) as a classifier to identify location and Environmental Health Data for each web source and Geocoding Web Services later generate coordinates for the identified location. In general, the Classifier examines every sentence and paragraph in the reports in order to match location name and Environmental Health categories against existing taxonomy of known patterns. This may cause multiple locations and multiple environmental health categories to be allocated to a single report.

Parser module uses a word-level N-gram approach (BodHuin & Totorella 2003; Caynar & Trenkle 1994) to match input against a dictionary of known patterns. After the initial data acquisition, the parser receives the input text, strips it of non-alphanumeric characters and splits it into word tokens. It then converts all capital letters to lowercase, except for those tokens that are only one or two characters in length. The parser then compares the input to its dictionary of place and environmental health category, mapping text patterns to the database IDs of all locations, environmental health categories, possible reactions and environmental dimensions known to the system. The dictionary patterns are stored in memory as a tree, where each node is a hash table that maps single tokens to either sub nodes or IDs (leaves), the system can look up each input token in constant time.

In News Feed Source, once the web sources are determined with location and environmental health data, the system stores them in a relational database (MySQL). User Request handling processes any request from public users whereas system request handling processes internal requests by the system.

System Implementation

The implementation uses Android integrated development environment software (IDE), which can be used to develop applications or plugs-ins. There are some major features in Android mobile-based environmental health information system: program startup, Google map view with three markers, web view output and list view output, and lastly search tab and setting tab.

Figure 4 shows the Android mobile-based environmental health information system program startup. The square highlighted icon represents the Android mobile application. With the MyEHMS Android SDK file, the public users can install the file into Android platform.

Figure 5 shows the Google map view with three markers. These three markers are defined in three colors: blue, red and green. Each of these colours represents different contexts. The red marker is the default marker when the user initiates the program with GPS switched on in the smartphone. It detects the current location of the user and returns the results with exact location. The blue marker is the default preference marker when the user initiates the program. It provides the environmental health information with user's location preference set up in the preference settings. Lastly, the green marker refers to the search results performed by user.

Figure 6 shows the web view output and list view output. As shown in Figure 5, there are three

Figure 4. Program startup

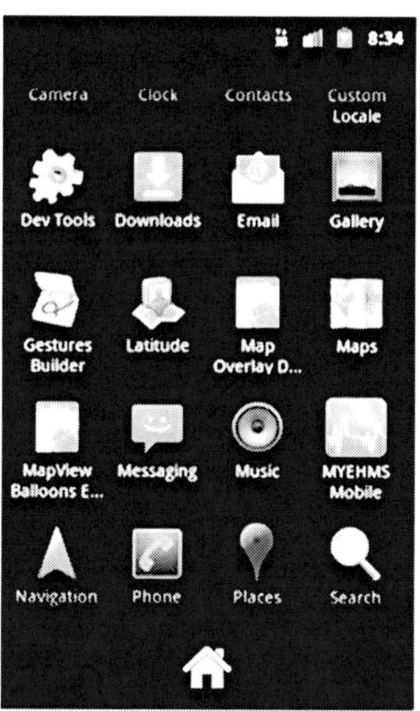

Figure 5. Google Map view with 3 markers

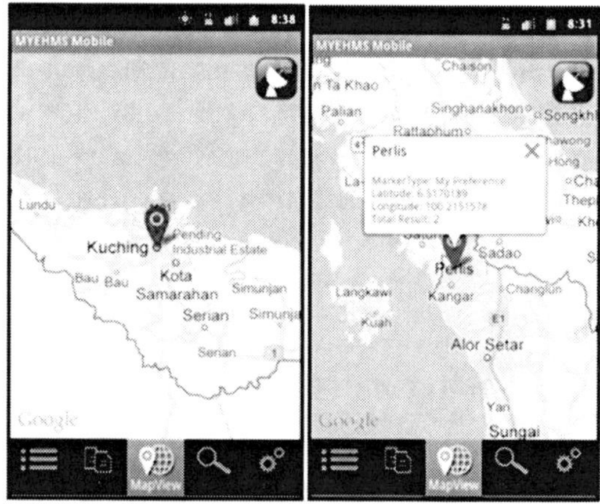
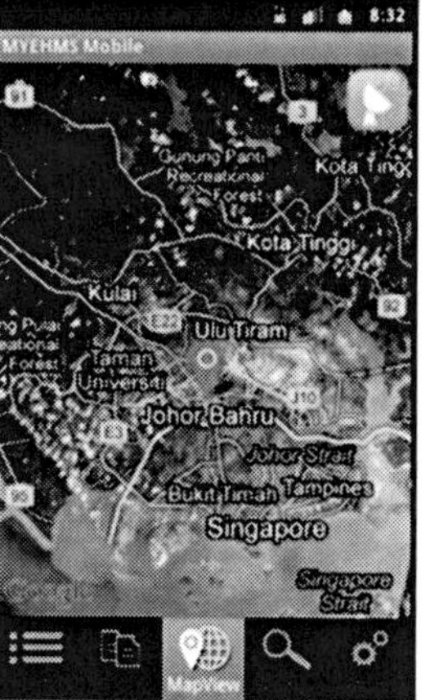

Figure 6. Web view output and list view ouput

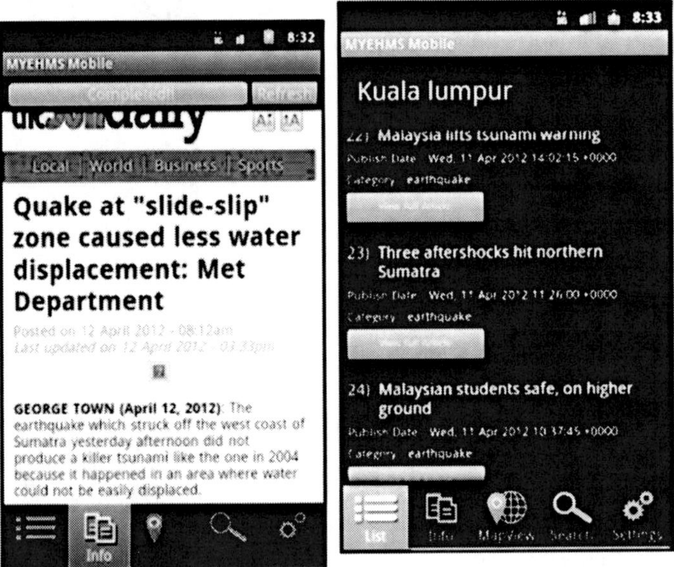

markers that are pinned on the map containing environmental health information. When the user clicks on the marker, it shows a list of environmental health information in that particular location, also known as list view output. If the users would like to view original source of environmental health information, the users can click on "view full article" to have web view output.

Figure 7 shows the search tab and setting tab. The search tab refers to a search form that allows the public user to select the state and city and environmental health category. This allows the user to freely and randomly choose the location and environmental health information category. The settings tab refers to user's preference settings of preferred location and preferred environmental

Figure 7. Search and settings tab

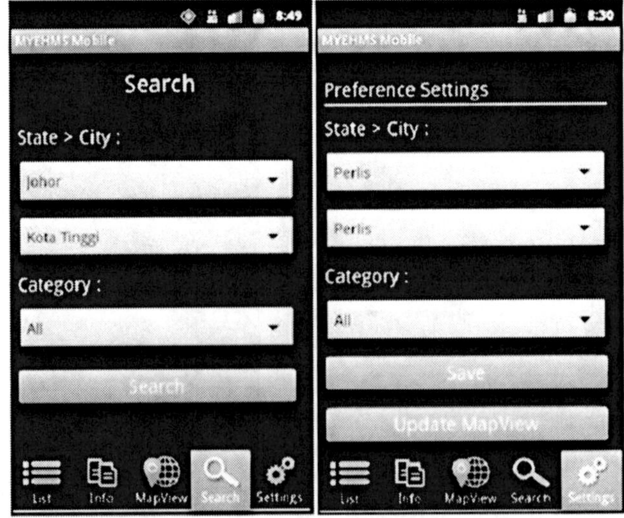

health information category. This allows the user to have easy access to the location and environmental health information for the next visit.

Figure 8 demonstrates how the public user can share, bookmark and comment the news. The public user is allowed to leave comments on the viewed alert page. Most importantly, the user is able to share and bookmark the alerts through multiple social media networks such as Twitter, Facebook and other popular social media sites.

System Accuracy Testing and Evaluation

The system's efficiency in retrieving the relevant environmental health data/keywords and location from news feed and matching against the known patterns of data/keywords in the proposed ontological model is tested. The system accuracy testing is divided into two parts:

- **Part 1:** Two selected social media networks – Facebook and Twitter profiles – would be created for testing purpose. These two social media networks required user registration on their sites before conducting the experiment. Some simple environmental health keywords and location were filled in to provide a platform on social media networks. For example, H1N1 – Kuala Lumpur. The challenge of part 1 is to locate the environmental health keywords and location from the self-created contents on social media network platforms. The result will be described in Figure 9.

- **Part 2:** Two selected real time platform of social media networks with existing environmental health websites – Facebook (MESYM) and Twitter (Ask.com). They are also known as Malaysia Environment Sustainability Youth Movement (MESYM) and Ask.com. These two original sites have synchronized their daily information in their social media networks. The challenge of part 2 is to locate the environmental health keywords and location among

Figure 8. Share, comment and bookmark news feed

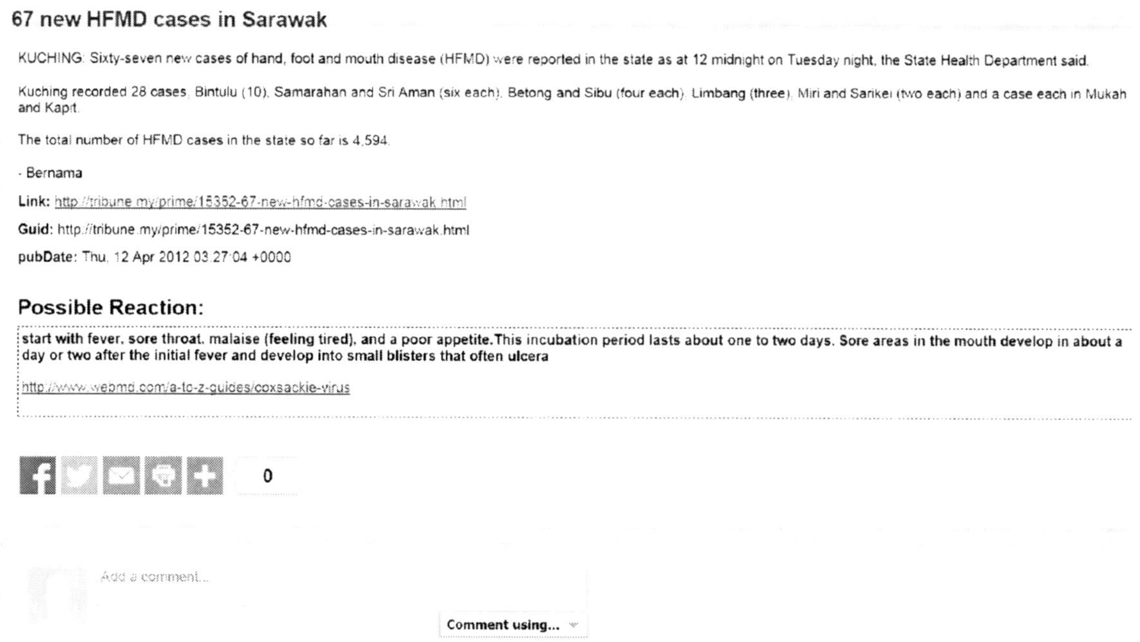

67 new HFMD cases in Sarawak

KUCHING: Sixty-seven new cases of hand, foot and mouth disease (HFMD) were reported in the state as at 12 midnight on Tuesday night, the State Health Department said.

Kuching recorded 28 cases, Bintulu (10), Samarahan and Sri Aman (six each), Betong and Sibu (four each), Limbang (three), Miri and Sarikei (two each) and a case each in Mukah and Kapit.

The total number of HFMD cases in the state so far is 4,594.

- Bernama

Link: http://tribune.my/prime/15352-67-new-hfmd-cases-in-sarawak.html

Guid: http://tribune.my/prime/15352-67-new-hfmd-cases-in-sarawak.html

pubDate: Thu, 12 Apr 2012 03:27:04 +0000

Possible Reaction:

start with fever, sore throat, malaise (feeling tired), and a poor appetite. This incubation period lasts about one to two days. Sore areas in the mouth develop in about a day or two after the initial fever and develop into small blisters that often ulcera

http://www.webmd.com/a-to-z-guides/coxsackie-virus

0

Add a comment...

Comment using... ▾

Figure 9. Social media networks simulation test

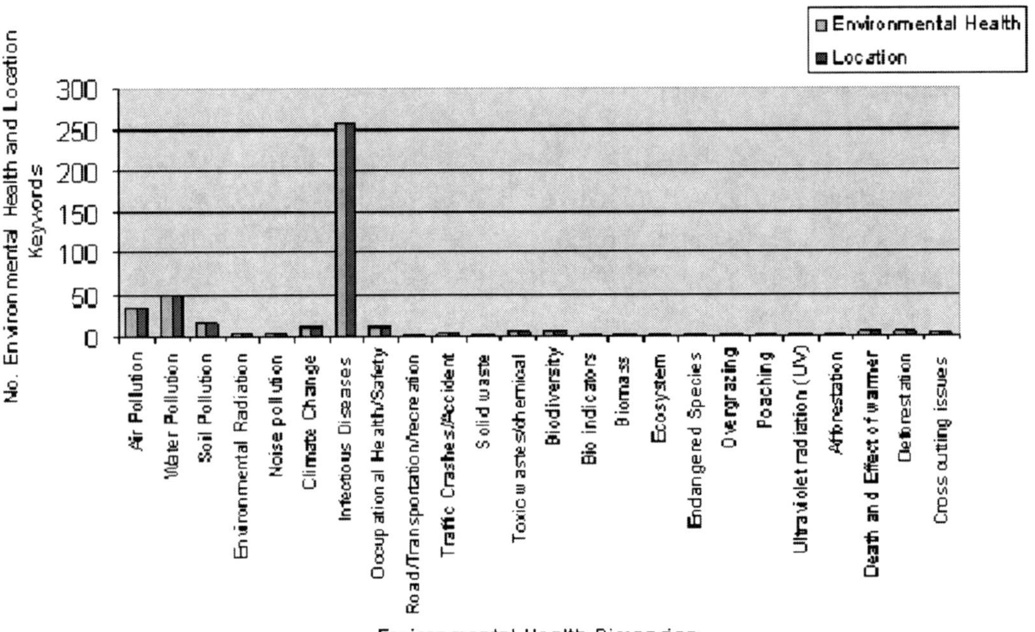

the complex vocabularies posted by existing environmental health parties in their own social media networks. The results retrieved by the system will be compared to original websites searched results as shown in Table 4.

Figure 9 shows the number of returned results is 100% (436 keywords for both environmental health and location keywords) from social media networks (Facebook and Twitter) simulation test (part 1) with no intervention of irrelevant keywords. With this simulation test (part 1), the system has indicated the readiness of the proposed ontological model to go further in the accuracy testing to access complicated news feeds such as with real time platform that may contain highly irrelevant vocabularies and alternative vocabularies. This has also proved that the methods used such as multi-tier architecture (Jain, Dahlin & Tewari 2005) and word-level N-gram approach (BodHuin & Totorella 2003; Caynar & Trenkle 1994) can efficiently read and parse the social media news

feed without error. This has also indicated that the proposed ontological model processed in stage 1, 2 and 3 is considered mature for accuracy testing.

Part 2 result is described in Table 4 and keyword refinement is part of the testing. The sources used for keyword refinement relies on the relevant keywords suggested by original websites and search engines. For example, MESYM and Ask.com used Facebook and Twitter as their alternatives in news publishing and besides they synchronized the latest articles and news in social media.

Table 4 shows that fewer keywords and locations were detected and retrieved by the system (before keyword refinement) from social media networks when compared to the returned results of original sites (No. of needed results). The number of returned results from the system is not consistent with the returned results from the original sites. This has indicated that those keywords structured in the proposed environmental health ontological model are not holistic enough to cope with the large amount of social media web sources. In order for the system to achieve

Table 4. Overview accuracy testing results of parsing social media networks

Environmental Health Dimensions	Environmental hazards, exposures and health	No. needed results	Before Keywords Refinement			After Keywords Refinement		List of Keywords refined and added to proposed ontological model
			No. news retrieved by MyEHMS	No. irrelevant news retrieved by MyEHMS	Accuracy in percentage (%)	No. news retrieved MyEHMS	Accuracy in percentage (%)	
Air pollution	Arsenic	14	12	0	86%	14	100%	rare earth, arsenic poisoning
	Dust	1	0	0	0%	1	100%	dusty
	Energy sector fly ash	1	0	0	0%	1	100%	fly ash
	Greenhouse gas	1	1	1	0%	1	100%	carbon footprint
	Lead	1	1	1	0%	1	100%	lead poisoning, lead emissions, heavy metal lead
	passive smoking	1	0	0	0%	1	100%	cigarettes, tobacco
	Slash-and-burn agriculture	1	0	0	0%	1	100%	slash and burn agriculture, slash and burn farming
	smoke/haze	1	0	0	0%	1	100%	smoky
	Trans-boundary air pollution	1	0	0	0%	1	100%	Trans-boundary haze pollution
Water Pollution	Arsenic	14	10	0	71%	14	100%	rare earth, arsenic poisoning
	deteriorating water quality	1	0	0	0%	1	100%	deteriorating water security
	Energy sector sludge disposal	1	0	0	0%	1	100%	sewage sludge
	rapid growth in water demand	1	0	0	0%	1	100%	Water Crisis
	Rural development sector drainage and flood control	18	0	0	0%	18	100%	Drainage, Floods
	Siltation caused by infrastructure development	1	0	0	0%	1	100%	siltation
	Siltation caused by logging	1	0	0	0%	1	100%	Siltation and logging

continued on following page

Table 4. Continued

Environmental Health Dimensions	Environmental hazards, exposures and health	No. needed results	Before Keywords Refinement			After Keywords Refinement		List of Keywords refined and added to proposed ontological model
			No. news retrieved by MyEHMS	No. irrelevant news retrieved by MyEHMS	Accuracy in percentage (%)	No. news retrieved MyEHMS	Accuracy in percentage (%)	
	Urban development sector drainage and flood control	18	0	0	0%	18	100%	Drainage, Floods
Soil Pollution	Energy sector sludge disposal	1	0	0	0%	1	100%	sewage sludge
	Slash-and-burn agriculture	1	0	0	0%	1	100%	slash and burn agriculture
	Soil degradation	5	2	0	40%	5	100%	environmental degradation
Climate Change	Droughts	7	0	0	0%	7	100%	drought
	Effects of Climate change	5	3	0	60%	5	100%	climate change
	flood	50	50	24	52%	50	100%	flash floods, flash flood, heavy flooding
Infectious Diseases	Avian Influenza	2	0	0	0%	2	100%	bird flu, avian flu, H5N1
	Hand, Foot and Mouth Disease	10	1	0	10%	10	100%	HFMD, Coxsackieviruses, Coxsackie A HFMD, Hand-foot-and-mouth, Coxsackie A, Coxsackie B, Pleurodynia, Bornholm disease
	Swine Flu H1N1	5	2	0	40%	5	100%	H1N1, Swine Flu, Swine Influenza A Virus
	Viral Hepatitis	1	0	0	0%	1	100%	Hepatitis A, Hepatitis B
Solid waste	Waste disposal	1	1	1	0%	1	100%	Industrial waste disposal
Biodiversity	number of species	1	0	0	0%	1	100%	Number of Orang Utan
Death and Effect of warmer temperature/ Global Warming	insect and mosquito-borne infections	1	0	0	0%	1	100%	mosquito borne, insect borne

continued on following page

Table 4. Continued

Environmental Health Dimensions	Environmental hazards, exposures and health	No. needed results	Before Keywords Refinement			After Keywords Refinement		List of Keywords refined and added to proposed ontological model
			No. news retrieved by MyEHMS	No. irrelevant news retrieved by MyEHMS	Accuracy in percentage (%)	No. news retrieved MyEHMS	Accuracy in percentage (%)	
Deforestation	Deforestation and destruction of biodiversity caused by logging	4	0	0	0%	4	100%	Forest clearing, Deforestation, Deforestation issues, deforestation rate
	Deforestation and destruction of biodiversity caused by conversion to other land use	4	0	0	0%	4	100%	Forest clearing, Deforestation, Deforestation issues, deforestation rate
Total	32 keywords being refined							61 new keywords

the same results made by different original sites search, alternative keywords would be added into the proposed ontological model to gain same amount of news returned by the original sites. In this accuracy testing, the improvements were made when there were irrelevant alerts retrieved by the system. The improvements were conducted by refining and adding more alternative keywords to the ontological model. About 60 keywords were updated accordingly to the ontological model. These newly added 60 keywords were discovered when conducting the manual search on original site such as MESYM and Ask.com. Search on these original sites may benefit the researcher to discover relevant news and keywords suggested by the search features.

In Table 4, the environmental health keywords under the air pollution, water pollution, soil pollution, and climate change tend to have low accuracy due to the high number of irrelevant results retrieved by MyEHMS. This has indicated that those environmental health keywords are very common and vague in most of the news written by publishers. Besides, some environmental health keywords under noise pollution, road/transportation/recreation safety, traffic crashes/accident, toxic wastes/chemical wastes/hazardous wastes, bio-indicators, biomass, ecosystem, endangered species, overgrazing, poaching, and ultraviolet radiation (UV) were not able to extract any news from original sites. This has again indicated that choosing the relevant news feed may achieve reliable results, especially the real-time platform that specializes in reporting specific environmental health topics. To date, it does not fail to retrieve relevant news with exact keywords matching.

Discussion

Table 4 shows the accuracy testing results of MyEHMS by retrieving from social media networks like Facebook and Twitter. It also indicates the comparative results before and after keyword refinement. Last but not least, it also shows a list of refined keywords that have been added to the proposed ontological model as improvements. It also indicates some environmental health dimensions and some environmental health hazards, exposures and health keywords that were successfully being improved in terms of keyword refinement. At this stage, there were nine environmental health dimensions and 32 environmental health hazards, exposures and health keywords. Accuracy testing of matching the social media networks – Facebook and Twitter – against the existing ontological model was calculated based on (100%/ no. needed results x no. news retrieved by MyEHMS). Before keyword refinement, there were only four keywords which achieved above 50% accuracy: Arsenic under air pollution (86%); Arsenic under water pollution (71%); effects of climate change under climate change (60%); and flood under climate change (52%). Besides, there were three keywords which achieved 10% to 40% accuracy: soil degradation under soil pollution (40%); Hand, foot, and mouth disease under infectious diseases (10%); and lastly Swine flu H1N1 under infectious diseases (40%).

The other 25 environmental health keywords were not successfully matched with any relevant news from social media networks. There were two reasons behind this: the different authors in social media networks may be using different vocabularies for the same topic. The vocabulary is not standardized in such an open platform and it may be difficult to find the exact keywords by the system. Therefore, keyword refinement was conducted on these 25 environmental health keywords in order to increase the number of retrieved results by the system.

FUTURE RESEARCH DIRECTIONS

This research has several areas for future improvement: user testing on the system effectiveness, prediction of environmental health patterns, integration with more healthcare-related systems, sorting and classification in environmental health ontological model at a deeper level.

- User testing on the system effectiveness.

One of the objectives in this research is to develop a comprehensive mobile-based environmental health information system that can serve public mobile users. Apart from accuracy testing, it is necessary to test the effectiveness of the system in improving the public health. Public health concerns for environmental health information system can be addressed in the evidence gathered regarding the performance of the system. Evidence of the system's performance must be viewed as credible. For example, the gathered evidence must be reliable, valid, and informative for its intended use. Many potential sources of evidence regarding the system's performance exist, including survey data collected from public users. This user testing involves reusing the accuracy testing records mentioned above and also identifying eligible stakeholders. Stakeholders refer to participants selected from random people with little knowledge of public health.

- Prediction on environmental health patterns through social media.

In future, investigation can be conducted by integrating more reliable medical sources supported by local and state level healthcare agencies. In knowledge discovery and data mining field, this is an essential element to develop a comprehensive environmental health management system that helps to predict the environmental health patterns. Prediction on environmental health patterns can be illustrated with a chart event. According to the collected data in MyEHMS, most of the environmental health information is considered post-event. Post-event refer to the incident that had already happened or just happened. In order to achieve the prediction concept, a forecasting model can be developed through integrating various valuable sources. For example, social media networks play a critical role to predict the environmental health patterns. Regular users of social media networks may post illness-related news. For example, a regular user makes a post that "today he is sick". With this, MyEHMS can collect and sort them into relevant groups and location. When the location and the particular disease are determined, it is assumed that the future incidents can be predicted. Apart from social media networks, weather forecast report may help to predict environmental health patterns. For example, 10% chance of showers today, but 70% chance of getting flu next month.

- Integrate with existing healthcare systems.

MyEHMS is only a prototype of tracking and monitoring environmental health issues in Malaysia. It is believed that the number of new diseases and toxic chemicals are growing every day. The growing number far exceeds the ability to test them on possible toxic effects on people, plants and animals in every place. It is unlikely for MyEHMS to detect all possible environmental health issues on a short term basis without improving the existing environmental health ontological model. However, it will be possible with support from other local healthcare-related systems from both private and public sector such as Total Hospital Information System (THIS), Personal Health Record (PHR), Teleprimary care, Clinical Information System (CIS), Oral Health Clinical Information System (OHCIS), and PrimaCare in Malaysia (Ministry of Health, 2012).

- Improve the Mobile-apps development.

More than ever, mobile apps are now looked upon as a robust tool that can make a big difference to tracking and monitoring environmental health issues. MyEHMS has a mobile-app version that allows tablet-users and mobile-users to keep track on environmental health issues in any places they want. The improvement shall be made when there is an opportunity to conduct user testing on the effectiveness of MyEHMS mobile-app. There is a

potential for MyEHMS to receive voice command and response with environmental health issues. Voice recognition in mobile may help those users to speak on phone while the phone can process the instruction and response with retrieved results from MyEHMS.

- Self-learning module.

The method of collecting the data, including numbers and types of reporting sources, and time spent on collecting data are critical for MyEHMS. Sometimes, mistakes cannot be made when reporting the environmental health information when it is critical. There is a potential for MyEHMS to get self-learning module such as keyword self-refinement or correction. Self-learning module refer to learning activities designed for MyEHMS to work independently when it meets suggested new keywords or alternative keywords in web sources. The research can be deployed state-of-art at self-learning algorithms that automatically figured out which keywords in the database of tweets were associated with elevated levels of diseases. The self-learning module is an essential element for MyEHMS to continually grow and serve not only public users but also patients and physicians. This may improve the availability and utility of existing data but also facilitate the creation of new data to ensure the accessibility of core and other environmental health related issues.

According to California Environmental Health Investigation Branch (2012), although the environment is known to play an important role in human health, no comprehensive, integrated, state or national system exists to track the countless hazards, exposures, and ensuing health effects that could be due to environmental factors. There are tens of thousands of chemicals, and researchers are still learning about the toxic effects of many of them (California Environmental Health Investigation branch, 2012). For example, when environment is broadly defined to include air pollution and infectious disease, we will be able to assess the status of local air as good, moderate, unhealthy, very unhealthy and hazardous (Malaysia Department of Environment, 2009), or we will be able to identify disease transmission through air, water, food or other communicable media. There is growing scientific evidence that environmental factors are strongly linked to many chronic diseases such as asthma, birth defects, and cancer (Center for Disease Control and Prevention, 2012). The current systems in Malaysia (Air Pollutant Index management and communicable disease control information system) are insufficient to track some hazards and chronic diseases.

In response to this challenge, many healthcare agencies and researchers have developed environment health surveillance systems that involve the on-going collection, integration, analysis, interpretation, and dissemination of data on environmental hazards; exposures to those hazards; and related health effects in their own countries. The goal of tracking is to provide information that can be used to plan, apply, and evaluate actions to prevent and control environmentally related hazards, exposures and health. Undeniably, the social media networks and mobile technologies now provide absolute alternatives for monitoring the environmental health effect. They have absolute means of instant information mobility, real time update, forecast visualization, and prevention role in environmental health disaster.

CONCLUSION

We have seen that the Android mobile-based environmental health information source is a research stepping-stone in utilizing the social media networks and mobile technologies as data inputs and sources to understanding the effect of environmental health issues. Based on the accuracy testing results, data shows that the system is able to match exact environmental health keywords after keyword refinement was conducted and improved. This has also indicated that part 2 testing is rather more complicated than part 1 when it comes to evaluating the accuracy of parsing news feed data. It is believed that in real time platform social media users tend to use different vocabularies on the same topic. The vocabulary is not standardized in such an open platform and it may be difficult for the system to find the exact keywords. Further research is needed to have better control of ambiguity environmental health information by integrating with existing surveillance systems and ontological models that are much more constructive.

REFERENCES

Android. (2013). *Android application*. Retrieved March 4, 2013, from http://www.Android.com/

Avnet, L. (2013). Twitter could be useful in tracking disease outbreaks, study suggest. *Mashable*. Retrieved February 5, 2013, from http://www.huffingtonpost.com/2013/01/24/twitter-disease-outbreaks_n_2543495.html

Bautista, C. (2013). Twitter can help health officials track outbreaks. *Mashable*. Retrieved March 5, 2013, from http://mashable.com/2013/01/24/twitter-can-track-disease-outbreaks/

BodHuin. T., & Totorella, M. (2003). Using grid technologies for web-enabling legacy systems. In *Proceedings of Eleventh Annual International Workshop on Software Technology and Engineering Practice (STEP'03)*, (pp. 186-195). STEP.

California Environmental Health Investigation Branch. (2012). California Environmental Health Tracking Program. *Environmental Health Investigation Branch*. Retrieved June 4, 2012, from http://www.ehib.org/project.jsp?project_key=EHSS01

Cayzer, S. (2004). Semantic blogging and decentralized knowledge management. *Communications of the ACM, 47*(12), 47–52. doi:10.1145/1035134.1035164

Celcom. (2012). Celcom focuses on innovative mobile healthcare solutions. *Celcom*. Retrieved July 8, 2012, from http://www.theborneopost. com/2012/06/08/celcom-focuses-on-innovative-mobile-healthcare-solutions/

Centres for Disease Control and Prevention. (2010). *National environmental public health tracking network*. Center for Disease Control and Prevention. Retrieved June 5, 2012, from http://ephtracking.cdc.gov/showLocationLanding.action

Chunara, R., Andrews, J. R., & Brownstein, J. S. (2012). Social and news media enable estimation of epidemiological patterns early in the 2010 Haitian cholera outbreak. *The American Journal of Tropical Medicine and Hygiene*, *86*(1), 39–45. doi:10.4269/ajtmh.2012.11-0597 PMID:22232449

Department of Environment. (2011). Air Pollutant Index Management System (APIMS). *Department of Environment Ministry of Natural Resources and Environment*. Retrieved June 5, 2011, from http://www.doe.gov.my/apims/

Department of Health New York. (2009). Glossary. *Department of Health*. Retrieved June 15, 2011, from http://www.health.ny.gov/environmental/public_health_tracking/about/glossary.htm

European Environment Agency (EEA). (2011). *Air Pollution monitoring system*. Retrieved June 8, 2011, from http://www.eea.europa.eu/maps/ozone/map

Facebook. (2013). Retrieved May 7, 2013, from https://www.facebook.com/

Factbrowser.com. (2012a). Malaysia has 34MM mobile subscribers and 17.5MM internet users. *Factbrowser*. Retrieved May 6, 2013, from http://www.factbrowser.com/facts/6143/

Factbrowser.com. (2012b). 87.9% of Malaysians on the Internet access Facebook. *Factbrowser*. Retrieved May 6, 2013, from http://www.factbrowser.com/facts/3404/

Factbrowser.com. (2012c). Malaysia's mobile penetration is more than 100%, compared to 59% for internet and 41% for social media. *Factbrowser*. Retrieved May 6, 2013, from http://www.factbrowser.com/facts/4159/

Firefly. (2013). Social animals on the move in Asia: A social media & mobile perspective. *Firefly*. Retrieved May 5, 2013, from http://www.fireflymb.com/Libraries/Papers_and_Presentations/FireflyMillwardBrown_AMAP_Social_Animals.sflb.ashx

Freifeld, C., & Brownstein, J. (2007). *HealthMap*. Retrieved June 7, 2011, from http://www.healthmap.org/about/

Garrett, J. J. (2005). Ajax: A New Approach to Web Applications. *Adaptive Path*. Retrieved July 12, 2011, from http://www.adaptivepath.com/ideas/ajax-new-approach-web-applications

Google. (2012). Google Flu Trends. *Google.org*. Retrieved August 25, 2011, from http://www.google.org/flutrends/about/how.html

Health Protection Agency. (2010). Introduction to environmental public health tracking. *Health Protection Agency*. Retrieved May 8, 2013, from http://www.hpa.org.uk/webc/HPAwebFile/HPAweb_C/1287143109858

Healthmap. (2012). Healthmap. *Boston Children Hospital*. Retrieved June 4, 2012, from http://healthmap.org/en/

Jain, N., Dahlin, M., & Tewari, R. (2005). TAPER: Tiered approach for eliminating redundancy in replica synchronization. In *Proceedings of the 4th conference FAST 2005 on USEUNIX Conference on File and Storage Technologies*. USEUNIX.

Laird, S. (2012). How social media is taking over the news industry. *Mashable*. Retrieved May 20, 2013, from http://mashable.com/2012/04/18/social-media-and-the-news/

Lemon, S. M., Hamburg, M. A., Sparling, P. F., Choffnes, E. R., & Mack, A. (2007). Global infectious disease surveillance and detection: Assessing the challenges – Finding solutions. *Forum on Microbial Threats*. Retrieved May 8, 2013, from http://www.ncbi.nlm.nih.gov/books/NBK52867/pdf/TOC.pdf

Lowensohn, J. (2008). Google now tracking flu trends via search. *CNET*. Retrieved August 18, 2011, from http://news.cnet.com/google-now-tracking-flu-trends-via-search/

Maxis. (2012). Maxis and IJN establish partnership to bring healthcare content and awareness to maxis customers. *Maxis*. Retrieved 15 May, 2013, from http://www.maxis.com.my/mmc/index.asp?fuseaction=home.article&aid=618&status=1

MedLinePlus Health. (n.d.). Environmental Health Ontology. *BioPortal*. Retrieved June 10, 2011, from http://bioportal.bioontology.org/search

Ministry of Health. (2007). Communicable Disease Control Information System. *Ministry of Health*. Retrieved July 15, 2011, http://www.unescap.org/idd/events/2007_REM-avian-influenza/Surveillance-of-infectious-diseases-in-Malaysia.pdf

Ministry of Health. (2013). MyHealth. *Ministry of Health*. Retrieved 8 May, 2013, from http://www.myhealth.gov.my/v2/

Mokhtar, M. B., & Murad, M. D. W. (2010). Issues and framework of environmental health in Malaysia. *The Free Library by Farlex*. Retrieved June 1, 2011, http://www.thefreelibrary.com/Issues+and+framework+of+environmental+healt h+in+Malaysia.-a0222252556

New York Department of Health. (2009). Glossary. *Environmental Health Tracking*. Retrieved May 20, 2013, from http://www.health.ny.gov/environmental/public_health_tracking/about/glossary.htm

Nsubuga, P., White, M. E., Thacker, S. B., Anderson, M. A., Blount, S. B., & Broome, C. V. … Trostle, M. (2006). *Public Health Surveillance: A tool for targeting and monitoring interventions disease control priorities in developing countries* (2nd ed.). Retrieved May 20, 2013, from http://www.ncbi.nlm.nih.gov/books/NBK11770/

O'Reilly, T. (2005). What is Web 2.0: Design patterns and business models for the next generation of software. *O'Reilly*. Retrieved July 16, 2011, from http://oreilly.com/web2/archive/what-is-web-20.html

Richards, T. B., Croner, C. M., Rushton, G., Brown, C. K., & Fowler, L. (1999). Geographical Information Systems and Public Health. *The Long Island Breast Cancer Study Project*. Retrieved March 10, 2011, from http://healthcybermap.org/HGeo/res/phr.pdf

Robertson, C., Sawford, K., Daniel, S. L. A., Nelson, T. A., & Stephen, C. (2010). *Mobile phone-based infectious disease surveillance system, Sri Lanka*. Retrieved May 13, 2013, from http://wwwnc.cdc.gov/eid/article/16/10/pdfs/10-0249.pdf

Schmidt, C. W. (2012). *Trending now: Using social media to predict and track disease outbreaks*. Retrieved May 15, 2013, from http://www.ncbi.nlm.nih.gov/pmc/articles/PMC3261963/

Sime Darby Healthcare. (2013). *Sime Darby Healthcare*. Retrieved May 15, 2013, from http://www.simedarbyhealthcare.com/

Taylor, C. (2013). *250,000 social media users in U.S. said they got the flu*. Retrieved May 18, 2013, from http://mashable.com/2013/01/16/facebook-twitter-flu/

Thesaurus, C. R. I. S. P. (2006). Environmental Health Ontology. *BioPortal*. Retrieved June 11, 2011, from http://bioportal.bioontology.org/search

Twitter. (2013). *Twitter Inc*. Retrieved May 18, 2013, from https://twitter.com/

Vodafone. (2012). *Disease outbreak*. Retrieved May 22, 2013, from http://mhealth.vodafone.com/solutions/access_to_medicine/disease_outbreaks/

Wisconsin Department of Health Services. (2011). *Wisconsin Environmental Public Health Tracking*. Retrieved June 8, 2011, from http://www.dhs.wisconsin.gov/epht/DataInfo.htm

Woodfin, G. (2011). *How to find your twitter RSS Feed & Profile ID Number*. Retrieved August 25, 2011, from http://www.glenwoodfin.com/rss/how-to-find-your-twitter-rss-feed-in-2011/

World Fact Book, C. I. A. (2012). The World Factbook Environment: Current issues. *Central Intelligence Agency*. Retrieved June 7 2011, from https://www.cia.gov/library/publications/the-world-factbook/fields/2032.html

World Health Organization. (2005). Malaysia Environmental Health Country Profile. *World Health Organization*. Retrieved June 8, 2011, from http://www.environment-health.asia/fileupload/malaysia_ehcp_07Oct2004.pdf

World Health Organization. (2008). *Foodborne disease outbreaks: Guidelines for investigation and control*. Retrieved August 29, 2011, from http://www.who.int/foodsafety/publications/foodborne_disease/outbreak_guidelines.pdf

Zhang, J., Shi, H., & Zhang, Y. (2009). Self-organizing map methodology and Google maps services for geographical epidemiology mapping. In *Proceedings of Digital Image Computing: Technique and Application 2009* (DICTA '09) (pp. 229-235). DICTA. doi:10.1109/DICTA.2009.46

KEY TERMS AND DEFINITIONS

Android: A type of operating system developed by Google for Mobile phones.

Environmental Health Surveillance/Information System: A surveillance system involving the collection, analysis, and dissemination of data for use in public health practices.

Environmental Health Tracking: The ongoing collection, integration, analysis, and interpretation of data about environmental hazards, exposure to environmental hazards and human health effects potentially related to exposure to environmental hazards.

Geocoding: A process of finding associated geographic coordinates (often expressed as latitude and longitude) from other geographic data.

Google Map: A web mapping service application and technology provided by Google.

Mobile Health Technologies: A term used for practice medicine and public health, supported by mobile devices.

Ontological Model: A domain ontology (or domain-specific ontology) models a specific domain, which represents part of the world.

RSS News Feed: A family of web feed formats used to publish frequently updated works such as blog entries, news headlines, audio and video.

Social Media: A media for social interaction, using highly accessible and scalable publishing techniques.

This work was previously published in Social Media and Mobile Technologies for Healthcare edited by Mowafa Househ, Elizabeth Borycki, and Andre Kushniruk, pages 173-200 copyright year 2014 by Medical Information Science Reference (an imprint of IGI Global).

Index

D

N

National Electronic-Health Transition Authority (NEHTA) 1444
National Health System (NHS) 376, 637, 1444, 1679
natural disasters 1271, 1273
neonatal health 1141, 1143, 1150
neurosurgery 1338-1340, 1342-1343, 1346-1347
non-adoption 391-392, 395-396, 400-401, 404-405, 407-408
Noncommunicable Chronic Diseases (NCD) 295
noncommunicable diseases 260, 267, 270, 281
norm analysis 26, 33, 35, 38, 41-42, 44, 329, 1059, 1066, 1070

O

ontological approach 445, 458-459
ontological model 32, 450, 578, 582-584, 586, 591-592, 595-597, 601
Operative Role Management (ORM) 1379-1381, 1384, 1388-1389, 1391, 1394
Opportunistic Mobile Networks (OMN) 1045
organizational learning 360-361, 366-367, 1537
organizational semiotics 26, 37, 45, 319-320, 328, 330, 332, 336, 341, 346, 363, 1059

P

palliative care 183-189, 191-196, 199
Parkinson's Disease (PD) 555, 694, 1174, 1635
participative health 1185
participatory mapping 1361, 1365, 1374-1375
pathology services 60-63
pathway knowledge 26, 32, 42, 45
patient monitoring 320-321, 323-324, 331, 336, 346, 469, 472, 475, 483, 551-553, 555-556, 567-570, 605-606, 736, 751-753, 787, 842, 854, 862, 874, 1017, 1019-1022, 1026-1027, 1029-1030, 1033, 1040-1041, 1552, 1606-1607, 1609-1610, 1624, 1626
patient outcomes 19, 25, 823-824, 843, 846, 848-851, 855, 863-864, 874, 903, 1103, 1121, 1187, 1507, 1691, 1697, 1709
patient safety 25-28, 30-35, 45, 63-65, 104, 120, 320-321, 346, 361-362, 365-367, 416, 531, 606, 821-825, 834, 841, 900-901, 903-904, 909, 918, 962, 1001, 1008, 1048-1049, 1062-1063, 1069, 1108, 1119, 1122, 1127, 1186-1187, 1198, 1223-1227, 1230-1232, 1234, 1238, 1244, 1338, 1347, 1398, 1442, 1445-1447, 1449, 1453-1456, 1493, 1510, 1536-1537, 1540, 1546, 1568-1569, 1579, 1593, 1600, 1668, 1695

patient-safety culture 26-27
patient view 1097, 1099, 1104, 1106, 1109, 1111, 1117, 1436
pay-as-you-go 710, 1414, 1427, 1431
pelvic floor muscle training 304, 317
perceived enjoyment 238, 241, 243, 248-249, 251-252, 257
perceived irritation 238, 242, 247, 257
perceived monetary value 238, 241, 248-249, 251, 257
perceived usefulness 49-52, 55-57, 195, 197, 241, 252, 686, 1555, 1557
performance dashboards 1135
perioperative process 1119-1125, 1127-1129, 1131, 1135
Personal Health Records (PHR) 490-491, 500-502, 509, 511-512, 521, 597, 962, 1073, 1079, 1081, 1083-1084, 1087-1088, 1096, 1246-1247, 1253, 1260, 1435, 1438, 1444, 1467, 1725
Personal Health Systems (PHS) 659, 1110, 1396, 1398, 1401, 1404
Personal Identifiable Information (PII) 510, 516, 521
personalized medicine 717, 842, 847, 857-859, 862, 864, 874, 962, 1246-1248, 1251-1252
Personally Controlled Electronic Health Records (PCEHR) 50, 980, 1320-1322, 1324, 1337, 1436, 1444
Personal Medical Device (PMD) 1087-1088, 1096
pervasive healthcare 319-324, 328, 330-332, 334, 337-342, 346, 1721
Pervasive Healthcare Information Provision (PHIP) 319-322, 324, 330-332, 334, 338-342, 346
PGOT framework 1511-1512, 1518, 1524, 1526
pharmaceutical care 1445-1447, 1455-1456, 1463
pharmaceutical protocols 641, 660
pharmaco-cybernetics 1445, 1447, 1449, 1452, 1455-1456, 1463
pharmaco-informatics 1447, 1463
physical therapy 298-299, 301-305, 312, 317
Platform-as-a-Service (PaaS) 563, 576
Platform for Privacy Preferences (P3P) 1442, 1444
political attitudes 822, 1207-1208, 1210-1214, 1218-1219
post-analytical 1223-1226, 1228, 1235, 1244
Post-Traumatic Stress Disorder (PTSD) 512, 1339, 1360, 1437
power outage 877-881, 883, 887-888, 1012
pre-analytical 1223-1226, 1228-1232, 1234-1238, 1244
price premium 846, 874
Principal Component Analysis (PCA) 1449, 1463
privacy rule 515, 1006-1007, 1432-1435, 1439, 1444

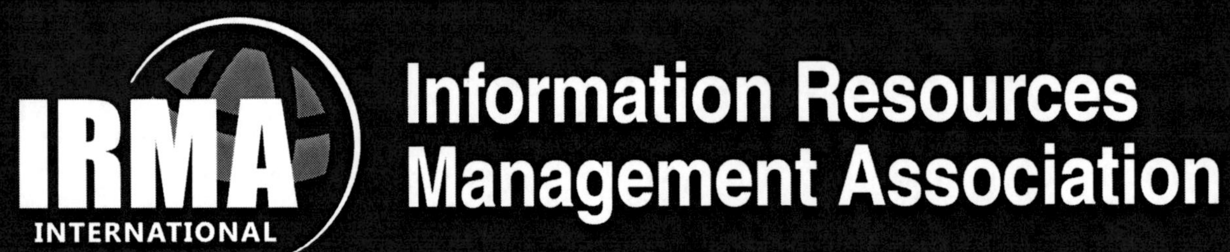

Become an IRMA Member

Members of the **Information Resources Management Association (IRMA)** understand the importance of community within their field of study. The Information Resources Management Association is an ideal venue through which professionals, students, and academicians can convene and share the latest industry innovations and scholarly research that is changing the field of information science and technology. Become a member today and enjoy the benefits of membership as well as the opportunity to collaborate and network with fellow experts in the field.

IRMA Membership Benefits:

- **One FREE Journal Subscription**

- **30% Off Additional Journal Subscriptions**

- **20% Off Book Purchases**

- Updates on the latest events and research on Information Resources Management through the IRMA-L listserv.

- Updates on new open access and downloadable content added to Research IRM.

- A copy of the Information Technology Management Newsletter twice a year.

- A certificate of membership.

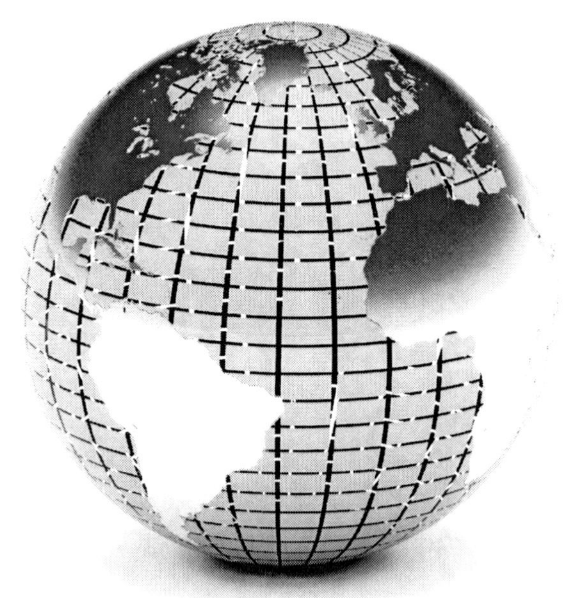

IRMA Membership $195

Scan code to visit irma-international.org and begin by selecting your free journal subscription.

Membership is good for one full year.

CPSIA information can be obtained at www.ICGtesting.com
Printed in the USA
LVOW09*0922160915

454396LV00013B/73/P